# LUNG GROWTH
# AND DEVELOPMENT

# LUNG BIOLOGY IN HEALTH AND DISEASE

*Executive Editor*

**Claude Lenfant**
*Director, National Heart, Lung and Blood Institute*
*National Institutes of Health*
*Bethesda, Maryland*

The opinions expressed in these volumes do not necessarily represent the views of the National Institutes of Health.

# LUNG GROWTH AND DEVELOPMENT

*Edited by*

## John A. McDonald

*Mayo Clinic Scottsdale*
*Scottsdale, Arizona*

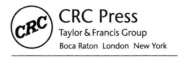

**CRC Press**
Taylor & Francis Group
Boca Raton London New York

CRC Press is an imprint of the
Taylor & Francis Group, an **informa** business

Informa Healthcare USA, Inc.
52 Vanderbilt Avenue
New York, NY 10017

International Standard Book Number-10: 0-8247-9772-8 (Hardcover)
International Standard Book Number-13: 978-0-8247-9772-0 (Hardcover)

Visit the Informa Web site at
www.informa.com

and the Informa Healthcare Web site at
www.informahealthcare.com

# INTRODUCTION

This title and this number are both a symbol and a celebration.

In 1770 Benjamin Franklin wrote:

> The rapid progress [that] science now makes occasions my regretting sometimes that I was born too soon. It is impossible to imagine the height to which we may be carried, in a thousand years, the power of man over matter. . . . All diseases may be prevented or cured not excepting that old age and our lives lengthened at pleasure even before the antediluvian standard.

Unquestionably, the same could be said today except that our imagination needs not stretch over a thousand years, but over only a few years and, in many instances, only a few months.

This book is a repository of what we know today about the growth and development of the lung and its many components. It is also a storehouse of ideas and challenges that, like a beacon, will attract and guide new investigations. But, in addition, it is a symbol of the growth of our knowledge about the functions of the lung in health and disease.

Remember! It was only in 1953 that Julius Comre asked his famous question "Does the lung have any other function?" (i.e., other than respiratory function). Sorokin's 1970 publication *The Cells of the Lungs* provided momentum for a voyage in lung biology that has been distinguished by remarkable progress and discoveries.

It was the consolidation of the huge body of knowledge about the lung that led to the initiation of the series of monographs Lung Biology in Health and Disease. A dozen or so volumes were envisioned when the first one appeared in 1976. No one at that time could imagine that so much would happen—so much growth in our knowledge—that 20 years later we would be celebrating the one-hundredth volume of the series. Furthermore, who would have thought that we would already by marching briskly into the second hundred!

Progress in understanding the biology of a mature organ is in part determined by our knowledge of its development. Thus, this volume is an important milepost for the continuation of our voyage into further discoveries. One of the earlier volumes in the series was titled *Development of the Lung*. Even the most casual comparison of its contents with those of this new volume beautifully illustrates the new heights we have reached in our knowledge of lung growth and development, and all of this was achieved not in a thousand years, but in less than two decades!

As the Executive Editor of the series of monographs, I felt privileged when Dr. McDonald accepted my invitation to revisit this fertile area of investigation. My advisors had all recommended him, but I knew that his schedule might preclude his acceptance. I was so pleased when he agreed to undertake this project and proceeded to assemble a group of well-recognized worldwide experts to develop the volume. Of course, when this started, we had no way of knowing that this important work would have the added distinction of being volume number one hundred. But, now that this is the case, I am indeed pleased and grateful that John McDonald and his authors are the architects of this exciting contribution, which symbolizes so much.

Claude Lenfant, M.D.
Bethesda, Maryland

# PREFACE

In this volume, a number of experts highlight new developments in diverse aspects of lung development. Basic scientists studying the lung will find valuable insights into basic concepts of lung development, comprehensive reviews of existing knowledge, comparative information regarding different species, and rich sources for further reading. Health care providers will gain insights into the pathophysiology of abnormalities in surfactant expression or metabolism, mucus hypersecretion, and compensatory lung growth.

The first four chapters deal with the essential question of how the lung forms. The structural aspects of this process, the role of transcription factors, and new developments in epithelial-mesenchymal interactions in lungs are discussed. Peter H. Burri provides a clear and well-illustrated overview of the structural changes occuring during pre- and postnatal lung development. Timely, new information on the role of transcription factors in regulation of epithelial cell gene transcription is covered in chapters from two groups at the forefront of this fast-moving area. Whitsett and Sever focus on essential roles of thyroid transcription factor-1 (TTF-1) and members of the forkhead family of transcription factors. Next, Hackett and Gitlin provide complementary information, emphasizing similarities and differences between the regulation of epithelial gene expression in the lung and other biological systems. Classic experimental embryological experiments and gene ablation studies demonstrate that highly orchestrated epithelial-mesenchymal interactions are absolutely essential for lung development. This topic is reviewed by Shannon and Deterding, whose careful experimental approaches have contributed much to this area. They provide a conceptual setting, followed by a comprehensive and informative discussion of important historical and recent work in this area. The role of structural molecules (e.g., extracellular matrix) as well as growth factors is covered.

Chapters 5–10 deal with cytodifferentiation and the development of specific lung tissues, including the conducting and alveolar epithelium, airway gland growth and differentiation, Clara cells, smooth muscle, vasculature, and innervation. Mallampalli, Acarregui, and Snyder provide an overview of the differentiation of the alveolar epithelium, describing the function, embryonic origin, and expression of cell-specific markers in alveolar types I and II cells. Basbaum and Li focus on a matter of critical importance to the clinician: regulation of airway gland growth and differentiation. They summarize the basic principles of airway gland growth gleaned from morphological observation and proceed to basic questions of gland development, including consideration of the role of progenitor cells, epithelial-mesenchymal interactions, growth factors, proteinases, and the regulation of expression of gland products including lysozyme and MUC 2. Plopper, who has contributed substantially to our understanding of the biology of the Clara cell, summarizes its developmental biology. A discussion of interspecies differences in Clara cell differentiation is particularly valuable to experimentalists working with different species. The expression of phenotypic markers and the regulation of Clara cell differentiation are also reviewed.

Another expert, Wu, reviews the growth and differentiation of tracheo-bronchial epithelial cells, arguing persuasively for a model of "epithelial failure" as a paradigm for lung cancer, mucus hypersecretion, and inflammation. The use of culture models for airway epithelial cell biology is covered in detail, and a model for autocrine/paracrine growth regulation is discussed. The critical role of vitamin A in tracheal epithelial integrity is also covered. Next, Dey reviews current concepts of the development of the innervation of human and animal lungs, including the embryonic origins of the nervous system, comparative studies in different animal modles, the ontogeny of specific neurotransmitters, and basic principles regulating interactions between the nervous system and target tissues. McCray and Nakamura review the development of airway smooth muscle protein expression, and the physiology of airway smooth muscle during development. The potential relationship between airway smooth muscle development and disease, including oxygen toxicity, bronchopulmonary dysplasia, and reversible airway obstruction in early childhood, is also discussed.

Chapters 11–18 deal with control of lung growth and cytodifferentiation, including specific critical biomaterials (elastin, laminin, collagens), and the role of neuropeptides, other hormones, and lung injury in modulating lung structure and function. Schuger, who has contributed much to our understanding of the role of laminin in lung development, reviews current data on its structure and function, and potential role in lung morphogenesis. Crouch, Mecham, Davila, and Noguchi review the structure, supramolecular organization, and expression of two major classes of lung extracellular matrix molecules—collagens and elastic fibers—in lung development. Roman reviews current concepts in cell-cell and cell-matrix interactions in vasculogenesis in the developing lung. Sunday, who has made major contributions to the field of neuropeptides and lung development, follows with a remarkably comprehensive chapter. Proper development of a functional surfactant system is critical to establishing respiration, and Odom and Ballard survey recent work on the development and hormonal regulation of the surfactant system. They focus on cellular and molecular regulatory mechanisms, and provide a thorough review of recent developments in this area. Horowitz and Davis provide information on mechanisms and consequences of lung injury associated with premature birth, integrating and correlating information presented in earlier chapters. Understanding of pathophysiological changes and of normal developmental processes requires in vitro models in which isolated cells or organ culture can be performed. Hilfer and Searls, pioneers in this area, review and integrate data into the context of such model systems. The advent of lung transplantation as a treatment for a variety of otherwise fatal lung diseases makes understanding of compensatory lung growth timely and important. Gilbert, Petrovic-Dovat, and Rannels review the history and current status of this area, and place experimental work into a clinical context.

**John A. McDonald**

# CONTRIBUTORS

**Michael J. Acarregui, M.D.**   Assistant Professor, Department of Pediatrics, University of Iowa College of Medicine, Iowa City, Iowa

**Philip L. Ballard, M.D., Ph.D.**   Professor of Pediatrics, Department of Pediatrics, University of Pennsylvania School of Medicine, The Children's Hospital of Philadelphia, Philadelphia, Pennsylvania

**Carol Basbaum**   Professor, Department of Anatomy and Cardiovascular Research Institute, University of California, San Francisco, California

**Peter H. Burri, M.D.**   Professor of Anatomy, and Chairman, Institute of Anatomy, University of Berne, Berne, Switzerland

**Edmond C. Crouch, M.D., Ph.D.**   Professor of Pathology, Department of Pathology, Washington University School of Medicine, St. Louis, Missouri

**Rosa M. Davila, M.D.**   Assistant Professor, Department of Pathology, Washington University School of Medicine, St. Louis, Missouri

**Jonathan M. Davis, M.D.**   Associate Professor of Pediatrics, Director of Neonatology, Co-Director, CardioPulmonary Research Institute, Department of Pediatrics, Winthrop-University Hospital, State University of New York at Stony Brook School of Medicine, Mineola, New York

**Robin R. Deterding, M.D.**   Assistant Professor, Section of Pulmonary Medicine, Department of Pediatrics, University of Colorado School of Medicine, Denver, Colorado

**Richard D. Dey, Ph.D.**   Professor, Department of Anatomy, West Virginia University, Morgantown, West Virginia

**Kirk A. Gilbert, Ph.D.**   Postdoctoral Fellow, Department of Cellular and Molecular Physiology, Pennsylvania State University College of Medicine, Hershey, Pennsylvania

**Jonathan D. Gitlin, M.D.**   Associate Professor of Pediatrics and Pathology, Department of Pediatrics, Washington University School of Medicine, St. Louis, Missouri

**Brian P. Hackett, M.D., Ph.D.**   Assistant Professor of Pediatrics, Department of Pediatrics, Washington University School of Medicine, St. Louis, Missouri

**S. Robert Hilfer, Ph.D.**   Professor of Biology, Department of Biology, Temple University, Philadelphia, Pennsylvania

**Stuart Horowitz, Ph.D.**   Director, CardioPulmonary Research Institute, Winthrop-University Hospital, State University of New York at Stony Brook School of Medicine, Mineola, New York

**Kuen-Shan Hung, Ph.D.**   Professor, Department of Anatomy and Cell Biology, University of Kansas Medical Center, Kansas City, Kansas

**J.-D. Li, M.D.**   Department of Anatomy, University of California, San Francisco, California

**Melissa Lim, M.D.**   Department of Anatomy and Cardiovascular Research Institute, University of California, San Francisco, California

**Rama K. Mallampalli, M.D.**   Assistant Professor, Department of Internal Medicine, University of Iowa College of Medicine, Iowa City, Iowa

**Paul B. McCray, Jr., M.D.**   Associate Professor, Department of Pediatrics, University of Iowa College of Medicine, Iowa City, Iowa

**Robert P. Mecham, Ph.D.**   Alumni Endowed Professor of Cell Biology and Medicine, Departments of Cell Biology and Medicine, Washington University School of Medicine, St. Louis, Missouri

**Kenneth T. Nakamura, M.D.**   Associate Professor of Pediatrics, Department of Pediatrics, Kapiolani Medical Center, John A. Burns School of Medicine, Honolulu, Hawaii

**Akihiko Noguchi, M.D.**   Cardinal Glennon Children's Hospital, St. Louis University Medical Center, St. Louis, Missouri

**Michael W. Odom, M.D.**   Assistant Professor, Department of Pediatrics, The University of Texas Health Science Center at San Antonio, San Antonio, Texas

**Lidija Petrovic-Dovat, M.D.**   Postdoctoral Fellow, Department of Cell and Molecular Physiology, Pennsylvania State University College of Medicine, Hershey, Pennsylvania

**Charles G. Plopper, Ph.D.**   Professor of Anatomy, Physiology and Cell Biology, School of Veterinary Medicine, University of California, Davis School of Veterinary Medicine, Davis, California

**D. Eugene Rannels, Ph.D.**   Distinguished Professor and Vice Chairman, Department of Cellular and Molecular Physiology, Pennsylvania State University College of Medicine, Hershey, Pennsylvania

**Jesse Roman, M.D.**   Chief, Pulmonary and Critical Care Medicine Section, Department of Medicine, Atlanta Veterans Affairs Medical Center, Decatur, and Assistant Professor of Medicine, Emory University School of Medicine, Atlanta, Georgia

**Lucia Schuger, M.D.**   Associate Professor, Department of Pathology, Wayne State University School of Medicine, Detroit, Michigan

**Robert L. Searls, Ph.D.**   Department of Biology, Temple University, Philadelphia, Pennsylvania

**Zvjezdana Sever**   Graduate Student, Division of Pulmonary Biology, Children's Hospital Medical Center, Cincinnati, Ohio

**John M. Shannon, Ph.D.**   Research Faculty, Department of Medicine, National Jewish Center for Immunology and Respiratory Medicine, and Associate Professor of Medicine, University of Colorado School of Medicine, Denver, Colorado

**Jeanne M. Snyder, Ph.D.**   Professor, Department of Anatomy, University of Iowa College of Medicine, Iowa City, Iowa

**Mary E. Sunday, M.D., Ph.D.**   Associate Professor, Harvard Medical School; Department of Pathology, Brigham and Women's Hospital; and Children's Hospital, Boston, Massachusetts

**Jeffrey A. Whitsett, M.D.**   Professor of Pediatrics, University of Cincinnati College of Medicine, and Director, Divisions of Neonatology and Pulmonary Biology, Department of Pediatrics, Children's Hospital Medical Center, Cincinnati, Ohio

**Reen Wu, Ph.D.**   Professor, California Regional Primate Research Center and Department of Internal Medicine, University of California at Davis, Davis, California

# CONTENTS

# LUNG GROWTH
# AND DEVELOPMENT

# 1

## Structural Aspects of Prenatal and Postnatal Development and Growth of the Lung

PETER H. BURRI

University of Berne
Berne, Switzerland

### I. Introduction

#### A. Overview

The development of the human lung encompasses a period starting with the first appearance of the tracheal bud in the developing embryo and ending somewhere in early childhood. Although birth represents an extremely important event for the individual and produces abrupt changes in the function of the respiratory organ, the development of the pulmonary structures is a relatively steady and continuous process. It is therefore difficult to assess the moment when lung development is completed—a subject of continuing debate.

There is good evidence that fetal breathing movements play a role in lung development (see review in ref. 1). There are also indications that the early onset of respiration in a prematurely born baby may speed up the functional maturation of the lung; it is surprising, however, that the effects on the lung tissue framework of the replacement of the lung fluid by air have never been studied in detail. Admittedly, the impact of birth at term on the pulmonary tissue framework is limited (and does certainly not represent a signal for the transition from one developmental stage to the next). Nevertheless, the importance of birth per se justifies to distinguish a prenatal and a postnatal period of lung development (Fig. 1).

*1*

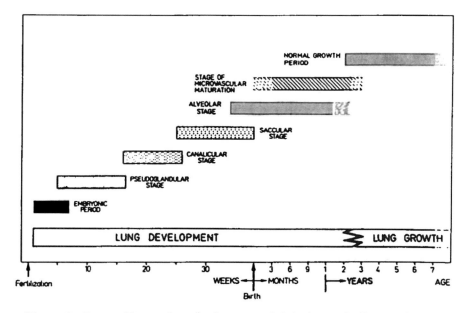

**Figure 1** Stages of human lung development and their time scale. Some periods are overlapping, particularly the alveolar stage and the stage of microvascular maturation. Open-ended bars indicate fuzzy boundaries of stages. (From ref. 75).

Evidently, such a distinction tacitly implies that the lung is not mature at birth; a fact, which has not been appreciated to its full extend until the 1960s or 1970s.

Regarding the onset of lung development, the phase of organogenesis occurs so early that it falls into the so-called "embryonic" period, which usually is defined as the first 5–7 weeks of development of the new organism.

This chapter presents a condensate of the various phases of lung development with emphasis on the structural alterations involved in transforming the lung from its glandular organization into the mature functional organ.

### B. The Human Lung and Animal Models

Although a large number of studies deal with the human lung, it is evident that our understanding of the developmental processes has gained more from the investigation of animal models, because they are experimentally accessible.

Fortunately, it appears that the major steps and mechanisms in lung development are well preserved from one species to the other. As expected, the schedule for the staging is different, as it is also for the timing of birth. This means, on a practical basis for lung research, that insights into developmental steps and events obtained from experimental animals may cautiously be used to interpret and analyze observations made in human lungs, and that experimentally established developmental mechanisms in animal models may with a critical mind be projected to occur also in the human lung.

Because tissue preservation is much better in animal lungs fixed under optimal conditions, the microphotographs of this chapter are often taken from rat lungs—a species in which the development has been very well investigated.

## II. Prenatal Lung Development

### A. Organogenesis, or the Embryonic Period (1–7 Weeks)

The embryonic period comprises the early phase of development of the new organism during which most organs are laid down. It is therefore not considered as a particular or specific phase of lung development. The lungs appear at gestation day 26 as a ventral outpouching of the foregut. Laterally on both sides, the laryngotracheal grooves appear, deepen, and start to separate the lung bud from the prospective esophagus in a caudocranial direction.

At the cranial end of the outpouching, a connection of the lung to the foregut is maintained, corresponding to the later hypopharynx with its entrance to the larynx. The lung bud elongates, soon divides dichotomously, and invades the surrounding mesenchyme. At the age of about 4.5 weeks, the lung anlage shows five tiny saccules, two on the left-hand side and three on the right-hand side, thus preforming the future lobar bronchi and the corresponding lung lobes. By successive dichotomous divisions, the complexity of what corresponds to the future airway tree increases rapidly. By the end of the 7th week, the latter is already preformed down to the subsegmental branches. It is important to point out that lung development is strongly determined by the interaction of the endodermally derived epithelial tubules and the mesenchymal structures which are of mesodermal origin. These interactions have been elegantly documented by the experiments of Alescio and Cassini (2), Taderera (3), Spooner and Wessells (4), and Wessells (5). If mesenchyme from the tip of a bud is transplanted to the side of the prospective tracheal tube, it induces there the outgrowth of a new bud. Alternatively, the mesenchyme alongside the prospective tracheal portion transplanted to the end tip of a bud prevents further branching. Furthermore, the branching type of the airway tree seems to be determined by the mesenchyme: Transplantation of chicken lung mesoderm close to mouse lung epithelium induced the latter to branch in an avian fashion.

Less spectacular, but nonetheless evident, are interactions during later stages of lung development, where it is known that cell to cell contacts and paracrine mechanisms between the alveolar epithelium and the pulmonary fibroblasts govern differentiation steps of the alveolar epithelial cells of type II and vice versa (6,7).

The vascular connections are also established in this early stage: The pulmonary arteries are derived from the sixth pair of aortic arches and the pulmonary vein appears as a small tubule growing out from the left atrial portion of the heart.

However, before these connections are set up, the first vascular plexus surrounding the foregut and the prospective trachea is of systemic nature. Its arterial supply originates from the prospective aorta and the blood is first drained into systemic veins. During further development, the single pulmonary vein stem divides and reaches the future lung tissue. While vascular connections are made, the stem and its two first-order branches are incorporated into the left atrium resulting in the latter having four vein orifices. This ontogenetic origin of the pulmonary veins explains why cardiac muscle can be found in the central branches of the pulmonary venous tree.

After the age of 7 weeks, the lung looks like a primitive small gland and has entered the pseudoglandular stage of development (Fig. 2).

## B.  Stages of Fetal Lung Development

### Pseudoglandular Stage (5–17 Weeks)

Some years ago, the pseudoglandular stage was usually been referred to as the bronchial phase of lung development. The opinion indeed prevailed that, as shown by Bucher and Reid (8), the complete set of generations of gas-conducting airways of the future lung was present by the end of this stage, and that from here onward the peripheral, or gas-exchanging, portions of the lung would develop (9).

Although this preforming of the bronchial tree is still accepted today, it represents only part of the truth.

It was previously been assumed that the peripheral portions of the airway tree contained, so to speak, the roots of the future gas-exchange tissue. Boyden (9) had claimed that the prospective acinus could be defined at the lung periphery at the end of the pseudoglandular stage: He formulated that the pseudoglandular stage ended with the birth of the acinus. Immunohistochemical techniques had also already proved many years ago that epithelial cells at the periphery of the airway tree were precursors of the later alveolar epithelium (10,11).

More recent morphological and morphometric findings obtained in the rat lung indicate that the amount of prospective parenchyma present during the pseudoglandular stage has probably been grossly underestimated so far (12,13). These studies revealed that half of the epithelial cell mass of the lung parenchyma present in the saccular stage just before birth (day 23) was already there in the late pseudoglandular stage (day 20). Furthermore, taking a completely different methodological approach, Kitaoka and co-workers (14) established that in the human lung all the airway divisions down to the level of the alveolar ducts were present toward the end of the pseudoglandular stage. They counted the number of end

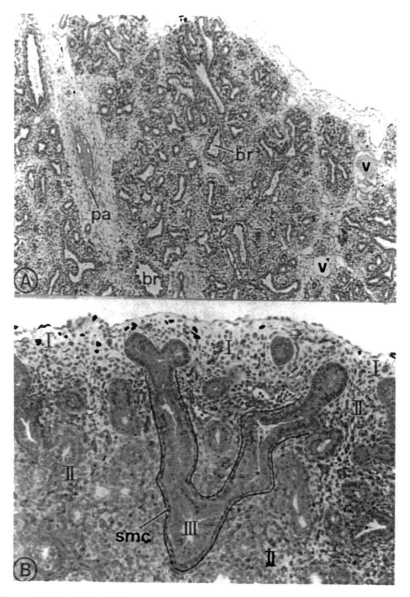

**Figure 2** Pseudoglandular stage of lung development. (A) Human fetal lung, gestational age about 15 weeks. Bright bands of loose mesenchyme containing veins (v) indicate subdivision of lung into segments and lobules. Denser mesenchyme surrounds the tubular sprouts. pa, pulmonary artery; br, bronchus. Light micrograph × 65. (B) Subpleural region of rat lung in pseudoglandular stage, gestational day 19. Zone I (I) is characterized by a loose arrangement of mesenchymal cells immediately below the pleura. In zone II (II) epithelial tubes are ensheated by a more densely packed network of interstitial cells. Zone I to zone II boundary is the site of formation, growth, and differentiation of gas exchange region. The future conductive airways are lying in zone III (III), which is characterized by epithelial tubes with an outer layer of smooth muscle cell precursors (smc). Light micrograph × 150.

segments in samples of three human lungs and calculated that more than 20 and 22 generations of air spaces were present in the pseudoglandular and canalicular stages, respectively. For comparison, the adult human lung contains on average 24 generations of airways inclusive of the trachea (15). Therefore, the view that the pseudoglandular stage is the stage of conducting airway development cannot further be maintained.

The proximal airway generations are lined by a very tall columnar epithelium. The height of the lining cells decreases with further branching to reach a cuboidal shape in the terminal branches.

Besides the standard equipment with the various cytoplasmic organelles, the epithelial cells are loaded with glycogen, which represents the fuel for the later cytodifferentiation—a fact already mentioned by Claude Bernard in 1859. Cell and tissue differentiation occur usually in a centrifugal manner during the whole lung development. So the first ciliated cells, and also the goblet and basal cells, appear in the central airways and are spread with time to the more peripheral tubules. Interestingly, however, the epithelial lining of the uttermost periphery is maintained, at least in part, in an undifferentiated state until the alveolar stage, as is documentated in Figure 3 in a postnatal human lung aged 26 days. Formation of cartilage is first found centrally before 10 weeks, in the segmental bronchi around week 12, and proceeds to the last bronchial generations until about week 25 according to Bucher and Reid (8). Regarding vascular development, which has been extensively and carefully investigated prenatally by Hislop and Reid (16–18), and postnatally by Haworth and Hislop (19), Haworth and co-workers (20,21) and Allen and Haworth (22), it is well known that the arterial tree as a rule branches in accord with the airways, whereas the veins run in between the airway branches in connective tissue septa extending between each generation of dichotomously branching airways as proposed by Verbeken and co-workers (23). Both these principles, however, undergo some specific variations. The arteries show additional branching: Besides the conventional branches running with the airways, there are so-called supernumerary branches, usually small, which supply the alveolar regions adjacent to the walls of the airways. The veins have to depart from their interaxial course in the central lung portions, where the larger branches must join the pulmonary hilum with the airways and arteries.

At the end of the pseudoglandular stage, the hierarchical pattern of the preacinar airways and blood vessels corresponds to that of the adult lung. Recent investigations by confocal microscopy have also shown that these structures, in particular the bronchial tree, are abundantly innervated from the very early stages of development (24).

### Canalicular Stage (16–26 Weeks)

According to the studies of Boyden (9), the transition of the pseudoglandular to the canalicular stage is marked by the "birth of the acinus"; that is, by the

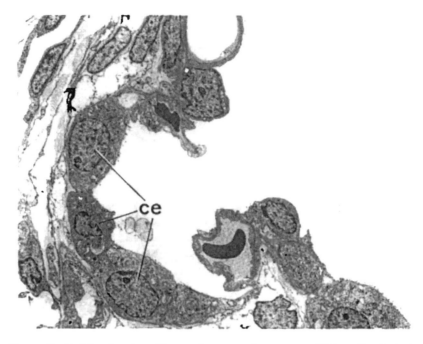

**Figure 3** Peripheral region of human lung parenchyma at age 26 days. End bud of an airway with cuboidal epithelial cells (ce) with some structural characteristics of type II pneumocytes. Electron micrograph × 2215.

prospective gas-exchanging tissue becoming visible in the light microscope. This early acinus consists of an airway stem and a spray of short tubules arranged in a cluster, with the whole structure being delineated by a sheath of loose mesenchyme.

This stage is called canalicular because the future lung parenchyma has become "canalized" by the multiplication of capillaries. Originally, therefore, the name of this stage had nothing to do with the widening of the air spaces in this stage—air spaces which have later sometimes been termed canaliculi. The growing capillaries form a three-dimensional loose network in the mesenchyme. With the expansion of the future air spaces, they come to lie closer to the epithelial layer and rearrange to form a peritubular network. Simultaneously, the cuboidal, glycogen-rich epithelial cells lining the tubules begin to flatten out, so that regions with a thin air-blood barrier appear. In the course of this differentiation, the interepithelial junctional complexes first situated around the apex of the cuboidal cells are shifted to the lower half of the intercellular clefts. Where this happens, the cuboidal cells will differentiate into type I epithelial cells, and into type II pneumocytes where this does not happen. It is presently unknown what governs this process of air-blood barrier formation. It is likely that we are facing here again an interaction between the mesodermally derived endothelium and the endodermally derived epithelium, but this remains an hypothesis. Following their differentiation, the type II cells start to accumulate lamellar bodies, which are often seen in association with multivesicular bodies and with membrane-bound granules containing electron-dense material. Lamellar bodies represent the intracellular storage form of components of the surfactant. Their appearance precedes, therefore, the presence of surface-active material in the air spaces. In most species, surfactant secretion occurs at about 80–85% of total gestation duration. In the human fetus surfactant is already present at only 60% of gestation time.

As Mercurio and Rhodin (25,26) have described, the undifferentiated epithelial cells contain few small lamellar bodies before they start actually to differentiate into either type I or type II cells. This makes it less surprising that in adult lungs the type II cell is considered as the stem cell for both cell lines.

In summary, the canalicular stage brings about important changes in lung structure, which have far-reaching significance for lung function. Indeed, the formation of a thin air-blood barrier and the secretion of surface-active material into the air spaces give a prematurely born baby a first chance to survive toward the end of this developmental stage.

### Saccular or Terminal Sac Stage (24 Weeks to Term)

At the transition of the canalicular stages to the saccular stage, the peripheral airways form typical terminal clusters of widened air spaces called saccules. By lenthening and widening of all air space generations distal to the terminal bronchioles and also by the addition of the last generations of air spaces, the prospective lung parenchyma (defined as the future gas-exchange region) increases massively in size. According to Boyden (9), the terminal sacs will give rise on average to three generations of prospective alveolar ducts and one generation of alveolar sacs. In the light of the findings of Kitaoka and co-workers (14), this increase in the number of generations could be more limited though.

Evidently, each newly formed generation of the airway tree originally has the shape of a blind-ending saccule. When it divides dichtomously, however, it becomes itself a tube giving rise to two new saccules. Even when all generations are formed, the shape of these tubes and saccules is further altered by alveolization. We have therefore suggested that these structures be called transitory ducts and transitory saccules, respectively, or more generally, transitory air spaces (27). Indeed, a transitory saccule becomes a transitory duct when dividing, the transitory duct an alveolar duct when alveoli are formed, and, finally, a transitory saccule is transformed into an alveolar sac, respectively.

As a result of the air space widening, the intervening interstitial tissue between the air spaces is "compressed" and its volume proportion markedly decreases. This in turn profoundly alters the three-dimensional structure of the pulmonary capillary bed and sets the stage for the coming formation of the alveoli.

The capillary networks surrounding neighboring transitory air spaces get closer together, so that the inter-air space walls appear to contain a double capillary network. As we shall discuss later, this septal structure represents a prerequisite for alveolar formation within the parenchyma.

### C. Concept of Fetal Lung Development as Derived from Experimental Work in Rats

In a study involving a light and electron microscopic morphological and quantitative analysis, we analyzed the prenatal phases of lung development in the rat and proposed a concept for the developmental events (12,13). On the grounds of purely morphological criteria, we distinguished in microscopic sections of developing lungs four distinct zones, which are diagrammatically illustrated in Figure 4. Primarily the zones define lung compartments as morphologically identifiable entities, the fate of which can be followed up during the stages of development. The zone concept represented an essential step for the morphometric analysis of prenatal lung development, because it allowed us to define reference spaces for quantitation.

In our model, zone I is characterized by a lighter staining in light and electron microscopic sections caused by the presence of a loose mesenchyme formed by primitive interstitial cells and by capillaries. From day 19 onward, it also contains the end tips of the epithelial tubules. Although the absolute volume of zone I increases till gestational day 21 (Fig. 5), its volume proportion or volume density is highest in the early pseudoglandular stage and decreases steadily until the end of the canalicular stage. Finally, zone I is no longer present in the saccular stage.

Zone II appears as a darker stained more centrally located area. It consists of a densely packed mesenchyme containing dark cells and small capillaries. This zone represents the prospective gas-exchanging parenchyma of the lung. Its volume is therefore increasing massively during development, with birth representing a marked step up due on the one hand to prenatal water loss and on the other hand to a rapid postnatal increase in air content.

Zones III and IV represent the prospective nonparenchymal structures; that is, the purely conducting, non–gas-exchanging portions of the newborn lung. In zone III, the branches of the airways and of the blood vessels are ensheathed by smooth muscle cell precursors; in zone IV, they are additionally enveloped by adventitial cells. Zone IV is not yet present in the early pseudoglandular stage.

From the morphological and quantitative findings, we developed the following understanding of lung development:

The processes of growth and differentiation in the prenatal lung occur in a centrifugal direction.

Zone I is a zone of organ growth. It forms a mantle of undifferentiated tissue around the lung kernel containing zones II–IV. While cells at the border of zone I/II differentiate and slip continuously into zone II, the mesenchymal and endo-

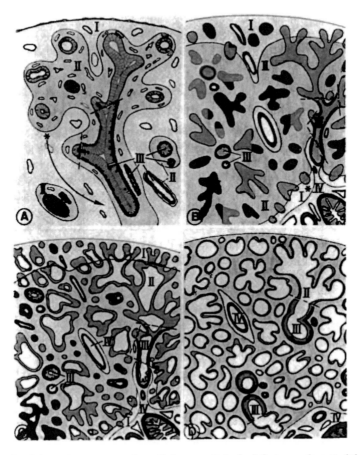

**Figure 4** Schematic representation of the morphological features characterizing the prenatal stages of lung development, according to the zone concept. (A) Early pseudoglandular stage, characterized by the fluid-filled, club-shaped tips of epithelial tubules in zone II and by the absence of zone IV. Note that zone I contains no epithelial tubules yet. For explanation of asterisk and arrow, see (B). (B) Late pseudoglandular stage. All four zones are now present owing to the transformation of proximal zone III into zone IV. Epithelial tubules have extended into zone I. As a result of the recurrent growth of zone II (see arrow in [A]), remnants of zone I form a thin sheath around zone IV structures (central airways and vessels). These portions of zone I represent the peribronchial and perivascular growth regions for the future gas-exchange parenchyma. The number of tubules in zone II has increased dramatically. (C) Canalicular stage. The airway lumina of zone III, the air spaces of zone II, and partially also the proximal portions of zone I tubules have widened. Distal tubules in zone I are still club shaped and lined with cuboidal epithelium. (D) Saccular stage. Zone I has completely disappeared, as have also all the tubular structures. Airway lumina and air spaces have undergone a marked widening. (From ref. 12.)

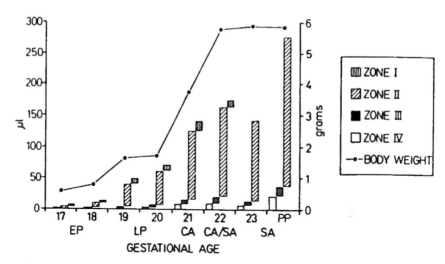

**Figure 5** Body weight curve in grams and absolute zone volumes in microliters of developing rat lung. Gestational age in days; PP, 20 hrs postpartum; EP, early pseudoglandular stage; LP, late pseudoglandular stage; CA, canalicular stage; CA/SA, overlapping of CA and SA stage; SA, saccular stage. (From ref. 12.)

thelial cells multiply at the periphery. This process is likely to go on until all generations of air spaces (except the alveoli) are formed. Zone I therefore disappears at the end of the saccular stage.

Zone II represents on the one hand the future gas-exchanging compartment. It increases in size through differentiation processes at the border I/II, where zone I cells are continuously shifted into zone II (see Fig. 2B). On the other hand, it also contains in its central portions the "germinal layer" for zone III. Here, mesenchymal cells differentiate into smooth muscle cell precursors which ensheath the future bronchi and blood vessels.

Zones III and IV contain the prospective purely conducting structures, the only difference between them being that zone IV elements already possess an adventitial layer. As explained above, zone III extends by differentiation processes taking place at the border III/III. Zone IV appears first in the late pseudoglandular stage when an adventitial layer becomes visible, which subsequently "grows" peripheralad by differentiation from proximal zone III.

Summarizing the zone concept by focusing on the fate of a single primitive zone I mesenchymal cell, we state that an early zone I cell and its descendants are likely to be successively integrated into zone II, III, or IV, because these zones extend peripheralad. A later zone I mesenchymal cell will only reach zone II and differentiate into an interstitial cell of the interalveolar septum. According to the volume proportions of the different zones, the latter situation will be the most frequent one. The fate of the endothelial and epithelial cells of zone I can be interpreted accordingly.

An interesting observation was the detection in zone I of rounded free cells as early as day 17. They were interpreted as histiocytes or histiocyte precursors.

The events that occur in the lung around the time of birth merit special attention. In the rat lung, the canalicular stage is of very short duration (1–2 days), whereas the saccular stage lasts 1–2 days before birth, but it goes on for about further 4 days after birth. As apparent from Figure 5, body weight does not increase over the birth period (days 22 to 1 day postpartum), whereas lung volume drops significantly prior to birth. This reduction in lung volume reflects mainly a sudden volume change in the prospective air space compartment. Rather than to attribute the observed loss of lung liquid to a fixation artefact, we concluded that the liquid secreted into the prospective air spaces, which greatly contributes to normal development of the lung by expanding it (28,29), is lost due to functional alterations (increase of elastic recoil, relaxation of the laryngeal sphincter, fetal breathing movements). The reduction in the septal tissue mass found after birth is also due to the ongoing dehydration of the interstitium. The turnover of lung liquid, its regulation and implications on lung development have recently been presented and discussed in excellent reviews by Strang (30) and by Hooper and Harding (31).

### D. The Lung at Birth

In contrast to the rat lung, the human lung is born in the phase of alveolization, which starts at around week 36 and lasts into early childhood. Since, however, over 85% of the alveoli are going to be formed after birth, we consider that alveolar formation is, in the human, a mainly postnatal event. It is assumed that at birth the human lung contains the complete set of airway generations with the most peripheral airways being relatively short however. Starting from the last generation of conducting airways, the lung parenchyma contains several genera-tions of transitory ducts and, as the last generation on each pathway, a transitory saccule. These structures are to be transformed into alveolar ducts and alveolar sacs, respectively, by a process of air space septation, which generates the alveoli.

## III. Postnatal Lung Development

### A. Alveolar Stage (Week 36 Preterm to 18 Months Postnatal)

In humans, the start, the duration, and the time-point of completion of alveolar formation have long been and (still are) a subject of debate. Between no alveoli at all at birth (9), 20 millions (32), and 50 millions (33), the reader has the choice in the literature of the past 25 years. A similar situation is found regarding the end of alveolization: 20 years (34), 8 years (35), and 2 years (33). The reasons for these seemingly erratic numbers are numerous:

1. The clear definition of an alveolus in a light microscopic section is difficult. Therefore, those investigators who have analyzed and compared the alveolar counting results on sections and on three-dimensional reconstructions found large discrepancies between the two approaches (36). During alveolization, this difficulty is even aggravated.
2. The stereological particle counting techniques used in earlier studies were not bias free; new counting procedures have since been elaborated like the dissector (37) and the selector (38), which allow an improved approach to the problem.
3. The final number of alveoli in the adult human lung varies considerably: range 212–605 × 106 millions, depending on body size (33).
4. There is a period of bulk alveolar formation, which probably shifts into a period of alveolar formation at a slow pace, the definitive end of which can hardly be assessed.

It is therefore not very likely that very reliable data as to the termination of the period of alveolization shall ever be obtained.

Nevertheless, with the above limitations in mind, we conclude on the basis of our morphological and quantitative investigations, using the lungs of seven children aged between 1 and 64 months and eight adult lungs, that alveolization is likely to be terminated by 18 or 24 months. Based on morphological criteria alone, we even suspect bulk alveolar formation to be completed by about 6 months of age.

What are the mechanisms of alveolar formation? Alveolization has extensively been investigated in the rat lung, where it can be followed easily in the light and the scanning electron microscopes (Fig. 6A–D). Alveolization starts with the appearance of low ridges along both sides of the saccular walls (Figs. 7 and 8). They incompletely subdivide the transitory channels and saccules of the saccular lung into smaller units, the alveoli, which appear first as shallow outpouchings on scanning electron micrographs (Fig. 7B). Through these events, the channels and saccules become alveolar ducts and alveoli or sacs, respectively. The new interalveolar walls have been designated as secondary septa, because they arise from the intersaccular walls, that is, the primary septa present at birth. In transsections, the secondary septa contain a central sheet of connective tissue, flanked on both sides by a capillary layer (Fig. 7C). Sometimes the latter are interconnected by capillary loops running over the free edge of the septum (Fig. 7D). At the tip of the crest or below the capillary loop, we find cross-sectioned fibers of elastin. Alveolar formation is closely linked to the deposition of elastin in the saccular lung: Already in 1936, Dubreuil and co-workers (39) had described in the human lung that interalveolar walls would appear where elastin had been deposited along the inter-air space wall. The ultrastructure of primary and secondary septa and their morphological interrelation strongly suggest that new alveoli are formed by the alternate upfolding of one of the two capillary layers on both sides of the primary septa (Fig. 9).

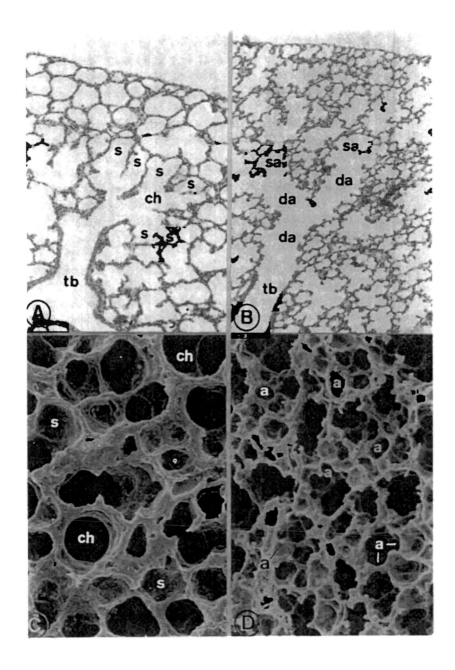

This mode of formation of alveolar walls has interesting and important implications.

1. During the process of alveolization, all the inner air space walls (i.e., primary and secondary septa) contain a capillary bilayer. This immature structure contrasts with the adult morphology of the interalveolar septum, where a single capillary layer occupies practically the whole width of the septum. We have therefore termed both the primary and secondary septa as primitive septa. This term defines their immature state. Primary and secondary septa are, however, different in one important respect. The two capillary layers of the primary septa possess many interconnections, because they originate from a primarily three-dimensional network. In secondary septa, however, the capillary networks are not interconnected except over the free edge, because they have been brought together by the upfolding of a flat sheet (Fig. 10). If, later in time, interconnections can be found at other places, these have been formed by the process of capillary fusioning described below.

2. Alveoli can only be formed where a capillary layer can be folded up. This is the case in all septa containing a double capillary layer (i.e., in the primitive septa) but is also possible where the most peripheral air spaces with only a coarse single capillary network (see p. 21) abut against the pleura or the adventitial layers of bronchi or larger vessels.

3. Following alveolar formation, the capillary networks of the pulmonary parenchyma have to undergo a process of capillary maturation to assume the adult morphology. These structural remodeling, which deeply affects the morphology of the parenchymal septa, represents the last step in lung development.

---

**Figure 6** Follow-up observation of alveolar formation in the rat lung as seen in light (A and B) and in scanning electron microscopy (C and D). (A) Subpleural portion of airways of a rat lung on day 1 postpartum. Terminal bronchiole (tb) divides into smooth-walled channels (ch) which end in saccules (s). No true alveoli are present. (B) Day 21 after birth, same magnification as (A). The corresponding structures in (A) can be directly compared and their maturation examined: The terminal bronchiole (tb) now opens into the formerly smooth-walled channels, which have elongated and have been transformed into alveolar ducts (da) (typical respiratory bronchioles are lacking in the rat lung). The saccules of (A) are partitioned into alveolar sacs (sa) surrounded by alveoli. Light micrographs × 95. (C) Day 1 postpartum. Large cavities correspond to the smooth-walled channels (ch) or saccules (s) in (A). No alveoli can be observed. (D) Day 21 after birth, same magnification as (C). Numerous small, polygonal outpouchings; that is, the alveoli (a) have been formed in the previously larger cavities. Scanning electron micrographs × 265.

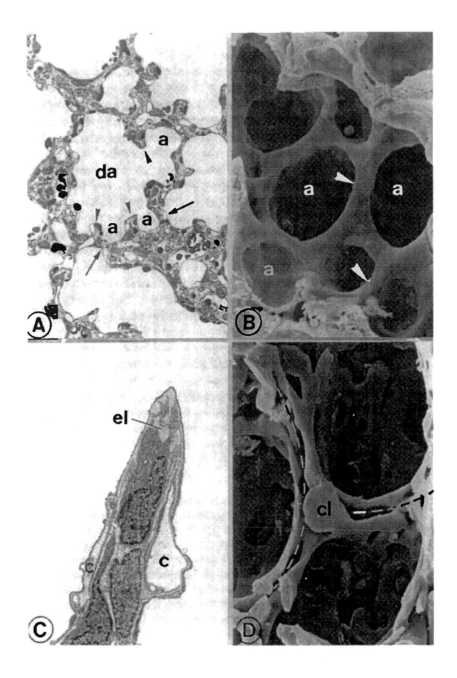

## B.  Stage of Microvascular Maturation

While bulk alveolar formation proceeds, the next developmental process becomes increasingly active: the transformation of the bilayered capillary network in the parenchymal septa into the typical single layered network found in the lung of the older child and of the adult (Figs. 11A and B).

Based on observations made in transmission electron microscopy, two processes are postulated for this maturation: capillary fusions and preferential growth.

### Capillary Fusions or Merging of Septal Capillary Networks

Morphometric analysis of the postnatal rat lung shows that the interstitial volume of the parenchymal septa is decreasing in absolute terms during the third postnatal week despite an increase in total lung volume of 20%. This means that the connective tissue layer separating the capillary networks thins out and that the capillaries of both sides of the septum get closer to each other. In transmission electron microscopy, a frequent observation is that the capillary lumina are merely separated by the cytoplasmic extension of a single endothelial cell. Although such pictures evidently represent the necessary intermediate step in the proposed fusion process, they have to be interpreted with caution, because they can also be obtained by sectioning simple capillary bifurcations. Scanning electron micrographs are, however, equally suggestive for a merging of the two capillary layers but cannot prove it either. There is, at present, no way to follow up the course of events by in vivo microscopy, but we can on the one hand attempt to interpret correctly the findings by fitting static observations into a dynamic process, and on the other hand accumulate further arguments in support of our interpretation. Two observations seem relevant in this respect.

(1) The capillary network of the gas-exchange tissue exhibits two distinct

**Figure 7**  Alveolar formation in the rat lung on day 7 illustrated by different imaging techniques. (A) Light micrograph illustrating numerous low ridges (arrowheads) originating from primary septa (arrows). The secondary septa confine shallow depressions which represent the new alveoli (a). The former saccules are subdivided into alveolar ducts (da). × 245. (B) Scanning electron micrograph showing formation of alveoli (a) by the outgrowth of secondary septa (arrowheads). × 460. (C) Electron micrograph of a secondary septum showing its central axis of connective tissue flanked by capillaries (c) on both sides. The tip of such a crest often contains fibers of elastin (el). × 3830. (D) Scanning electron micrograph of a Mercox cast of lung capillaries. Capillaries are located on both sides of assumed secondary septa (dotted lines). Capillary loop located at the tip of a secondary septum (cl). × 865.

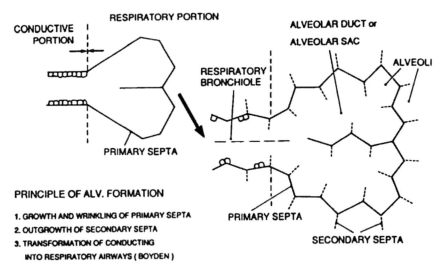

CONDUCTIVE PORTION

RESPIRATORY PORTION

RESPIRATORY BRONCHIOLE

ALVEOLAR DUCT or

ALVEOLAR SAC

ALVEOLI

PRIMARY SEPTA

PRIMARY SEPTA

SECONDARY SEPTA

PRINCIPLE OF ALV. FORMATION

1. GROWTH AND WRINKLING OF PRIMARY SEPTA
2. OUTGROWTH OF SECONDARY SEPTA
3. TRANSFORMATION OF CONDUCTING
   INTO RESPIRATORY AIRWAYS ( BOYDEN )

**Figure 8**   Schematic diagram of process of alveolar formation.

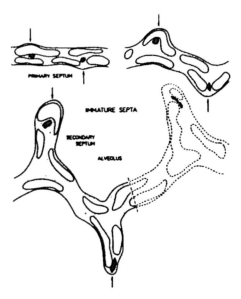

**Figure 9**   Principles of formation of secondary septa. Low ridges (arrows) are formed by lifting up one of the two capillary layers from a primary septum. The ridges grow into secondary septa which also have a bilayer of capillaries. Elastin depositions are closely related to the outgrowth of new septa. (From ref. 27.)

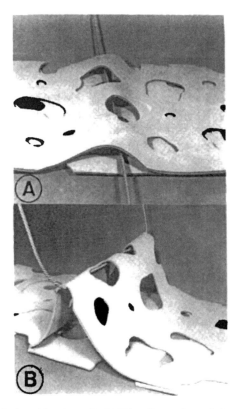

**Figure 10** Model of septal outgrowth. (A) Two flat perforated sheets, represent the two capillary layers; the wire represents elastic fibers. (B) Illustration of the upfolding process and formation of a secondary septum. Notice the capillary bilayer in secondary septum, which is not interconnected excepted over the tip.

patterns. It is relatively dense in the true interalveolar walls, whereas it is coarse where it is adjacent to nonparenchymal structures like the pleura or the peribronchial or perivascular sheaths (40,41). (2) The appearance of interalveolar pores of Kohn during the phase of septal restructuring (42).

Both of these observations can be explained on the grounds of a continuous ontogenic process affecting the mesenchyme intervening between the prospective air spaces. Indeed, the mesenchyme between the future air spaces undergoes a continuous reduction in mass during all the developmental stages. This leads first to the formation of the still relatively thick intersaccular walls with the capillary bilayer allowing for the alveolization. Then, as proved by morphometry, the volume reduction of the interstitium goes on resulting in intercellular contacts

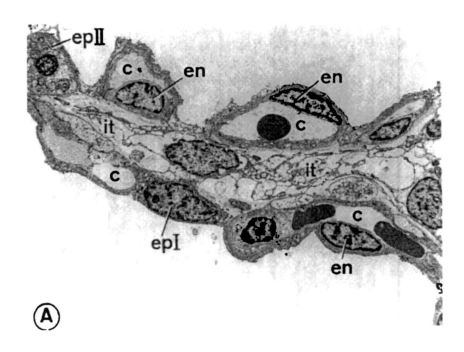

(A)

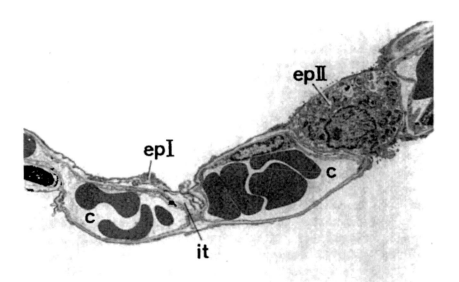

(B)

between endothelial cells of adjacent capillary layers. We recently obtained evidence for apoptosis being involved in this process (43). Where the lumina finally merge, the resulting network will have a capillary density twice as high as the original ones. Where the peritubular capillary networks abut to the pleura or to peribronchial or perivascular connective tissue, there will be nothing to merge with: The capillary network will remain coarse. When ultimately the interstitial layer further thins out, the epithelial layers of adjacent alveoli will come into direct cell to cell contact, "merge," and give rise to pores of Kohn. As we have recently shown, these contacts occur between type II and type I as well as between type I and type I pneumocytes (42). Depending on the extent of the interstitial tissue reduction, which is species dependent and may be genetically determined, the result will be a lung with few or with numerous interalveolar pores.

It has to be pointed out clearly, that the merging of the capillaries and the formation of the pores of Kohn do not necessitate merging or confluency of cells either endothelial or epithelial. What merges, in fact, are lumina (capillary or alveolar), and this is achieved by cell contacts followed by shifting and rearranging the cell junctions.

This succession of events affecting the interalveolar septum in our view strongly supports the concept that capillary merging represents a crucial step in septal transformation. However, since the merging will always be focally distributed, it must be extended by subsequent preferential growth.

### Preferential Growth of Merged Areas

Preferential growth represents a well-established mechanism in embryologic development (e.g., in heart septation) by which considerable morphological and structural alterations can be effected. We propose that preferential growth is likely to play a role in microvascular maturation: the areas where a focal merging has occurred would grow more rapidly than the immature portions of the septum and thus spread the mature condition over wide areas. Even if only one of the two networks would grow by increasing its number of meshes, septal morphology would be greatly altered. How capillary network growth is implemented in the lung is discussed below.

---

**Figure 11** Capillary arrangement in human interalveolar lung septa. (A) 26-day-old baby. Immature or so-called "primitive" septum with two capillary layers ensheathing the central interstitial tissue layer (it). Notice the thin air-blood barriers located on the air space sides of the septum. c, capillary; en, endothelial cell; ep I, pneumocyte type I; ep II, pneumocyte type II. Electron micrograph × 2560. (B) Adult situation. A single capillary layer within the septum. The markedly reduced interstitial tissue runs here on one side of the septum only. For labels, see (B). Electron micrograph × 2630.

## IV.  Disturbances of Alveolization

In the past 10 years, numerous reports have been published indicating that the stage of alveolization corresponds to a very critical period of lung development highly sensitive to all kinds of influences. In 1985, Massaro and co-workers (44) described that treatment of rat pups with minute quantities of dexamethasone from postnatal days 4 to 13 severely impeded the formation of alveoli. Subsequent work by Massaro and Massaro (45), by Blanco et al. (46), and by Sahebjami and Domino (47) confirmed and extended these findings. There is evidence that alveolar formation is not only disturbed by glucocorticoids but also by alterations in $O_2$ partial pressure of the inspired air. Exposure during the critical phase to either hypoxia or hyperoxia (48–53) impaired the alveolization of the lung.

Thyroid hormones seem to be heavily involved in the postnatal phase of lung development but in a reciprocal manner to the glucocorticoid action. Indeed, treatment with thyroxine from birth to 4 or 6 days increased the degree of parenchymal septation by day 5 or 7, whereas a treatment with propylthiouracil (PTU), an inhibitor of thyroid function from birth to the age of 13 days, impeded normal alveolar formation as estimated by mean chord lengths of the air spaces or by air space surface to volume ratios (54). Based on the assumption that alveoli can only be formed in the central parenchymal regions as long as septa contain a double capillary layer (i.e., are of a primitive structure), and on the fact that alveolar wall thinning was accelerated under glucocorticoid treatment, we hypothesized that dexamethasone would not inhibit septal outgrowth per se but rather lead to a precocious maturation of the capillary system.

We were recently able to provide evidence for this theory (55). In rats treated with 0.1 μg of Decadron (a registered trademark of Merck, Sharpe, and Dohme for dexamethasone) from postnatal days 2–15, alveolization was not only markedly impeded but the stage of microvascular maturation was already advanced on days 10 and 13, leading to a markedly increased septal maturation index (SMI).

The SMI was established by dividing the morphometrically measured alveolar surface area underlaid with a single capillary network by the area underlaid with a double capillary network. The SMI was 0.61 versus 0.47 on day 10 and 0.76 versus 0.57 for day 13 in Decadron-treated rats compared with controls.

An interesting and surprising observation was made on day 21; that is, 1 week after withdrawal of Decadron: The trend toward a precocious maturation of the lung appeared to be reversed. The interalveolar walls of the experimental animals were suddenly thicker and the arithmetic mean septal thickness higher than in the controls. Areas with a double capillary network were again more prominent and low secondary septa and also lipid-containing interstitial fibroblasts (which had prematurely disappeared under Decadron treatment) reappeared. On the whole, the pulmonary parenchyma seemed to have regressed in development. Our interpretation of this phenomenon was that we were facing a kind of rebound phenomenon. Morishige and Joun (56) had reported that lung fibroblasts, whose activity had been depressed by glucocorticoid treatment, exhibited a proliferative reaction when treatment was stopped, which resulted in a septal thickening. Interestingly, an analogous developmental rebound effect was recently described by Bruce and co-workers (57). In experiments involving exposure to 95% $O_2$ of rat pups between days 4 and 14, they observed by in situ hybridization a marked depression of the amount of tropoelastin mRNA levels in the lungs of exposed animals. These levels, however, peaked postexposure, whereas they had markedly fallen in the controls.

Our observations of compensatory late immaturity could explain the observation of Massaro and co-workers (44) that further alveoli had to be formed between ages 14 and 60 days. Because they assumed that alveolization could no more be achieved by the standard mode after 2 weeks of age, they postulated alveoli to be formed by other means than septation.

There are numerous reports that indeed further alveoli are formed after the second week in the rat lung under normal conditions.

As we have explained earlier in this chapter, on theoretical grounds the septation theory permits further and life-long alveolization at the uttermost limits of the lung parenchyma; that is, where the air spaces rest upon the connective tissue of pleura, bronchi, or arteries and veins. Hence, there are two possible mechanisms for the belated alveolization after glucocorticoid treatment: first, the ongoing septation in the most peripheral alveolar sacs, or second, a late further round of alveolization within the parenchyma made possible by the observed shift toward immaturity 1 week after cessation of glucocorticoid treatment.

Recently, Blanco (58) proposed that after septation of the existing saccules within the first 2 weeks, the further alveolization takes place by formation of new saccules which would in turn be septated. This interesting hypothesis is based on model assumptions and calculations. The questions of how and where the new saccules are formed remains, however, open.

Whatever the background for the postglucocorticoid treatment process may be, it is evident from all work published so far that following septation inhibition during the phase of bulk alveolar formation, the full complement of alveoli can no longer be produced. This is evidenced in the light micrographs of Figure 12, which compare the lung parenchyma of a control and a Decadron-treated rat at 60 days. The late manifestation of glucocorticoid administration early in life is a somewhat "emphysematous"-looking lung with fewer and larger air spaces.

## V. Growth of the Lung

### A. Growth of the Gas Exchange Tissues

It is evident that prenatally and during the first years of life lung growth occurs conjointly with lung development. Theoretically, the period of normal growth

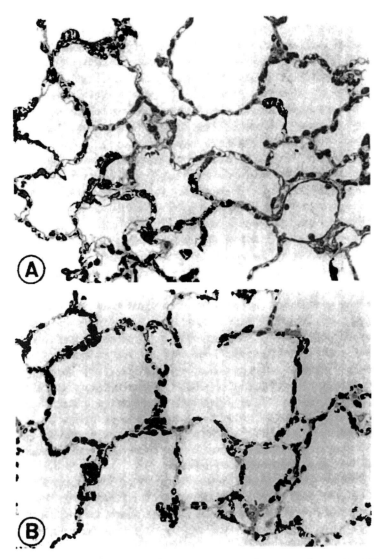

**Figure 12**  Late effects of dexamethasone treatment on lung parenchyma at age 60 days. (A) Control animal. (B) Animal treated with dexamethasone. The experimental animal shows enlarged air spaces compared to the control. In both groups the parenchyma looks mature. Light micrographs × 260.

proper starts when lung development is completed. The transition of development into "simple" growth is, however, imperceptible, as is the transition from growth into aging, where further structural modifications occur (59,60). Although many allometric relationships are close to one in the growth phase, full volume proportionality between lung compartments is not achieved. This means that even when development ends and growth takes over, there is no quantitatively constant tissue framework.

Morphometric data obtained from the lungs of seven children aged between 26 days and 5 years complemented by data from eight adult lungs allowed us to distinguish two phases of lung growth (61) (Fig. 13). The first phase corresponds to the period of alveolar development and of microvascular maturation. It is characterized by major shifts in the quantitative parameters of the parenchymal compartments, whereas the second phase represents a period of more equilibrated growth.

The most prominent changes during phase I are the overproportionate volume increases in the compartments involved in $O_2$ transport. Interestingly, the massive increase in capillary blood volume (see Fig. 13b) coincides with the stage of microvascular maturation, where the double capillary network is reduced to a single one. This indicates that capillary network transformation is associated with intense capillary growth—a further argument in favor of the preferential growth theory.

The volume of air in the lung increases more than lung volume and at the expense of septal volume (see Fig. 13a). Hence, the lung becomes more and more aerated with age. From the three tissue components forming the interalveolar walls, the epithelium and endothelium present a stable quantitative relationship during childhood, whereas the volume density of the interstitium decreases markedly (as was also found in the rat lung in the corresponding period) (62). This is due exclusively to a reduction in the interstitial cell compartment. The data suggest that the lung is born with a given amount of interstitial cells, which are then dispersed in the growing lung. During the same period, the absolute volume of the extracellular interstitium is increasing twofold. In the human lung, both type I and type II alveolar epithelial cells grow with septal volume to the power of one and hence maintain a stable volumetric relationship. In the rat, this was not the case. Type II cell volume augmented by a factor of six between days 4 and 21, whereas type I cell volume increased only twofold (63). This latter study also showed that the content of lamellated bodies in type II cells was quantitatively adapted to the growing gas exchange surface area: At each age investigated, the total lamellar body volume spread over the alveolar surface yielded a surfactant film of constant thickness. Increases in lamellar body volume densities were also reported by Massaro and co-workers (64) in the rat around birth and between postnatal days 10 and 60. These investigators also found a tendency for higher lamellar body surface to volume ratios with age, indicating that the average

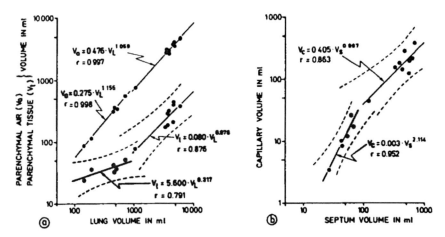

**Figure 13**  Double logarithmic plots of (a) parenchymal airspace ($V_a$) and parenchymal tissue volume ($V_t$) versus lung volume ($V_L$), respectively, and (b) capillary volume ($V_c$) versus septal volume ($V_s$). Regression lines are plotted separately for individuals younger and older than 18 months. The 95% confidence bands for the regression lines are limited by dashed lines. The confidence band for log Va is not drawn to avoid overcrowding of the figure; it is very narrow. (From ref. 61.)

lamellar body decreased in size with growth. The effective quantities of surfactant components like surfactant protein A (SP A) and saturated phosphatidylcholine (Sat PC) in relation to the gas-exchange surface area have recently been determined in the postnatal rat lung by Ohashi and co-workers (65). They demonstrated age-dependent changes in these parameters as well in alveolar washes as in total lung. SP A and Sat PC were highest per unit surface area on day 1, decreased with age, then peaked again on day 21 and fell toward day 50.

All these results indicate that owing to the complex function of surfactant, its quantity and composition in the alveoli do not directly reflect changes in other quantitive lung parameters like alveolar surface area, lung volume, or lamellar body volume.

In the second phase of growth, which (on the basis of the best fit of the growth curves) we postulated to start at the age of about 18 months, the lung volume and the lung compartments grow in a more proportionate way. They also increase to the power of one with body mass (see Fig. 13). For statistical reasons, this does not preclude slight shifts between compartments, as mentioned above.

Alveolar and capillary surface areas do not exhibit the biphasic pattern. Over the whole postnatal period until adulthood, they increase linearly with body weight, as also does the morphometrically calculated pulmonary diffusion capacity.

From these observations, we can conclude that the lung entering the second phase of growth may be considered as representing a miniaturized version of the adult lung.

### B. Growth of the Pulmonary Capillary Bed

In both the human and the rat lung, lung volume increases about 23 times between birth and adulthood (61). In the same period, capillary surface area increases by the same factor and capillary volume by over 35 times. From the investigation of casts of the rat lung microvasculature by scanning electron microscopy, it is evident that the capillary network is not just stretched to fit the growing gas-exchange surface, because the meshes of the network are smaller and denser in the adult that in the newborn lung. This means that new capillary segments have to be added within the capillary bed.

Usually, vascular network growth is assumed to be achieved by capillary sprouting. This means that at the side of a capillary either solid endothelial buds or hollow protrusions would grow into the surrounding connective tissue, contact a neighboring capillary wall, interconnect, and open up to the circulation. Based on light microscopic en face views of interalveolar walls Short (66) had proposed that the capillary network in interalveolar walls would grow by addition of new meshes. When studying the microvascular maturation in Mercox (a registered trademark of Japan Vilene Company, Tokyo, Japan, for a methyl-methacrylate) casts of rat lungs of various ages, we observed the presence of numerous tiny holes (diameter below 1.5 μm) in sheet-like areas of the capillary bed (Fig. 14A) (41). These holes were highly suggestive of newly formed intercapillary meshes, which would then increase in diameter. The iterative addition of such holes would allow the capillary network to grow without the need for sprouting.

In analogy to the growth of cartilage, we termed this process intussusceptional or intussusceptive microvascular growth* (IMG).

Evidently the holes in the cast must correspond to slender transcapillary tissue pillars in longitudinal or in cross sections of capillaries of the interalveolar walls (see Fig. 14B). By the electron microscopic investigation of serially sectioned interalveolar walls, we were able to demonstrate the existence of different types of pillars of required size (65). From the details of their ultrastructure (see Fig. 15), we tentatively proposed the following mode for their formation.

1. Formation across the lumen of a disk-like zone of contact between endothelial cells of opposite walls

---

*According to the *Merriam Webster Dictionary of the English Language*, *intussusception* means "the deposition of new particles of formative material among those already embodied in a tissue or structure."

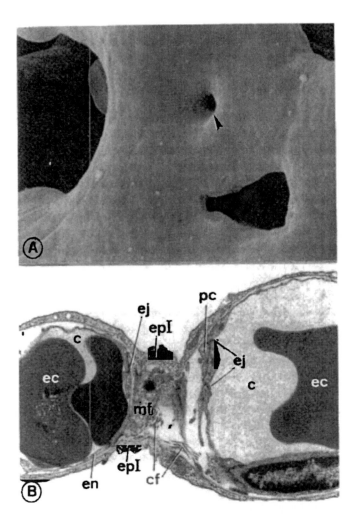

**Figure 14** Illustration of transcapillary tissue pillars related with intussusceptive capillary growth in rat lung parenchyma. (A) Mercox cast of the capillary bed. The pillar appears as a tiny hole of <1.5 μm diameter (arrowhead). Scanning electron micrograph × 8970. (B) Transsection of a fully developed transcapillary tissue pillar in phase IIIc (see Fig. 15). The pillar contains axially a cytoplasmic extension of a myofibroblast (mf) interconnecting the opposite epithelial layers (epI), a portion of a pericyte (pc) adjacent to the capillary endothelium (en), and a few collagen fibrils (cf). The diameter of the pillar is about 2.5 μm. c, capillary; ec, erythrocytes; ej, endothelial cell junctions. Electron micrograph × 10,800.

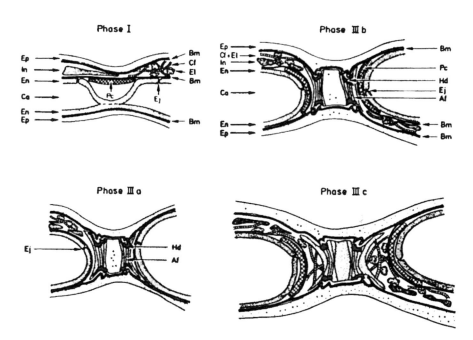

**Figure 15** Illustration of the concept of intussusceptive capillary growth derived from electron optical images. Phase I: Creation of an area of contact between opposite walls. Phase III: Formation of the interstitial core of the pillar. IIIa: Invasion by a cytoplasmatic process of a myofibroblast into the pillar. IIIb: Invasion by a cytoplasmatic process of a pericyte into the pillar. IIIc: Definitive stabilization of the pillar by connective tissue fibers. Af, actin filaments; Bm, basement membrane; Ca, capillary lumen; Cf, collagen fibrils; Ej, endothelial junction; El, elastin; En, endothelium; Ep, epithelium; Hd, hemidesmosome-like structures or attachment bodies; In, interstitium; Pc, pericyte. (From ref. 76.)

2. Formation of a tight junction between the contacting endothelial cells running around the disk
3. Thinning of the cytoplasmic extensions in the disk and rupturing of the disk membrane
4. Invasion of the disk core by interstitium: by cytoplasmic extensions of myofibroblasts, and then of pericytes
5. Stabilization of the pillar by collagen components and growth of the pillar to a normal sized capillary mesh

In the meantime, the presence of IMG has been documented in various species and organ systems and even in tumor growth (67–72). As depicted in Figure 16, some additional and alternative modes of formation could be detected. IMG appears to be an important mechanism of capillary network growth, which is

I. Formation of transcapillary tissue pillars

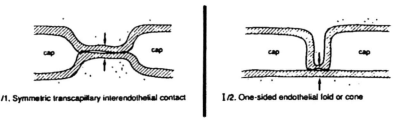

I/1. Symmetric transcapillary interendothelial contact | I/2. One-sided endothelial fold or cone

II. Thinning out of interluminal walls

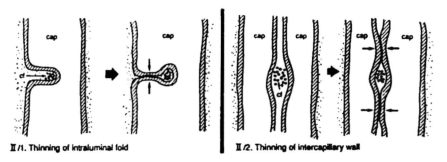

II/1. Thinning of intraluminal fold | II/2. Thinning of intercapillary wall

**Figure 16** Illustration of various modes of implementation of intussusceptive micro-vascular growth as observed in lung and in chicken chorioallantoic membrane. Transcapillary tissue pillars are either formed directly by zones of contact between opposite capillary walls, where the interstitial tissue breaks through the endothelium (arrows in I) or by a process where the capillary lumen breaks through the walls of intracapillary tissue folds (arrows in II/1 or of adjacent capillaries (arrows in II/2).

not only relevant to the lung but may represent a fundamental angiogenetic process in the organism.

## VI. Final Dimensions of the Adult Lung

The quantitative structural data of a standard adult human lung are summarized in Table 1. These dimensions represent, so to speak, the final goal the developmental processes and growth are aiming at. The data were obtained from eight human lungs (six male, two female) thoroughly investigated by light and electron micro-scopic morphometric techniques (61,73,74). When the adult human lung is compared with the one of a newborn baby, some interesting facts can be retained: Specific lung volume is 58 ml/kg body weight in the adult versus 47 ml/kg at 1 month of age, and the volume density of parenchymal air spaces reaches 86.5% in

**Table 1**  Average Dimensions of the Adult Human
Lung

| | |
|---|---|
| Body weight (kg) | 74 ± 4 |
| Lung volume (ml) | 4340 ± 285 |
| Parenchymal volume (ml) | 3907 ± 256 |
| Parenchymal air spaces (ml) | 3386 ± 243 |
| Parenchymal capillary blood (ml) | 213 ± 31 |
| Parenchymal tissue (ml) | 298 ± 36 |
|   alveolar epithelium | 85.7 ± 13.0 |
|   interstitium, cellular | 48.6 ± 5.5 |
|   interstitium, acellular | 107.9 ± 13.1 |
|   endothelium | 55.9 ± 6.1 |
| Air space surface area ($m_2$) | 143 ± 12 |
| Capillary surface area ($m_2$) | 126 ± 12 |
| Arithmetic mean barrier thickness ($\mu$m) | 2.2 ± 0.2 |
| Harmonic mean barrier thickness ($\mu$m) | 0.62 ± 0.04 |

the adult and only 74% around birth. Correspondingly, the figures for the septal volume density (made up of tissue and capillary volume) are 13.5 and 26%, respectively. The capillary blood volume proportion in the septum increases from about 16% to 42% at the sole expense of the interstitial volume density, which falls from 58% to only 30.5%.

The tissue changes are also reflected by the arithmetic mean thickness of the septum, which is a parameter obtained by dividing total tissue mass by alveolar surface area. This value decreases from 5.0 $\mu$m at birth to 2.5 $\mu$m in the adult lung. The harmonic mean thickness of the air-blood barrier, however, which represents an estimate of the resistance to gas diffusion remains astonishingly stable with values around 0.6 $\mu$m despite all the developmentally caused alterations in lung structures.

The gas-exchange surface areas (alveolar and capillary) and the diffusion capacity for $O_2$ increase linearly with body weight (61).

Summarizing these data, we conclude that the adult lung contains more parenchymal air, less tissue, but much more capillary blood than the newborn one. Furthermore, it appears that lung development and growth represent well-balanced processes which occur in keeping with the requirements of the organism for an adequate and undisturbed oxygen supply.

### Acknowledgments

Research was supported by grants from the Swiss National Science Foundation (Nrs. 3100-2775.89 and 3100-36530.92). The author gratefully acknowledges the assistance of Dr. S. Tschanz, Dr. J. Schittny, K. Wyler, B. Haenni, and K. Babl in preparing the manuscript.

### References

1.  Skinner SJM. Fetal breathing movements: a mechanical stimulus for fetal lung cell growth and differentiation. In: Gluckman PD, Johnston BM, Nathaniels PW, eds. Advances in Fetal Physiology. Ithaca, NY: Perinatology Press, 1989: 133–151.

2.  Alescio T, Cassini A. Induction in vitro of tracheal buds by pulmonary mesenchyme grafted on tracheal epithelium. *J Exp Zool* 1962; 150:83–94.

3.  Taderera JV. Control of lung differentiation in vitro. *Dev Biol* 1967; 16:489–512.

4.  Spooner BS, Wessells NK. Mammalian lung development: interactions in primordium formation and bronchial morphogenesis. *J Exp Zool* 1970; 175:445–454.

5.  Wessells NK. Mammalian lung development: Interactions in formation and morphogenesis of tracheal buds. *J Exp Zool* 1970; 175:455–466.

6.  Griffin M, Bhandari R, Hamilton G, Chan YC, and Powell JT. Alveolar type II cell-fibroblast interactions, synthesis and secretion of surfactant and type I collagen. *J Cell Sci* 1993; 105:423–432.

7.  Rannels DE, Rannels SR. Influence of the extracellular matrix on type 2 cell differentiation. *Chest* 1989; 96:165–173.

8.  Bucher U, Reid L. Development of the intrasegmental bronchial tree: The pattern of branching and development of cartilage at various stages of intra-uterine life. *Thorax* 1964; 16:207–218.

9.  Boyden EA. Development and growth of the airways. In: Hodson WA, ed. Lung Biology in Health and Disease. Development of the Lung. Vol. 6. New York: Dekker, 1977:3–35.

10. Ten Have Opbroek AAW. Immunological study of lung development in the mouse embryo II. First appearance of the great alveolar cell, as shown by immunofluorescence microscopy. *Dev Biol* 1979; 69:408–423.

11. Ten Have Opbroek AAW. The development of the lung in mammals: an analysis of concepts and findings. *Am J Anat* 1981; 162:201–219.

12. Burri PH, Moschopulos M. Structural analysis of fetal rat lung development. *Anat Rec* 1992; 234:399–418.

13. Moschopulos M, Burri PH. Morphometric analysis of fetal rat lung development. *Anat Rec* 1993; 237:38–48.

14. Kitaoka H, Burri PH, Weibel ER. Development of the human fetal airway tree—analysis of the numerical density of airway endtips. *Anat Rec* 1996; 244:207–213.

15. Weibel ER. Morphometry of the Human Lung. Heidelberg: Springer, 1963.

16. Hislop A, Reid L. Intra-pulmonary arterial development during fetal life—branching pattern and structure. *J Anat* 1972; 113:35–48.

17. Hislop A, Reid L. Pulmonary arterial development during childhood: branching pattern and structure. *Thorax* 1973; 28:129–135.

18. Hislop A, Reid L. Fetal and childhood development of the intrapulmonary veins in man—branching pattern and structure. *Thorax* 1973; 28:313–319.

19. Haworth SG, Hislop AA. Adaptation of the pulmonary circulation to extra-uterine life in the pig and its relevance to the human infant. *Cardiovasc Res* 1981; 15:108–119.
20. Haworth SG, de Leval M, Macartney FJ. Hypoperfusion and hyperperfusion in the immature lung. Pulmonary arterial development following ligation of the left pulmonary artery in the newborn pig. *J Thorac Cardiovasc Surg* 1981; 82:281–292.
21. Haworth SG, Hall SM, Chew M, and Allen K. Thinning of fetal pulmonary arterial wall and postnatal remodelling: ultrastructural studies on the respiratory unit arteries of the pig. *Virchows Arch A* 1987; 411:161–171.
22. Allen K, Haworth SG. Human postnatal pulmonary arterial remodeling. Ultrastructural studies of smooth muscle cell and connective tissue maturation. *Lab Invest* 1988; 59:702–709.
23. Verbeken EK, Cauberghs M, Van de Woestijne KP. Membranous bronchioles and connective tissue network of normal and emphysematous lungs. *J Appl Physiol* 1996 (in press).
24. Weichselbaum M, Everett AW, Sparrow MP. Mapping the innervation of the bronchial tree in fetal and postnatal pig lung using antibodies to PGP9.5 and SV2. *Am J Resp Cell Mol Biol* 1996; 15 (in press).
25. Mercurio AR, Rhodin JAG. An electron microscopic study on the type I pneumocyte in the cat: differentiation. *Am J Anat* 1976; 146:255–272.
26. Mercurio AR, Rhodin JAG. An electron microscopic study on the type I pneumocyte in the cat: pre-natal morphogenesis. *J Morphol* 1978; 156:141–156.
27. Burri PH. Pulmonary development and lung regeneration. In: Pulmonary Diseases and Disorders. Fishman AP, ed. Vol. 1. 2nd ed. New York: McGraw Hill. 1988:61–78.
28. Alcorn D, Adamson TM, Lambert TF, Maloney JE, Ritchie BRPM. Morphological effects of chronic tracheal ligation and drainage in the fetal lamb lung. *J Anat* 1977; 123:649–660.
29. Moessinger AC, Harding R, Adamson TM, Singh M, Kiu GT. Role of lung fluid volumen in growth and maturation of the fetal sheep lung. *J Clin Invest* 1990; 86:1270–1277.
30. Strang LB. Fetal lung liquid: secretion and reabsorption. *Physiol Rev* 1994; 71:991–1016.
31. Hooper SB, Harding R. Fetal lung liquid: a major determinant of the growth and functional development of the fetal lung. *Clin Exp Pharmacol Physiol* 1995; 22:235–247.
32. Davies G, Reid L. Growth of the alveoli and pulmonary arteries in childhood. *Thorax* 1970; 25:669–681.
33. Langston C, Kida K, Reed M, Thurlbeck WM. Human lung growth in late gestation and in the neonate. *Am Rev Respir Dis* 1984; 129:607–613.
34. Emery JL, Wilcock PF. The postnatal development of the lung. *Acta Anat* 1966; 65:10–29.
35. Dunnill MS. Postnatal growth of the lung. *Thorax* 1962; 17:329–333.
36. Hansen JE, Ampaya EP. Lung morphometry: a fallacy in the use of the counting principle. *J Physiol* 1974; 37:951–954.
37. Sterio DC. The unbiased estimation of number and sizes of arbitrary particles using the disector. *J Microsc* 1984; 134:127–136.

38. Cruz-Orive LM. Arbitrary particles can be counted using a disector of unknown thickness: the selector. *J Microsc* 1986; 145:121–142.
39. Dubreuil G, Lacoste A, Raymond R. Observations sur le développement du poumon humain. *Bull Histol Tech Microsc* 1936; 13:235–245.
40. Miller WS. The lung. 2nd ed. Springfield, IL: Thomas, 1947:74–88
41. Caduff JH, Fischer LC, Burri PH. Scanning electron microscopic study of the developing microvasculature in the postnatal rat lung. *Anat Rec* 1986; 216:154–164.
42. Weiss MJ, Burri PH. Formation of interalveolar pores in the rat lung. *Anat Rec* 1996; 244:481–489.
43. Schittny JC, Burri PH. A peak of programmed cell death appears during postnatal lung development. *J Cell Biochem* 1995; 19B:319 (abstract).
44. Massaro D, Teich N, Maxwell S, Massaro GD, Whitney P. Postnatal development of alveoli. Regulation and evidence for a critical period in rats. *J Clin Invest* 1985; 76:1297–1305.
45. Massaro D, Massaro GD. Dexamethasone accelerates postnatal alveolar wall thinning and alters wall composition. *Am J Physiol* 1986; 251:R218–R224.
46. Blanco LN, Massaro GD, Massaro D. Alveolar dimensions and number: developmental and hormonal regulation. *Am J Physiol* 1989; 257:L240–L247.
47. Sahebjami H, Domino M. Effects of postnatal dexamethasone treatment on development of alveoli in adult rats. *Exp Lung Res* 1989; 15:961–973.
48. Randell SH, Mercer RR, Young SL. Postnatal growth of pulmonary acini and alveoli in normal and oxygen-exposed rats studied by serial section reconstructions. *Am J Anat* 1989; 186:55–68.
49. Massaro GD, Olivier J, Dzikowski C, Massaro D. Postnatal development of lung alveoli: suppression by 13% $O_2$ and a critical period. *Am J Physiol* 1990; 258:L321–L327.
50. Blanco LN, Massaro D, Massaro GD. Alveolar size, number, and surface area: developmentally dependent response to 13% $O_2$. *Am J Physiol* 1991; 261:L370–L377.
51. Blanco LN, Frank L. The formation of alveoli in rat lung during the third and fourth postnatal weeks: effect of hyperoxia, dexamethasone, and deferoxamine. *Pediatr Res* 1993; 34:334–340.
52. Frank L, McLaughlin GE. Protection against acute and chronic hyperoxic inhibition of neonatal rat lung development with the 21-aminosteroid drug U74389F. *Pediatr Res* 1993; 33:632–638.
53. Thibeault DW, Heimes B, Rezaiekhaligh M, Mabry S. Chronic modifications of lung and heart development in glucocorticoid-treated newborn rats exposed to hyperoxia or room air. *Pediatr Pulmonol* 1993; 16:81–88.
54. Massaro D, Teich N, Massaro GD. Postnatal development of pulmonary alveoli: modulation in rats by thyroid hormones. *Am J Physiol* 1986; 250:R51–R55.
55. Tschanz SA, Damke BM, Burri PH. Influence of postnatally administered glucocorticoids on rat lung growth. *Biol Neonate* 1995; 68:229–245.
56. Morishige WK, Joun NS. Influence of glucocorticoids on postnatal lung development in the rat: possible modulation by thyroid hormone. *Endocrinology* 1982; 111:1587–1594.
57. Bruce MC, Bruce EN, Janiga K, Chetty A. Hyperoxic exposure of developing rat lung decreases tropoelastin mRNA levels that rebound postexposure. *Am J Physiol* 1993; 265:L293–L300.

58. Blanco LN. A model of postnatal formation of alveoli in rat lung. *J Theoret Biol* 1992; 157:427–446.
59. Escolar JD, Gallego B, Tejero C, Escolar MA. Changes occurring with increasing age in the rat lung: morphometrical study. *Anat Rec* 1994; 239:287–296.
60. Mizuuchi T, Kida K, Fujino Y. Morphological studies of growth and aging in the lungs of Fischer 344 male rats. *Exp Gerontol* 1994; 29:553–567.
61. Zeltner TB, Caduff JH, Gehr P, Pfenninger J, Burri PH. The postnatal development and growth of the human lung. I. Morphometry. *Respir Physiol* 1987; 67:247–267.
62. Burri PH, Dbaly J, Weibel ER. The postnatal growth of the rat lung. I. Morphometry. *Anat Rec* 1974; 178:711-730.
63. Vidic B, Burri PH. Morphometric analysis of the remodeling of the rat pulmonary epithelium during early postnatal development. *Anat Record* 1983; 207:317–324.
64. Massaro GD, Clerch L, Massaro D. Perinatal anatomic development of alveolar type 2 cells in rats. *Am J Physiol* 1986; 251:R470–R475.
65. Ohashi T, Pinkerton K, Ikegami M, Jobe AH. Changes in alveolar surface area, surfactant protein A, and saturated phosphatidylcholine with postnatal rat lung growth. *Pediatr Res* 1994; 35:685–689.
66. Short RHD. Alveolar epithelium in relation to growth of the lung. *Philos Trans Soc Biol* 1950; 235:35–87.
67. Patan S, Haudenschild C, Burri PH. Intussusceptive capillary growth plays a role in early development of the chicken vasculature (abstr). Proceedings of the International Symposium on Angiogenesis, St. Gallen, Switzerland, March 13–15, 1991.
68. Patan S, Alvarez MJ, Schittny JC, Burri PH. Intussusceptive microvascular growth: a common alternative to capillary sprouting. *Arch Histol Cytol* 1992; 55:65–75.
69. Patan S, Haenni B, Burri PH. Evidence for intussusceptive capillary growth in the chicken chorio-allantoic membrane (CAM). *Anat Embryol* 1993; 187:121–130.
70. Wilting J, Christ B, Bokeloh M, Weich HA. In vivo effects of vascular endothelial growth factor on the chicken chorioallantoic membrane. *Cell Tissue Res* 1993; 274:163–172.
71. Nagy JA, Morgan ES, Herzberg KT, Manseau EJ, Dvorak AM, Dvorak HF. Pathogenesis of ascites tumor growth: angiogenesis, vascular remodling, and stroma formation in the peritoneal lining. *Cancer Res* 1995; 55:376–385.
72. Patan S, Haenni B, Burri PH. Implementation of intussusceptive capillary growth in the chicken chorioallantoic membrane (CAM): 1. Pillar formation by folding of the capillary wall. *Microvasc Res* 1996; 51:80–98.
73. Gehr P, Bachofen M, Weibel ER. The normal human lung: ultrastructure and morphometric estimation of diffusion capacity. *Respir Physiol* 32:121–140.
74. Crapo JD, Barry BE, Gehr P, Bachofen M. Cell numbers and cell characteristics of the normal human lung. *Am Rev Respir Dis* 1982; 126:332–337.
75. Zeltner TB, Burri PH. The postnatal development and growth of the human lung. II. Morphology. *Respir Physiol* 1987; 67:269–282.
76. Burri PH, Tarek MR. A novel mechanism of capillary growth in the rat pulmonary microcirculation. *Anat Rec* 1990; 228:35–45.

# 2

# Respiratory Epithelial Cell Gene Transcription

**JEFFREY A. WHITSETT**

University of Cincinnati College of Medicine
Children's Hospital Medical Center
Cincinnati, Ohio

**ZVJEZDANA SEVER**

Children's Hospital Medical Center
Cincinnati, Ohio

## I. INTRODUCTION

Biochemical, genetic, and functional analyses of the promoter/enhancer regions of the genes encoding surfactant proteins A, B, C, and the Clara cell secretory protein (CCSP) have provided insight into the general mechanisms by which respiratory epithelial cell gene expression is determined. Interactions between nuclear transcription proteins and *cis*-acting elements in the 5'-flanking regions of these genes activate transcription in a respiratory epithelial cell–selective manner. The homeodomain containing DNA binding protein, thyroid transcription factor-1 (TTF-1) and members of the forkhead family of transcription factors (hepatocyte nuclear factors [HNF]-3α and [HNF]-3β and [HFH]-8) bind to DNA elements that stimulate or inhibit gene transcription in respiratory epithelial cells. TTF-1 and HNF family members are also likely to act during embryonic development, committing the foregut endoderm to form the respiratory epithelium. Later in development, these same transcription factors provide signals that regulate surfactant protein synthesis required for postnatal adaptation to air breathing and host defense. This chapter reviews recent experiments that have provided insight into the molecular mechanisms controlling gene expression in the respiratory epithelium.

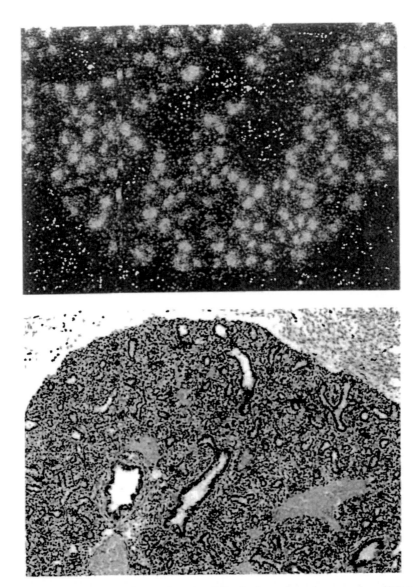

**Figure 1** In situ hybridization of SP-B mRNA in the embryonic mouse lung (PC day 13.5). Darkfield photomicrograph of SP-B mRNA is demonstrated by autoradiography of $^{35}$S-labelled SP-B antisense probe (top). Brightfield photomicrograph was prepared after staining with hemotoxylin-eosin (bottom).

## II. Regulation of Surfactant Protein Gene Expression

Surfactant proteins A, B, and C are abundant phospholipid-associated proteins that are expressed primarily in type II epithelial cells lining the alveolus of the lung (1,2). SP-C is expressed exclusively in type II epithelial cells in postnatal lung. SP-A and SP-B are expressed at high levels in type II cells, and both are also detected in subsets of nonciliated epithelial cells in tracheal-bronchial glands and in nonciliated cells of the conducting airways. Expression of each of these genes is extinguished when type II cells undergo terminal differentiation to type I cells that constitute most of the gas-exchange surface of the alveolus. SP-C mRNA is readily detected in respiratory epithelial cells of the embryonic lung buds, being detected as early as 10–11 days postconception (PC) in the fetal mouse lung (3). SP-B mRNA is first detected several days later in the epithelial cells of the lung buds (Fig. 1). The expression of all three proteins increases markedly between days 16–18 PC in the developing mouse embryo in association with increased synthesis of surfactant lipids required for postnatal lung function. SP-A, SP-B, and CCSP are also expressed in the conducting airway, being detected between days 16 and 17 PC by immunohistochemistry or in situ hybridization analysis of the developing mouse lung (3). CCSP is not readily detected in type II epithelial cells or type I cells and is expressed primarily in the Clara cells or nonciliated columnar cells lining the conducting airways beginning on PC days 17–18 in the mouse. The temporal-spatial pattern of expression of these lung epithelial cell proteins is overlapping but each has a distinct pattern during organogenesis of the lung. These findings provide support for the concept that gene expression in respiratory epithelial cells may be controlled by shared transcriptional elements that must be further modified to determine their unique temporal-spatial distributions in the developing and mature respiratory epithelium.

## III. The SP-B Gene as a Model System of Analysis of Lung Epithelial Gene Transcription and Function

Analysis of the surfactant protein B promoter demonstrated the important role of a nuclear transcription factor, thyroid transcription factor-1 (TTF-1), in surfactant protein gene expression (4). SP-B is a 79–amino acid amphipathic peptide associated with surfactant phospholipids in the alveolus (for review, see ref. 5). SP-B enhances the rate of spreading and stability of phospholipids critical to reducing surface tension during dynamic compression and expansion of the surfactant layers in the alveolus. The important role of SP-B in surfactant function is supported by numerous experimental lines, including the inhibitory effects of anti–SP-B antibodies on lung function in vivo (6), the finding that infants with genetic defects in the SP-B gene suffer from acute neonatal respiratory failure unresponsive to exogenous surfactant (7,8), and that homozygous transgenic mice bearing a null mutation in the SP-B gene fail to expand their lungs at birth (9). The distinctive type II cell organelles, lamellar bodies, and tubular myelin are absent in the type II cells of SP-B (−/−) knockout mice. SP-B deficiency also leads to the incomplete or aberrant processing of surfactant protein C. Similarly, both the SP-B–deficient mice and infants lack the active forms of both SP-B and SP-C (9,10). In the mouse and human, SP-B is expressed primarily in type II epithelial cells but is also detected in a subset of epithelial cells lining conducting airways (11,12). The temporal, spatial and humoral regulation of SP-B synthesis is controlled at both transcriptional and posttranscriptional levels (5). However, analysis of the mechanisms controlling surfactant protein B expression were initially complicated by the lack of differentiated cells that could be used to assess SP-B gene transcription in vitro.

## IV.  In Vitro Models for Analysis of Respiratory Epithelial Gene Transcription (MLE Cells)

Respiratory epithelial cells rapidly loose their differentiated phenotype in cell culture in association with the loss of synthesis of surfactant proteins. Likewise, pulmonary adenocarcinoma cell lines rarely express surfactant proteins, limiting their utility for the analysis of gene expression in vitro. Screening a large number of immortalized pulmonary adenocarcinoma cell lines led to the identification of cell line H441-4 that expressed both SP-A and SP-B (13). Subsequently, H441 cells have been used in the analysis of lung epithelial cell gene expression by numerous investigators. To establish a more complete repertoire of respiratory epithelial cell lines, transgenic mice were made in which the SV40 large T antigen (early region) was expressed under control of SP-C promoter, producing mice that reproducibly developed pulmonary adenocarcinomas before 5–6 months of age. Tumor cells (mouse lung epithelial, or MLE cells) derived from these mice were readily established in culture and clonal lines were developed for the study of epithelial cell function in culture (14). Of these, MLE-12, expressing SP-C and SP-B mRNAs; and MLE-15, expressing SP-A, SP-B and SP-C (and under some conditions, CCSP mRNAs) have been useful in the analysis of transcriptional elements regulating lung epithelial cell gene expression.

## V.  Genetic Analysis of the SP-B Promoter/Enhancer Elements

The SP-B gene comprises 11 exons and 10 introns which are located on human chromosome 2 in a site syntenic with that of the murine SP-B gene on chromosome 14 (15,16). The 5′-flanking region of the SP-B gene was sufficient to direct the expression of chimeric reporter genes in H441-4 cells in vitro (4,17) and in transgenic mice in vivo (R. Bohinski, and J.A. Whitsett, et al., unpublished observations). Deletion analysis of the human SP-B gene promoter demonstrated that the lung epithelial cell specificity of gene transcription of SP-B-CAT constructs was conferred by as little as −218 base pairs from the start of transcription (17). DNAse footprinting analysis of the region identified five readily discernible binding sites wherein nuclear proteins bound to the *cis*-acting elements in the proximal 5'-flanking region of the SP-B gene (Fig. 2a). Of these DNA binding protein sites, two sites binding lung cell–specific factors were chosen for further study using electromobility shift analysis (EMSA), site-specific mutagenesis, and transfection assays using H441 and MLE-15 cells. Distinct DNA-protein interactions were located in the SP-B promoter −70 to −110 base pairs from the start of transcription and were termed SP-B(F1) and SP-B(F2), respectively (4) (Fig. 2b). Other DNAse footprints present in this region were consistent with binding of SP-1 transcription factors and CAAT enhancer binding proteins that are found in many eukaroytic genes.

## VI. TTF-1 Binds to and Activates Transcription at the SP-B(F1) Binding Site

TTF-1 is a 38 kDa nuclear transcription protein previously identified in thyroid epithelial cells on the basis of its ability to bind to and activate the promoter elements of thyroperoxidase and thyroglobulin genes (for review, see ref. 18; 19). TTF-1 is a member of the NKx2.1 family of nuclear transcription factors initially identified in *Drosophila*. TTF-1 was identified by immunohistochemistry and in situ hybridization analysis in the developing rat brain, thyroid, and lung epithelium (20). Although a clear consensus binding site for TTF-1 in surfactant protein genes was not readily apparent, the presence of SP-B(F1) site, the high level of expression of TTF-1 in respiratory epithelial cells, and the apparent similarity of the nucleotides in the DNAse footprinted regions supported the possibility that TTF-1 might interact with the SP-B enhancer region. Bohinski et al. used EMSA, site-specific mutagenesis, transfection assays, and antibody shifts to demonstrate the TTF-1 protein binding sites in the SP-B gene (4) (see Fig. 2b). TTF-1 markedly activated the SP-B promoter by interacting with clearly defined sites in the proximal promoter region of the SP-B gene termed the SP-B(F1) site. TTF-1 binds to multiple, clustered sites in the proximal region of the SP-B promoter (F1) located between −80 and −100 base pairs (bp) from the start of transcription and to a more distal region located −331 to −439 bp from the start of transcription (4) (Fig. 3). These proximal sites are in close proximity to the *cis*-active element binding nuclear transcription factor HNF-3α or its related family members (4). Site-specific mutation of the TTF-1 or HNF binding sites markedly decreased

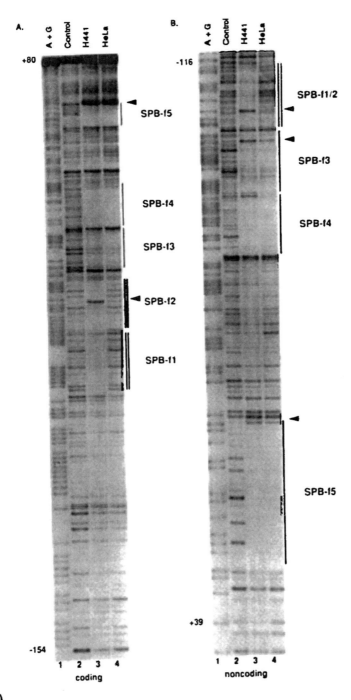

(a)

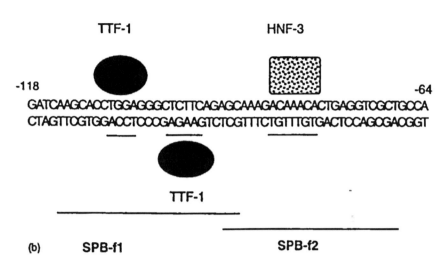

**Figure 2** (a) DNAse footprint analyses of the human SP-B gene promoter. Labeled SP-B gene DNA probes were incubated with nuclear extracts from H441 or HeLa cells and digested with DNAse I. Protected sites are indicated by side bars. Binding to SP-B(F1) and SP-B(F2) were detected in H441 but not HeLa cells (double bars) indicating lung cell-specific binding of nuclear proteins to the sites. Subsequent studies identified these proteins as TTF-1 and HNF-3α, respectively. (b) Organization of *cis*-acting elements SP-B(F1) and SP-B(F2) that bind lung cell-selective nuclear proteins TTF-1 and HNF-3α.

promoter activity in vitro, suggesting that cooperative interactions between TTF-1 and HNF family members are critical to the function of the SP-B promoter proximal regulatory element. The SP-B(F1) region determines lung epithelial specificity of the proximal promoter region from the SP-B gene but does not, by itself, serve as an enhancer capable of activating other gene promoters. In contrast, the cluster of TTF-1 binding sites in the more distal region of the SP-B gene ($-331$ to $-439$ bp) serves as a strong lung epithelial cell–specific enhancer that activates minimal viral promoters in a position-independent manner in H441 and MLE-15 cells (21). TTF-1 protein also forms sulfhydryl-dependent oligomers that bind to clustered sites such as those in the SP-B promoter and may therefore provide a highly organized, high-affinity DNA-protein binding complex that may influence the general transcription machinery of the SP-B promoter (22). The numerous TTF-1 binding sites, their distinct affinities, and their close apposition to other DNA binding motifs provides a variety of mechanisms by which complex and perhaps subtle cell-specific, temporal, spatial, and humoral regulation can be imparted to gene expression.

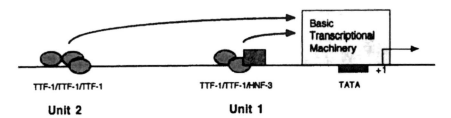

**Unit 2**                          **Unit 1**

**Figure 3**   Multiple TTF-1 binding sites interact with HNF binding sites in the human SP-B gene promoter. A distal TTF-1 cluster (Unit 2) further activates lung cell-specific activity directed by the proximal element located −64 to −118 (Unit 1).

## VII.  Regulation of TTF-1 Gene Expression

TTF-1 is expressed in the developing forebrain, thyroid, and respiratory epithelium (20). In the rodent lung, TTF-1 is first detected in respiratory epithelial cells at the time of lung bud formation (PC days 9–10 in the mouse) (20; L. Zhou and Whitsett, unpublished observations). Thereafter, TTF-1 is expressed abundantly in respiratory epithelial cells of the trachea, bronchi, and the developing respiratory tubules, being more robustly expressed in distal epithelial cells, the levels decreasing in the more proximal regions of the conducting airways (Fig. 4). In the postnatal lung, TTF-1 is expressed at lower levels, being restricted to the subsets of respiratory epithelial cells in the conducting airways and at highest levels in type II epithelial cells in the alveolar region. TTF-1 is undetectable in type I cells of the murine and human lung. Thus, the distribution of TTF-1 expression includes subsets of cells that express SP-A, SP-B, SP-C, and CCSP. Since the cell and sites of expression of these proteins include overlapping but distinct subsets of epithelial cells, TTF-1 appears to be required for their expression but does not determine the heterogeneity of distinct subsets of epithelial cells that express surfactant proteins and CCSP in the lung. TTF-1 mRNA is also expressed by a number of pulmonary adenocarcinoma cell lines, including H441, MLE-12, and MLE-15 cells (23).

## VIII.  TTF-1 Binds and Activates SP-A, SP-B, SP-C, and CCSP Promoter Elements

The overlapping expression of TTF-1, SP-A, SP-B, SP-C, and CCSP suggested that TTF-1 might play a critical role in the regulation of transcription of proteins expressed in the respiratory epithelium. Indeed, analysis of the promoter elements of SP-A, SP-C, and CCSP revealed consensus sequences for *cis*-active elements in the 5′ regions of each of the genes that bound TTF-1. EMSA, site-specific mutagenesis, transfection assays, and DNA footprint analysis identified transcrip-

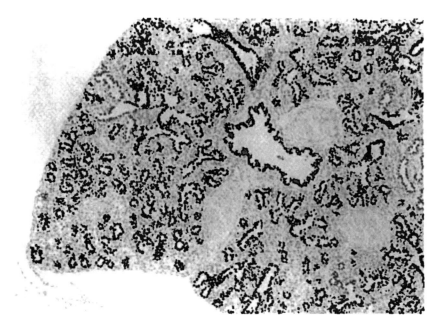

**Figure 4** Distribution of TTF-1 in the developing mouse lung (PC day 15). TTF-1 was detected by immunohistochemistry using anti-rat TTF-1 antiserum (kindly provided by Dr. R. DiLauro).

tionally active TTF-1 binding sites in each of the genes (24,25). Of critical interest was the observation that the expression of TTF-1 in HeLa cells (which do not express surfactant proteins or CCSP) with an expression plasmid directing the synthesis of TTF-1 strongly activated transcription of the promoter-CAT constructs derived from surfactant proteins A, B, C, and CCSP in vitro (4). Thus, in HeLa cells, TTF-1 alone was sufficient to confer transcriptional activation of each of the lung cell–specific genes. TTF-1 binding sites identified in the promoter enhancer regions of these genes are listed in Table 1. The early expression of TTF-1 in lung development and its role in the regulation of transcription of several respiratory epithelial cell genes supports its potential important role in lung morphogenesis and differentiation.

The sequence specific binding of TTF-1 is restricted to the 5' CAAG 3' motif as shown by the in vivo footprinting studies; however, the specificity of that recognition is determined by domains in the amino and carboxy regions of the TTF-1 molecule located outside the homeodomain (HD) itself (26,27). Although TTF-1-HD consists of a characteristic helix-turn-helix structure similar to other homeodomain-containing proteins (28), the TTF-1 gene is not located in the chromosome containing other known HOX genes and is not expressed in a typical

**Table 1**  TTF-1 Binding Sites in the Promoter Regions
of Surfactant Protein Genes as Identified by
Electromobility Shift Assay, DNAse Footprinting, or
Site-Specific Mutagenesis

| Promoter region | Distance from start transcription | |
|---|---|---|
| SPA-A (mouse) | C TCAAG | −255 to −57 |
| | T CTAAG | |
| | G TTAAG | |
| | C TGAAG | |
| SP-B(F1) (human) | C TGAAG | −70 to −100 |
| | T CCAGG | |
| SP-B distal (human) | C CGAAC | −439 to −410 |
| | C TCAAG | −417 to −390 |
| | C TCAAG | −396 to −267 |
| SP-C (mouse) | C CCAAG | −180 to −160 |
| | C CCAAG | −180 to −160 |
| SP-C (human) | G CCAAG | −180 to −160 |
| SP-B distal (mouse) | C TCAAG | −345 to −331 |
| | G TCAAG | −356 to −370 |
| | C ATAAG | −332 to −318 |
| | T AGAGA | −296 to −282 |
| SP-B proximal (mouse) | C TCAAG | −18 to −5 |

anteroposterior manner of this family of transcription activators. Recombinant
TTF-1-HD protein binds to the SP-B(F1) sites in vitro, resulting in an unique
spatial arrangement consisting of two TTF-1 proteins in a head to tail orientation
and separated by approximately one helical turn of the DNA molecule. TTF-1
binding sites are often found clustered in regulatory regions of the target genes
(4,26). Binding to these clustered sites is most likely facilitated by the formation
of TTF-1 protein inter- and intramolecular disulfide bonds (22). The location of
TTF-1 sites in the surfactant protein and CCSP-promoter elements, their numbers,
and relationships to other DNA-protein binding sites are unique to each of these
gene promoters and may therefore provide a mechanism by which the surfactant
genes and CCSP may be independently modulated.

## IX.  Role of HNF Family Members in the Regulation of Gene Expression in the Lung

HNF-3α, HNF-3β, and HNF-3γ were first described in homeotic mutations in
*Drosophila* and identified as positive transactivator of liver-specific genes in

mammals (for review, see ref. 29). Evidence has accumulated that this family of transcription proteins plays an important role in cell differentiation and pattern formation of cells and tissues originating from gut endoderm, including the lung. The determination of embryonic organ-specific expression is, at least in part, achieved by transcriptional regulation among HNF family members.

HNF-3 family members are sequence specific DNA binding proteins. Their binding domain is a nonclassic homeodomain motif with homology to the *Drosophila forkhead* gene product. A model of HNF-3γ protein with a consensus sequence from the liver-specific transthyretin promoter revealed that HNF-3γ binds DNA as a monomer (30). The polypeptide consists of three α-helices forming a hydrophobic core at the N-terminus with the third helix (H3) making direct contacts with the major groove of DNA. Although H3 contains evolutionary conserved residues that contact DNA sites, the recognition specificity of the protein-DNA contact is determined by the helix-2 turn and the N-terminus of the helix-3a (31). Recognition sites of the protein do not contact DNA directly but likely influence the ability of HNF-3γ to achieve a distinct conformation. HNF-3γ makes contacts with the DNA backbone using three loops that consist of connecting α-helices and/or three β-sheets. Consequently, intermolecular contacts are generated with both DNA strands. Because the DNA binding domain shared by all HNF-3 proteins resembles a butterfly, it is often referred to as the "winged helix" motif. An optimal site for HNF-3 DNA binding was determined by comparison of known promoter targets. The sequence of the consensus most common recognition site is TATTGA$^C/_T$TT$_A$/TG. In the lung, distinct binding motifs have been identified, as among diverse liver-specific genes. The TGT3 sequence is referred to as HNH-5 binding motif (HNF-3 homologue-5) to distinguish it from liver-specific motifs. In the human SP-B promoter, this consensus sequence differs by two nucleotides flanking the TGT3 core motif (4) and may comprise a weaker binding site for HNF-3 proteins than that in the liver.

## X. Regulation of HNF-3 Family Members Expression in Lung

The expression pattern of the HNF-3 family members revealed distinct distribution of their mRNAs in various tissues (32). HNF-3α mRNA was detected at highest level in the large intestine and stomach and lesser amounts were found in the liver, lung, and small intestine. HNF-3β mRNA was detected in the same tissues. However, HNF-3γ mRNA was not detected in the lung. In recent gene-targeting experiments in transgenic HNF-3β knockout mice, HNF-3β was identified as the important determinant of an embryonic floor plate organization and formation of the foregut endoderm (33). HNF-3β mRNA was detected in the Henson's node, through which cells migrate before separating into the three primitive germ layers. HFH-4 and HNF-3α were coexpressed in the bronchiolar epithelia of the rat lung, whereas HNF-3β transcripts were detected in the smooth muscle surrounding arterioles and bronchioles (34); the significance of which is at present not clear. On the other hand, type II cells derived from SV40 large T antigen–transformed cells (MLE-15) expressed both HNF-3α and HNF-3β mRNAs (23). Human pulmonary adenocarcinoma H441 cells produced HNF-3α, whereas A549 expressed only HNF-3β. Both HNF-3α and HNF-3β mRNAs were detected in bronchiolar epithelial cells by in situ hybridization, the signal being detected within cells with morphological and histological characteristics of Clara cells of the adult rat lung (35).

## XI. The Role of HNF-3 Family Factors in CCSP Gene Expression

CCSP is synthesized and secreted from nonciliated bronchiolar epithelial cells. Regulatory elements that determine lung cell selectivity are located in the 5'-flanking region (−2339 to +57 bp) of the gene as determined in transgenic animals (36). Transient transfection of H441 human cells with deletion constructs driven by the CCSP promoter were utilized to localize distinct regions of the gene that stimulated cell-specific CCSP transcription (37,38). Factors responsible for cell-specific expression in human H441 cell line and fetal sheep lung cells interact with the sequences −128 to −79 bp upstream from the transcriptional start site (region 1). This region binds ubiquitous octamer (Oct 1) and factors found in cell types other than lung, such as HNF family members and AP1. Mutually exclusive binding of AP1 and HNF-3β to the overlapping binding site in the region 1 cannot be recapitulated in the rat liver extracts which normally express both HNF-3β and AP1 transcription factors (37). Complex combinatorial and protein-protein or protein-DNA interactions are therefore likely to modulate cell-specific transcription of CCSP. However, the elimination of region I in the CCSP promoter did not abolish cell-specific expression in H441 cell line, suggesting that there are other regions or factors contributing to the lung epithelial cell specificity of transcription; such specificity is likely imposed by *cis*-acting elements binding TTF-1. Furthermore, cotransfection of TTF-1 expression vector transactivates CCSP promoter–driven CAT reporter in human HeLa cells (4).

These findings support a role for both TTF-1 and HNF-3 family members in the regulation of CCSP gene expression (36–38). The interaction between the two HNF binding sites, as well as exclusion of AP1 binding, appears to be positively regulated by the upstream *cis*-acting elements in region II of the CCSP promoter (39). Coexpression of HNF-3β cDNA expression vector in H441 cells inhibited CCSP promoter activity. On the other hand, coexpression of both HNF-3α and HNF-3β revealed that these factors have opposite effects on expression directed by region I of the CCSP promoter. Although HNF-3α is a strong stimulator, HNF-3β appears to inhibit the activity of this region of the CCSP gene in HeLa cells (39).

## XII. Regulation of TTF-1 by HNF-3 Family Members in Lung Epithelial Cells

Cotransfection experiments with HeLa and 3T3 cells demonstrated that the promoter of the TTF-1 gene was activated by another homeodomain containing protein, HoxB-3 (40). However, HoxB-3 is not expressed in the H441 cells or MLE cells (K. Ikeda et al., unpublished observation). Moreover, HoxB-3 is expressed in developing lung mesenchyme rather than in the respiratory epithelium (41). Thus the upstream regulators of the TTF-1 gene remain poorly defined. Recent work suggests that HNF-3 forkhead family members may be involved in the transcriptional regulation of TTF-1 in the lung epithelial cells. TTF-1 transcription was markedly activated by cotransfection of an expression vector directing the synthesis of HNF-3β in MLE-15 cells. On the other hand, HNF-α, and HFH-8 inhibited the HNF-3β–dependent activation of TTF-1 promoter constructs in vitro (23). Thus, interactions among HNF-3 family members may directly influence surfactant protein or CCSP gene expression by directly altering TTF-1 gene expression. In summary, distinct combinations of binding sites for TTF-1, HNF-3α, HNF-3β, and other HFH family members, variations in their levels of expression, and their interaction with other nuclear transcription proteins provide versatile mechanisms that may influence lung epithelial cell gene expression during development (Fig. 5).

## XIII. Summary

The respiratory epithelium is a complex cell surface that lines the conducting and gas-exchange regions of the lung. The differentiation of the respiratory epithelium is subjected to precise developmental, hormonal, and host defense signals required to maintain lung function, clear pathogens from its surface, and initiate proliferative responses following injury. Respiratory epithelial cells also synthesize a number of polypeptides critical to surfactant homeostasis (e.g., SP-B and SP-C) and host defense (e.g., SP-A and SP-D) that are subject to precise transcriptional controls. The differentiation of the respiratory epithelium is determined, at least in part, by nuclear transcription proteins that are likely to provide the molecular mechanisms by which the respiratory epithelial cells proliferate and differentiate during lung morphogenesis. Such processes are likely recapitulated during the recovery of the respiratory epithelium following injury. Elucidation of the mechanisms controlling respiratory epithelial cell gene transcription may

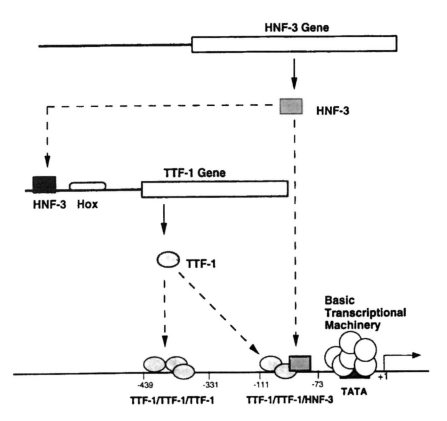

**Figure 5** Hierarchy of transcriptional mechanisms controlling lung epithelial cell gene expression. HNF-3β activates transcription of the TTF-1 gene by binding to a *cis*-acting elements in the promoter region of the TTF-1 gene, TTF-1 binds to the SP-B promoter at a number of sites, activating gene transcription in concert with HNF family members.

therefore provide important clues to the processes of lung morphogenesis and repair.

## Acknowledgments

The authors acknowledge support from the Cystic Fibrosis Foundation and the Center for Gene Therapy for CF and Other Lung Diseases, HL51832.

## REFERENCES

1. Weaver TE, Whitsett JA. Function and regulation of expression of pulmonary surfactant-associated proteins. Biochem J 1991; 273:249–264.
2. Kuroki Y, Voelker DR. Pulmonary surfactant proteins. J Biol Chem 1994; 42:25943–25946.
3. Wert SE, Glasser SW, Korfhagen TR, Whitsett JA. Transcriptional elements from the human SP-C gene direct expression in the primordial respiratory epithelium of transgenic mice. Dev Biol 1993; 156:426–443.
4. Bohinski RJ, DiLauro R, Whitsett JA. Lung-specific surfactant protein B gene promoter is a target for thyroid transcription factor 1 and hepatocyte nuclear factor 3 indicating common mechanisms for organ-specific gene expression along the foregut axis. Mol Cell Biol 1994; 14:5671–5681.
5. Whitsett JA, Nogee LM, Weaver TE, Horowitz AD. Human surfactant protein B structure, function, regulation and genetic disease. Physiol Rev 1995; 75:749–757.
6. Robertson B, Kobayashi T, Ganzuka M, Grossmann G, Li WZ, Suzuki Y. Experimental neonatal respiratory failure induced by a monoclonal antibody to the hydrophobic surfactant-associated protein SP-B. Pediatr Res 1991; 30(3):239–243.
7. Hamvas A, Cole FS, deMello D, Moxley M, Whitsett J, Colten HR, Nogee L. Surfactant protein-B deficiency: antenatal diagnosis and prospective treatment with surfactant replacement. J Pediatr 1994; 125:356–361
8. Nogee LM, deMello DE, Dehner LP, Colten HR. Brief report: deficiency of pulmonary surfactant protein B in congenital alveolar proteinosis. N Engl J Med 1993; 328:406–410.
9. Clark JC, Wert SE, Bachurski CJ, Stahlman MT, Stripp BR, Weaver TE, Whitsett JA. Targeted disruption of the surfactant protein B gene disrupts surfactant homeostasis, causing respiratory failure in newborn mice. Proc Natl Acad Sci USA 1995; 92:7794–7798.
10. Vorbroker DK, Profitt SA, Nogee LM. Whitsett JA. Aberrant processing of surfactant protein C (SP-C) in hereditary SP-B deficiency. Am J Physiol 1995; 268 (Lung Cell Mol Physiol):L647–L656.
11. Wikenheiser KA, Wert SE, Wispé JR, Stahlman M, D'Amore-Bruno M, Singh G, Katyal SL, Whitsett JA. Distinct effects of oxygen on surfactant protein B expression in bronchiolar and alveolar epithelium. Am J Physiol:(Lung Cell Mol Physiol). 1992; 262:L32–L39.

12. Khoor A, Stahlman MT, Gray ME, Whitsett JA. Temporal-spatial distribution of SP-B and SP-C proteins and mRNAs in the developing respiratory epithelium of human lung. J Histochem Cytochem 1994; 42:1187–1199.

13. O'Reilly MA, Gazdar AF, Morris RE, Whitsett JA. Differential effects of glucocorticoid on expression of surfactant proteins in a human lung adenocarcinoma cell line. Biochim Biophys Acta 1988; 970:194–204.

14. Wikenheiser KA, Vorbroker DK, Rice WR, Clark JC, Bachurski CJ, Oie HK, Whitsett JA. Production of immortalized distal respiratory epithelial cell lines from surfactant protein C/simian virus 40 large tumor antigen transgenic mice. Proc Natl Acad Sci USA 1993; 90:11029–11033.

15. Pilot-Matias TJ, Kister SE, Fox JL, Kropp K, Glasser SW, Whitsett JA. Structure and organization of the gene encoding human pulmonary surfactant proteolipid SP-B. DNA 1989; 8:75–86.

16. D'Amore-Bruno MA, Wikenheiser KA, Carter JE, Clark JC, Whitsett JA. Sequence, ontogeny and cellular localization of murine surfactant protein B mRNA. Am J Physiol (Lung Cell Mol Physiol) 1992; 262:L40–L47.

17. Bohinski RJ, Huffman JA, Whitsett JA, Lattier DL. Cis-active elements controlling lung cell-specific expression of human pulmonary surfactant protein- B gene. J Biol Chem 1993; 268(15):11160–11166.

18. Damante G, DiLauro R. Thyroid-specific gene expression. Biochim Biophys Acta 1994; 1218:255–266.

19. Civitareale D, Lonigro R, Sinclair AJ, DiLauro R. A thyroid specific nuclear protein essential for tissue specific expression of the thyroglobulin promoter. EMBO J 1989; 8:2573–2542.

20. Lazzaro D, Price M, De Felice M, DiLauro R. The transcription factor TTF-1 is expressed at the onset of thyroid and lung morphogenesis and in restricted regions of the foetal brain. Development 1991; 113:1093–1104.

21. Yan C, Sever Z, Whitsett JA. Upstream enhancer activity in the human SP-B gene is mediated by TTF-1. J Biol Chem 1995; 270:24852–24857.

22. Arnone MI, Zannini M, Di Lauro R. The DNA-binding activity and the dimerization ability of the thyroid transcription factor I (TTF-1) are redox regulated. J Biol Chem 1995; 270:12048–12055.

23. Ikeda K, Shaw-White J, Whitsett JA, HNF-3β activates transcription of TTF-1 in respiratory epithelial cells. Mol Cell Biol 1996; 16 (in press).

24. Bruno MD, Bohinski RJ, Huelsman KM, Whitsett JA, Korfhagen TR. Lung cell specific expression of the murine surfactant protein A gene is mediated by interactions between the SP-A promoter and thyroid transcription factor-1. J Biol Chem 1995; 270:6531–6536.

25. Kelly SE, Bachurski CJ, Burhans MS, Glasser SW. Transcription of the lung-specific surfactant protein C gene is mediated by thyroid transcription factor-1. J Biol Chem 1996; 27:6881–6888.

26. Damante G, DiLauro R. Several regions of Antennapedia and thyroid transcription factor 1 homeodomains contribute to DNA binding specificity. Proc Natl Acad Sci USA 1991; 88:5388–5392.

27. Damante G, Fabbro D, Pellizzari L, Civitareale D, Guazzi S, Polycarpou-Schwartz M, Cauci S, Quadrifoglio F, Formisano S, Di Lauro R. Sequence-specific DNA recogni-

tion by the thyroid transcription factor-1 homeodomain. Nucleic Acids Res 1994; 22:3075–3083.

28. Viglino P, Fogolari F, Formijano S, Bortolotti N, Damante G, DiLauro R, Esposito G. Structural study of rat thyroid transcription factor 1 homeodomain (TTF-1 HD) by nuclear magnetic resonance. FEBS 1993; 336:397–402.

29. Lai E, Clark KL, Burley SK, Darnell JE. Hepatocyte nuclear factor 3 forkhead or "winged helix" proteins: A family of transcription factors of diverse biologic function. Proc Natl Acad Sci USA 1993; 90:10421–10423.

30. Costa RH, Grayson DR, Darnell JE. Multiple hepatocyte-enriched nuclear factors in the regulation of transthyretin and α1-antitrypsin genes. Mol Cell Biol 1989; 9:1415–1425.

31. Overdier DG, Porecella A, Costa RH. The DNA-binding specificity of the hepatocyte nuclear factor 3/forkhead domain is influenced by amino acid residues adjacent to the recognition helix. Mol Cell Biol 1994; 14:2755–2766.

32. Kaestner KH, Hiemisch H, Luckow B, Schütz G. The HNF-3 gene family of transcription factors in mice: gene structure, cDNA sequence and mRNA distribution. Genome 1994; 20:377–385.

33. Sasaki H, Hogan BLM. HNF 3β as a regulator of fetal plate development. Cell 1994; 70:103–115.

34. Clevidence DE, Overdier DG, Peterson RS, Porcella A, Ye H, Paulson KE, Costa RH. Members of the HNF-3/forkhead family of transcription factors exhibit distinct cellular expression patterns in lung and regulate the surfactant protein B promoter. Dev Biol 1994; 166:195–209.

35. Bingle CD, Hackett BP, Moxley M, Longmore W, Gitlin JD. Role of hepatocyte nuclear factor-3α and hepatocyte nuclear factor-3β in Clara cell secretory protein gene expression in bronchiolar epithelium. Biochem J 1995; 308:197–202.

36. Stripp BR, Sawaya PI, Luse DS, Wikenheiser KA, Wert SE, Huffman JA, Lattier DL, Singh G, Katyal SL, Whitsett JA. Cis-acting elements that confer lung epithelial cell expression of the $CC_{10}$ gene. J Biol Chem 1992; 267:14703–14712.

37. Sawaya PL, Stripp BR, Whitsett JA, Luse DS. The lung-specific CC10 gene is regulated by transcription factors from the AP-1, octamer and HNF-3 families. Mol Cell Biol 1993; 13:3860–3871.

38. Bingle CD, Gitlin JD. Identification of hepatocyte nuclear factor-3 binding sites in the Clara cell secretory protein gene. Biochem J 1993; 295:227–232.

39. Sawaya PL, Luse DS. Two members of the HNF-3 family have opposite effects on a lung transcriptional element; HNF-3α stimulates and HNF-3β inhibits activity of region I from the Clara cell secretory protein (CCSP) promoter. J Biol Chem 1994; 269:22211–22216.

40. Guazzi S, Lonigro R, Pintonello L, Boncielli E, Di Lauro R, Mavilio F. The thyroid transcription factor-1 gene is a candidate target for regulation by Hox proteins. EMBO J 1994; 13:3339–3347.

41. Sham MH, Hunt P, Nonchev S, Papalopulu N, Graham A, Boncinelli E, Krumlauf R. Analysis of the murine Hox-2.7 gene: conserved alternative transcripts with differential distributions in the nervous system and the potential for shared regulatory regions. EMBO J 1992; 11:1825–1836.

# 3

# Role of Transcription Factors in the Development of the Pulmonary Epithelium

**BRIAN P. HACKETT and JONATHAN D. GITLIN**

Washington University School of Medicine
St. Louis, Missouri

## I. Introduction

An essential consideration in understanding vertebrate development is the nature of the molecular mechanisms regulating cellular differentiation. This process of differentiation requires the expression of a cell-specific array of genes that defines cell phenotype. Because only a small fraction of the genes available to a cell are expressed in the differentiated state, mechanisms for regulating gene expression are necessary to ensure that the correct complement of genes is expressed in a given cell. This cell-specific gene expression implies the existence of a hierarchy of regulatory molecules that activate or repress the expression of specific genes. Control of this complex regulation of gene expression may involve both passive and active mechanisms. Passive control results in the permanent inactivation of a gene and may involve epigenetic mechanisms. Active control involves conditional regulation of gene expression and, in general, entails the action of transcription factors that can stimulate or inhibit gene expression (1). The identification and characterization of molecules that regulate gene expression in invertebrates, such as *Drosophila* and *Caenorhabditis elegans*, has contributed greatly to understanding the molecular mechanisms of cellular differentiation in these organisms (2,3). The identification of homologous regulatory proteins in vertebrates is beginning to shed some light on how interactions between multiple regulatory molecules determine differentiation and cell-specific gene expression in these organisms as well.

The expression of any gene in a eukaryotic cell requires the activity of a group of proteins referred to as general transcription factors. These proteins, which include RNA polymerase II and the associated TFIIB, D, E, F, and H proteins, form a complex at the transcription initiation site that is required for the synthesis of mRNA (4). Although these general transcription factors ultimately mediate the temporal and spatial regulation of gene expression, the presence or absence of additional proteins is required for cell-specific gene expression. Such proteins include transcription factors which recognize and bind to unique DNA sequences within specific genes as well as coactivator proteins which guide protein-protein interactions between these specific and general transcription factors (5). Within any given gene there are multiple DNA sequence elements, both upstream and downstream from the transcription initiation site, which are recognized by a variety of specific transcription factors. It is the interplay between these multiple regulatory proteins and their cognate DNA sequences that ultimately determines the temporal and spatial pattern of cellular differentiation during development.

## II.  Cellular Differentiation During Development

### A.  Mechanisms of Cellular Differentiation: The Anterior Pituitary as a Paradigm

The development of the anterior pituitary gland serves as an ideal paradigm for the study of the role of transcription factors in development. Development of the anterior pituitary occurs in a well-defined temporal and spatial pattern. Five phenotypically distinct cell types all derive from Rathke's pouch ectoderm and appear in an ordered fashion during development: corticotropes first followed by thyrotropes, gonadotropes, somatotropes, and lactotropes. In addition, each of the five primary cell types within the anterior pituitary expresses a unique marker in the differentiated state that makes lineage analysis possible (6). The investigation of a *trans*-acting factor conferring cell-specific expression to the human growth hormone gene in the anterior pituitary resulted in the isolation and characterization of pit-1 (GHF-1), a transcription factor essential to differentiation of anterior pituitary cells (7-10). Sequence analysis of pit-1 indicates that it is a member of the POU domain family of transcription factors characterized by a conserved DNA binding domain termed the POU domain (10). Several lines of evidence suggest that pit-1 plays a critical role in the differentiation of cells in the anterior pituitary. Pit-1 is detected in a specific subpopulation of anterior pituitary cells just prior to the production of growth hormone and/or prolactin by these cells (11). Moreover, mutations in the *pit*-1 gene have been characterized in two dwarf mutant mouse strains, Snell and Jackson (12). These mice lack somatotropes, lactotropes, and thyrotropes and have a hypoplastic anterior pituitary gland (12). The expression of *pit*-1 prior to the differentiated state in these cell lineages and the absence of these lineages in mice with *pit*-1 mutations indicates an essential role for *pit*-1 in anterior pituitary differentiation.

### B. Mechanisms of Cellular Differentiation: The Lung as an Experimental System

The lung shares some of the attributes of the anterior pituitary gland that make it a suitable organ for studying the molecular mechanisms regulating cellular differentiation. First, as is discussed below, lung development proceeds in a well-defined temporal and spatial pattern. The various cell types which comprise the lung have been well defined in terms of their morphological and histological characteristics. Additionally, specific molecular markers have been characterized for at least some of the cell types in the lung and these can now be utilized to follow differentiation. Also, the ability to successfully culture lung explants allows for an in vitro approach to the study of lung development. As an example, the classic embryological experiments defining a role for the pulmonary mesenchyme in branching morphogenesis were performed with explanted, cultured embryonic lungs (13).

The lung, however, presents several daunting challenges to the investigator studying the molecular mechanisms regulating cellular differentiation. First, the number of differentiated cell types in the lung greatly exceeds the number of cell types found in the anterior pituitary. For example, at least 11 different epithelial cell types have been described in the conducting and respiratory portions of the lung (14). It is not at all clear what the lineage relationships are between all of these cell types and the existence and identity of stem cells has not been clearly delineated. Also, although unique molecular markers exist for some of the many pulmonary cell types, specific markers have not been identified for all of them. The lack of appropriate markers limits somewhat the ability to study fully cellular differentiation in the lung. Another disadvantage to the study of pulmonary differentiation is that the lung appears relatively late during the course of mammalian development. This limits the ability to use a gene knockout approach to study the role of potentially important regulatory molecules in the lung, as the knockout may be lethal prior to the appearance of the embryonic lung (15,16). This may necessitate the use of novel approaches, such as dominant negative mutations or somatic gene knockouts, to disrupt the function of regulatory proteins during lung development (17). On the other hand, the fact that the lung is not necessary for embryonic survival has some advantage. Experimental approaches that specifically disrupt normal lung development should not be lethal and the full lung phenotype can then be analyzed (17).

### C. Overview of Lung Development

*Lung Epithelial Differentiation*

The lung develops as an outpouching of the foregut endoderm into the mesenchyme of the fetal thorax. Proliferation of the primitive pulmonary epithelial cells results in a contiguous epithelium from the trachea to the acinus. In conjunction with this cellular proliferation, regional differentiation occurs along the length of the epithelium resulting in the formation of at least 11 differentiated epithelial cell types that in large part will determine lung function (14). Although there is some evidence from cell kinetic studies to suggest that basal cells, Clara cells and type II alveolar cells are the primary progenitor cells for the pulmonary epithelium, this is by no means an established point (18). These kinetic studies do not rule out the presence of a small population of as yet unidentified stem cells within the pulmonary epithelium. Lineage analysis with specific cellular markers or cell ablation studies will be required to identify stem cells in the pulmonary epithelium. Toxigenic cell ablation studies in transgenic mice expressing the diphtheria toxin A gene in type II alveolar cells, for example, have supported the concept of the type II cell as the progenitor of the type I alveolar cell (19).

Unlike some other organ systems, such as the gastrointestinal tract, proliferation and differentiation of lung cells is largely completed during the perinatal period and the mature epithelium is relatively quiescent (14). However, a variety of insults, including mechanical or chemical injury, infection, or neoplastic transformation, may alter the patterns of proliferation and differentiation in the mature lung resulting in changes in both lung structure and function (14). Thus, an elucidation of the mechanisms regulating cell proliferation and differentiation in the lung is important to understanding the development of normal pulmonary function and the pathophysiology of lung disease.

*Stages of Lung Development*

Although lung development is continuous during embryogenesis, several developmental periods have been delineated based on the anatomical and histological characteristics of the developing lung (Fig. 1). These stages of lung development are present in all mammalian species studied thus far, although the length of each stage is dependent on the specific length of gestation for each particular species. In addition to the histological features of the epithelium, specific molecular markers are now available for some epithelial cell types during lung development and these are noted in Figure 1 as well. In the discussion below where reference is made to the appearance of specific markers, unless otherwise stated, it is made to the mouse. Figure 1 also summarizes the temporal pattern of expression for some of the regulatory molecules discussed below.

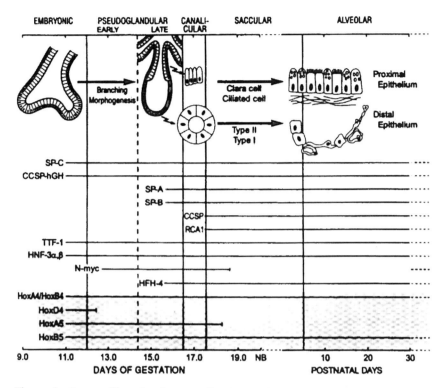

**Figure 1** Stages of lung development. The timing of each stage is based on gestation in the mouse. Horizontal lines indicate the temporal pattern of expression for each marker or transcription factor. The shaded region indicates genes expressed in the mesenchyme; all others are expressed in the epithelium.

## Embryonic Stage

During the initial period of lung development, which has been termed the embryonic stage, budding of the lung from the foregut endoderm and subsequent lobar division occur. During this stage, septation of the developing lung and esophagus also takes place (20). At this time during development, the pulmonary epithelium is columnar in appearance and the cells are multipotent. The first markers for pulmonary epithelial cells also make their appearance during this stage. Surfactant apoprotein C gene expression and expression of a Clara cell secretory protein (CCSP)–human growth hormone transgene are both detected in the pulmonary epithelium during this earliest stage of lung development. At this time, they appear to be expressed in the same population of cells (21,22).

### Pseudoglandular Stage

During the next stage of lung development, the pseudoglandular stage, branching morphogenesis results in the formation of air passages down to the level of the terminal bronchioles. It is during the late pseudoglandular stage that histological differences between proximal and distal pulmonary, epithelial cells first become apparent. The proximal primordial epithelium is characterized by columnar cells and the distal epithelial cells are cuboidal in shape (23). It is also during this stage that molecular markers specifying proximal and distal epithelium are first expressed in distinct populations of cells. Surfactant apoprotein C transcript is now detected in the distal epithelium and presumably identifies a population of primordial distal epithelial cells committed to the type II alveolar cell lineage (21). Expression of the recently described CCSP–human growth hormone transgene becomes restricted to the proximal primordial epithelium and presumably serves as a lineage marker for Clara cells (22). Expression of surfactant apoproteins A and B is also first detected in the late pseudoglandular stage [24,26]. These markers, however, are expressed in both distal and proximal epithelial cells (26,27).

### Canalicular Stage

During the canalicular stage of lung development, further development of the acinar portion of the lung occurs with the distal cuboidal cells forming the earliest components of the pulmonary acinus. Additionally, a decrease in mesenchymal tissue results in closer apposition of the pulmonary vasculature to the epithelium. In the rat, binding of *Ricinus communis* 1 agglutinin (RCA-1), a marker for type I alveolar cells, is first detected at the beginning of the canalicular stage. Binding of this agglutinin to apical surface glycoproteins is initially noted in undifferentiated distal cuboidal cells prior to the appearance of cells with structural characteristics of type I cells. Subsequently, this marker binds to the surface of fully differentiated type I cells (28). Also during the canalicular stage of lung development, expression of the endogenous CCSP gene is first detected in rats and mice in nonciliated bronchiolar epithelial cells termed Clara cells (22,29).

### Saccular Stage

The saccular stage of lung development is characterized by further changes in the acinar portion of the lung. This results in the appearance of respiratory saccules and alveolar ducts. Flattening of distal epithelial cells results in the appearance of cells with morphological characteristics of type I alveolar cells. Further thinning of the mesenchyme brings the pulmonary capillary bed into close approximation to the distal epithelium. It is also during the saccular period that increased production of surfactant components yields a potentially functional lung should birth occur.

### Alveolar Stage

The final stage of lung development, the alveolar stage, occurs primarily during postnatal life. During this period of time, further subdivision of the distal portion of the lung completes the process of alveolus formation.

## III. Transcription Factors in Developing Pulmonary Epithelium

Transcription factors that are potentially important in the developing pulmonary epithelium have been identified in several fashions, First, the recognition of known *cis*-acting elements in the regulatory regions of pulmonary genes has identified transcription factors important in cell-specific pulmonary epithelial gene expression. As an example of this, recognition of hepatocyte nuclear factor (HNF)–3 binding motifs in the CCSP promoter has led to the identification of members of this family of transcription factors as regulators of cell-specific CCSP gene expression (30,31). This suggests that members of the HNF-3 family may play a role in regulating differentiation of the pulmonary epithelium. The association between expression of a transcription factor in the pulmonary epithelium and developmental events has also identified potentially important regulatory molecules in the lung epithelium. The homeobox gene *TTF-1*, for example, is expressed in the developing pulmonary epithelium at the time of the initial branching of the lung bud from the foregut endoderm (32). This temporal pattern of expression is consistent with a role for *TTF-1* in the early differentiation of the pulmonary epithelium. Finally, a role for a known regulatory molecule in development of the pulmonary epithelium may be uncovered serendipitously. Targeted mutation of the N-*myc* gene by homologous recombination resulted in decreased expression of N-*myc* and pulmonary hypoplasia (33). Although the original aim of the experiment was to study the effect of a null mutation in the N-*myc* gene on embryonic development, this "partial knockout" reveals an important role for N-*myc* in lung epithelial development.

### A. Forkhead Domain Proteins (Winged helix)

#### HNF-3

CCSP gene expression is an informative developmental and cell-specific marker within the bronchiolar epithelium recapitulating cellular differentiation in the distal respiratory epithelium (29). In determining the mechanisms regulating cell-specific CCSP gene expression, it was established that 2.25 kilobases of the 5'-flanking region of the CCSP gene are sufficient to direct cell-specific expression of reporter genes to the bronchiolar epithelium of transgenic mice (34,35). Further evaluation of the CCSP promoter revealed a DNAse I footprinted region from −132 to −76 that contained a core binding motif for members of the HNF-3 family of transcription factors (30,31). Gel mobility shift assays with this foot-printed region using lung nuclear extract and specific antibodies revealed binding of both HNF-3α and HNF-3β with this sequence and mutagenesis of the HNF-3 sites abolished these interactions (30,31). Transient transfection of HNF-3α or HNF-3β expression vectors into a Clara cell-like cell line, H441 cells, in conjunction with various CCSP promoter constructs revealed that each of these transcription factors positively regulates CCSP gene expression and that the region from −132 to −76 is sufficient to mediate this effect (36,37). Consistent with this, recent studies reveal that this homologous region in the murine CCSP gene is sufficient to confer Clara cell specific gene expression in transgenic mice (38).

HNF-3α and HNF-3β belong to the forkhead family of transcription factors which was named for the mutation in a *Drosophila* family member that results in an embryo with a duplicated anterior pole (39). Since the isolation of the original family member, homologous proteins have been identified in a variety of meta-zoan organisms, including *Caenorhabditis elegans*, *Xenopus*, zebrafish, chickens, rodents, and humans (40). These DNA binding proteins have been shown to play an important role in cell fate determination and cell-specific gene expression (40). For example, mutation of the *C. elegans* forkhead gene *lin*-31 results in a loss of the normal differentiation of cell lineages required for vulval development (41). In the rodent liver, HNF-3α, HNF-3β, and HNF-3γ are involved in regulating the cell-specific expression of hepatic genes such as transthyretin and $\alpha_1$-antitryp-sin (42).

Proteins in the forkhead family are characterized by a conserved 100–amino acid DNA binding domain which has been termed the forkhead domain (40). X-ray crystallographic analysis of the HNF-γ forkhead domain complexed to DNA reveals a three-dimensional structure that includes three α-helices, three β-pleated sheets, and two wing-like loops (Fig. 2B) (43). Based on this three-dimensional structure, these proteins have also been termed winged-helix pro-teins. The primary site of contact between the DNA binding domain and the major groove of the target DNA is helix III (43). Binding specificity is determined by amino acid residues adjacent to helix III (44).

In the adult lung, expression of HNF-3α and HNF-3β is localized to the bronchiolar epithelium (37). During embryonic development, the patterns of expression of the three HNF-3 family members suggest that they may play important roles in regional differentiation of the gut endoderm and its derivatives which include the lung. (45–47). During early embryonic development, both HNF-3α and HNF-3β are expressed in the anterior region of the primitive streak and subsequently in the node which arises from this region. As invagination of the foregut begins, HNF-3α and HNF-3β expression is detected in the differentiating endoderm. Shortly thereafter, hindgut invagination begins and HNF-3α, HNF-3β, and HNF-3γ are all expressed in this posterior endoderm (45–47). By E9.0 of

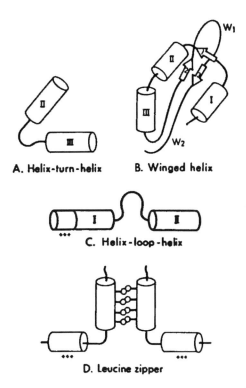

**Figure 2** Transcription factor DNA binding motifs. (A) Helix-turn-helix. Two α-helices are separated by a short turn of three amino acid residues. (B) Winged helix. A central core is formed by three α-helices and three β-pleated sheets; two loops of amino acids extend out from the central core. (C) Helix-loop-helix. Two α-helices are separated by a loop of amino acids. A basic region of amino acids may be associated with helix I. (D) Leucine zipper. The interaction between hydrophobic leucine side chains of α-helical domains allows dimerization to occur.

gestation in the mouse, distinct anterior boundaries of expression have been established for the three HNF-3 genes; HNF-3β has the most anterior boundary in the stomatadeum just anterior to the oral plate, HNF-3α expression extends up to the oral plate, and HNF-3γ has the most posterior domain extending to the junction of the liver diverticulum. Expression of all three genes extends posteriorly to the region of the hindgut (46). As organogenesis progresses along the length of the gut endoderm, HNF-3α and HNF-3β expression increases in the differentiating esophagus and laryngotracheal groove. Within the developing lung, expression is restricted to the bronchiolar epithelium (Fig. 3) (46,47). By E14.0 of gestation, HNF-3β expression is no longer detectable in the trachea or

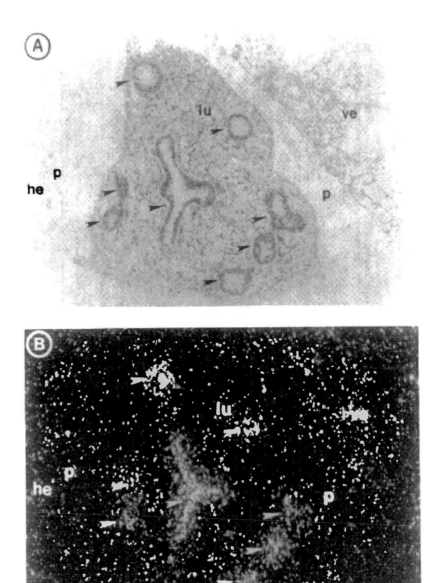

**Figure 3**   HNF-3 expression in the developing lung. In situ hybridization of E12.5 murine lung with a probe to HNF-3β DNA binding domain. Bright (A) and darkfield (B) views are shown. Transcript is detected in the epithelium of the developing bronchioles (arrowheads). No signal is seen in the surrounding mesenchyme. lu, lung; he, heart; ve, vertebrae; p, pleurae.

esophagus, whereas HNF-3α continues to be expressed in these developing organs (46). Both HNF-3α and HNF-3β continue to be expressed in the bronchiolar epithelium in the adult lung (37) (see Fig. 1).

Targeted disruption of the HNF-3β gene underscores the importance of this member of the family in embryogenesis (15,16). The resulting phenotype of the homozygous mutants is an embryonic lethal with failure of normal node and notochord development. Additionally, differentiation of the definitive endoderm is initiated but foregut development is arrested at an early stage. Consequently, there is no development of foregut derivatives such as the lung. The initiation of foregut development in the mutant mice suggests that other factors, perhaps HNF-3α, are capable of supporting the initial differentiation of the definitive endoderm, but that subsequent development requires the presence of HNF-3β (15,16). Because this phenotype is lethal prior to lung budding, it has not been instructive as to the role of HNF-3β in subsequent lung development.

In addition to the CCSP gene, HNF-3 binding sites have been identified in the promoter of the surfactant protein B gene (48). This site is located just upstream from two TTF-1 binding sites and mutation of the HNF-3 site results in reduced transcriptional activity of surfactant protein B constructs in transient transfection assays (48). It is interesting to note, as discussed below, that TTF-1 also transactivates the CCSP promoter (48). Thus at least two lung-specific genes exhibit regulation by both HNF-3 family members and TTF-1. This suggests coordinate regulation of lung-specific genes by these two transcription factors.

### Other Forkhead Proteins

From studies of the regulation of the CCSP gene, it has become clear that the HNF-3 proteins are not the only regulatory molecules required to direct the correct spatial and temporal pattern of CCSP gene expression (22,37). Since the original isolation of the vertebrate HNF-3 genes, a number of vertebrate genes with homologous DNA binding domains have been identified (49–53). Some of these newly identified forkhead proteins are expressed in the lung and may also be important regulators of cellular differentiation and cell-specific gene expression. The forkhead domain amino acid sequences of some of the forkhead proteins expressed in the lung are compared with the forkhead domain of HNF-3β in Table 1. None of these family members are exclusively expressed in the lung and interestingly, several (fkh-3, FREAC-1, and HFH-4) are expressed in both pulmonary and reproductive epithelium (50,51,53). Although these new members of the forkhead family show only 50–60% homology to the HNF-3β DNA binding domain, the regions of highest homology within the domains represent the α-helical regions of the domain (Table 1). Also, the homology between HFH-8 and FREAC-2 and FREAC-1 is 92 and 91%, respectively, suggesting that these genes are the human homologues of the murine HFH-8 gene.

**Table 1**  Comparison of Amino Acid Sequences of DNA Binding Domains of Forkhead Proteins Expressed in Lung

```
HNF-3β   H A K P P Y Y I S L I T M A I Q Q S P N K M L T L S E I Y Q W I M D L F P F Y
fkh-3    P T - - - - - - - - - - A - - A - - S - - G Q R A - - - G - - R Y - - G R - A - I -
HFH-8    P E - - - - - - - - - - A - - V - - S - - - - R - - - - - - - - F L O A R - - - F
FREAC-2  P E - - - - - - - - - - A - - V - - S - - - S - R - - - - - - - - F L Q A R - - - F
FREAC-1  P E - - - - - - - - - - A - - V - - S - - - T - R - - - - - - - - F L Q R S - - - F
HFH-4    - V - - - - - - - A T - - C - - M - A - K A T K I - - A - - - K - - T - N - C Y F

HNF-3β   R Q N Q Q R W Q N S I R H S L S F N D C F L K V P R A P D K P P G K G S F W T L H
fkh-3    - H - R P G - - - - - - - - L - E - - V - - - D D R - - - Y - - I D
HFH-8    - G A Y - G - K - - V - - - N - L - - E - I - L - K G L G R - - H Y - I D
FREAC-2  - G A Y - G - K - - V - - - N - L - - E - I - I - K G L G R - - H Y - I D
FREAC-1  - G S Y - G - K - - V - - - N - L - - E - I - I - K G L G R - - H Y - I D
HFH-4    - H A D P T - - - - - - - - N - L - K - I - - - E K - E - - G - - R I D

HNF-3β   P D S G N M F E N G C Y L R R Q K R F K C
fkh-3    - - C H D - - Q H - S F - - R R - T K          62%
HFH-8    - A - E E - - E - S F R - P R G - R R          56%
FREAC-2  - A - E F - - E - S F R - P R G - R R          55%
FREAC-1  - A - E F - - E - S F R - P R G - R R          55%
HFH-4    - O Y A E R L L S - A F K K - R L P P V H      48%
```

Dashes indicate conserved amino acid residues with respect to HNF-3β.

The patterns of expression for these recently identified forkhead genes in the developing lung have been fully described only for HFH-4 (53). HFH-4 expression is first detected in the murine lung at E14.5 of gestation during the late pseudoglandular stage (see Fig. 1). At this stage, its expression is confined to the developing proximal respiratory epithelium and remains so throughout subsequent lung development (Fig. 4). No expression is detected in the more distal pulmonary epithelium or mesenchyme (53). Expression in the adult lung is also associated with the bronchiolar epithelium (52,53). The timing of HFH-4 expression during development coincides with the initial morphological distinction between proximal columnar and distal cuboidal pulmonary epithelial cells and thus precisely demarcates the differentiation of proximal and distal respiratory epithelium (see Fig. 1) This timing suggests a role for HFH-4 in regulating the initial differentiation of these two distinct populations of pulmonary epithelial cells.

Based on the high degree of homology between their forkhead domains, the FREAC-1 and FREAC-2 proteins appear to be human homologues of murine HFH-8 (see Table 1). FREAC-1 and FREAC-2 expression has been detected in human fetal lung, although the precise timing and the cell specificity of expression have not yet been described (51). HFH-8 has been localized to the distal pulmonary epithelium in the adult murine lung (52). In contrast to HFH-4 then, these data suggest a role for this group of forkhead proteins in the developing distal pulmonary epithelium. Although recent data suggest that HFH-8 may play a role in activating the surfactant protein B gene promoter, surfactant protein B expression is also detected in the nonciliated bronchiolar epithelial cells where HFH-8 expression is not detectable (27,52). This suggests that different arrays of transcription factors may be regulating expression of the same gene in different cell types.

## B. Homeodomain Proteins (Helix-Turn-Helix)

Members of the homeodomain family of transcription factors were first identified as genes responsible for homeotic mutations in *Drosophila melanogaster* (54,55). Homeotic mutations were historically defined as mutations in which a normally formed body part develops in an abnormal location (e.g., a normally formed leg developing in the place of antenna in the Drosophila Antennepedia mutation) (2). Since the original description of these genes more than 10 years ago, homologous family members have been identified in all metazoan organisms examined (56). From a study of the function of these genes in *Drosophila, C. elegans*, and vertebrates, it has become clear that they are important determinants of body axis patterning and impart positional information to differentiating cells (2,57). In vertebrates, a group of these genes, the *Hox* family members, are arranged in four clusters on each of four chromosomes. They are aligned in the 3' to 5' direction

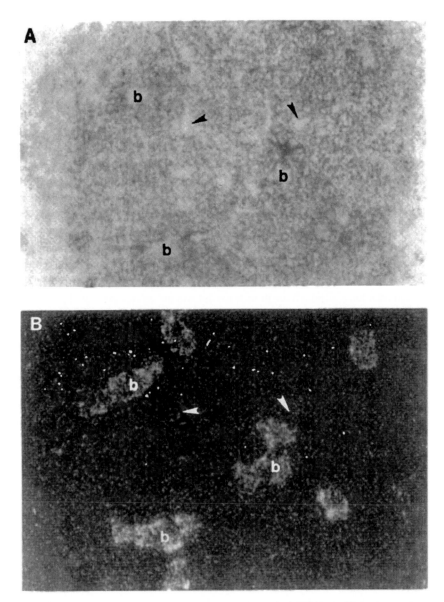

**Figure 4**   HFH-4 expression in the developing lung. In situ hybridization of E14.5 murine lung with a probe for HFH-4. Bright (A) and darkfield (B) views are shown. HFH-4 transcript is detected in the proximal epithelium of the developing bronchioles (b). Transcript is not detected in the developing acinar tubules (arrowheads) or surrounding mesenchyme.

within each cluster according to the anterior most boundary of their expression domain along the anterior-posterior body axis (57). Genes in the equivalent position in different clusters reveal the highest degree of homology and are referred to as paralogues. Thus far, 13 paralogous groups have been identified (57). The arrangement of the multiple *Hox* genes suggests that they arose by multiple duplications during the course of evolution from an ancestral gene (56). Homologous vertebrate homeodomain proteins outside of the *Hox* gene family have also been identified and characterized (58). The conserved homeodomain has also been observed in combination with other conserved domains in regulatory proteins such as pit-1 (10).

Members of the homeodomain family of transcription factors are characterized by a conserved 60–amino acid DNA binding domain termed the homeodomain. The 180 nucleotides encoding this domain are referred to as the homeobox (58). The homeodomain is characterized by four α-helical regions. Helices II and III are separated by a turn of three amino acids forming a characteristic helix-turn-helix motif that has also observed in prokaryotic gene–regulatory proteins (see Fig. 2A) (58). Helices III and IV provide the major contact points for binding in the major groove of the target DNA (58).

### TTF-1

Studies on the regulation of cell-specific gene expression in the thyroid gland have led recently to the isolation and characterization of a new homeodomain protein thyroid transcription factor-1 (TTF-1) (32,59–61). In addition to expression in the thyroid gland, TTF-1 is also expressed in the lung (59). The amino acid sequence of the TTF-1 homeodomain diverges from the conserved sequence of the *Hox* homeodomain proteins and the primary *Drosophila* homeotic genes and is more closely related to the *Drosophila* NK homeodomain proteins (59). The interaction between TTF-1 and DNA, however, still appears to involve contact between helix III of the helix-turn-helix DNA binding motif and the major groove of DNA (59). Also, the DNA sequences that most efficiently bind TTF-1 have a core recognition sequence with a 5'-CAAG-3' motif instead of the previously described 5'-TAAT-3' motif for homeodomain proteins (60).

During rat lung development, TTF-1 expression is first detected at E10.5 in the lung bud as it migrates ventrally from the foregut endoderm (Fig. 5; also see Fig. 1) (32). As lung development progresses, TTF-1 expression is detected in the primordial epithelium of the two primary branches of the initial lung bud on day E11.5 (Fig. 5) and continues to be expressed in the developing bronchiolar epithelium at least to day E15.5. Expression is restricted to the epithelium at all stages of development with no transcript noted in the surrounding fetal mesenchyme or in the foregut prior to lung budding (32). TTF-1 protein is also present in the developing lung bud at E10.5 as demonstrated by immunocytochemistry (32). The appearance of TTF-1 at the earliest point of lung budding suggests that it

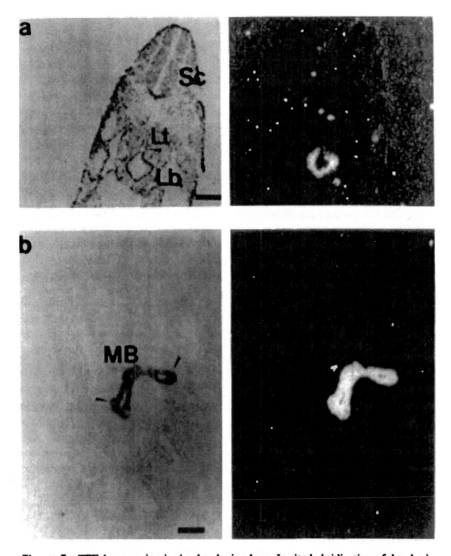

**Figure 5**  TTF-1 expression in the developing lung. In situ hybridization of developing rat lung with probe for TTF-1. (a) Bright (left) and darkfield views of transverse section of pharyngeal cavity from E10.5 day rat embryo. TTF-1 transcript is present in the epithelium of the budding lung (Lb). No transcript is detected in the laryngotracheal groove (Lt) or spinal cord (Sc). (b) Bright (left) and darkfield views of transverse section of pharyngeal cavity from E11.5 day rat embryo. TTF-1 transcript is identified in the epithelium of the two main bronchi (MB). (From Ref. 32; courtesy of The Company of Biologists Limited, Cambridge, United Kingdom.)

may play an important role in the initial differentiation of the lung epithelium from the foregut endoderm.

There is evidence to suggest that TTF-1 expression may be regulated by other homeobox genes. Cotransfection of HeLA cells or NIH3T3 cells with a TTF-1-luciferase chimeric gene and vectors expressing *Hox* gene cDNAs revealed that the human *HoxB3* gene transactivates the rat TTF-1 promoter (142 base pairs of 5'-flanking region) (61). No significant transactivation was observed with the other *Hox* genes tested (*HoxD3, HoxA4, HoxD4, HoxC5, HoxC8, HoxD8*) (61). Additionally, the TTF-1 promoter contains two 5'-ATTA-3' Hox core motifs that bind HoxB3 and when mutagenized inhibit transactivation by *HoxB3* (61). Although this evidence suggests a potential role for HoxB3 regulation of TTF-1 expression, unfortunately in the developing lung as well as in the thyroid, the two genes are expressed in different cell types: TTF-1 in the epithelium and *HoxB3* in the mesenchyme (32,62). It is difficult to reconcile this difference in expression pattern with a role for this particular *Hox* gene in regulation of TTF-1 expression, indicating that as yet unidentified homeobox genes may be involved in the regulation of TTF-1 expression.

In the thyroid gland, the thyroglobulin and thyroperoxidase genes are targets for TTF-1 regulation (59,63). Analysis of the surfactant apoprotein B gene promoter has indicated a potential role for TTF-1 in regulating lung-specific gene expression as well (48). Binding of TTF-1 to degenerate motifs in the surfactant protein B promoter has been identified and mutation of these sites results in decreased expression of surfactant protein B-CAT constructs in H441 cells (48). Also, cotransfection of HeLa cells (which do not express TTF-1 or surfactant B protein) with surfactant protein B-CAT constructs and vectors expressing TTF-1 results in transactivation of the surfactant protein B promoter (48). This same effect is observed with other lung-specific gene promoters, including CCSP and surfactant protein C. No transactivation is noted with a liver-specific promoter from transthyretin (48). These data illustrate the complexity of cell-specific gene regulation. First, although TTF-1 clearly is capable of transactivating the surfactant protein B gene, TTF-1 is expressed much earlier during lung development than surfactant protein B (25,32). This suggests that other elements, either positive or negative regulators, are required for the correct temporal pattern of gene expression during lung development. Also, although TTF-1 is capable of transactivating the CCSP and surfactant protein C genes as well as surfactant protein B in HeLa cells, the cell-specific pattern of expression for each of these genes is different (21,27,29). This again supports the view that other regulatory proteins are required for the correct spatial pattern of gene expression within the lung.

### Hox *Genes*

As discussed above, the vertebrate *Hox* genes are a group of homeobox genes arranged in four linear clusters along each of four chromosomes and exhibit the greatest sequence similarity to the eight primary homeotic genes of *Drosophila* (57). Analysis of the function of these genes during vertebrate development suggests that they are important determinants of the anterior-posterior body axis (57). The expression patterns of the *Hox* genes during lung development have not yet been completely described. In general, *Hox* gene expression during lung development is initially detected during early development (embryonic period or early pseudoglandular) and is localized to mesodermal cells. The role of these mesodermally expressed *Hox* genes in mediating mesodermal-epithelial interactions in the developing lung still needs to be explored. Although outside the scope of this chapter, the temporal patterns of expression for several of the *Hox* genes exhibiting expression in the pulmonary mesoderm during development have been included in Figure 1 for comparison (64–68).

### C. N-*myc* (Helix-Loop-Helix/Leucine Zipper)

N-*myc* belongs to a family of proto-oncogenes that includes c-*myc* and L-*myc*. N-myc was first identified from human neuroblastoma cells as a sequence homologous to the previously isolated c-myc (69). These proteins are characterized by conserved domains at their carboxyl end. A basic region in combination with a helix-loop-helix motif is located just upstream from a leucine zipper motif at the carboxyterminal (see Fig. 2C and 2D). The helix-loop-helix and leucine zipper motifs are thought to mediate homo- or heterodimerization of proteins with like motifs. The basic domain mediates binding to DNA target sequences. A domain required for transactivation is located in the aminoterminal region of these proteins (70). The Myc proteins appear to play important roles in regulating cell proliferation during normal development and neoplastic transformation. There is also evidence to suggest that downregulation of *myc* gene expression accompanies cellular differentiation (69)

The ability of the Myc proteins to form dimers appears to be important in regulating their activity. Another basic helix-loop-helix leucine zipper protein termed Max has been recently identified that is capable of forming heterodimers with all of the members of the Myc family (71). In fact, formation of Myc/Max heterodimers appears to be preferred over the formation of Myc/Myc homodimers. Such heterodimer formation is required for transcriptional activation by Myc (72). Two additional basic helix-loop-helix leucine zipper proteins, Mad and Mxi-1, have been identified that form heterodimers with Max, but do not dimerize with Myc (73,74). Mad and Myc thus compete for Max binding and the formation of Mad/Max dimers represses Myc activity (73). During cellular differentiation, *Mad* and *Mxi-1* expression is induced and the resulting heterodimer formation with Max antagonize Myc/Max activity (74,75).

During early embryonic development, N-*myc* expression is generally confined to the mesoderm of the developing embryo. N-*myc* expression is significant in the undifferentiated mesoderm of the anterior primitive streak, but as differentiation of this mesoderm occurs N-*myc* expression decreases (76). During later organogenesis, N-*myc* expression is detectable in a number of developing organs, including the lung. Expression in the murine lung is high at E12.5 and then declines during subsequent development (77,78). By in situ hybridization, this expression has been localized to the bronchiolar epithelium from E12.5 to E16.5 with no expression detectable by E18.5 (see Fig. 1). At these same stages of lung development, c-*myc* expression is restricted to the mesenchyme of the developing lung (78). The temporal pattern of N-*myc* expression in the lung is associated with the period of greatest pulmonary cell proliferation (78).

Targeted disruption of the N-*myc* gene results in embryonic lethality at E10.5–E12.5 of development (79–81). The fact that apparently normal embryonic development occurs up to day E10.5 suggests that N-*myc* expression is not essential for early embryogenesis. In homozygous embryos after E10.5, development is disrupted in a number of organ systems, including the nervous system, gastrointestinal system, genitourinary system, heart, and lung. This disruption appears to occur after the onset of organogenesis as the various organs are present, but show developmental abnormalities (79–81). Initial lung budding occurs in the homozygotes at E9.5 and there is no detectable difference between the lungs of homozygous and wild-type mice at this stage. By E10.5, however, there is a clear defect in branching morphogenesis and the homozygous lungs consist of only a trachea and mainstem bronchi with no distal branching (79,81). Culturing of the explanted lungs from the homozygous embryos in the presence of fetal calf serum stimulates branching to some degree, suggesting that serum components can at least in part overcome the lack of N-*myc* expression. Branching in these cultured lungs, however, is still reduced compared with explanted wild type lungs cultured in the presence of serum (81). Treatment of wild-type murine lungs explanted at E11.5 with transforming growth factor (TGF)–β1 results in an inhibition of branching morphogenesis and decreased expression of N-*myc*. The inhibition of N-*myc* expression was detectable prior to any observable change in lung morphology suggesting a mechanism for the TGF-β1 effect through its regulation of N-*myc* expression (82). It thus appears that with respect to lung development, N-*myc* expression is required for the continued proliferation of the partially differentiated pulmonary epithelium.

The importance of N-*myc* in proliferation of the pulmonary epithelium is confirmed by another targeted mutation in N-*myc* that results in reduced N-*myc* expression (33). Homologous recombination in this line of mice (N-*myc*$^{9a/9a}$) resulted in a "leaky" mutation that allows for reduced N-*myc* expression through alternative splicing. Homozygous mice die at birth of respiratory failure and the only significant abnormality is pulmonary hypoplasia. This defect appears to be primarily a defect in distal lung development with a reduced number of distal air spaces and apparently normal airway development. The defect in lung mor-

phogenesis is readily apparent by E12.5 with a reduction in lung size and decreased branching of the epithelium (Fig, 6). Measurement of N-*myc* mRNA
levels in homozygous animals revealed a 75% decrease in transcript abundance in
the lung compared with wild-type animals (33).

When heterozygous N-*myc*$^{9a/+}$ mice were bred with heterozygous mice
from one of the null allele lines (N-*myc*$^{BRP/+}$), the lungs of the compound heterozygous mice (N-*myc*$^{9a/BRP}$) were more severely affected than the lungs of homozygous 9a mice (83). The level of N-*myc* transcript and protein was reduced to an
even greater extent than in the 9a/9a mice, and although lung budding occurred,
branching morphogenesis was interrupted following the initial formation of the
mainstem bronchi. The distribution of *flk-1* and c-*myc* expression in the develop-

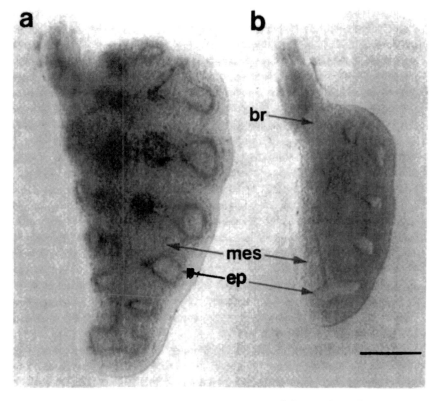

**Figure 6**  N-*myc* expression in wild-type (a) and N-*myc*$^{9a/9a}$ (b) mice. Whole-mount in
situ analysis was performed on E12.5 day murine lungs with a probe for N-*myc*. Expression
of N-*myc* is detected in the epithelium (ep) of the developing lung with decreased transcript
present in the 9a/9a lung. The 9a/9a lung is also smaller and shows less branching of the
developing epithelium. br, primary bronchus; mes, mesenchyme. (From Ref. 33; courtesy
of Cold Spring Harbor Laboratory Press, Cold Spring Harbor, New York.)

ing mesenchyme was unaffected in the compound heterozygous mice, suggesting that development of the mesenchymal components of the lung is not disrupted by the reduction in N-*myc* function (83).

## IV. Summary

The maturation of normal lung function relies on the correct temporal and spatial patterning of lung development. Moreover, the response of the lung to injury and to neoplastic transformation may involve a reenlistment of some of the same developmental programs which results in changes in lung structure and function. Regulation of these developmental programs requires the activities of multiple regulatory genes that mediate cellular proliferation and differentiation. At this time, we are just beginning to define the roles of the various regulatory molecules during lung development. Unlike the anterior pituitary where a single protein has been identified that appears to play a central role in the differentiation of some pituitary cell lineages, no such molecule has yet been identified in the lung. It may be that in the lung no such molecule exists and that the regulation of pulmonary growth and differentiation requires an interplay between multiple regulatory molecules. The molecules that have been identified as regulating lung development are not unique to the lung but also function in other developing organs. Some of these molecules, for example TTF-1 and the HNF-3 proteins, are clearly associated with the development of derivatives of the gut endoderm. A clearer delineation of the relationships between these various regulatory molecules and an identification of their targets is required for a fuller understanding of their roles in lung development and pathophysiology.

### Acknowledgments

The authors wish to thank Steven L. Brody and Colin D. Bingle for their helpful discussions and critical reading of the manuscript. The work described in this manuscript was supported in part by National Institute of Health Grants HL 41536 (J.D.G.) and R29 HL 52581 (B.P.H.).

### References

1. Blau HM. Differentiation requires continuous active control. Annu Rev Biochem 1992; 61:1213–1230.
2. Lawrence PA, Morata G. Homeobox genes: their function in *Drosophila* segmentation and pattern formation. Cell 1994; 78:181–189.
3. Salser S, Kenyon C. Patterning *C. elegans*: homeotic cluster genes, cell fates and cell migrations. Trends Genet 1994; 10: 159–164.

4.  Mitchell PJ, Tjian R. Transcriptional regulation in mammalian cells by sequence-specific DNA binding proteins. Science 1989; 245:371–378.
5.  Gstaiger M, Knoepfel L, Georgiev O, et al. A B-cell coactivator of octamer-binding transcription factors. Nature 1995; 373:360–362.
6.  Rhodes SJ, DiMattia GE, Rosenfeld MG. Transcriptional mechanisms in anterior pituitary cell differentiation. Curr Opin Genet Dev 1994; 4:709–717.
7.  Lefevre C, Imagawa M, Dana S, et al. Tissue-specific expression of the human growth hormone gene is conferred in part by binding of a specific trans-acting factor. EMBO J 1987; 6:971–981.
8.  Bodner M, Karin M. A pituitary-specific trans-acting factor can stimulate transcription from the growth hormone promoter in extracts of nonexpressing cells. Cell 1987; 50:267–275.
9.  Bodner M, Castrillo J-L, Theill LE, et al. The pituitary-specific transcription factor GHF-1 is a homeobox-containing protein. Cell 1988; 55:505–518.
10. Ingraham HA, Chen R, Mangalam HJ, et al. A tissue-specific transcription factor containing a homeodomain specifies a pituitary phenotype. Cell 1988; 55:519–529.
11. Simmons DM, Voss JW, Ingraham HA, et al. Pituitary cell phenotypes involve cell-specific pit-1 mRNA translation and synergistic interactions with other classes of transcription factors. Genes Dev 1990; 4:695–711.
12. Li S, Crenshaw III EB, Rawson EJ, et al. Dwarf locus mutants lacking three pituitary cell types result from mutations in the POU-domain gene *pit-1*. Nature 1990; 347: 528–533.
13. Wessels NK. Mammalian lung development: interaction in formation and morphogenesis of tracheal buds. J Exp Zool 1970; 175:455–466.
14. Ayers MM, Jeffery PK. Proliferation and differentiation in mammalian airway epithelium. Eur Respir J 1988; 1:58–80.
15. Ang S-L, Rossant J. *HNF-3β* is essential for node and notochord formation in mouse development. Cell 1994; 78:561–574.
16. Weinstein DC, Ruiz i Altaba A, Chen WS, et al. The winged-helix transcription factor *HNF-3β* is required for notochord development in the mouse embryo. Cell 1994; 78: 575–588.
17. Peters K, Werner S, Liao X, et al. Targeted expression of a dominant negative FGF receptor blocks branching morphogenesis and epithelial differentiation of the mouse lung. EMBO J 1994; 13:3296–3301.
18. Kauffman SL. Cell proliferation in the mammalian lung. Int Rev Exp Pathol 1980; 22:131–191.
19. Korfhagen TR, Glasser S, Wert S, et al. Cis-acting sequences from a human surfactant protein gene confer pulmonary-specific gene expression in transgenic mice. Proc Natl Acad Sci USA 1990; 87:6122–6126.
20. Sutliff KS, Hutchins GM. Septation of the respiratory and digestive tracts in human embryos: crucial role of the tracheoesophageal sulcus. Anat Rec 1994; 238:237–247.
21. Wert S, Glasser S, Korfhagen T, Whitsett, J. Transcriptional elements from the human SP-C gene direct expression in the primordial respiratory epithelium of transgenic mice. Dev Biol 1993; 156: 426–443.
22. Hackett BP, Gitlin JD. 5′ Flanking region of the Clara cell secretory protein gene

specifics a unique temporal and spatial pattern of gene expression in the developing pulmonary epithelium. Am J Respir Cell Mol Biol 1994; 11: 123–129.

23. Ten Have-Opbroek AAW. Lung development in the mouse embryo. Exp Lung Res 1991; 17:11–130.

24. Korfhagen TR, Bruno MD, Glasser SW, et al. Murine pulmonary surfactant SP-A gene: cloning, sequence and transcriptional activity. Am J Physiol 1992; 263:L546–L554.

25. D'Amore-Bruno MA, Wikenheiser KA, Carter JE, Clark JC, Whitsett JA. Sequence, ontogeny, and cellular localization of murine surfactant protein B mRNA. Am J Physiol 1991; 262:L40–L47.

26. Auten RL, Watkins PH, Shapiro DL, Horowitz S. Surfactant apoprotein A (SP-A) is synthesized in airway cells. Am J Respir Cell Mol Biol 1990; 3:491–496.

27. Wikenheiser KA, Wert SE, Wispé J, et al. Distinct effects of oxygen on surfactant protein B expression in bronchiolar and alveolar epithelium. Am J Physiol 1992; 262:L32–L39.

28. Joyce-Brady MF, Brody JS. Ontogeny of pulmonary alveolar epithelial markers of differentiation. Dev Biol 1990; 137:331–348.

29. Hackett BP, Shimizu N, Gitlin JD. Clara cell secretory protein gene expression in bronchiolar epithelium. Am J Physiol 1992; 262:L399–L404.

30. Sawaya PL, Stripp BR, Whitsett JA, Luse DL. The lung-specific *CC10* gene is regulated by transcription factors from the AP-1, octamer, and hepatocyte nuclear factor 3 families. Mol Cell Biol 1993; 13:3860–3871.

31. Bingle CD, Gitlin JD. Identification of hepatocyte nuclear factor-3 sites in the Clara cell secretory protein gene. Biochem J 1993; 295:227–232.

32. Lazzaro D, Price M, DeFelice M, DiLauro R. The transcription factor TTF-1 is expressed at the onset of thyroid and lung morphogenesis and in restricted regions of the foetal brain. Development 1991; 113:1093–1104.

33. Moens CB, Auerbach AB, Conlon RA, Joyner AL, Rossant J. A targeted mutation reveals a role for N-*myc* in branching morphogenesis in the embryonic mouse lung. Genes Dev 1992; 6:691–704.

34. Stripp BR, Sawaya PL, Luse DS, et al. Cis-acting elements that confer lung epithelial cell expression of the *CC10* gene. J Biol Chem 1992; 267:14703–14712.

35. Hackett BP, Gitlin JD. Cell-specific expression of a Clara cell secretory protein-human growth hormone gene in the bronchiolar epithelium of transgenic mice. Proc Natl Acad Sci USA 1992; 89:9079–9083.

36. Sawaya PL, Luse DS. Two members of the HNF-3 family have opposite effects on a lung transcriptional element; HNF-3α stimulates and HNF-3β inhibits activity of region I from the Clara cell secretory protein (CCSP) promoter. J Biol Chem 1994; 269:22211–22216.

37. Bingle CD, Hackett BP, Moxley M, Longmore W, Gitlin JD. Role of HNF-3α and HNF-3β in Clara cell secretory protein gene expression in the bronchiolar epithelium. Biochem J 1995; 308:197–202.

38. Ray MK, Magdalenos SW, Finegold MJ, DeMayo FJ. Cis-acting elements involved in the regulation of mouse Clara cell-specific 10-kDa gene. J Biol Chem 1995; 270: 2689–2694.

39.  Weigel D, Jürgens G, Küttner F, Seifert E, Jäckle H. The homeotic gene *fork head* encodes a nuclear protein and is expressed in the terminal regions of the *Drosophila* embryo. Cell 1989; 57:645–658.

40.  Lai E, Clark KL, Burley SK, Darnell Jr. JE. Hepatocyte nuclear factor 3/fork head or "winged helix" proteins: a family of transcription factors of diverse biologic function. Proc Natl Acad Sci USA 1993; 90:10421–10423.

41.  Miller LM, Galleagos ME, Morisseau BA, Kim SK. lin-31, a *Caenorhabditis elegans* HNF-3/fork head transcription factor homolog, specifies three alternative cell fates in vulval development. Genes Dev 1993; 7:933–947.

42.  Lai E, Prezioso VR, Tao W, Chen WS, Darnell Jr. JE, Hepatocyte nuclear factor 3α belongs to a gene family in mammals that is homologous to the *Drosophila* homeotic gene *fork head*. Genes Dev 1991; 5:416–427.

43.  Clark KL, Halay ED, Lai E, Burley SK. Co-crystal structure of the HNF-3/*fork head* DNA-recognition motif resembles histone H5. Nature 1993; 364:412–420.

44.  Overdier DG, Porcella A, Costa RH. The DNA-binding specificity. of the hepatocyte nuclear factor 3/forkhead domain is influenced by amino acid residues adjacent to the recognition helix. Mol Cell Biol 1994; 14:2755–2766.

45.  Sasaki H, Hogan BLM. Differential expression of multiple *fork head* related genes during gastrulation and axial pattern formation in the mouse embryo. Development 1993; 118:47–59.

46.  Monaghan AP, Kaestner KH, Grau E, Schütz G. Postimplantation expression patterns indicate a role for the mouse *forkhead/HNF-3α*, β and γ genes in determination of the definitive endoderm, chordamesoderm and neuroectoderm. Development 1993; 119:567–578.

47.  Ang S-L, Wierda A, Wong D, et al. The formation and maintenance of the definitive endoderm lineage in the mouse: involvement of HNF-3/forkhead proteins. Development 1993; 119:1301–1315.

48.  Bohinski RJ, DiLauro R, Whitsett JA. The lung-specific surfactant protein B gene promoter is a target for thyroid transcription factor 1 and hepatocyte nuclear factor 3, indicating common factors for organ-specific gene expression along the foregut axis. Mol Cell Biol 1994; 14:5671–5681.

49.  Clevidence DE, Overdier DG, Tao W, et al. Identification of nine tissue-specific transcription factors of the hepatocyte nuclear factor 3/forkhead DNA-binding domain family. Proc Natl Acad Sci USA 1993; 90:3948–3952.

50.  Kaestner KH, Lee K-H, Schlöndorff J, et al. Six members of the mouse *forkhead* gene family are developmentally regulated. Proc Natl Acad Sci USA 1993; 90:7628–7631.

51.  Pierrou S, Hellqvist M, Samuelsson L, Enerbäck S, Carlsson P. Cloning and characterization of seven human forkhead proteins: binding site specificity and DNA bending. EMBO J 1994; 13:5002–5012.

52.  Clevidence DE, Overdier DG, Peterson RS, et al. Members of the HNF-3/forkhead family of transcription factors exhibit distinct cellular expression patterns in lung and regulate the surfactant protein B promoter. Dev Biol 1994; 166:195–209

53.  Hackett BP, Brody SL, Liang M, et al. Primary structure of the HFH-4 gene and characterization of gene expression in the developing respiratory and reproductive epithelium. Proc Natl Acad Sci USA 1995; 92:4249–4253.

54. McGinnis W, Garber RL, Wirz J, Kuroiwa A, Gehring W. A homologous protein-coding sequence in Drosophila homeotic genes and its conservation in other metazoans. Cell 1984; 37:403–408.

55. Scott MP, Weiner AJ. Structural relationships among genes that control development: sequence homology between the Antennapedia, Ultrabithorax and fushi tarazu loci of *Drosophila*. Proc Natl Acad Sci USA 1984; 81:4115–4119.

56. Kenyon C. If birds can fly, why can't we? Homeotic genes and evolution. Cell 1994; 78:175–180.

57. Krumlauf R. *Hox* genes in vertebrate development. Cell 1994; 78:191–201.

58. Gehring WJ, Affolter M, Bürglin T. Homeodomain proteins. Annu Rev Biochem 1994; 63:487–526.

59. Guazzi S, Price M, DeFelice M, et al. Thyroid nuclear factor 1 (TTF-1) contains a homeodomain and displays a novel DNA binding specificity. EMBO J 1990; 9:3631–3639.

60. Damante G, Fabbro D, Pellizzari L, et al. Sequence-specific DNA recognition by the thyroid transcription factor-1 homeodomain. Nucleic Acids Res 1994; 22:3075–3083.

61. Guazzi S, Lonigro R, Pintonello L, et al. The thyroid transcription factor-1 gene is a candidate target for regulation by Hox proteins. EMBO J 1994; 13:3339–3347.

62. Sham MH, Hunt P, Nonchev S, et al. Analysis of the murine *Hox-2.7* gene: conserved alternate transcripts with differential distributions in the nervous system and the potential for shared regulatory regions. EMBO J 1992; 11:1825–1836.

63. Francis-Lana H, Price M, Polycarpou-Schwartz M, DiLauro R. Cell type-specific expression of the rat thyroperoxidase promoter indicates common mechanisms for thyroid-specific gene expression. Mol Cell Biol 1992; 12:576–588.

64. Gaunt SJ, Krumlauf R, Duboule D. Mouse homeogenes within a subfamily, *Hox-1.4*, *-2.6*, and *-5.1*, display similar anteroposterior domains of expression in the embryos, but show stage- and tissue-dependent differences in their regulation. Development 1989; 107:131–141.

65. Graham A, Papalopulu N, Lorimer J, et al. Characterization of a murine homeobox gene, *Hox 2.6*, related to the Drosophila Deformed gene. Genes Dev 1988; 2:1424–1438.

66. Dony C, Gruss P. Specific expression of the *Hox 1.3* homeo box gene in murine embryonic structures originating or induced by the mesoderm. EMBO J 1987; 6:2965–2975.

67. Krumlauf R, Holland PWH, McVey JH, Hogan BLM. Developmental and spatial patterns of expression of the mouse homeobox gene, *Hox 2.1*. Development 1987; 99:603–617.

68. Holland PWH, Hogan BLM. Spatially restricted patterns of expression of the homeobox-containing gene *Hox 2.1* during mouse embryogenesis. Development 1988; 102:159–174.

69. Marcu KB, Bossone SA, Patel AJ. Myc function and regulation. Annu Rev Biochem 1992; 61:809–860.

70. Lüscher B, Eisenman RN. New light on Myc and Myb. Part I. Myc. Genes Dev 1990; 4:2025–2035.

71. Blackwood EM, Eisenman RN. Max: a helix-loop-helix zipper protein that forms a sequence-specific DNA-binding complex with Myc. Science 1991; 251:1211–1217.
72. Amati B, Dalton S, Brooks MW, et al. Transcriptional activation by the human c-Myc oncoprotein in yeast requires interaction with Max. Nature 1992; 359:423–426.
73. Ayer DE, Kretzner L, Eisenman RN. Mad: a heterodimeric partner for Max that antagonizes Myc transcriptional activity. Cell 1993; 72:211–222.
74. Zervos AS, Gyuris J, Brent R. Mxi 1, a protein that specifically interacts with Max to bind Myc-Max recognition sites. Cell 1993; 72:223–232.
75. Ayer DE, Eisenman RN. A switch from Myc:Max to Mad:Max heterocomplexes accompanies monocyte/macrophage differentiation. Genes Dev 1993; 7:2110–2119.
76. Downs KM, Martin GR, Bishop JM. Contrasting patterns of c-*myc* and N-*myc* expression during gastrulation of the mouse embryo. Genes Dev 1989; 3:860–869.
77. Mugrauer G, Alt FW, Ekblom P. N-*myc* proto-oncogene expression during organo-genesis in the developing mouse as revealed by in situ hybridization. J Cell Biol 1988; 107:1325–1335.
78. Hirning V, Schmid P, Schulz WA, Rettenberger G, Hameister H. A comparative analysis of N-*myc* and c-*myc* expression and cellular proliferation in mouse organo-genesis. Mech Dev 1991; 33:119–126.
79. Stanton BR, Perkins AS, Tessarollo L, Sassoon DA, Parada LF. Loss of N-*myc* function results in embryonic lethality and failure of the epithelial component of the embryo to develop. Genes Dev 1992; 6:2235–2247.
80. Charron J, Malynn BA, Fisher P, et al. Embryonic lethality in mice homozygous for a targeted disruption of the N-*myc* gene. Genes Dev 1992; 6:2248–2257.
81. Sawai S, Shimono A, Wakamatsu Y, et al. Defects of embryonic organogenesis resulting from the targeted disruption of the N-*myc* gene in the mouse. Development 1993; 117:1445–1455.
82. Serra R, Pelton RW, Moses HL. TGFβ1 inhibits branching morphogenesis and N-*myc* expression in lung bud organ cultures. Development 1994; 120:2153–2161.
83. Moens CB, Stanton BR, Parada LF, Rossant J. Defects in heart and lung development in compound heterozygotes for two different targeted mutations at the N-*myc* locus. Development 1993; 119:485–499.

# 4

# Epithelial-Mesenchymal Interactions in Lung Development

JOHN M. SHANNON

National Jewish Center for Immunology
  and Respiratory Medicine
and University of Colorado School of
  Medicine
Denver, Colorado

ROBIN R. DETERDING

University of Colorado School of Medicine
Denver, Colorado

## I.  Introduction

The adult lung is a decidedly complex organ comprising at least 40 different cell types (1,2) that are involved in both respiratory and nonrespiratory functions. Despite this eventual complexity, the lung has ostensibly simple beginnings, originating as paired evaginations of the floor of the endodermal foregut into mesenchyme derived from the splanchnic mesoderm. These epithelial rudiments subsequently engage in a process commonly referred to as branching morphogenesis, in which the pulmonary tree and alveoli are generated by repetitive terminal and lateral branching of the epithelium. Concomitant with the extensive arborization of the pulmonary epithelium is the development of a highly ordered pulmonary vasculature. The parallel development of the pulmonary epithelium and vasculature in the embryo and fetus generate what will become the functional gas-exchange system.

The temporal and spatial coordination of pattern formation within the lung has been an area of interest for over 60 years. What has emerged from these studies, and is the topic of this chapter, is that interactions between the endodermally derived lung epithelium and the mesodermally derived mesenchyme are absolutely required for normal lung development to proceed. Understanding the basis for these interactions, which have been traditionally referred to as epithelial-mesenchymal interactions, has become an area of intense interest because of the possibility of developing new treatment strategies based on genetic manipulation. The alliance of classic methods in developmental biology with the increasingly powerful techniques of molecular biology has made elucidating the molecular basis of gene regulation during lung development a realistic possibility. In this chapter, we provide a historical perspective demonstrating the importance of epithelial-mesenchymal interactions to lung development and describe more recent data aimed at identifying candidate molecules critical to normal lung development.

## II. Concepts and Definitions

Epithelial-mesenchymal interactions are interactions that occur over short distances. They have been described in a variety of mammalian organs, including the lung, salivary gland (3,4), pancreas (5), mammary gland (6), kidney (7–9), tooth (10,11), limb (12), and urogenital derivatives (13). The vast majority of such studies have been done with the developing epithelium as the "responding" tissue. As described below, reciprocal interactions of the epithelium with the mesenchyme are also occurring, with the developing lung providing good evidence for this.

The interactions between epithelium and mesenchyme have been broadly divided into two types, permissive and instructive interactions. In permissive interactions, the responding tissue expresses genes inherent to that tissue in response to signals from the inducing tissue. These signals may take the form of hormones, growth factors, cytokines, or extracellular matrix molecules. The inducing tissue provides an environment that permits the responding tissue to express only those genes within its normal repertoire; no reprogramming of gene expression occurs. In instructive interactions, the inducing tissue causes the selective expression of new genes in the responding tissue that would never occur in the absence of the inducing tissue; that is, the inducing tissue instructs the responding tissue to reprogram its repertoire of gene expression. Wessells (14) has developed a useful set of criteria for defining instructive interactions:

1. In the presence of inducing tissue A, responding tissue B develops in specific way.
2. In the absence of tissue A, tissue B will not develop in that way.
3. In the presence of tissue A, tissue C, which normally develops differently, is altered to develop like tissue B (i.e., in the specific pattern associated with tissue A).
4. The responding tissue(s) does not respond in the specific pattern associated with tissue A when confronted with general, nonspecific stimuli.

Understanding instructive interactions is complicated further by the concept of competence, which is simply defined as the ability of a tissue to respond to an inducing signal. An inducing tissue may be producing instructive cues that effect a change in differentiation in one tissue, yet have no effect on another tissue, because it is not competent to respond to those cues. As is described below, competence is not a fixed property of a tissue and can change spatially and temporally over the course of development. Thus, competence itself can be viewed as a specific differentiated state within a tissue.

An additional concept is that of restriction, which is defined as the progressive loss in the ability of a cell/tissue to express a variety of different phenotypes. Restriction can occur quite early in development, as in the case of primordial germ cells, or much later, when processes of organogenesis are well underway. Restriction of a cell is thought to occur as the result of interaction(s) with other cells or cell products. Loss of competence can be viewed as a form of restriction.

## III. Epithelial-Mesenchymal Interactions in the Developing Lung

Initial observations documenting the importance of mesenchyme to embryonic lung development were made by Rudnick (15), in which embryonic chicken lung rudiments were grafted onto chorioallantoic membranes in ovo. The results showed that lung development usually proceeded in grafts in which the lung bud had just emerged, whereas a more consistent developmental response was seen if primary and secondary branches had been established in the grafts. If, however, the mesoderm surrounding the lung rudiment was removed prior to grafting, all further development ceased. The advent of suitable culture techniques for embryonic lung rudiments (see Chapter 17) allowed these observations to be confirmed and extended by others for both avian (16) and mammalian (17–20) species.

These studies were aided by two major technical advances now largely taken for granted. The first of these was the observation that the embryonic lung is able to sustain both branching morphogenesis and specialized lung cell differentiation in culture. These culture conditions have ranged from essentially undefined combinations of plasma and embryo extract to serum-free, hormonally defined media. The capability for continued lung development in vitro is true for even the earliest events in lung organogenesis. Spooner (19) demonstrated that primary lung buds would form in guts taken from embryos as early as the two-somite stage. These buds, however, would undergo further branching only if the guts were taken from embryos at the 25-somite stage, when the primary lung downgrowths have just emerged from the floor of the gut tube.

The second technical advance was the development of tissue recombination techniques. In these experiments, embryonic organ rudiments are isolated at a stage that allows clean separation of epithelium and mesenchyme, usually by a combination of enzymatic treatment followed by mechanical separation. The tissues can then be recombined and maintained in vitro or cultured by themselves. Particularly useful studies have compared the response of an epithelium to its own mesenchyme (homotypic recombinant) versus an unrelated mesenchyme (hetero-typic recombinant).

The results of numerous studies involving the separation, recombination, and culture of embryonic lung rudiments have led to several generally accepted principles concerning the role of epithelial-mesenchymal interactions in lung development. The first of these is the concept that embryonic lung epithelium will not survive for an extended period in the absence of mesenchyme. Second, branching morphogenesis of embryonic lung epithelium specifically requires an interaction with lung mesenchyme. Masters (20) demonstrated that embryonic mouse lung epithelium cultured in the absence of any mesenchyme underwent necrosis by 72 hr. A minimum amount of lung mesenchyme was required for branching to occur; further, the degree of epithelial cell cytodifferentiation was also correlated with the amount of lung mesenchyme that was present.

Embryonic lung epithelium appears to be able to survive in a heterotypic mesenchyme, although further proliferation and lung-like branching appear to be arrested. Dameron (16) demonstrated that the chick lung epithelial rudiment would survive when recombined with mesonephric, somitic, or chorioallantoic mesenchyme, but normal branching occurred only in the presence of lung mesen-chyme; limited branching was noted with metanephric mesenchyme. Using whole gut cultures, Spooner (19) showed that 25-somite (gestational day 9) mouse gut endoderm would form lung buds in response to salivary gland mesenchyme but would only branch in the presence of lung mesenchyme. The response of embry-onic lung epithelium to salivary gland mesenchyme is variable, apparently being dependent on the stage at which the epithelium is isolated. Epithelial lung rudi-ments isolated from day 12 mice or day 13 rats show no response when recom-bined with salivary gland mesenchyme, whereas epithelial rudiments isolated from lungs only 1 day older (when secondary branching has been initiated) show a limited branching response (21,22). Similarly, in recombinations of day 15 rat salivary gland mesenchyme with day 12 lung epithelium, Ball (23) observed an epithelial growth response in only 1 of 12 recombinants, and the one positive sample exhibited an aberrant gross morphology. An unanswered question in these experiments concerned the cytodifferentiated phenotype of the lung epithelial cells in response to recombination with salivary gland mesenchyme. When posi-tive responses were observed, the pattern of branching was specified by the mesenchyme; that is, like the salivary gland. Whether this mesenchyme was permissively supporting lung epithelial cell cytodifferentiation or instructively reprogramming the expression of a new phenotype is unknown. When recom-bined with mouse tracheal mesenchyme, mouse lung epithelium does not branch, and the number of cells containing osmiophilic lamellar bodies, the storage organelle of pulmonary surfactant, is reduced (24). Embryonic rat lung epithelium also forms a nonbranching cyst when recombined with rat tracheal mesenchyme of the same age (J.M. Shannon, unpublished observation).

The permissive effects of lung mesenchyme in stimulating lung epithelial proliferation, branching, and differentiation appear to be short range and mediated by a diffusible factor(s). This was demonstrated in transfilter tissue recombination experiments modeled after the pioneering studies done by Grobstein in the kidney and salivary gland (3,25). In this model system, isolated lung epithelial and mesenchymal rudiments are cultured in apposition to each other, with a Millipore filter interposed between them. These mesh-type filters, of 25 μm thickness and with nominal pore size of 0.45 μm, allow passage of macromolecules between the two tissue components but restrict direct cell-cell contact by virture of the tortuous pathways through the filter. Taderera (18) constructed transfilter recombinants using day 12 mouse lung epithelium and either day 12 mouse lung or day 5 chick lung mesenchyme. He observed that the epithelium did not branch in the absence of mesenchyme but simply spread over the surface of the plasma clot substratum. In the presence of lung mesenchyme, however, lung-like branching proceeded. An important observation in these experiments was that chick lung mesenchyme was as equally effective as mouse lung mesenchyme in supporting mouse lung epithelial branching, suggesting that the inductive molecule(s) involved in branching morphogenesis are evolutionarily conserved between birds and mammals. Wessells and Cohen (26) also used similar mouse lung epithelium/chick lung mesenchyme transfilter recombinants to demonstrate the involvement of collagen in the epithelial branching response and that this process requires the presence of mesenchyme. This conservation of permissive induction by lung mesenchyme from different species holds true for cytodifferentiation as well as branching: when day 16 mouse lung epithelium is directly recombined with chick lung mesenchyme, the epithelium branches over 2–5 days in culture, and the resultant epithelial cells contain copious numbers of lamellar bodies, indicating that type II cell differentiation has proceeded unabated (27).

The observation that embryonic lung epithelium has a very stringent requirement for lung mesenchyme in order for branching morphogenesis to progress suggests that specific factors provided by lung mesenchyme specify lung development. Several investigators have asked the question whether lung mesenchyme can act instructively on heterotypic epithelia. Recombinations of embryonic rat (21,23) or mouse (22) lung mesenchyme with salivary gland epithelium showed that lung mesenchyme could support robust branching of a heterotypic epithelium. This interaction was apparently a permissive one, since the induced epithelial cells contained abundant PAS-positive, amylase-resistant material consistent with salivary gland epithelial cell cytodifferentiation. An intriguing observation, however, was that tubules of parotid gland epithelium that formed in response to lung mesenchyme showed a marked accumulation of glycogen, whereas only trace amounts of glycogen were present in that epithelium in vivo or when it was recombined with salivary gland mesenchyme. Since glycogen serves as a major substrate for surfactant phospholipid biosynthesis in the fetal lung at the end of gestation (28), the possibility exists that some instructive influence of lung mesenchyme on parotid epithelium may have occurred.

A particularly useful system for studying the instructive capabilities of lung mesenchyme, as well as serving as a model for early events in lung development, is what we will refer to as the tracheal graft system. In this system, originally described by Alescio and Cassini (29), the embryonic (days 11–12 in the mouse) trachea had a portion of its own mesenchyme surgically removed and replaced by a heterotypic mesenchyme. When distal lung mesenchyme was grafted as the replacement mesenchyme, a remarkable response was observed: The lung mesenchyme induced the formation of a "supernumerary bud" from the wall of the tracheal epithelium that continued to branch in a pattern identical to that seen in the lung. Histochemically, the induced tracheal epithelial cells contained glycogen at a point in time after it had disappeared from uninduced cells and coincident with the high levels present in distal lung epithelial cells. These data were extended by Wessells (30), who showed that mesenchyme from the salivary gland, stomach, intestine, skin, and mammary gland could also induce the formation of a supernumerary bud when grafted onto denuded tracheal epithelium. Importantly, however, branching subsequent to initial bud formation only occurred when lung mesenchyme was grafted. Further, he demonstrated that tracheal mesenchyme inhibited branching of lung epithelium when grafted onto denuded lung epithelium. Thus, clearly important differences exist between lung and tracheal mesenchyme even though both have a similar spatial origin within the embryo.

A question arising from these studies concerned the cellular phenotype of the induced tracheal epithelium. This is because an alteration in pattern formation may not be accompanied by changes in cytodifferentiation. For example, when embryonic mouse mammary gland epithelium was recombined with salivary gland mesenchyme and maintained for several days in vitro, the epithelium proliferated readily and was induced to branch in a pattern consistent with salivary gland (31). However, when these recombinants were grafted under the kidney capsule of syngeneic females that were subsequently taken through a cycle of pregnancy and parturition, the epithelial cells synthesized milk proteins. Thus, although the salivary gland mesenchyme was permissive for the proliferation of mammary epithelium, and in fact specified epithelial patterning, no changes in the ultimate differentiated phenotype of the epithelial cells were induced. Furthermore, as noted above, the majority of the data derived from recombinants of embryonic lung mesenchyme and salivary gland epithelium appeared to support the concept that lung mesenchyme has only a permissive effect on this epithelium.

Thus, judicious selection of criteria for evaluating epithelial response is critical for the unambiguous interpretation of data generated in heterotypic tissue recombinants. This is an area that has benefited greatly from the advent of molecular techniques to detect expression of tissue-specific gene products.

To address the question of the instructive capabilities of embryonic lung mesenchyme on tracheal epithelium, we prepared tracheal grafts using tissues from day 13–14 fetal rats (32). Distal fetal rat lung mesenchyme grafted onto tracheal epithelium surgically denuded of its own mesenchyme induced a supernumerary bud that proceeded to branch in a lung-like pattern identical to prior studies in the mouse. When examined histochemically, the induced cells contained copious amounts of glycogen, and ultrastructural analysis revealed numerous lamellar bodies. These morphological criteria, however, may not be definitive of the distal lung epithelial cell phenotype. We therefore took advantage of the observation that surfactant protein C (SP-C) is a distal lung epithelial cell-specific marker in fetal rodents (33) and a type II cell specific marker in the adult rat (34). Epithelial cells of the trachea have never been shown to express SP-C at any point in development. We examined the branching structures induced in fetal tracheal epithelium by distal lung mesenchyme for the expression of SP-C mRNA and found that the induced epithelium exhibited intense concentrations of SP-C–positive cells in its most distal aspects; antibody staining for pro–SP-C protein demonstrated that this mRNA was indeed translated. This distal pattern of SP-C expression was identical to that seen in control cultures of intact lung explants from the same animals. This suggests that the tracheal epithelium had been induced to follow a spatial pattern of development specified by lung mesenchyme. The induction of tracheal epithelium to express SP-C occurred rapidly, since the induced tracheal epithelial cells of the primary supernumerary bud from tracheal epithelium 24 hr after were SP-C mRNA positive, whereas tracheal epithelial cells that remained associated with tracheal mesenchyme were SP-C negative. The sum of the molecular, histochemical, and ultrastructural data has led us to conclude that the lung mesenchyme is acting instructively on the tracheal epithelium; that is, the cells have been reprogrammed to express an entirely new phenotype that would they would not have done in the absence of lung mesenchyme.

Three other observations from these experiments warrant mention. The first is that the ability of tracheal epithelium to respond to the inductive cues produced by lung mesenchyme does not last indefinitely, since day 16 fetal rat tracheal epithelium was nonresponsive to day 13–14 lung mesenchyme; this temporal restriction of the epithelium was also noted in the mouse by Goldin and Wessells (35). Thus, the tracheal epithelium loses the competence to respond to the instructive cues provided by distal lung mesenchyme.

The second observation is that lung mesenchyme was unable to induce a supernumerary bud or branching when grafted onto day 13–14 esophageal or intestinal epithelia that had been denuded of their native mesenchymes. This suggests that restriction of these gut endodermal derivatives occurs earlier in development than in the trachea.

The third observation was that not all lung mesenchyme was equally effective in inducing the tracheal epithelium to express a lung epithelial cell phenotype. When mainstem bronchus mesenchyme was grafted onto denuded tracheal epithelium, a small, nonbranching supernumerary bud was the greatest response ever observed. These data suggest that proximal lung mesenchyme is somehow fundamentally different from distal lung mesenchyme. Whether this heterogeneity in the inductive capabilities of lung mesenchyme is due to different subsets of mesenchymal cells that exist in a precise spatial arrangement in the developing lung or to changes in the inductive capabilities of individual cells (perhaps as a result of their interaction with specific epithelial cells) is at present unknown.

In summary, lung epithelium has a highly specific, evolutionarily conserved requirement for lung mesenchyme in order for proliferation and branching morphogenesis to proceed. Whether heterotypic mesenchymes can permissively support lung epithelial cell differentiation in the absence of cell proliferation and branching is unknown. Lung mesenchyme can act permissively to support salivary gland morphogenesis and instructively in the reprogramming of tracheal epithelium. At the stages studied, only epithelium from the region of the gut destined to give rise to respiratory tissues is competent to respond to mesenchymal signals. Whether a more extensive region of the gut endoderm from younger embryos might respond to the same instructive cues remains to be determined.

We would be remiss not to address the issue of reciprocity in epithelial-mesenchymal interactions during lung development. As noted above, the factors produced by lung mesenchyme that support lung epithelial growth and branching are diffusible. Taderera (18) demonstrated that the ability of lung mesenchyme to support epithelial branching was maintained when a Millipore filter was interposed between the two tissues, when direct contact between the epithelium and mesenchyme was not discernible. Additional, and often overlooked, observations made by Taderera using the transfilter culture system concerned the effects of the epithelium on the mesenchyme. He observed that vascular and stromal cells only developed in the mesenchyme when it was cultured transfilter to lung epithelium, stating:

> In the absence of epithelium, lung mesenchyme fails to elaborate any of the characteristic pulmonary connective tissue histotypes. The inability of spinal chord and salivary epithelium to influence lung mesenchymal histogenesis seems to suggest that epithelial contribution to mesenchymal histogenesis is to some extent a specific one.

Although reagents and techniques available at the time did not allow a more precise identification of the cell types involved, these observations support the concept that development of the specialized cell types in the nonepithelial compartment of the lung is dependent on the presence of epithelium itself. Thus, a true reciprocity would exist in which epithelial proliferation and differentiation are induced by an as yet unidentified mesenchymal cell population. The induced epithelium (or a subpopulation thereof) in turn produces factors that stimulate mesenchymal cell proliferation, differentiation, and organization.

## IV. Molecular Mechanisms Mediating Epithelial-Mesenchymal Interactions in the Developing Lung

The mature lung is a multifunctional organ comprising many specialized cell types that arise in a highly specific spatial pattern during the course of development. It comes as no surprise, then, that the regulation of the events that specify the differentiation of this heterogeneous cell population during lung development is proving to be extremely complex. In this section, we present a brief overview of current information regarding the molecular mechanisms regulating lung development. We have separated these into two broad categories, the influence of extracellular matrix molecules and the influence of soluble factors, being mindful of the fact that these two categories are almost certainly inextricably related. We recognize that not all of these factors are necessarily mediators of epithelial-mesenchymal interactions, and where appropriate, we note the more likely candidate molecules.

## V. Influence of Extracellular Matrix

The extracellular matrix (ECM), whose importance in the generation and stabilization of tissue architecture was recognized long ago, has been shown in the last 25 years to play a central, dynamic role in many biological processes (for review, see ref. 36). The number of ECM-associated molecules, as well as isoforms of those molecules, continues to increase. The ECM affects cell activities in two ways. The first is the effects of the ECM molecules themselves, and the second is the ability of the ECM to serve as a reservoir for other molecules, notably growth factors (37). The influence of ECM on lung development has been an area of great interest in the past decade, and we are now just beginning to appreciate the interplay among various ECM components.

### A. Collagens

Branching of the lung endoderm requires repetitive cleft formation, which is the result of differential ECM formation at the interface between the epithelium and mesenchyme. The collagen family of ECM molecules, which comprises at least 15 members, plays an important role in this process. Collagens I, III (38), and IV

(39) have all been localized to the developing rodent lung. The integrin collagen receptors $\alpha_1\beta_1$ and $\alpha_2\beta_1$ have been localized to late-gestation fetal lung fibroblasts but not epithelial cells (40).

Using transfilter tissue recombinants, Wessells and Cohen (26) demonstrated that treatment of mouse lung epithelial rudiments with collagenase resulted in the removal of the basal lamina, the abrogation of branching, and spreading of the epithelium over the substratum; branching resumed when the collagenase was washed out and the cultures immediately provided with fresh mesenchyme. From these observations, they accurately predicted that "the basement lamina or associated materials is dependent upon some form of collagen for stability." The involvement of collagen in lung patterning was further emphasized by in vitro experiments showing that disruption of collagen synthesis and secretion severely retarded branching morphogenesis. Use of the proline analogue L-azetidine-2-carboxylic acid (41,42) resulted in significant inhibition of branching morphogenesis. Inhibition of collagen secretion with $\alpha,\alpha'$-dipyridyl also perturbed normal morphogenesis (42). Cross-linking of collagen, however, was apparently unnecessary for normal branching to occur, since $\beta$-aminoproprionitrile, a lathyrogen that inhibits extracellular collagen cross linking, had essentially no effect on lung development in vitro. The effects of disrupting collagen synthesis on lung development are not confined to those seen in vitro: Significant decreases in air sac development and type II cell differentiation were observed when *cis*-hydroxyproline (43) or L-azetidine-2-carboxylic acid (44) were injected into pregnant rats during the last days of gestation. Although the importance of collagen to normal lung development is apparent, the type(s) of collagen involved is not completely clear, since collagenase treatment would digest all collagens and the proline analogues used would disrupt synthesis of all collagens. Type I collagen is apparently not the critical form, however, since lung explants from homozygous Mov 13 mice, which carry a retroviral insertion in the $\alpha 1(I)$ collagen gene that completely blocks its transcription, branch identically in vitro to wild-type controls (45).

## B. Laminin

As noted above, normal branching of the lung epithelium in vitro requires an intact basement membrane, of which the glycoprotein laminin is a principal component. In the developing mouse lung, laminin is present as early as day 10 (the onset of organogenesis), progressively increases over the course of gestation, and persists through adulthood (46). Staining with polyclonal antibodies demonstrated that laminin is primarily localized to the basement membrane, although some diffuse staining could be detected during fetal development in the mesenchyme and around blood vessels as they emerged. A detailed study of the expression of the $\alpha$, $\beta$, and $\gamma$ chains of laminin in the developing fetal rabbit lung showed that the chains were differentially regulated (47). Interestingly, the peak levels of laminin expression, as well as spatial distribution of the α and β chains, coincided temporally with the onset of differentiation of the alveolar epithelium.

In a series of studies, Schuger has demonstrated the importance of laminin to normal branching morphogenesis. Polyclonal antibodies to laminin were shown to inhibit branching in vitro in a dose-dependent manner (48). A subsequent study (49), using site-directed monoclonal antibodies showed that an antibodies directed against the cross region of the laminin A chain and against the globular region of the B chain(s) had similar effects on inhibiting branching. The antibody against the cross region of the A chain inhibited epithelial and mesenchymal cell attachment and epithelial cell proliferation, whereas the antibody against the B chain inhibited epithelial cell polarity and basement membrane assembly (50). Thus, it appears that laminin plays a multifunctional role in mediating normal lung morphogenesis.

### C. Fibronectin

A second major adhesion glycoprotein, fibronectin, shows a varied pattern of expression during lung morphogenesis. In the mouse, Roman and McDonald demonstrated (51) that fibronectin is found in mesenchymal cells during the glandular stage of development and shows a prominent concentration at the epithelial-mesenchymal interface. Expression decreased somewhat during the canalicular stage, when fibronectin was also found in vessel walls. Unlike expression of laminin, which peaks during the period of alveolar development, fibronectin expression decreased significantly during late gestation; furthermore, immunodetectable fibronectin was found in airway epithelial cells. Heine et al. (38) have demonstrated a colocalizaton of fibronectin and collagen I and III throughout lung development, suggesting an interrelationship of these ECM molecules in the regulation of branching morphogenesis. The spatial distribution of the integrin $\alpha_5\beta_1$, which binds the central cell-binding domain of fibronectin (including the tripeptide RGD [Arg-Gly-Asp]), for the most part paralleled the expression of fibronectin (51). Incubation of glandular stage lung rudiments with an RGD-containing peptide, which could effectively compete with RGD-containing ECM molecules for binding of several integrins, inhibited but did not abolish lung branching (52).

Genetic manipulation of the fibronectin gene has provided some information about its role in lung development. Transgenic mice null for fibronectin gene expression showed numerous abnormalities by day 8 of gestation and died by day 10.5; however, heterozygous fetuses appeared to develop normally even though heterozygous adults had only 50% of the wild-type circulating level of fibronectin (53). Targeting the $\alpha_5$-integrin subunit gene by homologous recombinantion also resulted in embryonic lethality, although somewhat later (days 10–11) in development (54); unfortunately, no mention was made of whether lung development had been initiated. Thus elucidation of the role of fibronectin in lung development will require further study.

### D.  Glycosaminoglycans and Proteoglycans

Glycosaminoglycans (GAGs) and proteoglycans (PGs) have been shown to mediate many aspects of development in a variety of systems. GAGs are unbranched chains of repeating disaccharide units in which one of the disaccharide pair is always an amino sugar that is usually sulfated. This sulfation, combined with carboxyl groups on most of the sugar residues, give GAGs a highly negative charge. The high negative charge of GAG chains attracts a great number of cations, which in turn draws a large amount of water into the matrix by osmotic action. Four general groups of GAGs have been defined on the basis of the types of sugar residues, how these residues are linked, and the number and distribution of sulfate groups. These are (1) hyaluronan, (2) chondroitin sulfate and dermatan sulfate, (3) heparin and heparan sulfate, and (4) keratan sulfate.

Hyaluronan is an extremely large (MW $8 \times 10^6$) molecule that is unique in two ways: the disaccharide units are nonsulfated and the GAG chain is not attached to protein. By virtue of its hydrophilicity, secreted hyaluronan is thought to play a role in development by creating a cell-free space into which cells or sheets of cells can migrate. This is consistent with the observations of Bernfield (55), who demonstrated that hyaluronan was found over the entire epithelial-mesenchymal interface of day 11–13 mouse lungs but was more abundant at the distal tips of the epithelium, the site of greatest morphogenetic activity.

As noted above, nonhyaluronan GAGs do not exist free in nature but rather are attached to a core protein to form PGs. This accomplished through the use of a link tetrasaccharide (xylose-galactose-galactose-glucuronic acid) attached to core protein serine residues, which serve as primers for polysaccharide elongation. PGs have the capacity for seemingly limitless heterogeneity, based on differences in core proteins and the number, type, and degree of sulfation of the attached GAG chains. Along with serving a role as a structural component of the ECM, PGs have functional roles in cell behavior. This has been demonstrated by the ability of PGs to bind signaling molecules such as fibroblast growth factor (FGF) and transforming growth factor-$\beta$ (TGF-$\beta$) (56,57). Another potential function of PGs is to serve as a integrated cell surface coreceptors for growth factors such as FGF (58). One such molecule, syndecan, binds to FGF and presents it to FGF receptors on the same cell. Syndecan expression has been detailed during days 12–18 of mouse lung development (59). During early gestation (day 12), syndecan is primarily localized on epithelial cell surfaces and to a lesser extent in mesenchymal cells. Syndecan expression becomes restricted to the lateral surfaces of all epithelial cells on days 14–16. As the saccular stage of lung development begins on day 18, syndecan is detected in virtually all of the epithelial cells of the conducting airways but not in the flattened alveolar type I cells; at least some of the cuboidal cells in the presumptive air sacs (possibly alveolar type II cells) exhibited syndecan expression. These observations suggest that syndecan may play different roles at different times in lung development.

The importance of PGs to fetal lung differentiation have been demonstrated in studies using the drug p-nitrophenyl-β-D-xylopyranoside (β-xyloside), which disrupts PG biosynthesis by competing with xylosylated core protein at the level of the first galactosyltransferase. This results in core proteins that have no GAG chains, along with the synthesis of a large number of free GAG chains. Explants from the distal lungs of day 16 fetal mice cultured in the presence of β-xyloside exhibited a loss of alveolar maturation, inhibition of type II cell differentiation, and suppression of surfactant phospholipid biosynthesis (60). β-xyloside inhibited the synthesis of chondroitin sulfate PG and effected its redistribution from intracellular to extracellular, while heparan sulfate PG was redistributed from intracellular to membranes (61). Thus, it appears that one or more PGs are involved in various aspects of normal lung development. With the exception of syndecan, the identification of the specific PGs that are important in these processes is in its infancy.

### E. Tenascin

The tenascins are a family of large, multidomain ECM molecules that share structural and functional features with laminin and fibronectin (62). Three members of the tenascin family have been described to date, and they have been named tenascin-C (TN-C), tenascin-R (TN-R), and tenascin-X (TN-X). Only TN-C and TN-X have been localized to the developing mammalian lung. Young et al. (63) demonstrated that TN-C was concentrated at the epithelial-mesenchymal interface and was present between mesenchymal cells during glandular stage branching morphogenesis in fetal rats. Expression increased over the course of gestation, reached peak levels 7 to 10 days postnatally, and then declined to barely detectable levels in adults. Electron microscopic immunocytochemistry demonstrated that, unlike laminin, TN-C was not part of the basal lamina. Bristow et al. (64) demonstrated that TN-X mRNA is also present in the developing human lung; information on the spatial distribution of the TN-X mRNA, however, was not available. Zhao and Young (65) have recently shown that TN mRNA is present exclusively in mesenchymal cells in the pre- and postnatal rat lung.

How the tenascins are involved in lung development is not completely clear. Antiserum to TN-C inhibited branching morphogenesis in cultured fetal rat lung explants, whereas having no effect on their overall growth (63). Further, bacterially-expressed fragments comprising the different fibronectin type III domains present in the TN-C monomer were equally effective to the antiserum in inhibiting branching, whereas a fragment expressed from the C-terminal fibrinogen-like domain had no effects. This would suggest an important role for TN-C in lung patterning. However, transgenic mice null for TN-C expression have no gross abnormalities in lung development (66). This suggests that there may be some functional redundancy (perhaps by TN-X) that compensates for the loss of TN-C. An alternative explanation is that the effects of a null TN-C gene are subtle in normal animals, and that an overt phenotype may only be manifest under conditions of stress (63). It has also been suggested that TN-C may be a nonfunctional protein in the lung, even though it is expressed at a high level (62).

### F.  Nidogen

Nidogen, also known as entactin, is a single polypeptide chain of $M_r = 15 \times 10^4$ that appears to be a ubiquitous component of basement membranes. Nidogen binds the basement membrane ECM molecules laminin, collagen IV, and the proteoglycan perlecan and has also been shown to have cell binding sites. Although the precise role of nidogen is not yet completely defined, current evidence supports a role for nidogen in facilitating the supramolecular self-assembly of basement membranes, perhaps by serving as a bridge molecule between laminin and collagen IV. Nidogen has been shown by immunocytochemistry to co-distribute with laminin in the basement membranes of epithelial ducts and blood vessels in the developing lung (67). Although nidogen polypeptide appears concentrated at the basement membrane interface between epithelium and mesenchyme, nidogen mRNA is evenly expressed throughout the mesenchyme. Since soluble nidogen is highly susceptible to protease digestion (68), the complexing of nidogen into the basement membrane appears to stabilize the polypeptide. These data illustrate the cooperative nature of epithelial-mesenchymal interactions in promoting lung morphogenesis, where the mesenchyme-derived protein nidogen can complex with laminin from the epithelium to promote normal morphogenesis. The possible importance of nidogen to normal lung morphogenesis was demonstrated by experiments in which explants of day 11 fetal mouse lung were incubated with an antibody that blocked nidogen binding to laminin but did not interfere with normal laminin assembly. The results showed that branching morphogenesis was inhibited by this antibody but in a stage-specific manner, since the effects of the antibody on branching diminished with increasing gestational age. Taken together with the data for laminin (see above), these data emphasize the requirement for an intact basement membrane for normal branching morphogensis to occur.

## VI.  Soluble Factors as Mediators of Epithelial-Mesenchymal Interactions in the Developing Lung

The foregoing discussion makes it clear that the temporal and spatial production of ECM molecules by both the developing lung epithelium and mesenchyme imparts a high level of complexity to the regulation of lung morphogenesis and cyto-differentiation. The situation is complicated further when the effects of the different classes of soluble factors (hormones, growth factors, and cytokines) are considered. In this section, we discuss the potential impact of a number of soluble factors that may serve as mediators of epithelial-mesenchymal interactions. The list is not all inclusive and contains some omissions, with the most obvious being the glucocorticoid and thyroid hormones. Although it has been amply demonstrated that these hormones have significant effects on lung growth and differentiation (69–71), their site of synthesis is outside the lung; hence they cannot be considered direct mediators of epithelial-mesenchymal interactions. We have also not included a discussion of the effects of exogenous cyclic AMP added to lung explants in vitro, because of its role as a second messenger in a cascade signaled by other molecules.

### A. Fibroblast Growth Factors

The FGF family currently comprises nine related molecules (72,73) that affect both proliferation and differentiation of a variety of cell types. The FGFs are notable for their ability to bind heparin or heparin-like molecules, which are present in the form of heparan sulfate PGs both on cell surfaces and in the ECM. FGF signaling is transduced by a family of transmembrane receptor tyrosine kinases, which currently numbers four members. The FGF receptors (FGFRs) are characterized by the presence of extracellular immunoglobulin-like loops. The number of these loops, and splice variants within them, result in a number of FGFR isoforms that can exhibit striking differences in binding specificity (74). Dimerization of the FGFRs is required for their activation.

Studies detailing the localization of different members of the FGF family in the developing lung have been somewhat limited. Immunocytochemistry has localized basic FGF (bFGF) to the ECM (75) and epithelial cells of the trachea, bronchi, and distal airways in the fetal rat (76). The cellular localization of acidic FGF (aFGF) during fetal lung development is not known, although it has been localized by immunostaining postnatally to the ECM, as well as airway epithelial cells and alveolar type II cells. aFGF and bFGF are notable for their lack of a classic signal peptide, indicating that they are deposited in the ECM by a novel secretory mechanism.

Keratinocyte growth factor (KGF; FGF-7) has recently attracted much interest as a mediator of epithelial-mesenchymal interactions in the lung, as well as in other organs (77,78). KGF is an epithelial-specific mitogen (79), and its mRNA in the developing lung has been localized to the lung mesenchyme (72,80). The potential role of KGF as a mediator of cross-talk between the epithelium and mesenchyme is made more compelling when distribution of the KGF receptor (KGFR) is examined. Two splice variants of the FGFR-2 exist that differ only in

49 amino acids in the carboxyterminus of the third immunoglobulin loop. One is the KGFR, which will bind KGF and aFGF with high affinity and bFGF at low affinity. The second is the *bek* gene, which does not bind KGF at all but aFGF and bFGF with high affinity (80). In situ hybridization studies (81,82) have shown that the KGFR is present only in the epithelium of the developing lung. Since it is uncertain how aFGF is secreted, KGF, which has a signal peptide for secretion, becomes a likely candidate molecule for an epithelial-mesenchymal mediator. This candidacy was considerably strengthened by experiments in which the KGFR was specifically inactivated in the developing lung (83). This was accomplished by taking advantage of the observation that SP-C is expressed only in the most distal epithelial cells of the developing rodent lung (33,34). Using the strong SP-C promoter to drive dominant-negative expression of a mutant KGFR resulted in a complete abrogation of lung branching beyond the bifurcation of the trachea. The importance of KGF (and perhaps aFGF) to the normal proliferation of the early lung epithelium has also been demonstrated in vitro (see below). Elucidation of the roles of other members of the FGF family in lung development awaits experimentation.

### B. Epidermal Growth Factor and Transforming Growth Factor-α

We will consider epidermal growth factor (EGF) and TGF-α together, since they have been shown to signal through the same receptor (EGFR). EGF and TGF-α are members of a family of at least five molecules that are characterized by specific structural similarities. In the early mouse lung (days 13–16), EGF mRNA has been detected in mesenchymal cells (84), whereas EGF protein (or precursor protein) has been detected in both epithelial and mesenchymal cells as well as the ECM (85). TGF-α has been detected in the developing rat lung (86), peaking during late gestation; the tissue localization, however, was not determined. In human fetuses from 10–22 weeks of gestation, Strandjord et al. (87) demonstrated immunodetectable TGF-α in epithelial cells and arterial smooth muscle cells; TGF-α mRNA expression appeared to increase with increasing gestational age.

Examining distribution of the EGF binding in the developing mouse lung, Partanen and Thesleff (88) demonstrated that binding of $^{125}$I-EGF was most intense in the mesenchymal cells subtending epithelial tubules on day 13, although epithelial cells were also labeled. By day 14, overall binding had decreased, but the distribution had changed: labeling was most intense in the distal epithelium and its surrounding mesenchyme. Warburton and colleagues (85) have shown that EGFR colocalized with EGF expression in the mouse lung in vivo and in vitro.

EGF appears to influence a number of aspects of lung development. The effects on branching morphogenesis reported for EGF have been inconsistent. One study demonstrated that EGF inhibited in vitro branching morphogenesis in the early mouse lung (89), apparently by stimulating production of matrix-degrading metalloproteinases. Other studies, however, have shown that EGF stimulates an increase in the number of terminal branches in cultured lungs from embryos of the same age (85). Furthermore, addition of oligodeoxynucleotides coding for EGF antisense resulted in an inhibition of branching (90). In experiments analogous to the tracheal graft studies described above, Goldin and Opperman (91) were able to demonstrate that a piece of agarose saturated with EGF was able to induce a supernumerary bud when grafted onto tracheal epithelium denuded of its own mesenchyme; branching did not proceed beyond the initial bud.

EGF has also been shown to have positive effects on later aspects of lung epithelial cell development, since it accelerated fetal rabbit lung maturation when administered in vivo (92). EGF also increased the rate of surfactant phospholipid biosynthesis in cultured fetal rat lung explants (93) and the production of surfactant protein A (SP-A) in fetal human lung explants (94). It is possible that the effects of EGF on phospholipid biosynthesis may not be direct, since EGF has also been shown to accelerate the production of fibroblast pneumonocyte factor (FPF; see below), which itself stimulates maturation of the surfactant system (95).

The potential role of EGF in normal lung development has been addressed by genetic manipulation of TGF-α and the EGFR. Mice with a targeted disruption of the TGF-α gene developed normally, appeared healthy, and were capable of producing healthy litters; the only apparent phenotypic change was an alteration in skin architecture that resulted in waviness in the whiskers and fur (96,97). The engineered mice were shown to be homologues of the naturally mutated waved-1 (wa-1) strain (96). The notable lack of pathology in these mice was ascribed to a functional redundancy of TGF-α that could be provided by EGF or another EGF-like molecule.

Waved-2 (wa-2) mice have a point mutation in the tyrosine kinase domain of the EGFR that leads to a 5- to 10-fold decrease in autophosphorylation and a more than 90% reduction in phosphorylation of exogenous substrates in vitro (98). Since these mice develop normally, with the exception of wavy hair and attenuated lactation, the necessity of a fully functional EGFR in lung development was brought into question. Two recent experiments (99,100) involving the targeted disruption of the EGFR gene by homologous recombination have suggested a more important role for EGF in lung development. These animals exhibited several abnormalities, including significant respiratory distress, that led to neonatal mortality in the 8–20 days after birth. The lungs of these animals were characterized by atelectasis, septal thickening, and reduced epithelial cytodifferentiation as indicated by reduced immunostaining for SP-A and SP-C. Some of the animals exhibited dilated, unbranched terminal airways near the pleural surface. The extent of lung morphogenesis indicates that EGF may not be as fundamentally important to early branching morphogenesis as KGF/aFGF but rather may play an important role in saccular stage development and maturation of the surfactant system. Taken together, these data support a role for EGF in normal lung development, although it is difficult to separate lung-specific delays in development from the overall retardation of growth seen in EGFR null animals.

However, the genetic background on which the EGFR null mutation was expressed was important: Threadgill et al. (101) demonstrated that the EGFR null mutation on a CF-1 background resulted in peri-implantation lethality, whereas against a 129/Sv background, the fetuses died at mid gestation owing to placental defects. On a CD-1 background, the mice lived for up to 3 weeks postnatally before succumbing to a variety of abnormalities. These mice, however, showed no differences in the extent of lung development from normal littermates, including staining for pro–SP-B and pro–SP-C.

Although it seems likely that EGF or TGF-α will turn out to play a role in lung development, clearly more data are needed detailing their temporal and spatial expression. The necessity for proper developmental expression of TGF-α in the lung has been demonstrated by Korfhagen et al. (102), who constructed transgenic mice in which human TGF-α expression was driven by the robust human SP-C promoter. Resultant animals developed severe pulmonary fibrosis postnatally.

### C.  Platelet-Derived Growth Factor

Platelet-derived growth factor (PDGF), which serves as a mitogenic competence factor, is composed of two related polypeptide chains (termed A and B) that are linked by multiple disulfide bonds to form three isoforms (PDGF-AA, PDGF-AB, and PDGF-BB) (103). PDGF binds to specific tyrosine kinase receptors (PDGFRs) on the cell surface. Two types of PDGFR (α- and β-receptor), which dimerize to initiate cell signaling, have been described. The α-receptor will bind either A or B chains, whereas the β-preceptor will bind only B chains; thus dimerized α-receptors bind all three PDGF isoforms, dimerized β-receptors bind only PDGF-BB, and the heterodimeric receptor binds PDGF-AB and PDGF-BB (104,105).

PDGF-AA and PDGF-BB have been localized by immunostaining to both the epithelium and mesenchyme during rat lung development (76). The epithelium stained positive as early as day 12 of gestation, with the mesenchyme becoming positive 2 days later. Expression of both isoforms as detected by Western blotting peaked during the late glandular stage (days 16–17) then showed a progressive decrease until term. These observations correlated with those made for PDGF-A and PDGF-B chain mRNA expression (106). A rat fetal lung fibroblast cell line, however, was shown to express only PDGF-AA (107).

PDGF-AA and PDGF-BB appear to play different roles in early rat lung development. Treatment of day 12 lung explants with oligodeoxynucleotides coding antisense for PDGF-A or with neutralizing antibodies against PDGF-AA resulted in a reduction in lung size, DNA synthesis, and the number of terminal branch points (108). PDGF-A mRNA was present in the epithelium and PDGF α-receptor mRNA was present in the mesenchyme of day 12 lungs at the time of initiation of the cultures, suggesting the potential for cross-talk between the two tissues during the earliest period of lung organogenesis. The validity of this possibility was somewhat obscured by the fact that both mRNAs were expressed in the mesenchyme later in gestation. Similar experiments performed using antisense oligodeoxynucleotides for PDGF-B (109) also resulted in a reduction in explant size and DNA synthesis. The number of terminal branches, however, was not affected by PDGF-B antisense treatment, suggesting that PDGF-AA and PDGF-BB influence early lung development by different mechanisms. The effects of PDGF during late gestation may be different, since antisense PDGF-B, but not antisense PDGF-A, treatment reduced DNA synthesis in cultures of late-gestation fetal rat lung epithelial cells (110).

### D. Insulin-like Growth Factors

The insulin-like growth factors (IGF-I and IGF-II) are two related single-chain polypeptides that share structural homology with proinsulin. Two receptors (IGFR-1 and IGFR-2) for the IGFs have been demonstrated: IGFR-1 binds IGF-I with higher affinity than IGF-II, whereas IGFR-2 binds IGF-II with high and IGF-I with low affinity (111). IGFR-1 has been shown to be a tyrosine kinase receptor, whereas IGFR-2 has not yet been shown to activate any signaling pathway. The identification of IGFR-2 as the cation-independent mannose 6-phosphate receptor involved in lysosomal targeting (112,113) suggests that it may be involved in ligand clearance. Additionally, at least six IGF binding proteins (IGFBPs) have been described that have been shown to modulate IGF function in vitro (114–119).

The IGFs have been shown to be expressed in virtually every tissue examined, which has led to the hypothesis that they function as general autocrine or paracrine regulators of cellular function (111). IGF-I and IGF-II mRNAs have been described in the developing lungs of fetal rats as early as day 14 of gestation (120). The levels of IGF-I mRNA remained relatively constant, whereas those for IGF-II declined with increasing gestational age, becoming virtually undetectable postnatally (121). Spatial analysis of cells expressing IGF-I and IGF-II showed that although both epithelial and mesenchymal cells were positive, the predominant expression was in the mesenchyme (122,123).

The patterns of expression of IGFR-1 and IGFR-2 appear much more complex, since their levels of expression (121) and cellular distribution (120) vary with developmental stage. With the exception of IGFBP-1, all other IGFBP molecules are expressed in the developing lung. mRNAs for IGFBP-3, IGFBP-4, and IGFBP-5 show a similar pattern of expression in the rat, being relatively constant on days 16–19, decreasing on day 20, and then rising again until term (121). IFGBP-6 expression is low throughout most of gestation, rising only during the final 2 days. IGFBP-2 mRNA levels are constant through day 20, at which point levels progressively decrease until term. Klempt et al. (122) have shown that only the epithelium is positive for IGFBP-2 mRNA in the developing lung. Since IGFBP-2 preferentially binds IGF-II (124), this suggests a role for IGF-II in lung epithelial cell development.

The general importance of a functional IGF system in normal developmental processes has been demonstrated in transgenic mice. Animals homozygous for a targeted mutation in IGF-I were dwarfed and exhibited a variable neonatal lethality of unknown etiology (125). Animals with a targeted mutation for IGF-II also had retarded growth (60% of wild-type littermate body weights), but were viable and fertile (126). Double-mutant mice null for both IGF-I and IGF-II exhibited a compound phenotype that consisted of extremely retarded growth (30% of normal body weight) and neonatal lethality due to respiratory failure. Transgenic mice homozygous for a targeted mutation of the IGFR-1 gene also had retarded growth and died shortly after birth despite efforts to breathe. Histological examination revealed that the lungs were atelectatic, but the extent of branching did not appear compromised. Although the exact cause of respiratory failure in these animals (as well as the double mutants) remains undefined, the data as a whole suggest an important role for the IGF system in normal lung development.

### E. Hepatocyte Growth Factor

Hepatocyte growth factor (HGF), also known as scatter factor, is a pleiotropic heparin-binding growth factor that affects a variety of epithelial cells (127). The HGF receptor is a member of tyrosine kinase receptor family, and it has been shown to be identical to the c-*met* proto-oncogene (128). HGF mRNA has been shown to be present in the developing lung of humans (129), mice (130), and rats (131). Observations made in the mouse suggested that HGF was a good candidate molecule for mediating epithelial-mesenchymal interactions, because HGF mRNA was localized to mesenchymal cells, whereas mRNA for the c-*met* receptor was detected in the epithelium (131). This observation may reflect species specificity, since a study in the human fetal lung reported HGF mRNA in both mesenchymal and epithelial cells (129). The attractiveness of HGF as a potent growth factor in the lung was enhanced by the observation that HGF mRNA was upregulated during repair of lung injury induced by acid instillation (132). The role of HGF in lung development, however, has been brought into question by two separate studies (133,134) in which the HGF gene was disrupted by targeted homologous recombination. HGF null mice invariably died between days 13–16 of gestation; lung development in these fetuses, however, was identical to that seen in wild-type controls. Thus, HGF does not seem to be of primary importance in lung development at least up through the glandular stage. These data do not rule out a role for HGF later in gestation.

### F. Transforming Growth Factor-β

The TGF-β superfamily comprises a large group of at least 24 members that have been shown to be intimately involved in many key events of normal growth and development (for reviews, see refs. 135–137). There are currently five closely related isoforms (TGF-β1–5) of TGF-β. The 1–3 isoforms of TGF-β stimulate ECM deposition and inhibit epithelial cell proliferation. In the developing lung TGF-β1 has been immunolocalized to both epithelial and mesenchymal cells of the mouse on days 11–13 of gestation, with only epithelial cells staining positive on days 15–18 (38). Extracellular staining of TGF-β1 was seen throughout the stroma, but was predominant at the epithelial-mesenchymal interfaces in the clefts of developing branch points, colocalizing with fibronectin, and collagens I and III. These data suggest that TGF-β1 influences branching morphogenesis by modulating the production and deposition of ECM molecules. This possibility was strengthened by the observation that TGF-β1 can regulate production of tenascin in the fetal rat lung (138). The actual site of production of TGF-β in the fetal lung may not yet be resolved: studies in the adult rat and mouse have shown that although bronchial epithelial cells stain positive for TGF-β proteins, mRNA expression has been confined to fibroblasts just subtending the epithelial ducts and to smooth muscle cells (139), and fetal rat lung fibroblasts have been shown to synthesize and secrete TGF-β (140).

When added to explant cultures of early (day 11.5) mouse lungs, TGF-β1 caused a dose-dependent decrease in explant size and inhibition of branching morphogenesis that could be reversed by washing out the ligand (141). These effects coincided with a significant decrease in the expression of the N-*myc* protooncogene in the epithelium. Since it has been shown that targeted mutations of the N-*myc* locus resulted in severely compromised lung development (142–144), it was speculated that TGF-β1 acts on the lung epithelium by directly suppressing N-*myc* expression. TGF-β can also affect fetal lung epithelial cell differentiation, since treatment of human fetal lung explants with TGF-β inhibited expression of SP-A (145).

Manipulation of the TGF-β1 gene has not clarified its role in normal lung development. Prenatal lethality on day 10.5 occurred in 50% of fetuses homozygous for a targeted mutation in TGF-β1 owing to defects in hematopoiesis and vasculogenesis (146). Mice surviving to term died by 3–4 weeks of age from multifocal massive infiltration of inflammatory cells (147,148). The lungs of these animals showed normal epithelial development but were characterized by perivasculitis and pneumonia. The lack of an effect of the TGF-β1 null genotype on lung development may be due to a functional redundancy provided by other

TGF-β isoforms, although it has been suggested that the presence of TGFβ may be superfluous (149).

### G. Vascular Endothelial Growth Factor

As discussed above, a specific example of potential reciprocity between tissue compartments in the developing lung can be found in vasculogenesis. Vascularization can occur through two basic processes. The first, angiogenesis, is the process by which new capillaries sprout from preexisting vessels and invade a tissue. The brain, limb, and kidney are examples of organs that are vascularized by angiogenesis during development (for review, see ref. 150). The second process, vasculogenesis, results from the de novo proliferation and organization of endothelial precursor cells (angioblasts); this occurs in a variety of developing organs, including the lung (151). Angioblasts initially form a primary vascular plexus within the tissue, which eventually links up to the main circulation coming from the heart. The vascular bed in the embryonic lung is thought to arise by vasculogenesis. This has been most convincingly demonstrated in avian species using intracoelomic chimeric tissue recombinations between quail and chick embryonic lungs (152). In these experiments, chimeras were made by grafting prevascularized lung rudiments from quail embryos onto the embryonic chick lung, as well as the reciprocal of chick lung onto quail. A specific antibody against quail endothelial cells allowed determination of the species of origin of the vasculature. The results clearly showed that the endothelial cells that arose within the grafted lung came from the graft itself and not from angiogenic ingrowth from the host. Identical observations were made for other organs (stomach, pancreas, intestine) in which the epithelium is endodermally derived. From these observations, Pardanaud (152) hypothesized that the endoderm induces the emergence of endothelial cells in its associated mesoderm.

The relatively recently discovered vascular endothelial growth factor (VEGF) is a candidate molecule likely to play a major role in mediating epithelial-mesenchymal cross-talk during lung vascular development. VEGF is a member of the PDGF family that is identical to vascular permeability factor (153,154) and vasculotropin (155). VEGF is found in abundance in highly vascularized tissues such as the kidney, placenta, and lung. Unlike members of the FGF family, VEGF appears to be an endothelial-specific mitogen (for review, see ref. 156). VEGF also contains a signal peptide, which suggests that it is secreted by a classical pathway. All available data suggest that VEGF is involved in both vasculogenesis and angiogenesis (157). By antibody staining, VEGF is detected in epithelial cells in the glandular stage human fetal lung (158). In situ hybridization studies on the adult rat (154) and guinea pig (153) lung suggest that VEGF expression is primarily localized to the epithelium. Studies in the embryonic quail lung (159), however, show that mesenchymal cells may also express VEGF.

Two closely related receptor tyrosine kinases have been demonstrated to be receptors for VEGF. One is the *fms-like* tyrosine kinase (flt-1) (160). The other is the *fetal liver kinase* (flk-1, the murine homologue of the human KDR gene (161–163). Mutations in the mouse flt-1 and flk-1 genes generated by homologous recombination in embryonic stem cells gave very different results. Mice homozygous for a targeted mutation of the flt-1 gene had differentiated endothelial cells in both embryonic and extraembryonic regions, but these cells failed to assemble into normal vascular channels, and the embryos died at midsomite stages (164). The targeted mutation of the flk-1 gene also resulted in embryonic lethality due to a defect in the development of endothelial and hematopoietic cells themselves (165). flk-1 is expressed exclusively in the vascular endothelium in mouse embryos and is the earliest known marker for endothelium and endothelial cell precursors (159,166). flk-1 has been detected in the mouse lung as early as day 12.5 (glandular stage) of gestation (167). The importance of flk-1 (and hence VEGF) to vascularization has been demonstrated in experiments in which C6 glioblastoma tumor cells, which secrete VEGF, were subcutaneously cotransplanted with cells producing replication-defective retroviruses expressing a truncated form of flk-1 (168). The strategy was that the retroviruses would infect the endothelial cells (as well as other cells) and abrogate the signaling cascade initiated by VEGF by dominant-negative inhibition of flk-1. The results showed a drastic reduction in tumor growth, presumably due to the inability of the VEGF-secreting tumor cells to stimulate neovascularization in nonresponsive endothelial cells. The sum of these observations is that VEGF may play an instructive role in the induction and elaboration of the vasculature.

Thus, a situation exists in which development of the pulmonary vasculature depends on the interaction of epithelium and mesenchyme: the epithelium produces VEGF, a ligand that is absolutely required for normal vasculogenesis, whereas the responding endothelial cell precursor cells reside within the mesenchyme. The cross-talk between different cell types may not end there. The induced endothelium itself may then produce factors to recruit other mesodermal cells (e.g., smooth muscle cell precursors) necessary for the completion of vessel structure. Such a functional dependence on reciprocity among different cell types makes it easy to envision that an abnormality in either tissue compartment might have profound effects on the other. For example, an aberration in the ability of epithelial cells to elaborate vasculogenic factors could produce defects in vascular development. The ability of epithelium to specify patterns of development in mesenchymal cells has important implications for potential strategies for therapy (particularly gene therapy), since the lung epithelium provides a readily accessible target for manipulation.

### H. Bombesin-like Peptides

Production of bombesin-like peptides (BLPs) in the lung is localized to pulmonary neuroendocrine cells, which are present in high numbers in the epithelium of fetal and newborn lung (169–174). The preferential (>50%) localization of pulmonary neuroendocrine cells at epithelial branchpoints in early gestation suggested a developmental role for these cells, and hence BLPs, in mediating some aspects of lung patterning. This notion was reinforced by the demonstration that receptors for gastrin-releasing peptide (a BLP) were highest in mesenchymal cells at the clefts of airway and blood vessel branchpoints; furthermore, fibronectin, which accumulates at branchpoints in the developing lung (38), was shown to induce gastrin-releasing peptide in some undifferentiated cell lines (175).

Bombesin treatment of explant cultures has been demonstrated to affect branching morphogenesis in the mouse (176) and type II cell differentiation (177) in the mouse and human. Bombesin administered to pregnant mice during late gestation increased maturation of the surfactant system in the fetal lungs (178). Inhibition of the enzyme CD10/neutralendopeptidase 24.11 (NEP), which hydrolyzes BLPs and is found in the developing mouse and human lung, resulted in enhanced growth and differentiation (178,179). An attractive hypothesis arising from the sum of these data is that BLPs from the epithelium stimulate mesenchymal cells to elaborate ECM molecules that are then involved in directing branching morphogenesis. Further, the observation that ECM components can induce BLP expression suggests the possibility for a positive feedback loop.

### I. Fibroblast-Pneumonocyte Factor

Although glucocorticoids are not synthesized by the lung, an extensive literature documents their involvement in several aspects of lung development, particularly maturation of the pulmonary surfactant system in late gestation (for review, see refs. 70 and 71). A series of observations, originally made by Smith (180), have suggested that the effects of glucocorticoids on enhancing surfactant phospholipid biosynthesis are not due to the direct action of the hormone on presumptive alveolar type II cells but rather are mediated through the actions of a fibroblast-derived polypeptide that was named fibroblast-pneumonocyte factor (FPF). The bulk of the data on FPF has come from in vitro studies of late-gestation (day 20) fetal rat lung epithelial cells. It was shown that these cells increased synthesis of disaturated phosphatidylcholine, the major surfactant phospholipid, when cultured with medium conditioned by cortisol-stimulated fetal lung fibroblasts. Culture of the epithelial cells with cortisol alone had little effect on surfactant phospholipid synthesis. FPF acts by stimulating the activity of cholinephosphate cytidylyltransferase, which is the rate-limiting enzyme in phosphatidylcholine synthesis (181). FPF has been estimated to have a molecular mass of 5–15 kDa (180), and it is apparently quite stable (182). Although the precise identification and characterization of FPF have remained elusive, the data provide evidence that epithelial-mesenchymal interactions persist late into gestation and affect processes beyond lung patterning.

### J. Retinoic Acid

Although retinol (vitamin A) is not synthesized in the lung, fetal lung fibroblasts are capable of storing retinoids as retinyl esters (183,184). These are hydrolyzed to retinol, which is then serially oxidized to retinoic acid (RA), the most active form of the vitamin. RA (all-*trans* and 9-*cis* RA) exert their influence through receptors that are members of the steroid hormone receptor superfamily (185). Three RA receptor (RAR) and three retinoid X receptor (RXR) genes have been identified, each with multiple isoforms of differing affinities and specifities. This results in a potential for great diversity in cellular responses to RA. In addition to receptor molecules, there are cytoplasmic binding proteins for retinol (CRBP) and retinoic acid (CRABP), each of which has two isoforms. These may function as cytoplasmic chaperones for retinoids (either molecule) or modulate responsiveness to RA by preventing it from binding to nuclear receptors (CRABP) (for review, see ref. 186).

RA has been shown to be fundamentally involved in several developmental systems, and the lung appears to be no exception. RARs and retinoid binding proteins have been identified in the developing lung, with nonuniform patterns of distribution. Treatment of cultured lung explants from day 13.5 fetal rats with exogenous RA had profound effects on lung development (187). Not only was branching morphogenesis impeded at high ($10^{-6}$–$10^{-5}$ M) concentrations of RA, significant changes in epithelial cytodifferentiation also occurred. Expression of mRNAs for SP-A, SP-B, and SP-C, markers of distal lung epithelial differentiation, were downregulated in a dose-dependent fashion by RA. The results suggested that RA has the effect of inducing a more proximal epithelial cell phenotype, and that this may be mediated by differential regulation of spatial information provided by genes in the *Hox* family (188).

### VII. Proliferation and Differentiation of Lung Epithelial Cells in the Absence of Mesenchyme

As detailed above, all available data suggest that the interactions between epithelium and mesenchyme in lung development involve an interplay among components of the ECM and a number of soluble factors. Drawing on these studies, it seemed plausible that the requirement for mesenchyme in vitro might be supplanted by providing the epithelium with a complex culture environment that attempted to mimic that provided by pulmonary mesenchyme. To this end, we (189) initiated cultures of purified day 13–14 fetal rat distal lung epithelium in a reconstituted basement membrane extracted from the EHS tumor, which has been shown to support adult alveolar type II cell differentiation (190–192). The initial culture medium tested, which contained insulin, EGF, aFGF, cholera toxin, fetal bovine serum, and 15-fold concentrated bronchoalveolar lavage fluid (BALF), was chosen because it had been shown to support low-density proliferation of adult alveolar type II cells (193). The results were striking: Proliferation of the epithelial cells over the 5-day culture period resulted in very large, lobulated organoids. Furthermore, cytodifferentiation of the epithelial cells continued in culture, including the expression of surfactant proteins A, B, and C, as well as the formation of osmiophilic lamellar bodies and a basal lamina. In a subsequent study, we determined that the critical components of this complex medium were insulin, cholera toxin, and aFGF. KGF, which has a classic signal peptide, was able to replace aFGF, which will bind the KGF receptor. The effects of cholera toxin were shown to be independent of increasing intracellular cyclic AMP; the in vivo processes that stimulation with cholera toxin is mimicking is at present unknown. The importance of members of the FGF family in promoting mesenchyme-free epithelial growth has also been shown in the mouse (194). The number of different cell types that can arise in these cultures is still unclear, however, as is the assessment of whether their spatial distribution approximates that which occurs during normal lung organogenesis.

## VIII.  Summary and Conclusions

The studies discussed above make it clear that the mechanisms underlying the requirement for pulmonary mesenchyme in the generation of the lung architecture and specialized cell phenotypes involve a complex interplay of growth factors, hormones, cytokines, and ECM molecules. Thus, it seems unlikely that a single "lung morphogen" will be identified. The advent of molecular techniques has stimulated a renaissance of interest in lung developmental biology, which has resulted in new insights into the interactions between epithelium and mesenchyme. If the number of important observations that have been reported over the last several years is any indication, we are on the threshold of discovering some of the fundamental tenets governing lung development. While these will be of great interest at the level of basic biology, their importance to the development of new strategies for the prevention and treatment of pathologies resulting from lung immaturity cannot be overestimated.

### Acknowledgments

The authors wish to thank Mary Peterson for excellent secretarial assistance. Robin R. Deterding is a Parker B. Francis Fellow in Pulmonary Research.

### References

1.   Haies DM, Gil J, Weibel, ER. Morphometric study of rat lung cells. I. Numerical and

dimensional characteristics of parenchymal cell populations. Am Rev Respir Dis 1981; 123:533–541.

2. Crapo JD, Barry BE, Gehr P, Bachofen M, Weibel ER. Cell number and cell characteristics of the normal human lung. Am Rev Respir Dis 1982; 125:332–337.

3. Grobstein C, Cohen J. Collagenase: effect on the morphogenesis of embryonic salivary epithelium in vitro. Science 1965; 150:626–628.

4. Grobstein C. Mechanisms of organogenetic tissue interaction. Natl Cancer Inst Monogr 1967; 26:279–299.

5. Rutter WJ, Wessells NY, Grobstein C. Controls of specific synthesis in the developing pancreas. Natl Cancer Inst Monogr 1964; 13:51–65.

6. Kratochwil K. Organ specificity in mesenchymal induction demonstrated in the embryonic development of the mammary gland of the mouse. Dev Biol 1969; 20: 46–71.

7. Grobstein C. Inductive interaction in the development of the mouse metanephros. J Exp Zool 1955; 130:319–340.

8. Lehtonen E. Epithelio-mesenchymal interface during mouse kidney tubule induction in vivo. J Embryol Exp Morphol 1975; 34:695–705.

9. Saxén L, Lehtonen E, Karkinen-Jääskeläinen M, Nordling S, Wartiovaara J. Are morphogenetic tissue interactions mediated by transmissible signal substances or through cell contacts? Nature 1976; 259:662–663.

10. Kollar EJ, Baird G. Tissue interaction in developing mouse tooth germs. II. The inductive role of the dental papilla. J Embryol Exp Morphol 1970; 24:173–186.

11. Slavkin HC. Embryonic tooth formation: A tool for developmental, biology. In: Oral Sciences Reviews. Copenhagen: Munksgaard, 1974:

12. Harrison RG. Experiments on the development of the forelimb of Amblystoma, a self-differentiating equipotential system. J Exp Zool 1918; 25:413–461.

13. Cunha GR. Epithelial-stromal interactions in the development of the urogenital tract. Int Rev Cytol 1976; 47:137–194.

14. Wessells N. Tissue Interactions and Development. Meno Park, CA: Benjamin, 1977.

15. Rudnick, D. Developmental capacities of the chick lung in chorioallantoic grafts. J Exp Zool 1933; 66:125–154.

16. Dameron F. Etude de la morphogenese de la bronche de l'embryon de Poulet associee a differents mesenchymes en culture in vitro. Comput Rend Acad Sci 1961;

17. Sampaolo G, Sampaolo L. Observations histologiques sur le poumon de foetus de Cobaye, cultive in vitro. Comput Rend Assoc Anat 1959; 45:707–714.

18. Taderera JT. Control of lung differentiation in vitro. Dev Biol 1967; 16:489–512.

19. Spooner BS, Wessells N. Mammalian lung development: Interactions in primordium formation and bronchial morphogenesis. J Exp Zool 1970; 175:445–454.

20. Masters JRW. Epithelial-mesenchymal interaction during lung development: The effect of mesenchymal mass. Dev Biol 1976; 51:98–108.

21. Lawson KA. The role of mesenchyme in the morphogenesis and functional differentiation of rat salivary epithelium. J Embryol Exp Morphol 1972; 27:497–513.

22. Lawson KA. Mesenchyme specificy in rodent salivary gland development: the response of salivary epithelium to lung mesenchyme ini vitro. J. Embryol. Exp. Morphal 1974:32:46–493.

23. Ball W. D. Development of the rat salivary glands. III. Mesenchymal specificity in the morphogenesis of the embryonic submillary and sublinqual glands of the rat. J Exp Zool 1974; 188:277–288.

24. Hilfer S, Rayner R, Brown J. Mesenchymal control of branching pattern in the fetal mouse lung. Tissue Cell 1985; 17:523–538.

25. Grobstein C. Trans-filter induction of tubules in mouse metanephrogenic mesenchyme. Exp Cell Res 1956; 10:424–440.

26. Wessells N, Cohen J. Effects of collagenase on developing epithelia in vitro: Lung, ureteric bud, and pancreases Dev Biol 1968; 18:294–309.

27. Hilfer S, Rayner R, Brown J. Mesenchymal control of branching pattern in the fetal mouse lung. Tissue Cell 1985; 17:523–538.

28. Bourbon JR, Rieutort M, Engle MJ, Farrell PM. Utilization of glycogen for phospholipid synthesis in fetal rat lung. Biochim Biophys Acta 1982; 712:382–389.

29. Alescio T, Cassini A. Induction in vitro of tracheal buds by pulmonary mesenchyme grafted on tracheal epithelium. J Exp Zool 1962; 150:83–94.

30. Wessells N. Mammalian lung development: Interactions in formation and morphogenesis of tracheal buds. J Exp Zool 1970; 175:455–466.

31. Sakakura T, Nishizuka Y, Dawe CJ. Mesenchyme-dependent morphogenesis and epithelium-specific cytodifferention in mouse mammary gland. Science 1976; 194:1439–1441.

32. Shannon JM. Induction of alveolar type II cell differentiation in fetal tracheal epithelium by grafted distal lung mesenchyme. Dev Biol 1994; 166:600–614.

33. Wert SE, Glasser SW, Korfhagen TR, Whitsett JA. Transcriptional elements from the human SP-C gene direct expression in the primordial respiratory epithelium of transgenic mice. Dev Biol 1993; 156:426–443.

34. Kalina M, Mason RJ, Shannon JM. Surfactant protein C is expressed in alveolar type II cells but not in Clara cells of rat lung. Am J Respir Cell Mol Biol 1992; 6: 595–600.

35. Goldin GV, Wessells NK. Mammalian lung development: the possible role of cell proliferation in the formation of supernumerary tracheal buds and in branching morphogenesis. J Exp Zool 1979; 208:337–346.

36. Hay ED. Extracellular matrix alters epithelial differentiation. Curr Opin Cell Biol 1993; 5:1029–1035.

37. Vlodavsky I, Folkman J, Sullivan R, Friedman R, Ishai R, Sasse J, Klagsbrun M. Endothelial cell-derived basic fibroblast growth factor: synthesis and deposition into the subendothelial extracellular matrix. Proc Natl Acad Sci USA 1987; 84:2282.

38. Heine U, Munoz E, Flanders K, Roberts A, Sporn M. Colocalization of TGF-beta 1 and collagen I and III, fibronectin and glycosaminoglycans during lung branching morphogenesis. Development 1990; 109:29–36.

39. Chen J-M, Little C. Cellular events associated with lung branching morphogenesis including the deposition of collagen type IV. Dev Biol 1987; 120:311–321.

40. Caniggia I, Han R, Liu J, Wang J, Tanswell AK, Post M. Differential expression of collagen-binding receptors in fetal rat lung cells. Am J Physiol 1995; 268:L136–L143.

41. Alescio T. Effect of a proline analogue, azetidine-2-carboxylic acid, on the morphogenesis in vitro of mouse embryonic lung. J Embryol Exp Morphol 1973; 29: 439–451.

42. Spooner B, Faubion J. Collagen involvement in branching morphogenesis of embryonic lung and salivary gland. Dev Biol 1980; 77:84–102.

43. King G, Adamson I. Effects of cis-hydroxyproline on type II cell development in fetal rat lung. Exp Lung Res 1987; 12:347–362.

44. Adamson I, King G. L-azetidine-2-carboxylic acid retards lung growth and surfactant synthesis in fetal rats. Lab Invest 1987; 57:439–445.

45. Kratochwil K, Dziadek M, Lohler J, Harbers K, Jaenisch R. Normal epithelial branching morphogenesis in the absence of collagen I. Dev Biol 1986; 117:596–606.

46. Schuger L, Varani J, Killen PD, Skubitz APN, Gilbride K. Laminin expression in the mouse lung increases with development and stimulates spontaneous organotypic rearrangement of mixed lung cells. Dev Dyn 1992; 195:43–54.

47. Durham PL, Snyder JM. Characterization of $\alpha 1$, $\beta 1$, and $\gamma 1$ laminin subunits during rabbit fetal lung development. Dev Dyn 1995; 203:408–421.

48. Schuger L, O'Shea S, Rheinheimer J, Varani J. Laminin in lung development: Effects of anti-laminin antibody in murine lung morphogenesis. Dev Biol 1990; 137: 26–32.

49. Schuger L, Skubitz APN, O'Shea KS, Chang JF, Varani J. Identification of laminin domains involved in branching morphogenesis: effects of anti-laminin monoclonal antibodies on mouse embryonic lung development. Dev Biol 1991; 146:531–541.

50. Schuger L, Skubitz APN, De Las Morenas A, Gilbride K. Two separate domains of laminin promote lung organogenesis by different mechanisms of action. Dev Biol 1995; 169:520–532.

51. Roman J, McDonald JA. Expression of fibronectin, the integrin $\alpha 5$, and $\alpha$-smooth muscle actin in heart and lung development. Am J Respir Cell Mol Biol 1992; 6: 472–480.

52. Roman J, Little C, McDonald J. Potential role of RGD-binding integrins in mammalian lung branching morphogenesis. Development 1991; 112:551–558.

53. George EL, Georges-Labouesse EN, Patel-King RS, Rayburn H, Hynes RO. Defects in mesoderm, neural tube and vascular development in mouse embryos lacking fibronectin. Development 1993; 119:1079–1091.

54. Yang JT, Rayburn H, and Hynes R. Embryonic mesodermal defects in $\alpha 5$ integrin-deficient mice. Development 1993; 119:1093–1105.

55. Bernfield MR, Cohn RH, Banerjee SD. Glycosaminoglycans and epithelial organ formation. Am Zool 1973; 13:1067–1083.

56. Ruoslaht E, Yamaguchi Y. Proteoglycans as modulators of growth factor activities. Cell 1991; 64:867–869.

57. Flaumenhaft R, Rifkin DB. The extracellular regulation of growth factor action. Mol Biol Cell 1992; 3:1057–1065.

58. Rapraeger AC, Krufka A, Olwin, BB. Requirement of heparan sulphate for bFGF-mediated fibroblast growth and myoblast differentiation. Science 1991; 252:1705–1708.

59. Brauker JH, Trautman MS, Bernfield M. Syndecan, a cell surface proteoglycan, exhibits a molecular polymorphism during lung development. Dev Biol 1991; 147: 285–292.

60. Smith C, Hilfer S, Searls R, Nathanson M, Allodoli M. Effects of $\beta$-D-Xyloside on differentiation of the respiratory epithelium in the fetal mouse lung. Dev Biol 1990; 138:42–52.

61. Smith C, Webster E, Nathanson M, Searls R, Hilfer S. Altered patterns of proteoglycan deposition during maturation of the fetal mouse lung. Cell Diff Dev 1990; 32: 83–96.

62. Erickson HP. Tenascin-C, tenascin-R and tenascin-X: a family of talented proteins in search of functions. Curr Opin Cell Biol 1993; 5:869–876.

63. Young SL, Chang L-Y, Erickson HP. Tenascin-C in rat lung: distribution, ontogeny and role in branching morphogenesis. Dev Biol 1994; 161:615–625.

64. Bristow J, Tee MK, Gitelman SE, Mellon SH, Miller WL. Tenascin-X: a novel extracellular matrix protein encoded by the human XB gene overlapping p450c21B. J Cell Biol 1993; 122:265–278.

65. Zhao Y, Young SL. Tenascin in rat lung development: in situ localization and cellular sources. Am J Physiol 1995; 269:L482–L491.

66. Saga Y, Yagi T, Ikawa Y, Sakakura T, Aizawa S. Mice develop normally without tenascin. Genes Dev 1992; 6:1821–1831.

67. Ekblom P, Ekblom M, Fecker L, Klein G, Zhang H-Y, Kadoya Y, Chu ML, Mayer U, Timpl R. Role of mesenchymal nidogen for epithelial morphogenesis in vitro. Development 1994; 120:2003–2014.

68. Mayer U, Mann K, Timpl R, Murphy G. Sites of nidogen cleavage by proteases involved in tissue homeostasis and remodeling. Eur J Biochem 1993; 217:877–884.

69. Hitchcock KR. Lung development and the pulmonary surfactant system: hormonal influences. Anat Rec 1980; 198:13–34.

70. Ballard PL. Hormonal regulation of pulmonary surfactant. Endocrine Rev 1989; 10:165–181.

71. Post M, Smith BT. Hormonal control of surfactant metabolism. In: Pulmonary Surfactant: From Molecular Biology to Clinical Practice. Elsevier, 1992:379–424.

72. Moscatelli D. Fibroblast growth factors. In: Cytokines of the Lung. New York, Dekker, 1993:41–76.

73. Mason IJ, Fuller-Pace F, Smith R, Dickson C. FGF-7 (keratinocyte growth factor) expression during mouse development suggests roles in myogenesis, forebrain regionalisation and epithelial-mesenchymal interactions. Mechan Dev 1994; 45:15–30.

74. Givol D, Yayon A. Complexity of FGF receptors: genetic basis for structural diversity and functional specificity. FASEB J 1992; 6:3362–3369.

75. Gonzalez A-M, Buscaglia M, Ong M, Baird A. Distribution of basic fibroblast growth factor in the 18-day rat fetus: localization in the basement membranes of diverse tissues. J Cell Biol 1990; 110:753–765.

76. Han RNN, Mawdsley C, Souza P, Tanswell AK, Post M. Platelet-derived growth factors and growth-related genes in rat lung. III. Immunolocalization during fetal development. Pediatr Res 1992; 31:323–329.

77. Yan G, Fukabori Y, Nikolaropoulos S, Wang F, McKeehan WC. Heparin-binding keratinocyte growth factor is a candidate stromal to epithelial cell andromedin. Mol Endocrinol 1992; 6:2123–2128.

78. Alarid ET, Rubin JS, Young P, Chedid M, Ron D, Aaronson SA, Cunha GR. Keratinocyte growth factor functions in epithelial induction during seminal vesicle development. Proc Natl Acad Sci USA 1994; 91:1074–1078.

79. Rubin J, Osada H, Finch P, Taylor W, Rudikoff S, Aaronson S. Purification and

characterization of a newly identified growth factor specific for epithelial cells. Proc Natl Acad Sci USA 1989; 86:802–806.

80.  Finch PW, Cunha GR, Rubin JS, Wong J, Ron D. Pattern of keratinocyte growth factor and keratinocyte growth factor receptor expression during mouse fetal development suggests a role in mediating morphogenetic mesenchymal-epithelial interactions. Dev Dyn 1995; 203:223–240.

81.  Johnson DE, Lu J, Chen H, Werner S, Williams LT. The human fibroblast growth factor receptor genes: a common structural arrangement underlies the mechanisms for generating receptor forms that differ in their third immunoglobulin domain. Mol Cell Biol 1991; 11:4627–4634.

82.  Urtreger AO. Developmental localization of the splicing alternatives of fibroblast growth factor receptor-2 (FGFR2). Dev Biol 1993; 158:475–486.

83.  Peters K, Werner S, Liao X, Wert S, Whitsett J, Williams L. Targeted expression of a dominant negative FGF receptor blocks branching morphogenesis and epithelial differentiation of the mouse lung. EMBO J 1994; 13:3296–3301.

84.  Snead ML, Luo W, Oliver P, Nakamura M, Don-Wheeler G, Bessem C, Bell GI, Rall LB, Slavkin HC. Localization of epidermal growth factor precursor in tooth and lung during embryonic mouse development. Dev Biol 1989; 134:420–429.

85.  Warburton D, Seth R, Shum L, Horcher PG, Hall FL, Werb Z, Slavkin HC. Epigenetic role of epidermal growth factor expression and signalling in embryonic mouse lung morphogenesis. Dev Biol 1992; 149:123–133.

86.  Kubiak J, Mitr MM, Steve AR, Hunt JD, Davies P, Pitt BR. TGF-α gene expression in late gestation fetal rat lung. Pediatr Res 1992; 31:286–290.

87.  Strandjord TP, Clark JG, Hodson WA, Schmidt RA, Madtes DK. Expression of transforming growth factors-α in mid-gestation human fetal lung. Am J Respir Cell Mol Biol 1993; 8:266–272.

88.  Partanen AM, Thesleff I. Localization and quantitation of [125]I-epidermal growth factor binding in mouse embryonic tooth and other embryonic tissues at different developmental stages. Dev Biol 1987; 120:186–197.

89.  Ganser GL, Stricklin GP, Matrisian L. EGF and TGFα influence in vitro lung development by the induction of matrix-degrading metalloproteinases. Int J Dev Biol 1991; 35:453–461.

90.  Seth R, Shum L, Wu F, Wuenschell C, Hall FL, Slavkin HC, Warburton D. Role of epidermal growth factor expression in early mouse embryo lung branching morphogenesis in culture: antisense oligonucleotide inhibitory strategy. Dev Biol 1993; 158:555–559.

91.  Goldin G, Opperman L. Induction of supernumerary tracheal buds and the stimulation of DNA synthesis in the embryonic chick lung and trachea by epidermal growth factor. J Embryol Exp Morphol 1980; 60:235–243.

92.  Catterton WZ, Escobedo MB, Sexson WR, Gray ME, Sundell HW, Stahlman MT. Effect of epidermal growth factor on lung maturation in fetal rabbits. Pediatr Res 1979; 13:104–108.

93.  Gross I, Dynia D, Rooney S, Smart D, Warshaw J, Sissom J, Hoath S. Influence of epidermal growth factor on fetal rat lung development in vitro. Pediatr Res 1986; 20:473–477.

94. Whitsett J, Pilot T, Clark J, Weaver T. Induction of surfactant protein in fetal lung. Effects of cAMP and dexamethasone on SAP-35 RNA and synthesis. J Biol Chem 1987; 262:5256–5261.

95. Nielsen H. Epidermal growth factor influences the developmental clock regulating maturation of the fetal lung fibroblast. Biochim Biophys Acta 1989; 1012:201–206.

96. Luetteke NC, Qiu TH, Peiffer RL, Oliver P, Smithies O, Lee DC. TGFα deficiency results in hair follicle and eye abnormalities in targeted and waved-1 mice. Cell 1993; 73:263–278.

97. Mann GB, Fowler KJ, Gabriel A, Nice EC, Williams RL, Dunn AR. Mice with a null mutation of the TGFα gene have abnormal skin architecture, wavy hair, and curly whiskers and often develop corneal inflammation. Cell 1993; 73:249–261.

98. Luetteke NC, Phillips HK, Qiu TH, Copeland NG, Earp HS, Jenkins NA, Lee DC. The mouse waved-2 phenotype results from a point mutation in the EGF receptor tyrosine kinase. Genes Dev 1994; 8:399–413.

99. Miettinen PJ, Berger JE, Meneses J, Phung Y, Pedersen RA, Werb Z, Derynck R. Epithelial immaturity and multiorgan failure in mice lacking epidermal growth factor receptor. Nature 1995; 376:337–341.

100. Sibilia M, Wagner EF. Strain-dependent epithelial defects in mice lacking the EGF receptor. Science 1995; 269:234–238.

101. Threadgill DW, Dlugosz AA, Hansen LA, Tennenbaum T, Lichti U, Yee D, LaMantia C, Mourton T, Herrup K, Harris RC, Barnard JA, Yuspa SH, Coffey RJ, Magnuson T. Targeted disruption of mouse EGF receptor: effect of genetic background on mutant phenotype. Science 1995; 269:230–234.

102. Korfhagen TR, Swan RJ, Wert SE, McCarty JM, Kerlakian CB, Glasser SW, Whitsett JA. Respiratory epithelial cell expression of human transforming growth factor-α induces lung fibrosis in transgenic mice. J Clin Invest 1994; 93:1691–1699.

103. Fabisiak JP, Absher M, Evans JN, Kelley J. Spontaneous production of PDGF A-chain homodimer by rat lung fibroblasts in vitro. Am J Physiol 1992; 263: L185–L193.

104. Hammacher A, Mellström K, Heldin C-H, Westermark B. Isoform-specific induction of actin reorganization by platelet-derived growth factor suggests that the functionally active receptor is a dimer. EMBO J 1989; 8:2489–2495.

105. Seifert RA, Hart CE, Phillips PE, Forstrom JW, Ross R, Murray MJ, Bowen-Pope DF. Two different subunits associate to create isoform-specific platelet-derived growth factor receptors. J Biol Chem 1989; 264:8771–8778.

106. Buch S, Jones C, Sweezey N, Tanswell K, Post M. Platelet-derived growth factor and growth-related genes in rat lung. I. Developmental expression. Am J Respir Cell Mol Biol 1991; 5:371–376.

107. Fabisiak JP, Kelley J. Platelet-derived growth factor. In: Cytokines of the Lung. New York: Dekker, 1993:3–39.

108. Souza P, Kuliszewski M, Wang J, Tseu I, Tanswell AK, Post M. PDGF-AA and its receptor influence early lung branching via an epithelial-mesenchymal interaction. Development 1995; 121:2559–2567.

109. Souza P, Sedlackova L, Kuliszewski M, Wang J, Liu J, Tseu I, Liu M, Tanswell AK, Post M. Antisense ligodeoxynucleotides targeting PDGF-B mRNA inhibit cell proliferation during embryonic rat lung development. Development 1994; 120: 2163–2173.

110. Buch S, Jassal D, Cannigia I, Edelson J, Han R, Liu J, Tanswell K, Post M. Ontogeny and regulation of platelet-derived growth factor gene expression in distal fetal rat lung epithelial cells. Am J Respir Cell Mol Biol 1994; 11:251–261.

111. Stiles AD, Moats-Staats BM, Retsch-Bogart GZ. Insulin-like growth factors. In: Cytokines of the Lung. New York: Dekker, 1993:77–99.

112. Morgan DO, Edman JC, Standring DR, Fried VA, Smith MC, Roth RA, Rutter WJ. Insulin-like growth factor II receptor as a multifunctional binding protein. Nature 1987; 329:301–307.

113. Nissley P, Kiess W, Sklar MM. The insulin-like growth factor II/mannose 6-phosphate receptor. In: Insulin-like Growth Factors: Molecular and Cellular Aspects. Boca Raton, FL: CRC Press, 1991:111–150.

114. Brown AL, Chiariotti L, Orlowski CC, Mehlman T, Burgess WH, Ackerman EJ, Bruni CB, Rechler MM. Nucleotide sequence and expression of a cDNA clone encoding a fetal rat binding protein for insulin-like growth factors. J Biol Chem 1989; 264:5148–5154.

115. Albiston AL, Herington AC. Cloning and characterization of the growth hormone-dependent insulin-like growth factor binding protein (IGFBP-3) in the rat. Biochem Biophys Res Commun 1990; 166:892–897.

116. Murphy LJ, Seneviratne C, Ballejo G, Croze F, Kennedy TG. Identification and characterization of a rat decidual insulin-like growth factor-binding protein complementary DNA. Mol Endocrinol 1990; 4:329–336.

117. Shimasaki S, Uchiyama F, Smimonaka M, Ling N. Molecular cloning of the cDNAs encoding a novel insulin-like growth factor-binding protein from rat and human. Mol Endocrinol 1990; 4:1451–1458.

118. Shimasaki S, Gao L, Shimonaka M, Ling N. Isolation and molecular cloning of insulin-like growth factor-binding protein-6. Mol Endocrinol 1991; 5:938–948.

119. Shimasaki S, Shimonaka M, Zhang H-P, Ling N. Identification of five different insulin-like growth factor binding proteins (IGFBPs) from adult rat serum and molecular cloning of a novel IGFBP-5 in rat and human. J Biol Chem 1991; 266:10646–10653.

120. Maitre B, Clement A, Williams MC, Brody JS. Expression of insulin-like growth factor receptors 1 and 2 in the developing lung and their relation to epithelial cell differentiation. Am J Respir Cell Mol Biol 1995; 13:262–270.

121. Moats-Staats BM, Price WA, Xu L, Jarvis HW, Stiles AD. Regulation of the insulin-like growth factor system during normal rat lung development. Am J Respir Cell Mol Biol 1995; 12:56–64.

122. Klempt M, Hutchins A-M, Gluckman PD, Skinner SJM. IGF binding protein-2 gene expression and the location of IGF-1 and IGF-II in fetal rat lung. Development 1992; 115:765–772.

123. Wallen LD, Han VKM. Spatial and temporal distribution of insulin-like growth factors I and II during development of rat lung. Am J Physiol 1994 267:L531–L542.

124. Forbes B, Szabo L, Baxter RC, Ballard FJ, Wallace JC. Classification of the insulin-like growth factor binding proteins into three distinct categories according to their binding specificities. Biochem Biophys Res Commun 1988; 157:196–202.

125. Liu J-P, Baker J, Perkins AS, Robertson EJ, Efstratiadis A. Mice carrying null mutations of the genes encoding insulin-like growth factor 1 (*Igf-1*) and type 1 IGF receptor (*Igf1r*). Cell 1993; 75:59–72.

126. DeChiara TM, Efstratiadis A, Robertson EJ. A growth-deficiency phenotype in heterozygous mice carrying an insulin-like growth factor II gene disrupted by targeting. Nature 1990; 345:78–80.

127. Rubin JS, Chan, AM-L, Bottaro DP, Burgess WH, Taylor WG, Cech AC, Hirschfield DW, Wong J, Miki T, Finch PW, Aaronson SA. A broad-spectrum human lung fibroblast-derived mitogen is a variant of hepatocyte growth factor. Proc Natl Acad Sci USA 1991; 88:415–419.

128. Bottaro DP, Rubin JS, Faletto DL, Chad AM-L, Kmiecik TE, Vande Woude GF, Aaronson SA. Identification of the hepatocyte growth factor receptor as the c-*met* proto-oncogene product. Science 1991; 251:802–804.

129. Wang J, Souza P, Kuliszewski M, Tanswell AK, Post M. Expression of surfactant proteins in embryonic rat lung. Am J Respir Cell Mol Biol 1994; 10:222–229.

130. Degen SJF, Stuart LA, Han S, Jamison CS. Characterization of the mouse cDNA and gene coding for a hepatocyte growth factor-like protein: expression during development. Biochemistry 1991; 30:9781–9791.

131. Sonnenberg E, Meyer D, Weidner KM, Birchmeier C. Scatter factor/hepatocyte growth factor and its receptor, the c-met tyrosine kinase, can mediate a signal exchange between mesenchyme and epithelia during mouse development. J Cell Biol 1993; 123:223–235.

132. Yanagita K, Matsumoto K, Sekiguchi K, Ishibashi H, Niho Y, Nakamura T. Hepatocyte growth factor may act as a pulmotrophic factor on lung regeneration after acute lung injury. J Biol Chem 1993; 268:21212–21217.

133. Schmidt C, Bladt F, Goedecke S, Brinkmann V, Zschiesche W, Sharpe M, Gherardi E, Birchmeier C. Scatter factor/hepatocyte growth factor is essential for liver development. Nature 1995; 373:699–702.

134. Uehara Y, Minowa O, Mori C, Shiota K, Kuno J, Noda T, Kitamura N. Placental defect and embryonic lethality in mice lacking hepatocyte growth factor/scatter factor. Nature 1995; 373:702–705.

135. Kelley J. Transforming growth factor-β. In: Cytokines of the Lung. New York: Dekker, 1993:101–137.

136. Kingsley DM. The TGF-8 superfamily: new members, new receptors, an new genetic tests of function in different organisms. Genes Dev 1994; 8:133–146.

137. Wall NA, Hogan BLM. TGF-β related genes in development. Curr Opin Genet Dev 1994; 4:517–522.

138. Zhao Y, Young SL. TGF-β regulates expression of tenascin alternative-splicing isoforms in fetal rat lung. Am J Physiol 1995; 268:L173–L180.

139. Pelton RW, Johnson MD, Perkett EA, Gold LI, Moses HL. Expression of transforming growth factor-$\beta_1$, -$\beta_2$, and -$\beta_3$ mRNA and protein in the murine lung. Am J Respir Cell Mol Biol 1991; 5:522–530.

140. Kelley J, Fabisiak JP, Hawes K, Absher M. Cytokine signaling in lung: transforming growth factor-$\beta$ secretion by lung fibroblasts. Am J Physiol 1991; 260:L123–L128.

141. Serra R, Pelton RW, Moses HL. TGF$\beta$1 inhibits branching morphogenesis and N-*myc* expression in lung bud organ cultures. Development 1994; 120:2153–2161.

142. Moens CB, Auerbach AB, Conlon RA, Joyner AL, Rossant J. A targeted mutation reveals a role for N-*myc* in branching morphogenesis in the embryonic mouse lung. Genes Dev 1992; 6:691–704.

143. Moens CB, Stanton BR, Parada LF, Rossant J. Defects in heart and lung development in compound heterozygotes for two different targeted mutations at the N-*myc* locus. Development 1993; 119:485–499.

144. Sawai S, Shimono A, Wakamatsu Y, Palmes C, Hanaoka K, Kondoh H. Defects of embryonic organogenesis resulting from targeted disruption of the N-*myc* gene in the mouse. Development 1993; 117:1445–1455.

145. Whitsett J, Weaver T, Lieberman M, Clark J, Duagherty C. Differential effects of epidermal growth factor and transforming growth factor-$\beta$ on synthesis of Mr = 35,000 surfactant-associated protein in fetal lung. J Biol Chem 1987; 262:7908–7913.

146. Dickson MC, Martin JS, Cousins FM, Kulkarni AB, Karlsson S, Akhurst RJ. Defective haematopoiesis and vasculogenesis in transforming growth factor-$\beta$1 knock out mice. Development 1995; 121:1845–1854.

147. Shull MM, Ormsby I, Kier AB, Pawlowski S, Diebold RJ, Yin M, Allen R, Sidman C, Proetzel G, Calvin D, Annunziata N, Doetschman T. Targeted disruption of the mouse transforming growth factor-$\beta$1 gene results in multifocal inflammatory disease. Nature 1992; 359:693–699.

148. Kulkarni AB, Huh, C-G, Becker D, Geiser A, Lyght M, Flanders KC, Roberts AB, Sporn MB, Ward JM, Karlsson S. Transforming growth factor $\beta$1 null mutation in mice causes excessive inflammatory response and early death. Proc Natl Acad Sci USA 1993; 90:770–774.

149. Erickson HP. Gene knockouts of c-*src*, transforming growth factor $\beta$1, and tenascin suggest superfluous, nonfunctional expression of proteins. J Cell Biol 1993; 120:1079–1081.

150. Risau W. Vasculogenesis, angiogenesis and endothelial cell differentiation during embryonic development. In: The Development of the Vascular System. Basel: Karger, 1991: 58–68.

151. Sherer GK. Vasculogenic mechanisms and epithelio-mesenchymal specificity in endodermal organs. In: The Development of the Vascular System. Basel: Karger, 1991:37–57.

152. Pardanaud L, Yassine F, Dieterlen-Lievre F. Relationship between vasculogenesis, angiogenesis and haemopoiesis during avian ontogeny. Development 1989; 105:473–485.

153. Berse B, Brown LF, Van De Water L, Dvorak HF, Senger DR. Vascular permeability

factor (vascular endothelial growth factor) gene is expressed differentially in normal tissues, macrophages, and tumors. Mol Biol Cell 1992; 3:211–220.

154. Monacci WT, Merrill MJ, Oldfield EH. Expression of vascular permeability factor/ vascular endothelial growth factor in normal rat tissues. Am J Physiol 1993; 264: C995–C1002.

155. Plouet J, Schilling J, Gospodarowicz D. Isolation and characterization of a newly identified endothelial cell mitogen produced by AtT-20 cells. EMBO J 1989; 8:3801.

156. Ferrara N. Vascular endothelial growth factor. The trigger for neovascularization in the eye. Lab Invest 1995; 72:615–618.

157. Ferrara N, Houck K, Jakeman L, Leung DW. Molecular and biological properties of the vascular endothelial growth factor family of proteins. Endocrine Rev 1992; 13:18–32.

158. Shifren JL, Doldi N, Ferrara N, Mesiano S, Jaffe RB. In the human fetus, vascular endothelial growth factor is expressed in epithelial cells and myocytes, but not vascular endothelium: Implications for mode of action. J Clin Endocrinol Metab 1994; 79:316–322.

159. Flamme I, Breier G, Risau W. Vascular endothelial growth factor (VEGF) and VEGF receptor 2 (flk-1) are expressed during vasculogenesis and vascular differentiation in the quail embryo. Dev Biol 1995; 169:699–712.

160. Shibuya M, Yamaguchi S, Yamane A, Ikeda T, Tojo A, Matsushime H, Sato M. Nucleotide sequence and expresison of a novel human receptor-type tyrosine kinase gene (flt) closely related to the fms family. Oncogene 1990; 5:519–524.

161. Matthews W, Jordan CT, Gavin M, Jenkins NA, Copeland NG, Lemischka IR. A receptor tyrosine kinase cDNA isolated from a population of enriched primitive hematopoietic cells and exhibiting close genetic linkage to *c-kit*. Proc Natl Acad Sci USA 1991; 88:9026–9030.

162. Terman BI, Dougher-Vermazen M, Carrion ME, Dimitrov D, Armellino DC, Gospodarowicz D, Böhlen P. Identification of the KDR tyrosine kinase as a receptor for vascular endothelial cell growth factor. Biochem Biophys Res Commun 1992; 187: 1579–1586.

163. Quinn TP, Peters KG, De Vries C, Ferrara N, Williams LT. Fetal liver kinase 1 is a receptor for vascular endothelial growth factor and is selectively expressed in vascular endothelium. Proc Natl Acad Sci USA 1993; 90:7533–7537.

164. Shalaby F, Rossant J, Yamaguchi TP, Gertsenstein M, Wu X-F, Breitman ML, Schuh AC. Failure of blood-island formation and vasculogenesis in Flk-1–deficient mice. Nature 1995; 376:62–66.

165. Fong G-H, Rossant J, Gertsenstein M, Breitman ML. Role of Flt-1 receptor tyrosine kinase in regulating the assembly of vascular endothelium. Nature 1995; 376:66–70.

166. Yamaguchi TP, Dumont DJ, Conlon RA, Breitman ML, Rossant J. *flk*-1, An *flt*-related receptor tyrosine kinase is an early marker for endothelial cell precursors. Development 1993; 118:489–498.

167. Millauer B, Wizigmann-Voos S, Schnürch H, Martinez R, Moller NPH, Risau W, Ullrich A. High affinity VEGF binding and developmental expression suggest Flk-1 as a major regulator of vasculogenesis and angiogenesis. Cell 1993; 72:835–846.

168. Millauer B, Shawver LK, Plate KH, Risau W, Ullrich A. Glioblastoma growth inhibited in vivo by a dominant-negative Flk-1 mutant. Nature 1994; 367:576–579.

169. Cutz E, Chan W, Track NS. Bombesin, calcitonin and leuenkephalin immunoreactivity in endocrine cells of the human lung. Experientia 1981; 37:765–767.
170. Johnson DE, Lock JE, Elde RP, Thompson TR. Pulmonary neuroendocrine cells in hyaline membrane disease and bronchopulmonary dysplasia. Pediatr Res 1982; 16:446–454.
171. Track NS, Cutz E. Bombesin-like immunoreactivity in developing human lung. Life Sci 1982; 30:1553–1556.
172. Stahlman MT, Kasselberg AG, Orth D, Gray ME. Ontogeny of neuroendocrine cells in human fetal lung: II. An immunohistochemical study. Lab Invest 1985; 52:52–60.
173. Spindel ER, Sunday ME, Hofler H, Wolfe HJ, Habener JF, Chin WW. Transient elevation of mRNAs encoding gastrin-releasing peptgide (GRP), a putative pulmonary growth factor, in human fetal lung. J Clin Invest 1987; 80:1172–1179.
174. Li H, Witte DP, Branford WW, Aronow BJ, Weinstein M, Kaur S, Singh G, Schreiner CM, Whitsett JA, Scott WJ Jr, Potter SS. Gsh-4 encodes a LIM-type homeodomain, is expressed in the developing central nervous system and is required for early postnatal survival. EMBO J 1994; 13:2876–2885.
175. King KA, Torday JS, Sunday ME. Bombesin and [Leu$^8$]phyllolitorin promote fetal mouse lung branching morphogenesis via a receptor-mediated mechanism. Proc Natl Acad Sci USA 1995; 92:4357–4361.
176. Aguayo SM, Schuyler WE, Murtagh JJ Jr, Roman J. Regulation of lung branching morphogenesis by bombesin-like peptides and neutral endopeptidase. Am J Respir Cell Mol Biol 1994; 10:635–642.
177. Sunday M, Hua J, Dai H, Nusrat A, Torday J. Bombesin increases fetal lung growth and maturation *in utero* and in organ culture. Am J Respir Cell Mol Biol 1990; 3:199–205.
178. Sunday ME, Hua J, Torday JS, Reyes B, Shipp MA. CD10/neutral endopeptidase 24.11 in developing human fetal lung. Patterns of expression and modulation of peptide-mediated proliferation. J Clin Invest 1992; 90:2517–2525.
179. King KA, Hua J, Torday JS, Drazen JM, Graham SA, Shipp MA, Sunday ME. CD10/neutral endopeptidase 24.11 regulates fetal lung growth and maturation in utero by potentiating endogenous bombesin-like peptides. J Clin Invest 1993; 91:1969–1973.
180. Smith B. Lung maturation in the fetal rat: acceleration by injection of fibroblast-pneumonocyte factor. Science 1979; 204:1094–1095.
181. Post M, Barsoumian A, Smith B. The cellular mechanism of glucocorticoid acceleration of fetal lung maturation. J Biol Chem 1986; 261:2179–2184.
182. Floros J, Post M, Smith B. Glucocorticoids affect the synthesis of pulmonary fibroblast-pneumonocyte factor at a pretranslational level. J Biol Chem 1985; 260:2265–2267.
183. Blomhoff R, Green MH, Berg T, Norum KR. Transport and storage of vitamin A. Science 1990; 250:399–404.
184. Tsutsumi C, Okuno M, Tannous L, Piantedosi R, Allen M, Goodman DS, Blaner WS. Retinoids and retinoid-binding protein protein expression in rat adipocytes. J Biol Chem 1992; 267:1805–1810.
185. De Luca LM. Retinoids and their receptors in differentiation, embryogenesis, and neoplasia. FASEB J 1991; 5:2924–2933.

186. Chytil F. The lungs and vitamin A. Am J Physiol 1992; 262:L517–L527.
187. Cardoso WV, Williams MC, Mitsialis SA, Joyce-Brady M, Rishi AK, Brody JS. Retinoic acid induces changes in the pattern of airway branching and alters epithelial cell differentiation in the developing lung in vitro. Am J Respir Cell Mol Biol 1995; 12:464–476.
188. Bogue CW, Gross I, Vasavada H, Dynia DW, Wilson CM, Jacobs HC. Identification of *Hox* genes in newborn lung and effects of gestational age and retinoic acid on their expression. Am J Physiol 1994; 266:L448–L454.
189. Deterding RR, Shannon JM. Proliferation and differentiation of fetal rat pulmonary epithelium in the absence of mesenchyme. J Clin Invest 1995; 95:2963–2972.
190. Rannels SR, Yarnell JA, Fisher CS, Fabisiak JP, Rannels DE. Role of laminin in maintenance of type II pneumocyte morphology and function. Am J Physiol 1987; 253:C835–C845.
191. Shannon JM, Mason RJ, Jennings SD. Functional differentiation of alveolar type II epithelial cells in vitro: effects of cell shape, cell-matrix interactions, and cell-cell interactions. Biochim Biophys Acta 1987; 931:143–156.
192. Shannon JM, Emrie PA, Fisher JH, Kuroki Y, Jennings SD, Mason RJ. Effect of a reconstituted basement membrane on expression of surfactant apoproteins in cultured adult rat alveolar type II cells. Am J Respir Cell Mol Biol 1990; 2:183–192.
193. Leslie CC, McCormick-Shannon K, Mason RJ, Shannon JM. Proliferation of rat alveolar epithelial cells in low density primary culture. Am J Respir Cell Mol Biol 1993; 9:64–72.
194. Nogawa H, Ito T. Branching morphogenesis of embryonic mouse lung epithelium in mesenchyme-free culture. Development 1995; 121:1015–1022.

# 5

# Differentiation of the Alveolar Epithelium in the Fetal Lung

RAMA K. MALLAMPALLI, MICHAEL J. ACARREGUI, and JEANNE M. SNYDER

University of Iowa College of Medicine
Iowa City, Iowa

## I. Introduction

Approximately 90% of gestation is required for the human fetal lung to develop the capacity for efficient respiration. Although the fetal lung is an organ without any apparent physiological purpose, it is by no means quiescent. As with other organs, tremendous growth and differentiation occurs in the lung during fetal life. Although alveolarization is primarily a postnatal process in most mammalian species, it is during gestation that the alveolar epithelium commences differentiation and begins to function. Cell-specific markers of type I and type II alveolar epithelial cells are expressed in undifferentiated pulmonary epithelium by mid-gestation, which is suggestive that cell fate in the future alveolus is determined relatively early, whereas morphological characteristics of type I and type II alveolar epithelial cells are not identified until much later in gestation.

### A. Physiological Role of the Alveolar Epithelium

The epithelial lining of the distal lung plays an important role in lung development. As previously reviewed by Strang (1), Bland and Nielson (2), and O'Bro-dovich (3), the precursor fetal lung alveolar epithelium changes from a fluid-secreting epithelium to a predominately fluid-adsorbing epithelium late in gestation. Lung liquid secretion by the distal fetal pulmonary epithelium is essential for normal lung growth and development (4,5). The movement of water that accompanies active chloride secretion by the primitive respiratory epithelium results in the accumulation of fluid within the lung lumina and large quantities of active fluid secretion from the lung into the amniotic fluid. Studies in chronically instrumented fetal lambs have demonstrated fluid flow rates ranging from 4.3 to 5.8 ml/kg/hr (6–8), which is an amount equivalent to the daily production of 8.4 L of fluid by an average adult's lungs (3). The primary purpose of the fetal lung liquid is to maintain the internal volume of the developing lung and to exert a hydrostatic pressure, which is estimated to be ~2.0 mm Hg, on the developing pulmonary airways and saccules (9). Experiments by Alcorn et al. demonstrated that draining lung liquid results in arrested lung growth (4). Conversely, both Alcorn et al. (4) and Moessinger et al. (5) found lung hyperplasia occurred after ligation of the major airways in the fetal lung, a condition which resulted in overdistention of the lung. Interestingly, indices of type II differentiation in the hyperplastic and hypoplastic lungs were not different from controls, suggesting that maintenance of internal lung volume by lung liquid is important for structural growth of the lung but apparently has little effect on alveolar epithelial cell differentiation.

Late in gestation, and just several days before the onset of labor in sheep, the rate of lung liquid secretion declines and active lung liquid absorption begins, presumably in order to clear the lung of fluid at the onset of air breathing (7,10). Lung fluid absorption, which increases during spontaneous labor in the fetal sheep, is inhibited by amiloride, an inhibitor of sodium ion transport, and occurs independent of $\beta$-adrenergic blockade (11). Lung liquid absorption has been shown to be associated with active transepithelial transport of sodium ions by alveolar epithelial cells with subsequent transfer of fluid into the interstitium of the lung and thence into the vasculature (3). Hormonal changes which occur in the fetus just before and during labor may be responsible for both the decrease in epithelial chloride ion secretion and the increase in sodium ion adsorption that are characteristic of the period around birth. Catecholamines such as epinephrine, acting via the stimulation of cAMP pathways, both inhibit fetal lung fluid secretion and augment fluid reabsorption during late gestation (12) and parturition (10). Other factors which have been implicated in adsorption of fetal lung fluid include arginine vasopressin (13), atrial naturetic peptide (14), epidermal growth factor (15), and prostaglandin $E_2$ (16).

The mature alveolar epithelium is composed of type I and type II cells (Fig. 1). Type I cells function to facilitate diffusion of gases between the alveolar air-liquid interface and blood flowing through subjacent capillaries. In the human, type I cells cover 93% of the alveolar surface area. Type II cells occupy the remaining 7% of the alveolar surface area but account for two-thirds of alveolar epithelial cell numbers (17). The percentage of alveolar surface area occupied by type I and type

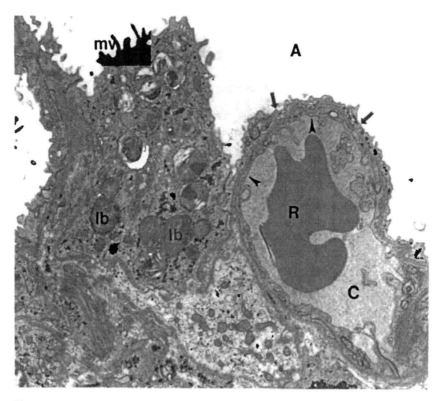

**Figure 1** Electron micrograph of lung tissue from a human newborn. The alveolar type II cell is filled with lamellar bodies. The thin cytoplasm of an alveolar type I cell covers the basement membrane that is shared with a capillary endothelial cell. R, red blood cell; A, alveolar lumen; C, capillary lumen; lb, lamellar body; mv, microvilli; thick arrow, type I cell cytoplasm; arrowhead, endothelial cell cytoplasm. (13,500×)

II cells varies slightly by species (18). As reviewed by Matalon (19) and more recently by Saumon and Basset (20), fluid homeostasis in the mature alveolar lumen is maintained by the active absorption of sodium ions by alveolar type II cells.

In addition to clearing lung fluid through active sodium ion transport, the type II alveolar epithelial cell secretes surfactant. This complex proteolipid mixture is essential for preventing alveolar collapse at end expiration and is therefore required for survival after birth when respiration commences. Surfactant secretion is stimulated in vivo by a number of factors, including air expansion of the lung (21,22) and agents which stimulate cAMP pathways (21). Alveolar type II cells maintained in vitro secrete surfactant when stimulated by agents which activate either cAMP (23–25) or protein kinase C–mediated pathways (23,26).

Additional properties of mature alveolar type II cells involve participation in host defense against infectious and noninfectious pathological agents (for review, see ref. 27). The alveolar lung-lining fluid, which contains many proteins and lipids secreted by alveolar type II cells, has antibacterial activity (28). For example, the surfactant fraction of bronchoalveolar lavage has been reported to enhance phagocytosis of *Staphylococcus aureus* by human alveolar macrophages (29,30). The major surfactant-associated protein, SP-A, has a structure homologous to complement factor C1q and can enhance FcR- and CR1-mediated phagocytosis of erythrocytes by cultured blood monocytes (31). SP-A also activates the opsonization of *S. aureus* (30) and herpes virus (32) by alveolar macrophages. The surfactant-associated protein SP-D has structural homology to SP-A, is produced and secreted by alveolar type II cells, and may also play a role in host defense (33). In addition to surfactant-associated proteins, mature alveolar type II cells secrete other proteins involved in host defense. These include complement factors (34), interferon (35), and an unidentified factor that kills *Pneumocystis carinii* in vitro (36).

Another function of mature type II alveolar epithelial cells is to act as progenitor cells in response to lung injury (37,38). When the lung alveolar epithelium is damaged by oxidant or chemical injury, alveolar type II cells divide and repopulate the damaged area within a few days and then differentiate into type I alveolar epithelial cells; thus restoring the respiratory function of the lung alveolus.

Whereas alveolar type II cells, through surfactant secretion, are responsible for preventing alveolar collapse, the alveolar type I cell participates in the actual gas-exchange function of the respiratory epithelium. Morphologically distinct, the large, flattened type I cells cover the vast majority of the alveolar surface area in the human (17). Type I cells are contiguous with one another and form a barrier to fluid, ions, and organisms. This barrier is composed of the thin type I cell, a common basement membrane and a capillary endothelial cell. The 0.6-$\mu$m mean thickness of this barrier permits passive diffusion of oxygen and carbon dioxide between the alveolar lumen and the capillary blood (39). Owing to difficulties in maintaining type I cells in culture, it is unclear if these cells have functions beyond that of gas diffusion and the creation of barriers. The absence of secretory granules within the cytoplasm of the type I cell suggests that the cell may lack secretory function. However, the presence of antigens specific for alveolar type I cells on rat alveolar type II epithelial cells which have flattened and dedifferentiated in culture (40), coupled with the demonstration of active sodium transport by these cells (41), suggests a possible role for alveolar type I cells in maintaining fluid homeostasis in the alveolus. Future information regarding type I cell function is likely to be obtained in studies involving molecular probes and antibodies to markers for specific type I alveolar cell functions such as ion transport.

## II.  Morphological Aspects of the Differentiation of the Alveolar Epithelium

### A.  Origin of the Lung

The mammalian lung originates as an endoderm-lined diverticulum from the ventral aspect of the foregut (42). After formation, the respiratory diverticulum grows into the splanchnic mesoderm that surrounds the primitive gut tube. The epithelium and submucosal glands associated with the respiratory system are derived from foregut endoderm, whereas the connective tissue elements of the respiratory system are derived from the splanchnic mesoderm associated with the respiratory diverticulum (43). The respiratory diverticulum and its associated mesoderm will subsequently give rise to the trachea, bronchi, bronchioles, and alveoli. There is abundant experimental evidence that splanchnic mesoderm induces the formation of the respiratory diverticulum and also directs the branching morphogenesis that occurs during early lung development (44–47).

In the human species, the respiratory diverticulum first appears at about 26 days of development (48). It is customary to divide lung development into four stages based on the morphological characteristics of the fetal lung tissue (49). The first stage, the embryonic stage, occurs from the time of appearance of the respiratory diverticulum to about 7 weeks of development. During this period, the original respiratory diverticulum lengthens to form the presumptive larynx and presumptive trachea and divides at its most caudal aspect to form the lung buds (43,48). In addition, the lung buds themselves undergo branching divisions during the embryonic stage of development to give rise to the first few orders of the presumptive bronchial tree, generally to the level of the future subsegmental bronchi (48). During the next phase of lung development, the pseudoglandular phase, which occurs from the 7th to the 16th week of gestation, the presumptive bronchial tree undergoes further branching, from 16 to 26 divisions, to form the basis of the future bronchial tree (Fig. 2A) (50). The next phase of lung development, the canalicular phase, occurs from the 16th to the 24th week of gestation, and it is the maturational phase when the differentiation of the epithelium of the distal lung begins to occur (Fig. 2B) (51). The final stage of fetal lung development, the terminal sac phase, extends from the 24th week of gestation to term, and it is the period in which true alveoli begin to be formed (Fig. 3C) (52,53). Lung development continues after birth and growth of the lung does not end until late adolescence (54,55).

The appearance of the lung diverticulum occurs at a much relatively earlier

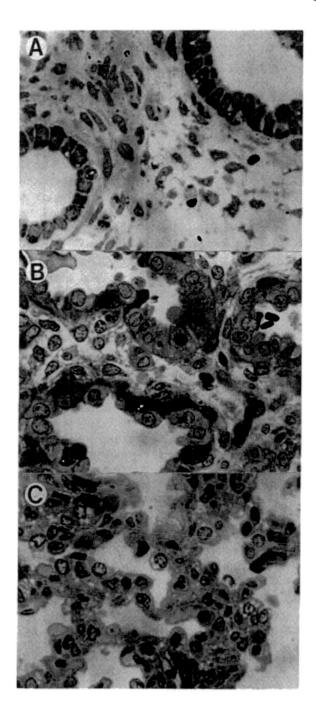

time point in the human species than in rodents (56). As pointed out by Ten Have-Opbroek and Plopper, in the human species, the lung diverticulum appears after ~9% of gestation has transpired, whereas in rodents such as the mouse and rat, the lung diverticulum does not appear until almost 50% of gestation has passed (56). The timing of the initiation of alveolar epithelial cell differentiation also differs significantly between primates and rodents, commencing much earlier in relative terms; that is, at about 50% of the length of gestation in the primate versus at about 75% of gestation in rodents. These observations are also suggestive that the period of alveolar differentiation occupies a much longer relative period of gestation in the primate (~50% of gestation) than in the rodent (~25% of gestation).

### B. Characteristics of the Progenitor Epithelial Cell in the Fetal Lung

The endoderm-derived epithelial cells that line the respiratory diverticulum early in lung development (i.e., during the embryonic period) have relatively few distinctive ultrastructural characteristics (42,57). The epithelial cells lining the primitive duct system are columnar in shape, usually contain pools of glycogen, and form a psuedostratified epithelium (Fig. 3). The epithelial cells in the embryonic lung epithelium are adherent to adjacent epithelial cells by cell junctions at the apical portion of their lateral plasma membranes (57). The primitive epithelium-lined ducts are surrounded by a cuff of mesenchymal cells frequently consisting of several layers of cells oriented perpendicular to the epithelium (58,59). Physical interactions between epithelial cells and the subjacent mesenchymal cells at these early stages of lung development have been frequently described (58,60,61).

During the process of lung development, the differentiation of the epithelium in the conducting portion of the respiratory tract (i.e., the trachea and the

---

**Figure 2**  Light micrographs of methylene blue-stained, epoxy sections of human fetal lung tissue at different stages of development. (500×) (A) Lung tissue from a 14-week-gestational-age fetus. Lung tissue in the pseudoglandular stage of lung development is characterized by abundant connective tissue and a few branching ducts that are lined by a columnar epithelium. There are very few capillaries in the tissue and none are associated with the ductal epithelium. (B) Lung tissue from a 24-week-gestational-age fetus. At the canalicular stage of development, the ducts are more numerous and their epithelial cells are cuboidal. Capillaries are more numerous than in previous stages and are closely associated with the ductal epithelium. Differentiated type II cells are first observed at this stage of development in the human fetus. (C) Lung tissue from a 40-week-gestational-age fetus. In the terminal sac stage of lung development, the number of capillaries is greatly increased and the relative amount of connective tissue greatly decreased when compared to previous stages of lung development.

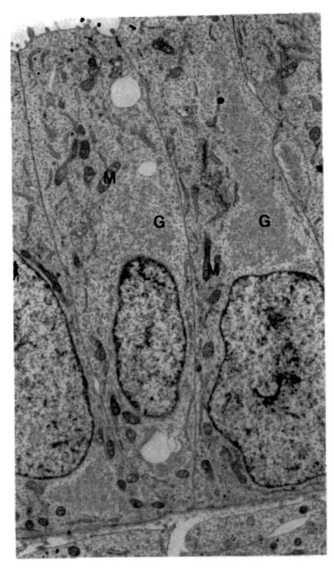

**Figure 3**    An electron micrograph of rabbit fetal lung epithelial cells at the pseudoglandular stage of development. This tissue was obtained at 19 days of gestation (term is 31 days in the rabbit). The cells contain large glycogen pools (G) and mitochondria (M). There is sparse rough endoplasmic reticulum, no Golgi apparatus, few multivesicular bodies, and no lamellar bodies in the cells. The cells are tall columnar in shape. (7800×) (From Ref. 82.)

future bronchi and bronchioles) begins first prior to the commencement of differentiation of the more distal respiratory portion of the lung (62). Ciliated cells have been observed in the proximal portions of the primitive duct system in the fetal lung as early as 10 weeks of gestation in the human, and most of the major bronchi have ciliated cells by 13 weeks of gestation (62). Submucosal glands begin developing at about 13 weeks of development in the proximal branches of the bronchial tree in the human fetus (62). Pulmonary neuroendocrine cells are detectable in the presumptive airways even earlier at 8 weeks of gestation (63). The differentiation of the conducting airway respiratory epithelium generally occurs in a proximal to distal pattern, with differentiation of the epithelium in terminal and respiratory bronchioles occurring last (64).

During the late pseudoglandular and early canalicular stages of lung development, the epithelial cells of the distal region of the respiratory tree change in shape and become cuboidal as compared with the columnar shape of the cells that line the more proximal portions of the lung (65–67). It has been hypothesized that this change in the morphological characteristics of the fetal lung epithelial cells, which is quite abrupt, demarks the separation of the developing respiratory tract into the future conducting (bronchi and bronchioli) and respiratory (respiratory bronchioles, alveolar ducts and sacs, and alveoli) portions (65). Thus, prior to this time, it is hypothesized that cells lining the respiratory tree may be multipotent and capable of differentiating into conducting airway epithelial cell types as well as into the cell types that line the respiratory portion of the lung. In addition to morphological evidence, the results of studies using cell-specific markers are also supportive of this concept. For example, the mRNA for SP-C, a surfactant-associated protein, has been detected in all epithelial cells of the fetal lung from the time the lung buds appear (68). Then, as lung development proceeds, the SP-C mRNA expression pattern becomes increasingly restricted until finally only alveolar type II cells express SP-C mRNA in the fetal lung prior to birth (Fig. 4) (69). The potential function of the SP-C protein at the very early embryonic stages of lung development is not known (70). Together these data are suggestive that a multipotent lung epithelial cell present in the very early lung gradually becomes committed to a specific cell lineage, based on its proximal to distal relative position in the respiratory tree, broadly considered either conducting airway epithelium or alveolar epithelium. A similar pattern of early widespread expression of a marker in the fetal lung epithelium followed by increasing restriction of expression during development has been described for a 40- to 42-kDa protein characteristic of differentiated alveolar type I cells which was detected using a monoclonal antibody (71). This antigen and its mRNA are detected in the epithelial cells lining the respiratory tree of the very early lung. Thereafter during lung development, its expression becomes restricted to alveolar type I cells (72,73). Overall, these observations suggest that the best source of a true multipotent lung epithelial cell may be in the epithelium present in the very early embryonic lung.

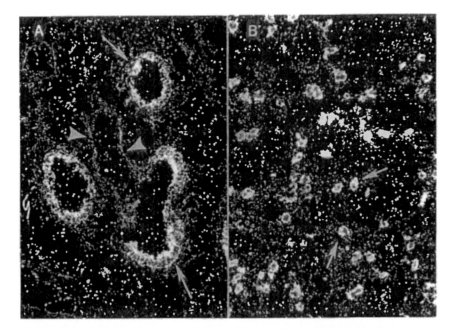

**Figure 4** In situ hybridization of surfactant protein C (SP-C) mRNA in rabbit fetal lung tissue. (A) SP-C mRNA is present uniformly in all distal duct epithelial cells (arrows) in day 19 gestational age fetal rabbit lung tissue (pseudoglandular stage). No SP-C mRNA was present in presumptive bronchiolar epithelial cells (arrowheads). (B) SP-C mRNA is restricted to alveolar type II cells (arrows) in adult rabbit lung tissue. Type I cells do not contain SP-C mRNA. A and B are printed at the same magnification. (From Wohlford-Lenane CL, et al. (cover illustration), 1992, with permission.)

The studies described above do not address how the positional information present in the primitive respiratory tree is perceived by the epithelial cells present at different levels of the branching tree. Because there are many studies suggestive that the fetal lung mesenchyme regulates lung morphogenesis and epithelial cell differentiation, the connective tissue elements adjacent to the epithelium are a likely source of the signals that convey positional information to the epithelium (44–47). However, how the mesenchyme associated with the developing respiratory tree differs at various levels and exactly what interactions direct branching morphogenesis and the differentiation of the epithelial cells in the conducting and respiratory portion of the lung are still unknown. Possible pathways of regulation include the production of growth factors, the assembly of a unique extracellular matrix in the basement membrane underlying the epithelium, and direct physical contact between the mesenchymal and epithelial cells. There is evidence for the importance of all of these pathways of interaction in the fetal lung (44–47,73–76).

## C. Differentiation of the Alveolar Type II Cell in the Fetal Lung

The best-characterized differentiated function of the alveolar type II cell is the synthesis of pulmonary surfactant (77). The morphological feature of the type II cell indicative of the production of surfactant is the appearance of lamellar bodies, which are the intracellular organelles in which surfactant is stored (77). Lamellar bodies are first observed in the human species within distal lung epithelial cells at 20–24 weeks; that is, during the canalicular stage of fetal lung development (66,67,78). As the lung matures, more type II cells differentiate and even later in gestation surfactant begins to be secreted into the alveolar lumen (78,172). The surfactant-associated proteins SP-A and SP-B are present in differentiated alveolar type II cells and in some bronchiolar epithelial cells (79). Studies in which the surfactant proteins SP-A and SP-B and their mRNAs have been localized in fetal lung tissue are suggestive that the epithelial cells in this region of the developing lung may be committed to the type II cell pathway of development prior to the appearance of lamellar bodies, because the surfactant protein mRNAs can be detected prior to the appearance of lamellar bodies in the fetal lung tissue (79,80,81).

In addition to the appearance of lamellar bodies, other cytological changes occur in the precursor fetal lung epithelial cell during the process of type II cell differentiation. One very characteristic ultrastructural event that occurs prior to the appearance of lamellar bodies in the undifferentiated precursor cell is the accumulation of large intracellular glycogen stores (57). The epithelial cell present in the very early lung is always characterized by the presence of glycogen pools (66,67). However, immediately prior to the commencement of surfactant lipid synthesis, these pools become even larger and then decrease in size as lamellar bodies accumulate in the cell. This morphological event has been quantitatively evaluated in the rabbit fetal lung tissue during gestation (Fig. 5A) (82). It was determined that the glycogen pools occupy ~15% of the cell volume in epithelial cells of the distal rabbit fetal lung on day 19 of gestation, which is a week prior to any evidence of type II cell differentiation (term in the rabbit is 31 days; alveolar type II cells are first observed on day 26 of gestation). Two days prior to the first appearance of intracellular lamellar bodies, the precursor alveolar epithelial cells accumulate glycogen in pools that occupy up to 30% of the total cell volume. Thereafter, a decline in glycogen pool volume density in the epithelial cells is inversely correlated with an increase in lamellar body volume density (Fig. 5B) (82). It has been postulated that the intracellular glycogen is a precursor in the synthesis of surfactant phospholipids in the type II cell (83).

Another important morphological event that occurs in the precursor fetal

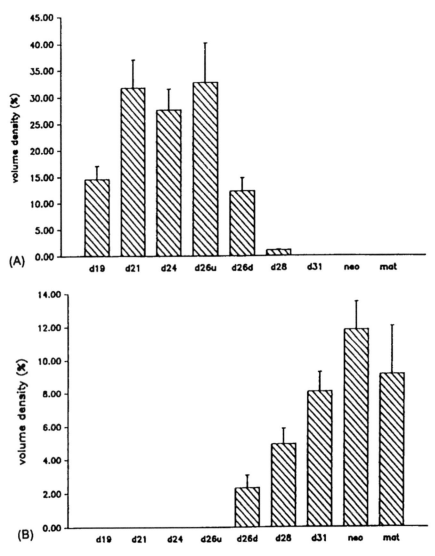

**Figure 5** Morphometric analysis of rabbit fetal, neonatal, and adult lung epithelial cells at the ultrastructural level. The data are expressed as the mean plus or minus the error of the mean. The volume densities are expressed as the percentage of the cell cytoplasmic volume that is occupied by glycogen pools (A) or lamellar bodies (B). Measurements were made in fetal lung epithelial cells at days 19 to 31 of gestation (d19 to d31), in neonatal lung (neo), and in adult lung tissue (mat). (Adapted from Figs. 3 and 5 in ref. 82.)

lung alveolar epithelial cell during development is a change in cell size and shape (82). The undifferentiated precursor epithelial cell in the fetal lung is relatively large and columnar in shape. Starting 5 days prior to the appearance of lamellar bodies in the differentiated rabbit fetal lung type II cell (i.e., on day 21 of gestation), the epithelial cells lining the distal tubules in the fetal lung decrease in size by more than 50% (82). Interestingly, the size of the cell nucleus also decreases at about the same time. Later, 2 days prior to the appearance of lamellar bodies, the columnar shape of the precursor epithelial cell changes to a cuboidal shape (82). These size and shape parameters then remain relatively constant in the late fetal, newborn, and adult lung alveolar type II cell. Finally, the average distance between distal epithelial cells in the fetal lung and the subjacent connective tissue cells decreases by almost 50% at the time differentiated type II cells are first identifiable (i.e. day 26 of gestation) (82). Together these morphometric data show that the undifferentiated presumptive alveolar epithelial type II cell undergoes many morphological changes prior to the appearance of lamellar bodies in the cell and thus is probably committed to this line of differentiation well before the commencement of surfactant synthesis (82).

Another aspect of the undifferentiated fetal lung alveolar epithelial cell that changes during development is its physical interaction with other cells and with the extracellular matrix. It has long been appreciated that the mesenchyme surrounding the primitive ducts present in the early fetal lung has a profound regulatory effect on the pattern of differentiation of the epithelium (44–47). In addition, physical interactions between fetal lung epithelial cells and subjacent connective tissue cells via foot processes have been described by many investigators (58,60,61,84–87). These foot processes have been shown to change in number in the fetal lung during development and also in several physiological states (58,60,61,84–87). Cell adhesion molecules such as cadherins have also been shown to be present in embryonic lung epithelial cells and to be involved in lung development (88). There is increasing evidence that cell-cell adhesion and cell adhesion to the extracellular matrix can cause second-messenger generation, activate a variety of second-messenger kinases, and change the structure of the cytoskeleton within the epithelial cell (89). Thus, the interactions of the fetal lung epithelial cell with other cells and with its extracellular environment may be profoundly important in directing the pathway of epithelial cell differentiation in the fetal lung (90).

Type II cells tend to be localized in the corners of the alveoli, bulge into the lumen, and are in close proximity to connective tissue cells lying beneath the epithelium (91). Although the proportion of type I and type II cells is roughly similar in most species, the surface area of the alveolus that is lined by the two alveolar epithelial cell types is profoundly different (18). In humans, almost 93% of the alveolar surface is covered by the thin flattened type I cell, whereas only about 7% of the surface area is occupied by alveolar type II cells. How this unique structure is achieved and maintained in the differentiated lung alveolus is not known. Differences in the extracellular matrix underlying the two cell types have been described and may be involved in achieving and maintaining the different phenotypes of the alveolar epithelial cells (92). In addition, although interactions of the type II cell with connective tissue cells have been reported, type I cells apparently form no interactions with connective tissue cells and only interact with subjacent endothelial cells via their shared basement membrane.

In the differentiated lung, the bronchiolar portion of the airway tree ends in a terminal bronchiole which channels inhaled air into a respiratory bronchiole, which is a structure whose wall is interrupted with alveoli, hence the term *respiratory bronchiole* (93). The epithelium of the terminal and respiratory bronchioles differs from that of the typical respiratory epithelium present in the remainder of the conducting portion of the lung (i.e., mucus-secreting cells are frequently absent), the proportion of ciliated cells is decreased, and the overall height of the epithelium is frequently decreased in this region of the lung (93). Another major difference in the epithelium that lines this transitional region of the lung is the presence of Clara cells (94). The Clara cell is characterized by a protrusion of its apical surface into the lumen of the bronchiole and by the presence of electron-dense secretory granules within the cell. The function of the Clara cell is unknown, although it is thought to secrete a serous fluid and has been shown to contain large amounts of cytochrome P450s, which is biochemical evidence of a role for the Clara cell in detoxifying harmful substances at the level of the bronchiole (95). The Clara cell, the nonciliated cell of the terminal and respiratory bronchiole, may also be present in the lung epithelium at higher levels in the bronchial and bronchiolar trees in some species (96). Some investigators have hypothesized that the Clara cell is a progenitor cell for the bronchiolar epithelium (97).

## D.  Differentiation of Alveolar Type I Cells

The morphological characteristics of the differentiated alveolar type I cell are unique. The cell is large, quite flattened, and relatively devoid of organelles (94). Alveolar type I cells do not contain a unique subcellular organelle such as the lamellar body and relatively few alveolar type I cell–specific markers have been identified. This lack of a biochemical or ultrastructural marker has greatly inhibited the study of this important cell type. In addition, the isolation of purified populations of type I cells has proven to be quite difficult (99,100).

Two monoclonal antibodies have been described that specifically stain type I cells in the mature lung (40,71–73). In both cases, the functional nature of the type I cell–specific antigens is not known. It has been determined that both type I cell–specific antigens are expressed in fetal lung precursor epithelial cells prior to differentiation of the alveolar epithelium. These data are suggestive that the precursor cell present in the distal tubules of the fetal lung respiratory tree may express characteristics of both alveolar epithelial cell types prior to commitment along one lineage pathway; that is, the alveolar epithelial type I or type II cell pathway. In addition, these data are indicative that the undifferentiated fetal lung alveolar epithelial cell may transduce some of the functions of the differentiated alveolar epithelium (e.g., with respect to fluid balance) prior to differentiation. These issues will require further study to identify unique functions of the type I cell and to link these functions with molecules that can be studied in model systems. The difference in the state of knowledge about the two alveolar epithelial cell types is striking. In light of the large surface area covered in the alveolus by the alveolar type I cell, the need for further information about this important cell type is great.

Initially, the fetal lung is relatively avascular and the connective tissue between the primitive epithelium-lined respiratory tree is relatively abundant (Fig. 6) (60). As lung development proceeds, the relative amount of vascular elements in the tissue increases and, as the endoderm-lined ducts in the fetal lung tissue divide and multiply rapidly, the relative amount of epithelium increases (Fig. 6) (101). The increase in volume density of capillaries in the fetal lung tissue during development is accompanied by a migration of the capillaries to locations immediately beneath the epithelium in the most distal aspects of the fetal lung. The epithelial cells overlying these capillaries become thinner and take on the morphological appearance of alveolar type I cells. Thus, morphological evidence is suggestive that the capillary induces the overlying distal fetal lung epithelial cell to differentiate along the type I cell phenotype. A continuing controversy in the literature is whether the fetal lung epithelium first differentiates into an epithelium composed entirely of type II cells followed by the further differentiation of some of these alveolar type II cells into alveolar type I cells or if the undifferentiated precursor cell can differentiate directly into either cell type. The evidence is quite strong that, in the adult lung, the alveolar type II cell is a stem cell for the repair of the alveolar epithelium and the generation of new alveolar type I and II alveolar epithelial cells (102,103). In lung injury, the damaged alveolar type I cells undergo cell death and are shed from the epithelium leaving a denuded basement membrane. Thereafter, the remaining type II cells in the region undergo cell division and reconstitute the epithelium with type II cells, some of which subsequently undergo differentiation into alveolar type I cells. One hypothesis is that a similar scenario may occur in the fetus; that is, an epithelium of alveolar type II cells gives rise to some cells that differentiate into alveolar type I cells. The available evidence is also consistent with the hypothesis that there is a stem cell in the fetus that gives rise to either cell type and that the undifferentiated stem cell is not obligated to go through the alveolar type II cell differentiation phenotype prior to differentiating into an alveolar type I cell. Resolution of this issue will require a better understanding of the biology of the alveolar type I epithelial cell so that markers for its differentiation can be evaluated in the fetal lung.

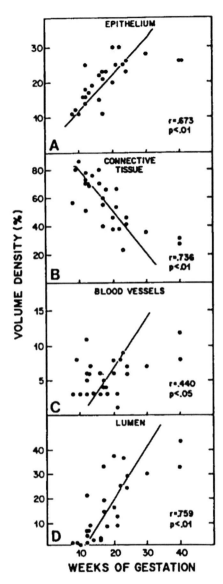

**Figure 6**  Morphometric analysis of structural changes in human fetal lung tissue during development in vivo. Representative tissue sections obtained throughout gestation in the human were analyzed using point-counting methods to determine the volume density occupied by epithelium (A), connective tissue (B), blood vessels (C), and the ductal lumina (D). Approximately 40 different samples were analyzed.

## III. Biochemical Aspects of the Differentiation of the Alveolar Epithelium

### A. Type I Cell Proteins

Aside from its premier role in barrier function within the alveolus, there is limited information available concerning other differentiated functions of the alveolar epithelial type I cell. Accordingly, there is a paucity of type I cell biochemical markers (Table 1), and identification of the type I cell phenotype has relied primarily on its distinctive morphology as a flattened cell when viewed under the light or electron microscope (103). It has been reported that type I cells, but not type II cells, express cell surface saccharide structures which bind *Ricinus co-munis I* (RC1), a lectin specific for β-galactose residues (104). Moreover, type II cells bind the lectin *Maclura pomifera* (MPA), a lectin specific for α-galactose residues, then gradually lose the MPA lectin-binding characteristic with time in culture, and acquire RC1 binding, a characteristic of the type I cell phenotype (104). These data suggest that at least in vitro, the type I cell might be derived from a type II cell precursor. Other in vitro studies using type I cell–specific monoclonal antibodies (40) as well as in vivo autoradiographic studies (103,105,

**Table 1**   Type I Alveolar Epithelial Cell–Associated Markers

| Marker | Description | Type II cells | Lung specific | References |
|---|---|---|---|---|
| Morphology | Flat, elongated | No | No | 102 |
| *Ricinus comunis* binding | Lectin for β-galactose | No | No | 104,108 |
| Monoclonal antibodies: | | | | |
|   SF-1 | Antibody to 40- to 42-kDa apical antigen | No | Yes | 71,72 |
|   Mab 411-52 | Antibody to postnatal murine antigen | No | ? | 107 |
|   II F1/VIII B2 | Antibodies to apical cell surface protein | No | Yes | 40 |
| ICAM-1 | Cell adhesion molecule | | | |
|   rat | | No | No | 109 |
|   human | | Yes | No | 110 |
| Carboxypeptidase M | Cell surface protease of vasoactive peptides | No | No | 111 |

SF-1, monoclonal antibody to type I cell membrane protein; Mab 411-52, monoclonal antibody to type I cell murine protein; II F1/VIII B2, monoclonal antibodies to type I cell membrane proteins; ICAM-1, intracellular adhesion molecule-1.

106) provide additional evidence in support of the premise that the alveolar type II cell serves as a stem cell for the alveolar type I cell.

Dobbs, Williams, and coworkers generated a cell- and tissue-specific monoclonal antibody to a 40- to 42-kDa apical membrane protein of rat alveolar type I cells (71). By comparing immunofluorescent labeling of lung tissues using the type I cell–specific monoclonal antibody to a type II cell marker (MPA lectin binding) at different stages of rat lung development, the investigators demonstrated that the type I cell marker was expressed as early as day 15, which is well before the morphological appearance of type I cells (72). Further, both the type I cell and type II cell markers were distributed extensively during mid gestation (days 19–20), and it appeared that many epithelial cells coexpressed both cell markers. Postnatally, these epithelial cell markers became more restricted to cells of the alveolar type I and type II morphological phenotype, respectively.

More recently, a rat monoclonal antibody has been generated which detects a cell surface epitope present in alveolar type I cells in neonatal and adult mouse lung (107). However, unlike RC1, which is expressed in fetal lung tissue (108), the use of this monoclonal antibody may be limited to the study of the generation of type I cells later in development or in the setting of lung injury, since the antigen recognized by the rat monoclonal antibody is expressed only in neonatal or adult mouse lung tissue. In addition, Christensen et al. have reported that another cell surface protein, intercellular adhesion molecule-1 (ICAM-1), appears to be expressed at much higher levels in differentiated rat alveolar type I cells when compared with alveolar type II cells (109). ICAM-1 and related proteins are involved in the migration of leukocytes to areas of inflammation. By using immunofluorescent labeling, expression of ICAM-1 was not detected in freshly isolated alveolar type II cells, but it increased as the cells were maintained in monolayer culture and gradually attained the morphological phenotype of alveolar type I cells. Other studies, however, using adult human lung tissue have demonstrated the presence of ICAM-1 on the majority of alveolar type II cells (110). The discrepancies between these two studies may be attributable to species differences and will require further investigation. The developmentally related expression of ICAM-1 in the fetal lung remains to be investigated. Finally, recent investigations have shown that the alveolar type I cell selectively expresses carboxypeptidase M, an enzyme that belongs to a large family of membrane-bound proteins which are involved in proteolytic cleavage of inflammatory proteins such as bradykinin and anaphylatoxins (111). Although the investigators did not report the developmental expression of this enzyme in the fetal lung, the detection of carboxypeptidase M in the alveolar type I cell appears to represent the first enzymatic marker of this cell type. Additional studies using type I cell–specific markers will be required to understand better the basic mechanisms involved in the differentiation of the alveolar type I cell.

### B. Type II Cell Proteins

As the cytodifferentiation of lung alveolar epithelium proceeds during development, some biochemical markers which are expressed relatively early in alveolar development in the undifferentiated epithelium become more restricted to the alveolar type II cell population. For example, the binding of the lectin MPA to alveolar type II cells, which occurs via a 200- to 230-kDa glycoprotein, is observed in the rat at 16 days of gestation, which is 3–4 days before the morphological identification of mature alveolar type II cells (112,113). The expression of MPA may not be limited to developing type II cells in mid gestation fetal rat lung (72,113). Ultimately, however, this marker becomes restricted to mature type II cells in late gestation, neonatal, and adult lung (112). A somewhat different pattern of expression has been reported for two related type II cell glycoproteins, pneumocin and gp 330 (114,115). The ontogeny of pneumocin in fetal rat lung correlates with the morphological appearance of mature type II cells, and this antigen is expressed by both alveolar type II cells and Clara cells but not by alveolar type I cells (114). The developmental expression of the apical surface protein gp 330 in the lung has not been examined, although it is present in the alveolar type II cell and in kidney epithelial cells (115) and is expressed early during embryogenesis of the nephron (116).

The temporal and spatial expression of several alveolar type II cell biochemical markers differ during lung development. For example, the hydrophobic surfactant associated protein SP-C, as well as SP-C mRNA, is detected well in advance of the morphological appearance of alveolar type II cells in rabbit and human fetal lung distal epithelium (69,70). By contrast, the detection of SP-A protein and mRNA in human, rabbit, and rat fetal lung tissue and of SP-B protein and mRNA in rat and rabbit fetal lung tissue generally coincides with or slightly precedes the morphological differentiation of type II cells (117–119). The expression of SP-B protein and mRNA in the human lung, however, is observed several weeks in advance of the induction of surfactant lipid synthesis and the appearance of differentiated type II cells (120). Interestingly, the expression of SP-D protein and mRNA in the rat lung occurs well after the morphological differentiation of type II cells (121).

Cytoskeletal components are another important class of type II alveolar cell-associated proteins. Tsilibary and Williams identified microfiliamentous structures in type II cells as actin by demonstrating binding to the S1 fragment of myosin to the microfilaments and their disruption by cytochalasin D (122). The microfilaments were especially concentrated in areas where lamellar bodies were associated with the apical membrane, suggesting a role for actin in lamellar body secretion. The alveolar type II cells contained greater concentrations of the actin microfilaments than type I cells. Type II cells also express cytokeratins, a class of intermediate filaments present in cells of epithelial origin. Paine et al. reported that undifferentiated fetal rat lung epithelial cells at day 18 gestation contain cytokeratin types 7, 8, and 18, whereas freshly isolated type II cells from adult lung contain cytokeratin type 19 (123). Moreover, when immature fetal epithelial cells were cultured on an extracellular matrix (Engelbreth-Holm-Swarm extract), which is known to promote the differentiation of type II cells, the fetal type II cells acquired the morphological features and pattern of cytokeratin expression typical of the more mature, adult type II cells. These data are suggestive that changes in the composition of the cytoskeleton may accompany the differentiation of alveolar type II cells from an undifferentiated precursor cell.

A number of enzymatic markers that are directly related to alveolar type II cell metabolism have also been identified (Table 2). Alkaline phosphatase appears to be a fairly specific phenotypic marker for alveolar type II cells, since alveolar type I cells or alveolar macrophages in adult lung tissue do not contain this enzyme as determined by histochemical staining (124). Alkaline phosphatase activity increases in fetal rat lung several fold during mid gestation, and the increase coincides temporally with the induction of surfactant lipid synthesis

**Table 2**   Type II Alveolar Epithelial Cell–Associated Markers

| Marker | Description | Type I cells | Lung specific | References |
|---|---|---|---|---|
| Morphology | Cuboid shape, apical microvilli lamellar bodies | No | No | 102 |
| *Maclura pomifera* binding | Lectin for α-galactose | No | No | 72,112,113 |
| Pneumocin | 165-kDa Apical surface sialoglycoprotein | No | No | 114 |
| gp330 | 330-kDa Apical surface glycoprotein | No | No | 115,116 |
| SP-C | Surfactant apoprotein | No | Yes | 69 |
| Cytokeratin type 19 | Intermediate filament | No | No | 123 |
| Enzymes | | | | |
| alkaline phosphatase | Intracellular phosphatase | No | No | 124,125 |
| P450b | Monoxygenase | No | No | 126 |
| γ-glutamyl-transferase | Metabolism of glutathione | No | No | 127 |
| Aminopeptidase N | Cell surface protease | No | No | 128,129 |
| Na$_+$-K$_+$ ATPase | Ion transporter | No | No | 148 |

gp330, a type II cell membrane glycoprotein; SP-C, surfactant apoprotein C; P450b, cytochrome monooxygenase; Na$_+$-K$_+$ ATPase, sodium potassium ATPase.

(124). Histochemical studies have further demonstrated this marker in isolated alveolar type II cells from fetal rat lung as early as day 19 gestation (125). Isolated type II cells maintained in culture exhibit a time-dependent decrease in alkaline phosphatase activity which is consistent with the loss of other differentiated functions of alveolar type II cells when the cells are maintained in vitro. Other biochemical markers of alveolar type II cells include cytochrome P450b (126) and $\gamma$-glutamyltransferase (127), enzymes which are detected in alveolar type II cells but not type I cells. Unlike alkaline phosphatase, limited attention has been given to the expression of cytochrome P450b and $\gamma$-glutamyltransferase in developing lung tissue. It is notable, however, that these enzymes are not only identified in alveolar epithelia but are also secreted by the type II cell and have been detected extracellularly in association with alveolar surfactant. The extracellular location of these enzymes has raised speculation that surfactant may serve as a vehicle in the distribution of several enzymes to gas-exchange areas of the lung (127).

Another enzymatic marker of type II cells is aminopeptidase N, a member of a class of cell surface proteins called ectopeptidases, which are enzymes that are involved in proteolytic cleavage of peptides. Funkhouser et al. demonstrated that aminopeptidase N, initially identified as a 146-kDa antigen, is expressed on the microvillous apical surface of alveolar type II cells in rat fetal lung as early as 14 days of gestation, which is well before the differentiation of type II cells (128,129). Thereafter, the enzyme is detected in a subset of cuboidal cells at day 19 of gestation, which is coincident with the morphological appearance of type II cells and is restricted to alveolar type II cells in adult lung tissue. It will be important to determine the significance of aminopeptidase N as it relates both to alveolar epithelial cell differentiation and type II cell physiology, since ectopeptidases have diverse biological functions, including the activation of proproteins, regulation of autocrine and paracrine factors, and the generation of antimicrobial peptides (130).

Several additional enzymes have been described in alveolar type II cells, but there is limited information with regard to their ontogeny, cell specificity, or biological role in the alveolar type II cell. For example, several studies are suggestive that alveolar type II cells are more resistent to oxidant injury than alveolar type I cells (131), and that this is the consequence of their high content of many antioxidant enzymes (132). A developmental increase in the expression of fetal lung antioxidant enzymes occurs during the latter part of gestation, possibly to prepare the fetus for exposure to the higher ambient oxygen tension which commences with extrauterine breathing (133). The specific activity of some type II cell antioxidant enzymes such as catalase decreases in isolated alveolar type II cells with time in culture as they lose an alveolar type II cell phenotype and acquire an alveolar type I cell phenotype (131). Conversely, the activity of other, unrelated enzymes, such as urokinase-type plasminogen activator (134) and phospholipase $A_2$ (135), increase in cultured alveolar type II cells as these cells gradually lose their differentiated function with time in culture. However, the presence of urokinase-type plasminogen activator and phospholipase $A_2$ enzymes in alveolar type I epithelial cells in situ has not yet been demonstrated.

It has been shown in biochemical studies that lysozyme (136), protein kinase C (137), cyclic AMP–dependent protein kinase (137), urokinase-plasminogen activator inhibitor-1 (138), and vitamin K–dependent carboxylase (139) are all present in alveolar type II cells. These enzymes may be also expressed by other lung cell types, including alveolar type I cells, and cannot as yet be considered reliable markers of the alveolar type II cell phenotype. Lysozyme is detected in fetal rat lung as early as day 20 of gestation, and the amount of this enzyme increases gradually with lung development reaching the highest levels in adult lung (136). By contrast, cyclic AMP–dependent protein kinase activity in the rat lung decreases just prior to birth, peaks in the neonatal period, and subsequently declines in the adult (140). Limited information is available regarding the ontogeny of protein kinase C, urokinase-plasminogen activator-1, and vitamin K–dependent carboxylase in the lung, although studies suggest that the specific activity of protein kinase C is also developmentally regulated with activities in adult lung greater than those observed in the newborn period (141). Enzymes involved in fatty acid and phospholipid metabolism, many of which are required for surfactant lipid synthesis, have also been characterized in fetal alveolar type II cells (142,143). The specific activities of some of these key surfactant lipid enzymes, including cholinephosphate cytidylyltransferase and fatty acid synthase, also increase during the mid and latter stages of lung development coincident with the induction surfactant synthesis (143). In addition, immunohistochemical studies have identified several lamellar body–associated hydrolases and proteases in alveolar type II cells, including acid phosphatase, aryl sulfatase, β-N-acetyl-glucosaminidase, cathepsin H, and γ-enolase (144–146). The developmental expression of these enzymes in the lung as well as their significance and specificity in alveolar type II cells is unknown. However, the detection of these proteins within lamellar bodies raises the possibility that enzymatic modulation of surfactant lipid or protein synthesis might occur within these organelles.

## C.  Other Alveolar Epithelial Cell Proteins

One important function of the alveolar epithelium is to serve as a physiological barrier that prevents the leakage of fluid from the interstitium into the alveolus, thereby maintaining an optimal gas-exchange surface. Alveolar type II cells in fetal lung are actively involved in the transport of sodium and chloride ions and therefore help regulate alveolar liquid accumulation (147). By using immunocytochemistry, Schneeberger and McCarthy detected a sodium-potassium ATPase transporter on the cytosplasmic surface of basolateral membranes of alveolar type

II cells; no transporter was observed in alveolar type I cells (148). Recently, Kemp et al. have identified a chloride-selective channel in alveolar type II cells isolated from the fetal guinea pig that was inhibited by GTP-binding proteins (149). The investigators did not evaluate if these channels were present in alveolar type I cells, but similar chloride channels have not been previously identified in adult type II epithelial cells. As the lung matures, evidence suggests that other transporters, including sodium-glucose (150), sodium–amino acid (151,152) sodium–hydrogen (153), chloride-bicarbonate (147), and potassium transporter (154) systems, also contribute physiologically to the maintenance of normal fluid, pH, and ionic properties of the alveolar-air fluid interphase and within the alveolar epithelium. The pattern of induction of these important proteins in the developing lung remains to be elucidated.

In addition to the regulation of alveolar fluid balance, there is increasing evidence that the alveolar type II cell is also involved in a wide array of inflammatory and immune defense processes in the lung. The major histocompatibility class (MHC) antigens represent a group of cell surface adhesion proteins that are presented to T lymphocytes and have considerable importance in eliciting an immune response. Freshly isolated adult type II cells express class II (Ia) MHC antigen but not class I MHC antigen; however, the expression of class I MHC antigen in type II cells increases with time in culture (155). The expression of Ia antigen is absent in the fetal lung but can be induced in cultured alveolar type II cells by γ-interferon (156), silica (157), and bleomycin (158). Furthermore, adult human alveolar type II cells express cell surface adhesion proteins such as ICAM-1 and integrins, which are proteins involved in the recruitment of leukocytes to sites of inflammation (110). Alveolar type II cells have been shown to secrete immunoglobulin (Ig) A, which is a product also secreted by the tracheobronchial epithelium (159). Several inflammatory products, including complement components (34), γ-interferon (160), monocyte chemotactic polypeptide-1 (MCP-1 [161]), interleukin-3 (162), interleukin-6 (163), nitric oxide (164), and granulocyte-macrophage colony-stimulating factor (GM-CSF, [162]), are secreted by type II cells maintained in vitro. In addition, an anti-inflammatory protein, lipocortin I, is synthesized in alveolar epithelial cells (165). This protein appears to mediate, in part, the actions of corticosteroids. Finally, recent attention has also been directed at the role of pulmonary surfactant proteins in type II cell–mediated host defense. In particular, SP-A and SP-D have been demonstrated to enhance the phagocytosis of *S. aureus*, *Pneumocystis carinii*, and some viral pathogens (30,33,166). Thus, alveolar type II cells in the mature lung may serve in a protective capacity as well as play a significant role in contributing to alveolar inflammatory processes. Much work, however, is needed to determine if, when, and where many of these important proteins are expressed in developing fetal lung tissue.

### D.  Surfactant Secretion and Recycling

The latter stages of alveolar development in the fetal and newborn human lung are characterized by a linear increase in alveolar volume and surface area (167). In order to maintain this expanding alveolar air-surface interface during perinatal development and permit effective gas exchange, a crucial and distinctive role of the differentiated type II alveolar epithelial cell is its ability to actively engage in the biosynthesis, secretion, and recycling of surfactant. An understanding of surfactant metabolism and its intracellular and extracellular processing is especially important in view of the fact that such knowledge might directly impact the development of newer therapies for disorders associated with surfactant deficiency. In this regard, surfactant-replacement therapy has had a major impact in the treatment of the neonatal respiratory distress syndrome (168). In addition, the administration of exogenous surfactant is currently under investigational use for the treatment of adult lung disorders that are also characterized by a functional deficiency of surfactant (169,170). Thus, the regulation of surfactant secretion and recycling by the alveolar type II epthelial cell has been an area of significant research interest in recent years.

Pulmonary surfactant is a lipoprotein mixture consisting of phospholipids, proteins, and neutral lipids. Disaturated phosphatidylcholine (DSPC) is the major surface-active phospholipid component of surfactant that is synthesized, stored, and secreted by the alveolar type II cell. Evidence to date indicates that DSPC is synthesized in the endoplasmic reticulum and stored within lamellar bodies prior to secretion from the type II cell. Lamellar bodies are concentric, lamellated organelles containing proteins and phospholipids; the phospholipid composition of these structures resembles that of alveolar surfactant (171). The protein components of surfactant also include several acid hydrolases, proteases, and enzymes involved in phospholipid metabolism (172). The absence within lamellar bodies of certain key enzymes involved in phospholipid synthesis indicates that these organelles are probably not active sites for surfactant lipid synthesis (173). In addition to a variety of enzymes, lamellar bodies also contain the surfactant apoproteins. The major apoprotein component of surfactant is SP-A, which is a glycosylated, collagen-like protein with diverse functions that is highly conserved between species. Other surfactant-associated proteins include SP-B and SP-C, hydrophobic proteins which facilitate the adsorption and spreading of surfactant lipid to the alveolar surface, and SP-D, which appears to share some structural and functional properties with SP-A (121,174). Both SP-B and SP-C are detected within lamellar bodies; however, in a recent study, SP-D was not immuno-localized within these organelles (175). The intracellular storage site of SP-A and the pathway of SP-A secretion remain controversial. Some investigators have detected high levels of SP-A protein within lamellar bodies (176). Other reports are suggestive that the lamellar body contains small amounts of this protein (177).

Indeed, by comparing the kinetics of phospholipid and SP-A secretion, recent studies, both in vivo and in vitro, have provided evidence that secretion of SP-A occurs via a route independent of the pathway used for phospholipid secretion (178,179). Moreover, the observation that SP-A secretion is not responsive to known secretogogues for surfactant phospholipids lends additional support to the proposition that the secretion of SP-A may be primarily constitutive and occurs independent of lamellar body secretion (180). Together, these observations suggest that the surfactant phospholipids, the hydrophobic surfactant-associated proteins, and some SP-A may be assembled together within lamellar bodies prior to secretion into the alveolus. The secretion of SP-A, however, may also be a continous process that follows an independent route of exit from the type II cell. Whether the secretion of surfactant in the fetal lung involves the same mechanisms present in the adult lung alveolar type II cell remains to be determined (181).

The secretion of lamellar bodies occurs by the process of exocytosis (Fig. 7). This involves fusion of the outer membrane of the lamellar body with the plasma membrane at the apical surface of the alveolar type II cell (182,183). The molecular and cellular events which influence the exocytosis of lamellar bodies are not well understood. The possibility that the cytoskeleton is involved in lamellar body exocytosis is supported by prior observations that cytoskeletal elements like actin and microtubules have been detected in close proximity to lamellar bodies (122). In addition, in some systems, the effect of agonists that increase surfactant secretion is blocked when cells are treated with agents which disrupt the actin or microtubular cytoskeletal framework (184,185). It has also been shown that actin is a substrate in fetal lung tissue for cAMP-dependent protein kinase, which is an intracellular enzyme which mediates the effect of several surfactant secretogogues (186). Other studies are suggestive that surfactant secretogogues alter cytoskeleton-associated proteins such as spectrin, perhaps via activation of intracellular calcium-dependent proteases (187). Clearly additional studies are needed to determine the specific role of the cytoskeleton in lamellar body secretion in fetal and mature alveolar type II cells.

Two major physiological factors that increase surfactant secretion in vivo are labor and ventilation. The levels of surfactant obtained in lung lavage increase significantly in fetal lungs obtained during late gestation and rise even further shortly after birth (188). When comparing the levels of surfactant secreted in lungs of fetal rabbits that underwent cesarean section with animals that progressed through labor, Rooney et al. observed that labor increased the secretion of surfactant (189). This effect of labor was hypothesized to be mediated by prostaglandins and β-adrenergic agonists, both of which stimulate surfactant secretion in vitro and are normally induced during labor (190). Ventilation or lung distention is another physiological stimulus which may contribute to increased surfactant secretion in the newborn period. Wirtz and Dobbs reported a direct relationship

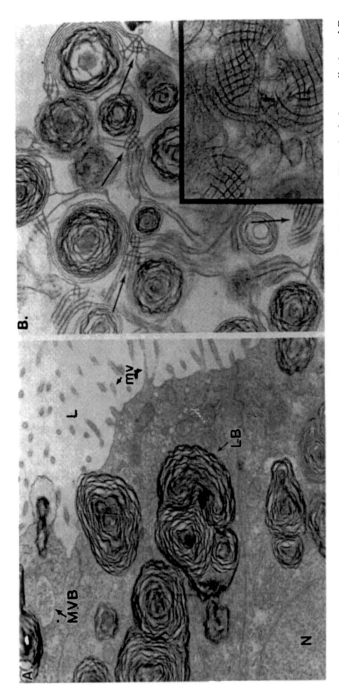

**Figure 7**  Electron micrographs of human fetal lung type II cells (A) and of secreted lamellar bodies (B) and tubular myelin (panel B, insert). In panel A, the apical surface of the type II cell is covered with microvilli (mv) and the cells are filled with lamellar bodies (LB). A multivesicular body, which may participate in the endocytosis and reutilization of surfactant, is labeled (MVB). N, nucleus, L, lumen. (45,000×) In panel B, secreted lamellar bodies, present in the lumen, are shown unwinding and transforming into the lattice-like tubular myelin (arrows). (42,000×) In the insert, a higher magnification of tubular myelin is shown. (85,000×) (From Mendelson CR, Boggaram V, Trends Endocrinol Metab, 1989; 1:20–25.)

between the degree of cellular stretch and the release of surfactant lipid in isolated alveolar type II cells that were cultured and stretched on an elastic membrane (191). Surfactant secretion from type II cells stimulated by stretch was preceded by a rise in intracellular calcium. Other studies are suggestive that distention-associated surfactant release is attenuated by β-adrenergic blockers, anticholinergic agents, or intracellular acidosis (192,193). Thus, both mechanical forces and chemical factors appear to mediate the effects of ventilation on surfactant secretion. All of these mechanisms can potentially affect the fetal lung at the time of birth.

The influence of labor and ventilation on surfactant secretion has led to the further study of the physiological and biochemical mechanisms whereby phospholipid secretion is regulated. Several physiological agents have been reported to stimulate surfactant secretion (Table 3). These agents will be summarized here, and the reader is also referred to more comprehensive discussions in several recent reviews (174,183,194). Studies using secretogogues have been performed in fetal and adult type II cells, and it is apparent that some developmental differences may exist in terms of the responsiveness of type II cells to these secretogogues (181). As shown in Table 3, the secretion of surfactant phospholipids is stimulated by β-adrenergic agents, purinoceptor agonists, agents which activate protein kinase

**Table 3**  Factors Which Increase Surfactant Secretion

| Modulator | Mediators | References |
|---|---|---|
| Labor | ? β-agonists, prostaglandins | 189,190 |
| Ventilation/lung distention | Chemical and mechanical factors | 191,192,193 |
| β-Agonists | cAMP | 174,183,197 |
| Purinoreceptor agonists | | |
|   $P_1$-$A_2$ receptor | cAMP | 174,183 |
|   $P_2$ | cAMP, PPI-PLC, calcium, DAG, PKC, and PLD | 174,198 |
| Phorbol esters | PKC | 137,216 |
| Vasopressin | PKC, calcium | 203 |
| Prostaglandins | cAMP? | 199 |
| Leukotrienes | ? | 199,205 |
| Methylxanthines | cAMP? | 206 |
| Histamine | Histamine receptor–mediated increase in cAMP | 207 |
| Lipoproteins | ? IP3, calcium, and PKC | 208 |
| Endothelin-1 | ? Calcium, DAG, and PKC | 209 |

cAMP, cyclic adenosine monophosphate; PKC, protein kinase C; DAG, 1,2-diacylglycerol; IP3, inositol 1,4,5-trisphosphate.

**Table 4**  Factors Which Decrease
Surfactant Secretion

| Modulator | References |
|---|---|
| SP-A | 210,211 |
| Surfactant phospholipids | 211,212 |
| Lectins | 213 |
| Neuropeptides | 214 |
| Cytoskeletal inhibitors | 184,185 |
| Purinoceptor inhibitors | 215,216 |
| Disulfonates | 217 |

SP-A, surfactant protein A.

C, and agents which increase intracellular calcium. The adrenergic system may be especially important during the perinatal period, because there is a developmental increase in the expression of β-adrenergic receptors in the lung (195). The actions of terbutaline, isoproterenol, and isoxaprine have been well studied in both fetal and adult lung tissue and are associated with activation of β-adrenergic receptors which in turn are coupled to adenylate cyclase by G-proteins. Thus, the stimulation of β-adrenergic receptors by these agents leads to an increase in intracellular cyclic AMP (cAMP) via the activation of adenylate cyclase. Cellular increases in cAMP activate cAMP-dependent protein kinase, which may ultimately lead to phosphorylation of cytoskeletal or other proteins which facilitate exocytosis of lamellar bodies from the cell. Forskolin, which directly increases cAMP, as well as cholera toxin or mastoparon, which activate G-proteins, have also been shown to increase surfactant phospholipid secretion (25,196,197).

Purinoceptor agonists, including adenosine, ATP, ADP, and AMP, stimulate surfactant release via activation of $P_1$ or $P_2$ receptors. The $P_1$ or $P_2$ receptors differ in their responses to the various purinoceptor agonists. For example, adenosine and AMP are $P_1$ agonists which specifically stimulate the $P_1$-$A_2$ receptor, whereas ATP is a $P_2$ receptor agonist. Unlike the $P_1$-$A_1$ agonists, the $P_1$-$A_2$ agonists increase cAMP and via activation of adenylate cyclase act in a manner similar to β-adrenergic agonists (183). The $P_2$ agonists appear to be more potent secretogogues for surfactant release than $P_1$ agonists (198). The effects of $P_2$ agonists like ATP appear to be mediated by multiple mechanisms, including activation of phosphoinositide-specific phospholipase C (PPI-PLC), elevation of cellular cAMP and calcium, stimulation of protein kinase C activity, and possibly phospholipase D activation (174). Adenosine and other purinoceptor agonists may also have physiological significance in the newborn lung, since the normal increases in surfactant secretion following term delivery in vivo may be inhibited by pretreatment with inhibitors of the purinoceptors (199).

Evidence also exists that surfactant secretion can be regulated by activation of protein kinase C and a rise in intracellular calcium. For example, tetradeca-noyl-13-phorbol acetate (TPA), a phorbol ester which activates protein kinase C, increases phospholipid secretion from type II cells (137). Stimulation of surfactant secretion also occurs after exposure of cells to ionomycin or A23187, which are agents that raise intracellular calcium levels (200,201). Conversely, lanthanum, which inhibits calcium entry into cells, diminishes surfactant secretion in newborn animals (202). The effects of some surfactant secretogogues may involve signaling via both protein kinase C and calcium signaling pathways. Vasopressin, for example, increases phospholipid secretion from type II cells, but these effects are blocked by tetracaine, a protein kinase C inhibitor, and also by $LaCl_3$, an agent which alters the intracellular distribution of calcium (203). As stated above, the actions of ATP also involve mobilization of calcium and activation of protein kinase C. Activation by ATP leads to the generation of inositol 1,4,5-trisphosphate ($IP_3$) and diacylglycerol. Diacylglycerol activates protein kinase C, and $IP_3$ in turn mobilizes calcium within the cell. Calcium can then activate a calcium-calmodulin–dependent protein kinase (Ca-CM-PK); the observation that A23187 induced secretion of surfactant in fetal type II cells is blocked by a Ca-CM-PK inhibitor supports the role of a calmodulin-type protein in regulating surfactant secretion in the fetal lung (204). Finally, other reported but less well-characterized surfactant secretogogues include leukotrienes (199), prostaglandins (205), methylxanthines (206), histamine (207), low-density lipoproteins (208), and endothelin-1 (209). Their role in surfactant secretion by the fetal and newborn lung remains to be elucidated.

Factors that inhibit phospholipid secretion may also be physiologically important in controlling the intra-alveolar pool size of surfactant in the fetus, newborn, and adult. These agents include surfactant apoprotein A (210,211), surfactant phospholipids (211,212), the lectins *Maclura pomifera* and concanavalin A (213), neuropeptides (214), cytoskeletal inhibitors (184,185), selective adenosine $A_1$ and $P_2$ antagonists (215,216), and disulfonates (217). The inhibitory effect of SP-A on phospholipid secretion appears to be greater than the inhibitory effect of surfactant phospholipid components, and this is observed both in cultured adult lung type II cells and in the intact newborn lung (210,218). SP-A inhibits basal as well as agonist-induced surfactant secretion. Interestingly, this inhibitory effect of SP-A is blocked by SP-D (210,219). Furthermore, the effects of SP-A appear to be mediated by high-affinity binding to receptors on type II cells (220,221). Recently, Oosting and Wright demonstrated that the SP-A receptor exhibited ligand specificity for SP-A and that binding is not mediated via the collagen-like or carbohydrate portions of SP-A (222). These findings suggest that surfactant components like SP-A inhibit secretion of phospholipid in vivo and in vitro via specific receptors and thus may provide an important feedback control mechanism in the developing lung.

The intra-alveolar pool of surfactant is dynamic and is regulated in part by ongoing secretion from alveolar type II cells, but it also represents the sum of other complex processes including intra-alveolar degradation, movement up the conducting airways, and recycling within the alveolus. Following secretion from type II cells, lamellar bodies rapidly unravel on the alveolar surface into tubular myelin, which is a structural form of surfactant believed to represent the precursor to the surfactant film (see Fig. 7) (223). This transformation process appears to be regulated by calcium (224). The surfactant monolayer film is highly enriched in DSPC, a situation which is presumed to result from the squeeze-out of apoproteins and other nonphospholipid components from the film during respiration (225). The majority of surfactant phospholipid and apoprotein components eventually reenter the type II cell; other potential pathways for clearance of surfactant include intra-alveolar degradation, proximal transport via the conducting airways, and phagocytosis by alveolar macrophages with subsequent degradation (194).

Studies in animal models have demonstrated developmental differences in surfactant metabolism, including differences in alveolar pool sizes and the capacity of the lung to secrete and recycle surfactant phospholipid. For example, the 3-day-old rabbit has a five-fold greater intra-alveolar pool size of surfactant phosphatidylcholine compared with the mature adult rabbit lung (226,227). Further, evidence gathered from in vivo pulse-labeling studies suggest that the time interval between the synthesis and transit of phospholipid to lamellar bodies and subsequent secretion of surfactant into the alveolar space is more delayed in the newborn lamb and 3-day-old rabbit compared with adult animals (228). It has also been demonstrated that the clearance mechanisms in developing animals may be more efficient than in adult animals. For example, the recycling of surfactant phosphatidylcholine is estimated to be 85% efficient in the 3-day-old rabbit compared with about 50% in adult rabbit lungs (194,229). Perhaps this recycling pathway is important in developing lungs in order to effectively maintain the large intra-alveolar pool size and also to compensate for the relatively delayed capacity of the alveolar type II cell to produce and secrete surfactant.

Studies involving the use of radiolabeled lipids and morphometric analysis indicate that uptake of surfactant lipid into the cytoplasmic compartment of type II cells occurs within minutes, with a subsequent time-dependent increase in the accumulation of phospholipid within lamellar bodies (230). Other organelles, such as lysozyme-containing dense multivesicular bodies and lysosomes, also participate in recycling of surfactant phospholipids, although these structures appear to exhibit lower levels of phospholipid accumulation than lamellar bodies (230,231). Wright et al. (232) and Rice et al. (233) have further demonstrated that surfactant phospholipid uptake by isolated type II cells is enhanced by SP-A, SP-B, and SP-C. Thus, surfactant phospholipid uptake is regulated by these surfactant apoproteins and the majority of lipid is directly reincorporated into lamellar bodies where it can be reutilized by the type II cell for surfactant secretion.

Similar to phospholipids, the surfactant apoproteins are also reutilized by type II cells. Recent studies indicate that SP-A is internalized by endocytosis with transfer to endosomes, multivesicular bodies, and lamellar bodies (234,235). However, unlike surfactant lipids, SP-A is not detected in the electron-lucent–type multivesicular bodies which lack lysosomal enzymes (230). Therefore, the route for SP-A recycling may be different from that of phospholipids, with limited intracellular degradation. Breslin and Weaver reported that SP-B binding may occur by a receptor-independent process (236), although other studies suggest that binding of SP-B by type II cells might be mediated by high-affinity surface receptors when SP-B is presented to cells in association with phospholipid (237). Preliminary evidence indicates that SP-D binding to macrophages might involve interaction with cell surface receptors (238); however, receptor-mediated uptake has not yet been demonstrated for SP-C or SP-D by alveolar type II cells.

## IV. Summary

The developing alveolar epithelium is capable of a variety of physiological functions. Lung fluid secretion throughout the majority of gestation results in optimal lung growth with generation of an adequate alveolar surface area for gas exchange at birth. The ultimate function of alveolar epithelium is gas exchange. The type I and type II alveolar cells which are responsible for facilitating gas exchange and maintaining lung function are derived from the undifferentiated epithelial cells which line the primitive respiratory tract. Although evidence exists to suggest that alveolar type I cells are derived from differentiated alveolar type II cells, other data suggest that type I cells differentiate directly from epithelial stem cells present in the distal fetal lung. A variety of markers for both alveolar type I and type II cells have recently been described. It is hoped that further characterization of such markers will generate important information regarding the cell lineage and function of both alveolar cell types. Such information will be especially interesting with regard to type I cells, which occupy greater than 90% of the alveolar surface area but about which relatively little is known.

### Acknowledgment

Supported by NIH HDHL 32650 (J.M.S.), HD 27748 (M.J.A.), HL 55584 (R.K.M.), and the Veterans Administration (R.K.M.).

### References

1. Strang LB. Fetal lung liquid: secretion and reabsorption. Physiol Rev 1991; 71:991–1016.

2. Bland RD, Nielson DW. Developmental changes in lung epithelial ion transport and liquid movement. Annu Rev Physiol 1992; 54:373–394.

3. O'Brodovich H. Epithelial ion transport in the fetal and perinatal lung. Am J Physiol 1991; 261:C555–C564.

4. Alcorn D, Adamson TM, Lambert TF, et al. Morphological effects of chronic tracheal ligation and drainage in the fetal lamb lung. J Anat 1977; 123:649–660.

5. Moessinger AC, Harding R, Adamson TM, et al. Role of lung fluid volume in growth and maturation of the fetal sheep lung. J Clin Invest 1990; 86:1270–1277.

6. Cassin S, Gause G, Perks AM. The effects of bumetanide and furosemide on lung liquid secretion in fetal sheep. Proc Soc Exp Biol Med 1986; 181:427–431.

7. Kitterman JA, Ballard PL, Clements JA, et al. Tracheal fluid in fetal lambs: spontaneous decrease before birth. J Appl Physiol 1979; 47:985–989.

8. Lawson EE, Brown ER, Torday JS, et al. The effect of epinephrine on tracheal fluid flow and surfactant efflux in fetal sheep. Am Rev Respir Dis 1978; 118:1023–1026.

9. Vilos GA, Liggin GC. Intrathoracic pressures in fetal sheep. J Dev Physiol 1982; 4:247–256.

10. Brown MJ, Olver RE, Ramsden CA, et al. Effects of adrenaline and of spontaneous labour on the secretion and absorption of lung liquid in the fetal lamb. J Physiol 1983; 344:137–152.

11. Chapman DL, Carlton DP, Nielson DW, et al. Changes in lung liquid during spontaneous labor in fetal sheep. J Appl Physiol 1994; 76(2):523–530.

12. Walters DV, Olver RE. The role of catecholamines in lung liquid absorption at birth. Pediatr Res 1978; 12:239–242.

13. Cassin S, Perks AM. Amiloride inhibits arginine vasopressin-induced decrease in fetal lung liquid secretion. J Appl Physiol 1993; 75(5):1925–1929.

14. Castro R, Ervin MG, Ross MG, et al. Ovine fetal lung fluid response to atrial natriuretic factor. Am J Obstet Gynecol 1989; 161:1337–1343.

15. Kennedy KA, Wilton P, Mellander M, et al. Effect of epidermal growth factor on lung liquid secretion in fetal sheep. J Dev Physiol 1986; 8:421–433.

16. Kitterman JA. Fetal lung development. J Dev Physiol 1984; 6:67–82.

17. Crapo JD, Barry BE, Gehr P, et al. Cell number and cell characteristics of the normal human lung. Am Rev Respir Dis 1982; 126:332–337.

18. Crapo JD, Young SL, Fram EK, et al. Morphometric characteristics of cells in the alveolar region of mammalian lungs. Am Rev Respir Dis 1983; 128:542–546.

19. Matalon S. Mechanisms and regulation of ion transport in adult mammalian alveolar type II pneumocytes. Am J Physiol 1991; 261:C727–C738.

20. Saumon G, Basset G. Electrolyte and fluid transport across the mature alveolar epithelium. J Appl Physiol 1993; 74:1–15.

21. Oyarzun MJ, Clements JA. Control of lung surfactant by ventilation, adrenergic mediators, and prostaglandins in the rabbit. Am Rev Respir Dis 1978; 117:879–891.

22. Hildebran JN, Goerke J, Clements JA. Surfactant release in excised rat lung is stimulated by air inflation. J Appl Physiol: Respir Environ Exercise Physiol 1981; 51:905–910.

23. Mason RJ. Surfactant synthesis, secretion, and function in alveoli and small airways.

Review of the physiologic basis for pharmacologic intervention. Respiration 1987; 515:3–9.

24. Brown LA, Longmore WJ. Adrenergic and cholinergic regulation of lung surfactant secretion in the isolated perfused rat lung and in alveolar type II cell in culture. J Biol Chem 1981; 256:66–72.

25. Rice WR, Hull WM, Dion CA, et al. Activation of cAMP dependent protein kinase during surfactant release from type II pneumocytes. Exp Lung Res 1985; 9: 135–149.

26. Chander A, Sen N, Wu AM, et al. Protein kinase C in ATP regulation of lung surfactant secretion type II cells. Am J Physiol 1995; 268:L108–L116.

27. Sherman MP, Ganz T. Host defense in pulmonary alveoli. Annu Rev Physiol 1992; 54:331–350.

28. Jonsson S, Musher DM, Goree A, et al. Human alveolar lining material and antibacterial defenses. Am Rev Respir Dis 1986; 133:136–140.

29. O'Neill SJ, Lesperance E, Klass DJ. Human lung lavage surfactant enhances staphylococcal phagocytosis by alveolar macrophages. Am Rev Respir Dis 1984; 130:1177–1179.

30. van Iwaarden F, Welmers B, Verhoef J, et al. Pulmonary surfactant protein A enhances the host-defense mechanism of rat alveolar macrophages. Am J Respir Cell Mol Biol 1990; 2:91–98.

31. Tenner AJ, Robinson SL, Borchelt J, et al. Human pulmonary surfactant protein (SP-A), a protein structurally homologous to C1q, can enhance FcR- and CR1-mediated phagocytosis. J Biol Chem 1989; 264:13923–13928.

32. van Iwaarden JF, van Strijp JA, Ebskamp MJ, et al. Surfactant protein A is opsonin in phagocytosis of herpes simplex virus type I by rat alveolar macrophages. Am J Physiol 1991; 261:L204–L209.

33. Deterding RR, Shimizu H, Fisher JH, et al. Regulation of surfactant protein D expression by glucocorticoids *in vitro* and *in vivo*. Am J Respir Cell Mol Biol 1994; 10:30–37.

34. Strunk RC, Eidlen DM, Mason RJ. Pulmonary alveolar type II epithelial cells synthesize and secrete proteins of the classical and alternative complement pathways. J Clin Invest 1988; 81:1419–1426.

35. Hahon N, Castronova V. Interferon production in rat type II pneumocytes and alveolar macrophages. Exp Lung Res 1989; 15:429–445.

36. Pesanti EL. Interaction of cytokines and alveolar cells with *Pneumocystis carinii in vitro*. J Infect Dis 1991; 163:611–616.

37. Castranova V, Rabovsky J, Tucker JH, et al. The alveolar type II epithelial cell: a multifunctional pneumocyte. Toxicol Appl Pharm 1988; 93:472–483.

38. Witschi H. Role of the epithelium in lung repair. Chest 1991; 99(suppl):22S–25S.

39. Gehr P, Bachofen M, Weibel ER. The normal human lung: ultrastructure and morphometric estimation of diffusion capacity. Respir Physiol 1978; 32:121–140.

40. Danto SI, Zabski SM, Crandell ED. Reactivity of alveolar epithelial cells in primary culture with type I cell monoclonal antibodies. Am J Respir Cell Mol Biol 1992; 6:296–306.

41. Russo RM, Lubman RL, Crandell ED. Evidence for amiloride-sensitive sodium channels in alveolar epithelial cells. Am J Physiol 1992; 262:L405–L411.

42. O'Rahilly R. The early prenatal development of the human respiratory system. In: Nelson GH, ed. Pulmonary Development. Transition from Intrauterine to Extrauterine Life. New York: Dekker, 1985:27:3–18.

43. Sadler TW (ed.) Langman's Medical Embryology. Baltimore: Williams & Wilkins, 1990:228–236.

44. Hilfer SR, Rayner RM, Brown JW. Mesenchymal control of branching pattern in the fetal mouse lung. Tissue Cell 1985; 17:525–538.

45. Masters JRW. Epithelial-mesenchymal interactions during lung development: the effect of mesenchymal mass. Dev Biol 1976; 51:98–108.

46. Spooner BS, Wessells NK. Mammalian lung development: interactions in primordium formation and bronchial morphogenesis. J Exp Zool 1970; 175:445–454.

47. Alescio T, Cassini A. Induction *in vitro* of tracheal buds by pulmonary mesenchyme grafted on tracheal epithelium. J Exp Zool 1962; 150:83–94.

48. O'Rahilly R, Boyden EA. The timing and sequence of events in the development of the human respiratory system during the embryonic period proper. Z Anat Entw 1973; 141:237–250.

49. Commission on Embryological Terminology. In: Arey LB, Mossman HW, eds. Nomina Embryologica. Lenningrad, Bethesda, MD: Fed Am Soc Exp Biol, 1970.

50. Bucher U, Reid L. Development of the intrasegmental bronchial tree: the pattern of branching and development of cartilage at various stages of intra-uterine life. Thorax 1961; 16:207–218.

51. Boyden EA. The mode of origin of pulmonary acini and respiratory bronchioles in the fetal lung. Am J Anat 1974; 141:317–328.

52. Hislop A, Reid L. Development of the acinus in the human lung. Thorax 1974; 29:90–94.

53. Langston C, Kida K, Reed M, et al. Human lung growth in late gestation and in the neonate. Am Rev Respir Dis 1984; 129:607–613.

54. Davies G, Reid L. Growth of the alveoli and pulmonary arteries in childhood. Thorax 1970; 25:669–681.

55. Boyden EA. Development and growth of the airways. In: Hodson WA, ed. Development of the Lung. New York: Dekker, 1977:6:3–35.

56. Ten Have-Opbroek AAW, Plopper CG. Morphogenetic and functional activity of type II cells in early fetal Rhesus monkey lungs. A comparison between primates and rodents. Anat Rec 1992; 234:93–104.

57. Snyder JM, Mendelson CR, Johnston JM. The morphology of lung development in the human fetus. In: Nelson GH, ed. Pulmonary Development. Transition from Intrauterine to Extrauterine Life. New York: Dekker, 1985:27:19–45.

58. Bluemink JG, Van Maurik P, Lawson KA. Intimate cell contracts at the epithelial/mesenchymal interface in embryonic mouse lung. J Ultrastruc Res 1976; 55:257–270.

59. Wessells NK. Mammalian lung development: Interactions in formation and morphogenesis of tracheal buds. J Exp Zool 1970; 175:455–466.

60. Riso J. Morphology of epithelio-mesenchymal interaction during lung development of the mouse. Cell Diff 1983; 13:309–318.

61. Jaskoll TF, Slavkin HC. Ultrastructural and immunofluorescence studies of basal lamina alterations during mouse-lung morphogenesis. Differentiation 1984; 28: 36–48.

62. Jeffrey PK, Reid LM. Ultrastructure of airway epithelium and submucosal gland during development. In: Hodson WA, ed. Development of the Lung. New York: Dekker, 1977:6:87–134.

63. Cutz E, Conen PE. Endocrine-like cells in human fetal lungs: an electron microscopic study. Anat Rec 1972; 173:115–122.

64. Plopper CG, et al. Development of airway epithelium: patterns of expression for markers of differentiation. Chest 1992; 101:25–55.

65. Ten Have-Opbroek AAW. The development of the lung in mammals: an analysis of concepts and findings. Am J Anat 1981; 162:201–219.

66. Hage E. The morphological development of the pulmonary epithelium of human foetuses studied by light and electron microscopy. Z Anat Entw 1973; 140:271–279.

67. McDougall J, Smith JF. The development of the human type II pneumocyte. J Pathol 1975; 115:245–251.

68. Wert SE, Glasser SW, Korfhagen TR, et al. Transcriptional elements from the human SP-C gene direct expression in the primordial respiratory epithelium of transgenic mice. Dev Biol 1993; 156: 426–443.

69. Wohlford-Lenane CL, Durham PL, Snyder JM. Localization of surfactant-associated protein C (SP-C) mRNA in fetal rabbit lung tissue by *in situ* hybridization. Am J Res Cell Mol Biol 1992; 6:225–234.

70. Khoor A, Stahlman MT, Gray ME, et al. Temporal-spatial distribution of SP-B and SP-C proteins and mRNAs in developing respiratory epithelium of human lung. J Histochem Cytochem 1994; 42:1187–1199.

71. Dobbs LG, Williams MC, Gonzalez R. Monoclonal antibodies specific to apical surfaces of rat alveolar type I cells bind to surfaces of cultured, but not freshly isolated, type II cells. Biochim Biophys Acta 1988; 970:146–156.

72. Williams MC, Dobbs LG. Expression of cell-specific markers for alveolar epithelium in fetal rat lung. Am J Respir Cell Mol Biol 1990; 2:533–542.

73. Brody JS, Williams MC. Pulmonary alveolar epithelial cell differentiation. Annu Rev Physiol 1992; 54:351–371.

74. King RJ, Jones MB, Minoo P. Regulation of lung cell proliferation by polypeptide growth factors. Am J Physiol 1989; 257:L23–L38.

75. Kelley J. Cytokines of the lung. Am Rev Respir Dis 1990; 141:765–788.

76. McGowan SE. Extracellular matrix and the regulation of lung development and repair. FASEB J 1992; 6:2895–2904.

77. Dobbs LG. Pulmonary surfactant. Ann Rev Med 1989; 40:431–446.

78. Williams MC, Mason RJ. Development of the type II cell in the fetal rat lung. Am Rev Respir Dis 1977; 115:37–47.

79. Weaver TE, Whitsett JA. Function and regulation of expression of pulmonary surfactant-associated proteins. Biochem J 1991; 273:249–264.

80. Wohlford-Lenane CL, Snyder JM. Localization of surfactant-associated proteins SP-A and SP-B mRNA in rabbit fetal lung tissue by in situ hybridization. Am J Respir Cell Mol Biol 1992; 7:335–343.
81. Khoor A, Gray ME, Hull WM, et al. Developmental expression of SP-A and SP-A mRNA in the proximal and distal respiratory epithelium in the human fetus and newborn. J Histochem Cytochem 1993; 41:1311–1319.
82. Snyder JM, Magliato SA. An ultrastructural morphometric analysis of rabbit fetal lung type II cell differentiation *in vivo*. Anat Rec 1991; 229:73–85.
83. Bourbon JR, Rieutort M, Engle MJ, et al. Utilization of glycogen for phospholipid synthesis in fetal rat lung. Biochim Biophys Acta 1982; 712:382–389.
84. Grant MM, Cutts NR, Brody JS. Alterations in lung basement membrane during fetal growth and type 2 cell development. Dev Biol 1983; 97:173–183.
85. Grant MM, Cutts NR, Brody JS. Influence of maternal diabetes on basement membranes, type 2 cells, and capillaries in the developing rat lung. Dev Biol 1984; 104:469–476.
86. Leung CKH, Adamson IY, Bowden DH. Uptake of $^3$H-prednisolone by fetal lung explants: role of intercellular contacts in epithelial maturation. Exp Lung Res 1980; 1:111–120.
87. Ryan U, Slavkin H, Revel JP, et al. Conference report: cell to cell interactions in the developing lung. Tissue Cell 1984; 16:829–841.
88. Hiray, et al. Expression and role of E- and P-cadherin adhesion molecules in embryonic histogenesis. Development 1989; 105:263–270.
89. Juliano RL, Hoskill S. Signal transduction from the extracellular matrix. J Cell Biol 1993; 120:577–585.
90. Sannes PL. Structural and functional relationships between type II pneumocytes and components of extracellular matrices. Exp Lung Res 1991; 17:639–659.
91. Young SL, Fram EK, Craig BL. Three-dimensional reconstruction and quantitative analysis of rat lung type II cells: a computer-based study. Am J Anat 1985; 174:1–14.
92. Sannes PL. Differences in basement membrane-associated microdomains of type I and type II pneumocytes in the rat and rabbit lung. J Histochem Cytochem 1984; 32:827–833.
93. Fawcett DW. Bloom and Fawcett. A Textbook of Histology. Philadelphia: Saunders, 1986:731–754.
94. Plopper CG, Mariassy AT, Hill LH. Ultrastructure of the nonciliated bronchiolar epithelial (Clara) cell of mammalian lung. III. A study of man with comparison of 15 mammalian species. Exp Lung Res 1980; 1:171–180.
95. Plopper CG, Cranz DL, Kemp L, et al. Immunohistochemical demonstration of cytochrome p450 monooxygenase in Clara cells throughout the tracheobronchial airways of the rabbit. Exp Lung Res 1987; 13:59–68.
96. Broers JLV, Jensen SM, Travis WD, et al. Expression of surfactant associated protein-A and Clara cell 10 kilodalton mRNA in neoplastic and non-neoplastic human lung tissue as detected by *in situ* hybridization. Lab Invest 1992; 66:337–346.
97. Brody AR, Hook GE, Cameron GS, et al. The differentiation capacity of Clara cells isolated from the lungs of rabbits. Lab Invest 1987; 57:219–229.

98. Crapo JD, Barry BE, Gehr P, et al. Cell number and cell characteristics of the normal human lung. Am Rev Respir Dis 1982; 125:332–337.

99. Picciano P, Rosenbaum RM. The type I alveolar lining cells of the mammalian lung. I. Isolation and enrichment from dissociated adult rabbit lung. Am J Pathol 1978; 90:99–122.

100. Weller NK, Karnovsky MJ. Isolation of pulmonary type I cells from adult rats. Am J Pathol 1986; 124:448–456.

101. Snyder JM, O'Brien JA, Rodgers HF. Localization and accumulation of fibronectin in rabbit fetal lung tissue. Differentiation 1987; 34:32–39.

102. Adamson IY, Bowden DH. The type 2 cell as progenitor of alveolar epithelial regeneration. A cytodynamic study in mice after exposure to oxygen. Lab Invest 1974; 30:35–42.

103. Adamson IYR, Bowden DH. Derivation of type 1 epithelium from type 2 cells in the developing rat lung. Lab Invest 1975; 32:736–745.

104. Dobbs LG, Williams MC, Brandt AE. Changes in biochemical characteristics and pattern of lectin binding of alveolar type II cells with time in culture. Biochim Biophys Acta 1985; 846:155–166.

105. Evans MJ, Cabral LJ, Stephens RJ, et al. Renewal of alveolar epithelium in the rat following exposure to $NO_2$. Am J Pathol 1973; 70:175–198.

106. Evans MJ, Cabral LJ, Stephens RJ, et al. Transformation of alveolar type 2 cells to type 1 cells following exposure to $NO_2$. Exp Mol Pathol 1975; 22:142–150.

107. Hotchkiss JA, Kennel SJ, Harkema JR. A rat monoclonal antibody specific for murine type 1 pneumocytes. Exp Mol Pathol 1992; 57:235–246.

108. Joyce-Brady MF, Brody JS. Ontogeny of pulmonary alveolar epithelial markers of differentiation. Dev Biol 1990; 137:331–348.

109. Christensen PJ, Kim S, Simon RH, et al. Differentiation-related expression of ICAM-1 by rat alveolar epithelial cells. Am J Respir Cell Mol Biol 1993; 8:9–15.

110. Guzman J, Izumi T, Nagai S, et al. ICAM-1 and integrin expression on isolated human alveolar type II pneumocytes. Eur Respir J 1994; 7:736–739.

111. Nagae A, Abe M, Becker RP, et al. High concentration of carboxypeptidase M in lungs: presence of the enzyme in alveolar type I cells. Am J Respir Cell Mol Biol 1993; 9:221–229.

112. Marshall BC, Joyce-Brady MF, Brody JS. Identification and characterization of the pulmonary alveolar type II cell *Maclura pomifera* agglutinin-binding membrane glycoprotein. Biochim Biophys Acta 1988; 966:403-413.

113. Honda T, Schulte BA, Fazel AR, et al. Lectin binding beneath the epithelium and in smooth muscle cells in the developing bronchial tree. Cell Diff Dev 1990; 31:31-42.

114. Lwebuga-Mukasa JS. Identification of pneumocin, a developmentally regulated apical membrane glycoprotein in rat lung type II and Clara cells. Am J Respir Cell Mol Biol 1991; 4:489–496.

115. Chatelet F, Brianti E, Ronco P, et al. Ultrastructural localization by monoclonal antibodies of brush border antigens expressed by glomeruli. Am J Path 1986; 122:512–519.

116. Sahali D, Mulliez N, Chatelet F, et al. Comparative immunochemistry and ontogeny of two closely related coated pit proteins. The 280-kd target of teratogenic antibodies

and the 330-kd target of nephritogenic antibodies. Am J Pathol 1993; 142:1654–1667.

117. Ballard PL, Hawgood S, Liley H, et al. Regulation of pulmonary surfactant apoprotein SP 28-36 gene in fetal human lung. Proc Natl Acad Sci 1986; 83:9527–9531.

118. Schellhase DE, Emrie PA, Fisher JH, et al. Ontogeny of surfactant apoproteins in the rat. Pediatr Res 1989; 26:167–174.

119. Boggaram VK, Qing K, Mendelson CR. The major apoprotein of rabbit pulmonary surfactant. Elucidation of primary sequence and cyclic AMP and developmental regulation. J Biol Chem 1988; 263:2939–2947.

120. Liley HG, White RT, Warr RG, et al. Regulation of messenger RNAs for the hydrophobic surfactant proteins in human lung. J Clin Invest 1989; 83:1191–1197.

121. Crouch E, Rust K, Marienchek W, et al. Developmental expression of pulmonary surfactant protein D (SP-D). Am J Respir Cell Mol Biol 1991; 5:13–18.

122. Tsilibary EC, Williams MC. Actin in peripheral rat lung: S1 labeling and structural changes induced by cytochalasin. J Histochem Cytochem 1983; 31:1289–1297.

123. Paine R, Ben-Ze'ev A, Farmer SR, et al. The pattern of cytokeratin synthesis is a marker of type 2 cell differentiation in adult and maturing fetal lung alveolar cells. Dev Biol 1988; 129:505–515.

124. Edelson JD, Shannon JM, Mason RJ. Alkaline phosphatase: a marker of alveolar type II cell differentiation. Am Rev Respir Dis 1988; 138:1268–1275.

125. Post M, Smith BT. Histochemical and immunocytochemical identification of alveolar type II epithelial cells isolated from fetal rat lung. Am Rev Respir Dis 1988; 137:525–530.

126. Serabjit-Singh CJ, Nishio SJ, Philpot RM, et al. The distribution of cytochrome P-450 monooxygenase in cells of the rabbit lung: an ultrastructural immunocytochemical characterization. Mol Pharmacol 1988; 33:279–289.

127. Joyce-Brady M, Takahashi Y, Oakes SM, et al. Synthesis and release of amphipathic gamma-glutamyl transferase by the pulmonary alveolar type 2 cell. Its redistribution throughout the gas exchange portion of the lung indicates a new role for surfactant. J Biol Chem 1994; 269:14219–14226.

128. Funkhouser JD, Cheshire LM, Ferrara TB, et al. Monoclonal antibody identification of a type II alveolar epithelial cell antigen and expression of the antigen during lung development. Dev Biol 1987; 119:190–198.

129. Funkhouser JD, Tangada SD, Jones M, et al. p146 type II alveolar epithelial cell antigen is identical to aminopeptidase N. Am J Physiol 1991; 260:L274–L279.

130. Funkhouser JD, Tangada SD, Peterson RD, et al. Ectopeptidases of alveolar epithelium: candidates for roles in alveolar regulatory mechanisms. Am J Physiol 1991; 260:L381–L385.

131. Simon RH, Edwards JA, Reza MM, et al. Injury of rat pulmonary epithelial cells by $H_2O_2$: dependence on phenotype and catalase. Am J Physiol 1991; 260:L318–L325.

132. Forman HJ, Fisher AB. Antioxidant enzymes of rat granular pneumocytes. Constitutive levels and effect of hyperoxia. Lab Invest 1981; 45:1–6.

133. Walther FJ, Wade AB, Warburton D, et al. Ontogeny of antioxidant enzymes in the fetal lamb lung. Exp Lung Res 1991; 17:39–45.

134. Gross TJ, Simon RH, Sitrin RG. Expression of urokinase-type plasminogen activator by rat pulmonary alveolar epithelial cells. Am J Respir Cell Mol Biol 1990; 3:449–456.

135. Peters-Golden M, Feyssa A. Augmented expression of cytosolic phospholipase A2 during phenotypic transformation of cultured type II pneumocytes. Am J Physiol 1994; 266:C382–C390.

136. Singh G, Katyal SL, Brown WE, et al. Pulmonary lysozyme—a secretory protein of type II pneumocytes in the rat. Am Rev Respir Dis 1988; 138:1261–1267.

137. Sano K, Voelker DR, Mason RJ, et al. Involvement of protein kinase C in pulmonary surfactant secretion from alveolar type II cells. J Biol Chem 1985; 260:12725–12729.

138. Parton LA, Warburton D, Lang WE. Plasminogen activator inhibitor type 1 production by rat type II pneumocytes in culture. Am J Respir Cell Mol Biol 1992; 6: 133–139.

139. Wallin R, Rannels SR. Identification of vitamin K–dependent carboxylase activity in lung type II cells but not in lung macrophages. Biochem J 1988; 250:557–563.

140. Whitsett JA, Matz S, Darovec-Beckerman C. cAMP-dependent protein kinase and protein phosphorylation in developing rat lung. Pediatr Res 1983; 17:959–966.

141. Malkison AM, Girard PR, Kno KF. Strain-specific postnatal changes in the activity and tissue levels of protein kinase C. Biochem Biophys Res Commun 1987; 145: 733–739.

142. Zimmermann LJ, Hogan M, Carlson KS, et al. Regulation of phosphatidylcholine synthesis in fetal type II cells by CTP:phosphocholine cytidylyltransferase. Am J Physiol 1993; 264: L575–L580.

143. Rooney SA. Fatty acid biosynthesis in developing fetal lung. Am J Physiol 1989; 257: L195–L201.

144. DiAugustine RP. Lung concentric laminar organelle. Hydrolase activity and compositional analysis. J Biol Chem 1974; 249:584–593.

145. Haimoto H, Takahashi Y, Koshikawa T, et al. Immunohistochemical localization of gamma-enolase in normal human tissues other than nervous and neuroendocrine tissues. Lab Invest 1985; 52:257–263.

146. Ishii Y, Hashizume Y, Watanabe T, et al. Cysteine proteinases in bronchalveolar epithelial cells and lavage fluid of rat lung. J Histochem Cytochem 1991; 39:461–468.

147. Lubman RL, Danto SI, Chao DC, et al. Cl-HCO₃ Exchanger isoform AE2 is restricted to the basolateral surface of alveolar epithelial cell monolayers. Am J Respir Cell Mol Biol 1995; 12:211–219.

148. Schneeberger EE, McCarthy KM. Cytochemical localization of Na-K-ATPase in rat type II pneumocytes. J Appl Physiol 1986; 60:1584–1589.

149. Kemp PJ, MacGregor GG, Olver RE, et al. G protein-regulated large-conductance chloride channels in freshly isolated fetal type II alveolar epithelial cells. Am J Physiol 1993; 265:L323–L329.

150. O'Brodovich H, Hannam V, Rafii B. Sodium channel but neither Na⁺-H⁺ nor Na⁺-glucose symport inhibitors slow neonatal lung water clearence. Am J Respir Cell Mol Biol 1991; 5:377–384.

151. Brown SE, Kim KJ, Goodman BE, et al. Sodium-amino acid cotransport by type II alveolar epithelial cells. J Appl Physiol 1985; 59:1616–1622.
152. Hautamaki RD, Greene B, Souba WW. Characterization of L-glutamine transport by type II alveolar cells. Am J Physiol 1992; 262:L459–L465.
153. Nord EP, Brown SE, Crandall ED. Characterization of $N^+$-$H^+$ antiport in type II alveolar epithelial cells. Am J Physiol 1987; 252:C490–C498.
154. DeCoursey TE. State-dependent inactivation of K currents in rat type II alveolar epithelial cells. J Gen Physiol 1990; 95:617–646.
155. Rochat TR, Casale JM, Hunninghake GW. Characterization of type II alveolar epithelial cells by flow cytometry and fluorescent markers. J Lab Clin Med 1988; 112:418–425.
156. McCarthy KM, Gong JL, Telford JR, et al. Ontogeny of Ia accessory cells in fetal and newborn rat lung. Am J Respir Cell Mol Biol 1992; 6:349–356.
157. Struhar DJ, Harbeck RJ, Gegen N, et al. Increased expression of class II antigens of the major histocompatibility complex on alveolar macrophages and alveolar type II cells and interleukin-1 secretion from alveolar macrophages in an animal model of silicosis. Clin Exp Immunol 1989; 77:281–284.
158. Struhar D, Greif J, Harbeck RJ. Class II antigens of the major histocompatibility complex are increased in lungs of bleomycin-treated rats. Immunol Lett 1990; 26:197–201.
159. Haimoto H, Nagura H, Imaizumi M, et al. Immunoelectronmicroscopic study of the transport of secretory IgA in the lower respiratory tract and alveoli. Virchows Arch (Pathol Anat Histopathol) 1984; 404:369–380.
160. Hahon N, Castranova V. Interferon production in rat type II pneumocytes and alveolar macrophages. Exp Lung Res 1989; 15:429–445.
161. Paine R, Rolfe MW, Standiford TJ, et al. MCP-1 expression by rat type II alveolar epithelial cells in primary culture. J Immunol 1993;150:4561–4570.
162. Blau H, Riklis S, Kravtsov V, et al. Secretion of cytokines by rat alveolar epithelial cells: possible regulatory role for SP-A. Am J Physiol 1994; 266:L148–L155.
163. Crestani B, Cornillet P, Dehoux M, et al. Alveolar type II epithelial cells produce interleukin-6 *in vitro* and *in vivo*. Regulation by alveolar macrophage secretory products. J Clin Invest 1994; 94:731–740.
164. Punjabi CJ, Laskin JD, Pendino KJ, et al. Production of nitric oxide by rat type II pneumocytes: increased expression of inducible nitric oxide synthase following inhalation of pulmonary irritant. Am J Respir Cell Mol Biol 1994; 11:165–172.
165. Ambrose MP, Hunninghake GW. Corticosteroids increase lipocortin I in alveolar epithelial cells. Am J Respir Cell Mol Biol 1990; 3:349–353.
166. Seeger W, Gunther A, Walurath HD, et al. Alveolar surfactant and adult respiratory distress syndrome. Pathogenetic role and therapeutic prospects. Clin Invest 1993; 71:177–190.
167. Hislop AA, Wigglesworth JS, Desai R, et al. Alveolar development in the human fetus and infant. Early Hum Dev 1986; 13:1–11.
168. Avery ME, Merritt TA. Surfactant replacement therapy. N Engl J Med 1991; 324:910–911.

169. Spragg RG, Gilliard N, Richman P, et al. Acute effects of a single dose of porcine surfactant on patients with the adult respiratory distress syndrome. Chest 1994; 105:195–202.

170. Kurashima K, Ogawa H, Ohka T, et al. A pilot study of surfactant inhalation in the treatment of asthmatic attack. Arerugi–Jpn J Allergol 1991; 40:160–163.

171. Rooney SA. Phospholipid composition, biosynthesis, and secretion. In: Parent RA, ed. Comparative Biology of the Normal Lung. Boca Raton, FL: CRC Press, 1992: 511–544.

172. Rooney SA. The surfactant system and lung phospholipid biochemistry. Am Rev Respir Dis 1985; 131:439–460.

173. Garcia A, Sener SF, Mavis RD. Lung lamellar bodies lack certain key enzymes of phospholipid metabolism. Lipids 1976;11:109–112.

174. Rooney SA, Young SL, Mendelson CR. Molecular and cellular processing of lung surfactant. FASEB J 1994; 8:957-967.

175. Voorhout WF, Veenendaal T, Kuroki Y, et al. Immunocytochemical localization of surfactant protein D (SP-D) in type II cells, Clara cells, and alveolar macrophages of rat lung. J Histochem Cytochem 1992; 40:1589–1597.

176. Alcorn JL, Mendelson CR. Trafficking of surfactant protein A in fetal rabbit lung in organ culture. Am J Physiol 1993; 264:L27–L35.

177. Froh D, Ballard PL, Williams MC, et al. Lamellar bodies of cultured human fetal lung: content of surfactant protein A (SP-A), surface film formation and structural transformation *in vitro*. Biochim Biophys Acta 1990; 1052:78–89.

178. Ikegami M, Lewis JF, Tabor B, et al. Surfactant protein A metabolism in preterm ventilated lambs. Am J Physiol 1992; 262:L765–L772.

179. Froh D, Gonzales LW, Ballard PL. Secretion of surfactant protein A and phosphatidylcholine from type II cells of human fetal lung. Am J Respir Cell Mol Biol 1993; 8:556–561.

180. Rooney SA, Gobran LI, Umstead TM, et al. Secretion of surfactant protein A from rat type II pneumocytes. Am J Physiol 1993; 265:L586–L590.

181. Griese M, Gobran LI, Rooney SA. Ontogeny of surfactant secretion in type II pneumocytes from fetal, newborn, and adult rats. Am J Physiol 1992; 262:L337–L343.

182. Ryan US, Ryan JW, Smith DS. Alveolar type II cells: studies on the mode of release of lamellar bodies. Tissue Cell 1975; 7:587–599.

183. Chander A, Fisher AB. Regulation of lung surfactant secretion. Am J Physiol 1990; 258:L241–L253.

184. Delahunty TJ, Johnston JM. The effect of colchicine and vinblastine on the release of pulmonary surface active material. J Lipid Res 1976; 17:112–116.

185. Brown LA, Pasquale SM, Longmore WJ. Role of microtubules in surfactant secretion. J Appl Physiol 1985; 58:1866–1873.

186. Whitsett JA, Hull W, Dion C, et al. cAMP dependent actin phosphorylation in developing rat lung and type II epithelial cells. Exp Lung Res 1985; 9:191–209.

187. Zimmerman UJ, Speicher DW, Fisher AB. Secretagogue-induced proteolysis of lung spectrin in alveolar epithelial type II cells. Biochim Biophys Acta 1992; 1137:127–134.

188. Rooney SA, Wai-Lee TS, Gobran L, et al. Phospholipid content, composition and biosynthesis during fetal lung development in the rabbit. Biochim Biophys Acta 1976; 431:447–458.

189. Rooney SA, Gobran LI, Wai-Lee TS. Stimulation of surfactant production by oxytocin-induced labor in the rabbit. J Clin Invest 1977; 60:754–759.

190. Marino PA, Rooney SA. The effect of labor on surfactant secretion in newborn rabbit lung slices. Biochim Biophys Acta 1981; 664:389–396.

191. Wirtz HRW, Dobbs LG. Calcium mobilization and exocytosis after one mechanical stretch of lung epithelial cells. Science 1990; 250:1266–1269.

192. Chander A. Regulation of lung surfactant secretion by intracellular pH. Am J Physiol 1989; 257:L354–L360.

193. Wright JR, Clements JA. Metabolism and turnover of lung surfactant. Am Rev Respir Dis 1987; 136:426–444.

194. Wright JR. Clearance and recycling of pulmonary surfactant. Am J Physiol 1990; 259:L1–L12.

195. Whitsett JA, Darovec-Beckerman C, Pollinger J, et al. Ontogeny of beta-adrenergic receptors in the rat lung: effects of hypothyroidism. Pediatr Res 1982; 16:381–387.

196. Mescher EJ, Dobbs LG, Mason RJ, et al. Cholera toxin stimulates secretion of saturated phosphatidylcholine and increases cellular cyclic AMP in isolated rat alveolar type II cells. Exp Lung Res 1983; 5:173–182.

197. Joyce-Brady M, Rubins JB, Panchenko MP, et al. Mechanisms of mastoparan-stimulated surfactant secretion from isolated pulmonary alveolar type 2 cells. J Biol Chem 1991; 266:6859–6865.

198. Rice WR, Singleton FM. $P_2$-purinoceptors regulate surfactant secretion from rat isolated alveolar type II cells. Br J Pharmacol 1986; 89:485–491.

199. Rooney SA, Gobran LI. Adenosine and leukotrienes have a regulatory role in lung surfactant secretion in the newborn rabbit. Biochim Biophys Acta 1988; 960:98–106.

200. Dobbs LG, Gonzalez RF, Marinari LA, et al. The role of calcium in the secretion of surfactant by rat alveolar type II cells. Biochim Biophys Acta 1986; 877:305–313.

201. Pian MS, Dobbs LG, Duzgunes N. Positive correlation between cytosolic free calcium and surfactant secretion in cultured rat alveolar type II cells. Biochim Biophys Acta 1988; 960:43–53.

202. Corbet A, Owens M. Lanthanum inhibits surfactant secretion stimulated by lung distension in newborn rabbits. Pediatr Res 1991; 30:190–192.

203. Brown LA, Wood LH. Stimulation of surfactant secretion by vasopressin in primary cultures of adult rat type II pneumocytes. Biochim Biophys Acta 1989; 1001:76–81.

204. Hill DJ, Wright TC Jr., Andews ML, et al. Localization of calmodulin in differentiating pulmonary type II epithelial cells. Lab Invest 1984; 51:297–306.

205. Gilfillan AM, Rooney SA. Arachidonic acid metabolites stimulate phosphatidylcholine secretion in primary cultures of type II pneumocytes. Biochim Biophys Acta 1985; 833:336–341.

206. Ekelund L, Enhorning G. Pulmonary surfactant release in fetal rabbits as affected by enprofylline. Pediatr Res 1985; 19:1000–1003.

207. Chen M, Brown LA. Histamine stimulation of surfactant secretion from rat type II pneumocytes. Am J Physiol 1990; 258:L195–L200.
208. Voyno-Yasenetskaya TA, Dobbs LG, Erickson SK, et al. Low density lipoprotein- and high density lipoprotein-mediated signal transduction and exocytosis in alveolar type II cells. Proc Natl Acad Sci 1993; 90:4256–4260.
209. Sen N, Grunstein MM, Chander A. Stimulation of lung surfactant secretion by endothelin-1 from rat alveolar type II cells. Am J Physiol 1994; 266:L255–L262.
210. Dobbs LG, Wright JR, Hawgood S, et al. Pulmonary surfactant and its components inhibit secretion of phosphatidylcholine from cultured rat alveolar type II cells. Proc Natl Acad Sci USA 1987; 84:1010–1014.
211. Kuroki Y, Mason RJ, Voelker DR. Pulmonary surfactant apoprotein A structure and modulation of surfactant secretion by rat alveolar type II cells. J Biol Chem 1988; 263:3388–3394.
212. Suwabe A, Mason RJ, Smith D, et al. Pulmonary surfactant secretion is regulated by the physical state of extracellular phosphatidylcholine. J Biol Chem 1992; 267: 19884–19890.
213. Rice WR, Singleton FM. Regulation of surfactant phospholipid secretion from isolated rat alveolar type II cells by lectins. Biochim Biophys Acta 1988; 958: 205–210.
214. Rice WR, Singleton FM. Regulation of surfactant secretion from isolated type II pneumocytes by substance P. Biochim Biophys Acta 1986; 889:123–127.
215. Gobran LI, Rooney SA. Adenosine A1 receptor-mediated inhibition of surfactant secretion in rat type II pneumocytes. Am J Physiol 1990; 258:L45–L51.
216. Rice WR, Singleton FM. Reactive blue 2 selectively inhibits $P_{2y}$-purinoceptor-stimulated surfactant phospholipid secretion from rat isolated alveolar type II cells. Br J Pharmacol 1989; 97:158–162.
217. Chander A, Sen S. Inhibition of phosphatidylcholine secretion by stilbene disulfonates in alveolar type II cells. Biochem Pharmacol 1993; 45:1905–1912.
218. Corbet A, Bedi H, Owens M, et al. Surfactant protein-A inhibits lavage-induced surfactant secretion in newborn rabbits. Am J Med Sci 1992; 304:246–251.
219. Kuroki Y, Shiratori M, Murata Y, et al. Surfactant protein D (SP-D) counteracts the inhibitory effect of surfactant protein-A (SP-A) on phospholipid secretion by alveolar type II cells. Interaction of native SP-D with SP-A. Biochem J 1991; 279:115–119.
220. Kuroki Y, et al. Alveolar type II cells express a high-affinity receptor for pulmonary surfactant protein A. Proc Natl Acad Sci USA 1988; 85:5566–5570.
221. Wright JR, Borchelt JD, Hawgood S. Lung surfactant apoprotein SP-A (26-36 kDa) binds with high affinity to isolated alveolar type II cells. Proc Natl Acad Sci 1989; 86:5410–5414.
222. Oosting RS, Wright JR. Characterization of the surfacant protein A receptor: cell and ligand specificity. Am J Physiol 1994; 267:L165–L172.
223. Williams MC. Conversion of lamellar body membranes into tubular myelin in alveoli of fetal rat lungs. J Cell Biol 1977; 72:260–277.
224. Sanders RL, Hassett RJ, Valter AE. Isolation of lung lamellar bodies and their conversion to tubular myelin figures *in vitro*. Anat Rec 1980; 198:485–501.

225. Clements JA. Composition and properties of pulmonary surfactant. In: Villee CA, Villee DB, Zuckerman J, eds. Respiratory Distress Syndrome. New York: Academic Press, 1973:77–95.

226. Jacobs H, Jobe A, Ikegami M, et al. Surfactant phosphatidylcholine sources, fluxes, and turnover times in 3-day old, 10-day old, and adult rabbits. J Biol Chem 1982; 257:1805–1810.

227. Ennema JJ, Reijngoud DJ, Wilderuur CR, et al. Effects of artificial ventilation on surfactant phospholipid metabolism in rabbits. Respir Physiol 1984; 58:15–28.

228. Jobe A, Ikegami M. Surfactant for the treatment of respiratory distress syndrome. Am Rev Respir Dis 1987; 136:1256–1275.

229. Lewis JF, Jobe AH. Surfactant and the adult respiratory distress syndrome. Am Rev Respir Dis 1993; 147:218–233.

230. Young SL, Fram EK, Larson E, et al. Recycling of surfactant lipid and apoprotein-A studied by electron microscopic autoradiography. Am J Physiol 1993; 265:L19–L26.

231. Rider ED, Pinkerton KE, Jobe AH. Characterization of rabbit lung lysosomes and their role in surfactant dipalmitoylphosphatidylcholine catabolism. J Biol Chem 1991; 266:22522–22528.

232. Wright JR, Wager RE, Hawgood S, et al. Surfactant apoprotein Mr=26,000-36,000 enhances uptake of liposomes by type II cells. J Biol Chem 1987; 262:2888–2894.

233. Rice WR, Sarin VK, Fox JL, et al. Surfactant peptides stimulate uptake of phosphatidylcholine by isolated cells. Biochim Biophys Acta 1989; 1006:237–245.

234. Ryan RM, Morris RE, Rice WR, et al. Binding and uptake of pulmonary surfactant protein (SP-A) by pulmonary type II epithelial cells. J Histchem Cytochem 1989; 37:429–440.

235. Young SL, Wright JR, Clements JA. Cellular uptake and processing of surfactant lipids and apoprotein SP-A by rat lung. J Appl Physiol 1989; 66:1336–1342.

236. Breslin JS, Weaver TE. Binding, uptake, and localization of surfactant protein B in isolated rat alveolar type II cells. Am J Physiol 1992; 262:L699–L707.

237. Bates SR, Beers MF, Fisher AB. Binding and uptake of surfactant protein B by alveolar type II cells. Am J Physiol 1992; 263:L333–L341.

238. Miyamura K, Leigh LE, Lu J, et al. Surfactant protein D binding to alveolar macrophages. Biochem J 1994; 300:237–242.

# 6

## Airway Gland Growth and Differentiation

**CAROL BASBAUM, J.-D. LI, and MELISSA LIM**

University of California
San Francisco, California

## I. Introduction

Very little investigative effort has been directed at the mechanisms mediating growth of airway submucosal glands. This is surprising in view of substantive evidence linking gland growth with hypersecretion both in chronic bronchitis (1,2) and cystic fibrosis (3). The existing information on airway gland growth is almost exclusively confined to morphological descriptions. These focus on human (4–9), rat, dog, sheep (10) opossum (11), monkey (12), and ferret (13). Basic principles of gland growth garnered from the descriptive studies are summarized below. Left unanswered are questions concerning the identity of the gland progenitor cell, the identity of growth factors controlling gland growth, the identity of enzymatic mechanisms permitting gland invasion of connective tissue, and the nature of epithelial-mesenchymal interactions controlling cell differentiation. In this chapter, literature from other fields is brought to bear on these questions and our own recent data are summarized where appropriate.

## II.  Basic Principles of Gland Growth

### A.  Morphological Descriptions of Airway Gland Formation

Formed from the lateral wall of the foregut (14), the presumptive airways are lined by endodermal cells that are morphologically indistinguishable from each other and resemble the lining cells of the adjacent developing esophagus. These primitive cells eventually differentiate into a variety of cell types within the airway surface epithelium and give rise to airway submucosal glands.

Glands first appear in the rostral human trachea at 10 weeks of fetal life. They later appear more caudally, reaching the carina by 11 weeks (7). During the next few weeks, glands appear in the bronchi (15), where they are more abundant proximally than distally, and are especially concentrated at bifurcations. New gland formation terminates in the middle of the 23rd week, with essentially all of the approximately 5000 glands of adult airways being present before birth. The increase in gland volume in adults is attributable to increasing growth of existing glands (16).

Gland formation occurs via a series of predictable events similar in all species so far examined. First, gland buds arise intraepithelially through the repeated mitosis of progenitor cells. Next, gland buds invade the lamina propria and grow into solid cylinders. Soon after, the solid cylinders develop lumina that communicate with the airway lumen. Finally, the tubes undergo branching and within them mucous and serous cell differentiation occurs.

### B.  What Is the Gland Progenitor Cell?

Because the airway glands are cellularly heterogeneous, consisting of serous, mucous, and myoepithelial cells, it is not apparent whether there is one or more progenitor cells. A similar question was recently resolved experimentally in the case of the gastric gland (17). Like the airway gland, the gastric gland consists of several cell types. Using a two-strain mouse chimera (C3H-BALB/c) and a strain-specific antibody, it was found that each gastric gland in the chimeric mice was composed entirely of either strain-specific antigen-positive or antigen-negative cells; no mixed glands were found. This stongly suggested that individual glands are derived from single pluripotential cells that differentiate into several gland phenotypes. In the absence of information of this kind for the airway glands, it can only be speculated that they too are formed from a single pluripotential progenitor cell. This view is consistent with histological images of solitary nests of dividing cells within the developing epithelium suggestive of clonality.

If we postulate the existence of a single theoretical progenitor cell, it remains to determine the identity of this cell. It was initially suggested that the progenitor for the glands was the airway epithelial basal cell (4,18). This was based on light microscopic images and was influenced by work in other tissues such as the skin showing that basal cells were reponsible for population and renewal of the epithelium as a whole. Recent studies showing that both basal and columnar cells are capable of cell division in the airway epithelium (19,20) have raised the question of which cells are progenitors for which other cells. Electron microscopic analysis of gland formation in the rhesus monkey (12) suggested, in contrast to conclusions reached by earlier light microscopic studies, that columnar cells were progenitor cells for the airway glands. In both the light and electron microscopic studies, hypotheses regarding the identity of the progenitor cell were based on subjective considerations. Definitive identification of the gland cell progenitor awaits double-labeling experiments in which immunochemical phenotype markers (21) and markers of cells undergoing proliferation (22) are used simultaneously.

### C. What Are the Growth Factors Controlling Gland Development?

Like the growth of other epithelial tissues, the growth of airway submucosal glands requires cell division. It has been established that the ordered sequence of events underlying cell division can be set in motion by peptide growth factors. Although the details of the control mechanisms remain poorly understood, it is clear that growth factors exert their effects by binding to, and thereby activating, cell surface receptors, many of which have tyrosine kinase activity (23). These receptor kinases catalyze the phosphorylation of tyrosine residues both within their own polypeptide chains and elsewhere in the cell (24). One important consequence of growth factor-receptor interaction appears to be activation of the synthesis of cyclins, which are proteins that are rate limiting for the activation of p34cdc2 protein kinase (25). It is believed that cdc2 kinase orchestrates cell division by phosphorylating an array of cellular proteins necessary for mitosis.

Growth factors (GFs) usually either affect early $G_0/G_1$ events (competence factors) or later events (progression factors) (26). In most cases, a single growth factor is not able to induce a quiescent cell to pass through $G_1$ and on to mitosis, but rather it acts in concert with other GFs. For example, fibroblast GF (FGF) and platelet-derived GF (PDGF), which normally function as competence factors, might act in concert with epidermal GF (EGF) or insulin-like GF (IGF), which normally function as progression factors. Based on their demonstrated ability to stimulate proliferation of tracheobronchial epithelial cells, EGF, transforming growth factor-$\alpha$ (TGF-$\alpha$), IGF, and keratinocyte G-F (KGF) are more likely than other factors to directly stimulate mitosis in the gland progenitor cells (27–31). EGF is of particular interest, because it has been localized to developing human bronchial submucosal glands by immunocytochemistry (32). Our own recent studies have revealed a peak of KGF RNA during gland development in the 7–14 postnatal day rat trachea. In situ hybridization revealed KGF RNA in the lamina propria at this time period.

### D.  What Is the Identity of Enzymes Permitting Gland Invasion of Connective Tissue?

Like other developmental processes, the growth of airway submucosal glands requires the migration of epithelial cells across basement membranes and through the interstitium. It is assumed that this migration involves proteolytic degradation of extracellular matrix components. Based on previous investigations of other invasive phenomena (33–37), the two major classes of proteinases likely to participate in such a process are the metalloproteinases and the serine proteinases. Both attack collagen, which is a major structural protein of the basement membrane and interstitium and one of the most important targets for proteolysis.

### Metalloproteinases

The metalloproteinases are a family of $Ca^{2+}$- and $Zn^{2+}$-dependent enzymes capable of degrading diverse components of the extracellular matrix. They contain the zinc-chelating motif VAAHExGH as well as the 5′ sequence PRCGxPDV critical to activation of the proenzymes. The metalloproteinase known as interstitial collagenase has a single specific cleavage site in native collagens I and III (38). The metalloproteinases known as gelatinases degrade native collagen (IV, V, VII, and X) to some extent, but they are more active against the denatured form of collagen known as gelatin (39). The major gelatinases are a 72-kDa form (gelatinase A) and a 92-kDa form (gelatinase B). It is likely that these gelatinases act synergistically with interstitial collagenase to degrade collagen in vivo. Other members of the metalloproteinase family degrade not only collagen but also other components of the extracellular matrix. Stromelysin and putative metalloproteinase (PUMP) (now known as matrilysin), for example, can degrade proteoglycans, gelatin, fibronectin, laminin, and elastin (40).

Our early in vitro observations revealed that bovine tracheal gland (BTG) cells, but not bovine tracheal surface epithelial cells, secreted a 72-kDa metalloproteinase (41). The purified proenzyme could be converted to an active 65-kDa form which was highly effective in degrading denatured collagen (gelatin) and also degraded native type I and IV collagens but with much less avidity. In immunoblots, the enzyme was recognized by an antibody directed against human gelatinase A, the 72-kDa gelatinase. Using immunocytochemistry, we showed that the purified enzyme disrupted type IV collagen of the gland basal lamina in situ, and that the gelatinase itself was present in tissue sections at the periphery of some tracheal gland acini in adult cows. These findings led us to explore the potential functions of the 72-kDa gelatinase during gland development.

Rat tracheal glands develop between postnatal days 7 and 28. Gland buds are present by day 7, there is active invasion of the connective tissue between days 7 and 21, and there is additional enlargement of the glands until day 28. Zymography and immunocytochemistry showed that the 72-kDa gelatinase is induced in and near submucosal glands during the invasive phase of their development. That this induction is at least partly controlled at the level of steady state mRNA was indicated by semiquantitative polymerase chain reaction (PCR) analysis of gland-enriched, microdissected tissue samples taken before, during, and after the completion of gland growth. In situ hybridization of tissue samples taken at the same time points revealed that at the peak of the invasive stage of development, the cognate mRNA was present in both epithelial cells of the early postnatal glands and in surrounding fibroblasts. Noninvasive adult glands and the surface epithelium did not contain the 72-kDa gelatinase mRNA. These findings show that the 72-kDa gelatinse is developmentally regulated in airway glands at the level of mRNA and suggest that this enzyme plays a role in the degradation of extracellular matrix during airway gland morphogenesis.

We do not know the mechanism by which the 72-kDa gelatinase gene is activated during airway gland development. Unlike the interstitial collagenase gene, that encoding the 72-kDa gelatinase has not been shown to be induced by cytokines, phorbol esters, growth factors, glucocorticoids, retinoids, or interactions with the extracellular matrix (38), although cell-specific expression is present. Analysis of the interaction of the 72-kDa gelatinase promoter with nuclear proteins before and after activation in the developing glands may shed light on the mechanisms by which the gene is activated.

Metalloproteinases are not only regulated at the level of transcription but may also be regulated at the level of activation of the secreted proenzyme (by proteolytic exposure of the $Zn^{2+}$ binding site) and by the extracellular inhibition of secreted enzyme by specific inhibitors. All three regulatory mechanisms may operate during gland growth. Regulation at the level of activation of the proenzyme can occur for some metalloproteinases through cleavage of the propeptide by plasmin or other proteinases. The mechanism by which the 72-kDa gelatinase is activated in vivo is unknown, although it is recognized that activation can be induced by agents including concanavalin A, phorbol esters, and the growth factor TGF-β (42,43). It is not known whether the activator is itself a proteinase or merely binds the 72-kDa gelatinase to trigger autocatalytic cleavage.

Regulation at the level of extracellular inhibition can occur in response to $\alpha^2$-macroglobulin, although this enzyme has poor access to lytic sites owing to its large size (780 kDa). Probably more biologically significant is inhibition by a family of metalloproteinase-specific inhibitors known as the tissue inhibitors of metalloproteinases (TIMPs). These are produced by many cell types, including connective tissue cells. Of the four members of the TIMP family, two have been well characterized. These have similar structures and functions. TIMP 1 is a 30-kDa glycoprotein (44) and TIMP 2 a 23-kDa unglycosylated protein (45). Both inhibitors form 1:1 complexes with metalloproteinase molecules. The precise mechanism of inhibition is not yet understood.

### Serine Proteinases

The serine proteinases known to play a role in extracellular matrix degradation are those of the plasminogen activator/plasmin system. Plasminogen activators cleave the inactive proenzyme plasminogen to the active proteinase plasmin. Two distinct plasminogen activators exist: tissue-type plasminogen activator (tPA; 70 kDa), which is largely involved in the regulation of clotting, and urokinase-type plasminogen activator (uPA; 50 kDa), which is involved in fibrinolysis as well as in tissue remodeling (38). Both tPA and uPA are secreted as single-chain forms. They differ, however, in that the single-chain form of tPA is active, whereas that of uPA is not (46). Immunocytochemistry has shown that uPA is widespread, being particularly prominent in fibroblasts of the gastrointestinal (GI) tract, trachea, kidney, and placenta (47). That fibroblasts have been seen to contain uPA (37,47) and epithelial cells have been shown to contain the uPA receptor (uPAr [48]) suggests that uPA-mediated invasive activity may occur in a paracrine manner, whereby epithelial cells induce local fibroblasts to produce uPA, bind the secreted enzyme to their own surfaces, and use the focalized enzyme for invasive behavior. The possibility that the uPA-plasmin system plays a role in airway gland growth is supported by our zymography data showing increased uPA activity in the region and time of gland growth. At the same time points, immunocytochemistry reveals uPA in basal cells of the developing surface epithelium and in cells of the developing glands. To help determine whether uPA at these sites is synthesized in the epithelial cells or merely bound via epithelial cell surface receptors, we are performing in situ hybridzation analysis for uPA and uPAR RNA. In vitro gland growth systems are available for determining whether inhibition of uPA impedes the ability of glands to penetrate underlying connective tissue.

Like the regulation of metalloproteinases, that of the plasminogen activators is exerted at three distinct levels: gene transcription, activation, and inhibition. One or more may operate during airway gland growth. Regulation at the level of transcription is modulated by a variety of agents such as phorbol esters, growth factors, peptide and steroid hormones, and retinoids and can be mediated through protein kinase C, cAMP, or tyrosine kinase specific signal transduction pathways (46). Specific growth factors influencing transcription of plasminogen activators include EGF (49), basic FGF (bFGF) (50,51), and PDGF (52). Although the growth factor effects are usually accompanied by cell division, uPA mRNA has also been seen to rise in nondividing cells (53). Regulation at the level of activation is achieved for uPA by cleavage of the single-chain proform, by an unknown activator, to an active two-chain disulfide-linked form. It has been shown that the single-chain pro-uPA is converted to the active two-chain form on binding to the cell surface, presumably to the uPA receptor (54,55). Regulation at the level of inhibition is achieved by the binding of PAs to the specific plasminogen activator inhibitors PAI-1 (45-kDa [56]), PAI-2 (60-kDa [57]), and protease nexin (58). A fourth inhibitor, PAI-3, reacts at a considerably slower rate (46). All are members of the serine protease inhibitor (serpin) superfamily and are found in connective tissue as well as in plasma (46).

### E. Serous and Mucous Cell Differentiation

Differentiation can be defined as the selective activation of specific genes in specific cells. Most eukaryotic genes are inactive in most cells, becoming active during the differentiation of only those cell types whose function requires their expression. Typically, gene activation is mediated by critical changes in chromatin structure, nucleotide methylation, or activation of DNA-binding proteins. These changes are in turn mediated by intracellular signaling pathways triggered by stimuli in the cell's environment. The subset of genes selectively expressed in serous cells is generally concerned with bacteriostatic and antiprotease activity. The subset of genes expressed in mucous cells is generally concerned with the elaboration of gel-forming mucins. The mechanisms mediating the activation of mucous cell–specific and serous cell-specific genes are poorly understood.

#### Epithelial-Mesenchymal Interactions Mediating Cell Differentiation

It has long been recognized that the cellular and biochemical composition of the underlying mesenchyme plays a critical role in the differentiation of epithelial cells (59–69). Heterotypic recombination experiments, in which epithelial and mesenchymal tissues taken from developmentally selected timepoints are apposed in vitro, have shown that the expression of transcription factors controlling differentiation of tooth epithelium (msx 1 and msx 2 [70]), hepatic epithelium (HNF3a and eH-TF [59,71,72]), and prostatic epithelium (testosterone-receptor complexes [73]) does not occur in the absence of mesenchyme taken from the appropriate anatomical location and developmental time point. The observation that airway gland formation and differentiation occur almost exclusively in regions overlying cartilage plates (12) suggests that cartilage-derived molecules control both gland morphogenesis and the differentiation of gland cells. Evidence supporting an instructive role for human fetal fibroblasts in airway gland morphogenesis (74) has already been obtained.

Extracellular signals affecting epithelial cell differentiation correspond not only to diffusible molecules released by mesenchymal cells but also to basement membrane molecules secreted by the epithelial cells themselves. For example, it has been found that β–casein expression in mammary epithelial cells requires the interaction of laminin with appropriate epithelial cell receptors; that is, the β1-integrins (75). The effect is regulated transcriptionally by a response element in the 5' flanking region of the β-casein gene (76,77). Airway gland cells are similarly responsive to signals transmitted by basement membrane components through β1-integrins (68). Details of the regulatory mechanism are currently unknown.

### Transcription Factors

Of particular interest to any discussion of cell differentiation is the subclass of transcription factors that do not merely control the transcription of one or a few specific genes but are able to influence overall patterns of cell differentiation. This is achieved through the binding of the transcription factor to the promoters of multiple tissue-specific target genes. Examples include the myogenic basic helix-loop-helix transcription factors (MyoD, myogenin, Myf-5, and herculin [78]), the hepatogenic transcription factors HNF 1–4 (79), and the pituitary-specific transcription factor pit-1 (80). Typically, in addition to activating tissue-specific genes (e.g., muscle filament proteins in myocytes), these master regulatory genes are active early in development (81–83), are evolutionarily conserved (81,82), and positively regulate their own transcription or that of other regulatory genes (84,85).

In the case of skeletal muscle, evidence for the existence of a master regulator gene emerged from experiments in which an embryonic fibroblast cell line (10T1/2) was subjected to demethylation by use of the agent 5-azacytidine (86). The high frequency of conversion to the myogenic phenotype suggested that the conversion was achieved by the activation of only a few genes. Later, experiments showed that the aza-myoblasts, but not the parental 10T1/2 cells, were able to drive the promoters of cloned muscle-specific genes on transfection (87). This indicated that demethylation by 5-azacytidine had activated the expression of muscle-specific transcription factors in the fibroblast cell line. The identification of these transcription factors was achieved using a subtractive hybridization approach using RNA from both aza-myoblasts and the parental cell line (88). Forced expression of one of these, MyoD, was sufficient to convert 10T1/2 cells to determined myoblasts. This approach has been used in subsequent studies to induce expression of other differentiation-associated genes (89–93).

Transcription factors, whether involved in the hierarchical control of phenotype or the control of a single tissue-specific gene, are among the most intriguing elements regulating gene expression (94). These proteins are crucial links in the transduction of extracellular signals to the cell nucleus, permitting cells to respond to changing environmental signals. The usual strategy for identifying transcription factors controlling gene activity involves (1) transfection analysis to identify DNA regulatory regions, (2) gel shift and footprinting analysis to localize protein binding sites, and (3) affinity isolation of binding proteins. This is our primary strategy in the determination of mechanisms controlling serous and mucous cell differentiation. Progress with respect to the serous cell gene lysozyme and the mucous cell gene mucin is outlined below.

### Lysozyme: Transcriptional Regulation of a Serous Cell Marker Gene

Lysozyme (also known as muramidase [EC 3.2.1.17]) is an enzyme catalyzing the hydrolysis of (1–4) glycosidic bonds between N-acetylmuramic acid and N-acetyl-D-glucosamine, constituents of the cell walls of most bacteria. Its antibacterial properties render it an important participant in mucosal defense at body surfaces and in leukocytes (95–97). Lysozyme is a differentiation marker for serous cells in the airway glands because it is selectively expressed by serous cells and not by mucous cells (98). We recently showed (99) that this selective expression of lysozyme is attributable to regulatory mechanisms controlling steady-state mRNA.

A common mechanism by which cells control steady state levels of specific mRNAs is through protein-DNA interactions occurring in the 5'-flanking region of a gene. With respect to lysozyme, this type of interaction has so far been analyzed only in the myeloid cell lineage and oviduct of the chicken (100–105).

Our analysis of mechanisms regulating lysozyme transcription in the serous cell began in the cow because of the quality and abundance of starting material for cell isolation from that species. Because at least 10 lysozyme genes exist in the cow (106), however, identification of *lys 5a* as the principal lysozyme gene expressed by cow serous cells was a necessary first step (107).

To identify DNA regulatory elements and transcription factors controlling *lys 5a* transcription, we characterized the regulatory activity and DNA-protein interactions of the 5'-flanking region of this gene. Although approximately 94 bp of 5'-flanking DNA were necessary for high-level expression in transient transfection assays, an evolutionarily conserved promoter within 66 bp of the transcription start site was sufficient to confer serous cell–specific expression. Farther upstream, within 6.1 kb of the 5'-flanking region, were four silencers. Analysis of the serous cell–specific lysozyme promoter by electrophoretic mobility shift assay (EMSA) revealed the presence of binding sites for three serous cell nuclear proteins, which were designated LSF1, LSF2, and LSF3. Binding of LSF2 and LSF3 was localized to a 20-mer subdomain (-50/-30) of the cell-specific promoter using binding competition assays. More accurate identification of the protein binding site(s) was achieved through the use of mutagenesis, which implicated the motif 5'AAGGAAT3' (-46/-40) in both protein binding and serous cell–specific transcriptional activity. This motif has previously been identified as a binding site for ets protein transcription factors, suggesting that serous cell–specific regulation of *lys 5a* transcription is partly controlled by the binding of ets-like protein(s) to the motif 5'AGGAAGT 3'. That the promoters of other serous cell–specific genes also contain ets binding sites suggests that ets proteins may control the establishment of the serous cell phenotype as a whole. Experiments examining the synthesis and activation of ets proteins at the time of lysozyme gene activation in tracheal gland development should elucidate the role of ets proteins in the developmental control of lysozyme transcription in serous gland cells.

### Mucin: Transcriptional Activation of a Mucous Cell Marker Gene

Mucin is a glycoprotein, the polypeptide portion of which is encoded by a gene family presently including eight members, MUC 1-8 (108-116). Among these, the most extensively studied and the only ones for which the aminoterminal sequence is known are MUC 1 (117), MUC 2 (118,119), and MUC 7 (115). Whereas MUC 1 encodes a cell surface glycoprotein and MUC 7 encodes a small salivary glycoprotein unlikely to contribute to airway obstruction, MUC 2 encodes a secreted mucin that could participate in airway obstruction if overproduced.

The human MUC 2 gene, although originally isolated from the intestine, encodes mucins synthesized in several organs, including the airway (120). To facilitate our studies of mucin gene activation in airway gland development and disease, we have established experimental models in the rat, necessitating the isolation of rat mucin cDNAs and genomic clones. To obtain these, we first screened a rat intestinal cDNA library using an upstream nontandem repeat cDNA fragment of the human MUC 2 gene (SMUC 313 [118]). Three cDNAs were isolated: 1-1, 8-1, and 21-1. A translation start site was found in cDNA 21-1. Combined nucleotide sequence for the three cDNAs contained an open reading frame spanning 4546 bp (119). This aminoterminal sequence contained a nontandem repeat domain enriched in cysteine (1392 residues) followed by an irregular tandem repeat domain (123 residues). Identity between this "rat MUC 2" gene and the human gene is about 80% in the nontandem repeat domain and about 35% in the irregular tandem repeat domain. Northern analysis showed expression of cognate RNA in the intestine and airway but not heart and spleen.

To obtain genomic clones containing the gene promoter, we screened a rat genomic library with the 5'-most region of cDNA 8-1, resulting in the isolation of an 18-kb genomic clone. Restriction mapping and sequencing identified a 1.4-kb subfragment containing the entire first exon and 5'-flanking sequence. Analysis of products of S1 nuclease protection assays and primer extension indicated that the major transcription start site was 28 bp upstream of the Kozak-associated ATG codon in our cDNA sequence.

Sequencing has so far provided the sequence of the 5'-flanking region extending to bp -1113. Computer subsequence analysis revealed the presence of potential transcriptional regulatory elements within this region including a TATA box, NFκB, AP1, SP1, PEA3 sites and an E box. To identify DNA sequences responsible for gland cell-specific MUC 2 transcription, we performed transient transfection assays using a series of plasmids containing variable length fragments of the rat MUC 2 5'-flanking sequence fused to a CAT expression unit. Plasmids were transfected into (1) SPOC 1, a spontaneously transformed rat tracheal epithelial cell line that forms glands when seeded onto denuded tracheal grafts (121); (2) HM 3, a high mucin–secreting human colon carcinoma cell line; and (3) NIH 3T3 mouse fibroblasts. The ongoing analysis of deletion mutants in these cell lines has so far revealed SPOC 1–specific transcriptional elements in fragment (-98/+7) and HM-3–specific elements in fragment (-295/-186). Still in its early stages, this work is being extended to define more accurately the motifs responsible for airway gland cell–specific expression of MUC 2.

The most significant information that could potentially arise from this type of analysis would be information suggesting the mechanisms by which serous and mucous cells differentiate from a common progenitor cell. Our work on the lysozyme promoter (see above) has revealed a transcription factor binding motif responsible for serous cell–specific lysozyme transcription that is also present in the promoters of multiple serous cell–specific genes (122). Our work on the mucin promoter, although less advanced, has revealed the presence of potential binding sites for AP 2 and HNF 5 also present in promoters of cytokeratin 19 and β1–4-galactosyltransferase (genes coexpressed in mucous cells). The existence of these shared motifs is consistent with the possibility that serous and mucous cell differentiation from a common progenitor cell are controlled by master regulatory genes or a hierarchy of several such genes. If so, knowledge of the gene regulatory pathways could potentially facilitate drug discovery efforts to selectively control differentiation and ensure an optimal balance of serous and mucous cells in the glands.

### References

1. Reid L. Measurement of the bronchial mucous gland layer: a diagnostic yardstick in chronic bronchitis. Thorax 1960; 15:132–141.
2. Snider G. Pathogenesis of emphysema and chronic bronchitis. Med Clin North Am 1981; 65:647–665.
3. Oppenheimer EH, Esterly JR. Pathology of cystic fibrosis: review of the literature and comparison with 146 autopsied cases. Perspect Pediatr Pathol 1975; 2:241–278.
4. Bucher U, Reid L. Development of the mucus-secreting elements in human lung. Thorax 1961; 16:219–225.
5. Thurlbeck W, Benjamin B, Reid L. Development and distribution of mucous glands in the fetal human trachea. Brit Dis Chest 1961; 55:54–64.
6. Tos M. Distribution and situation of the mucous glands in the main bronchus of human foetuses. Anat Anz Bd 1968; 123:481–495.
7. Tos M. Development of the tracheal glands in man. Acta Pathol Microbiol Scand 1966; 68(suppl 185):1–129.
8. Tos M. Development of the mucous glands in the human main bronchus. Anat Anz Bd 1968; 123:376–389.

9.  Lamb D, Reid L. Acidic glycoproteins produced by the mucous cells of the bronchial submucosal glands in the fetus and child: a histochemical autoradiographic study. Br J Dis Chest 1972; 66:248–253.

10. Smolich JJ, Stratford BF, Maloney JE, Ritchie BC. New features in the development of the submucosal gland of the respiratory tract. J Anat 1978; 127:223–238.

11. Sorokin SP. On the cytology and cytochemistry of the opossum's bronchial glands. J Anat 1965; 117:311–338.

12. Plopper CG, Weir AJ, Nishio SJ, Cranz DL, St. George JA. Tracheal submucosal gland development in the rhesus monkey, Macaca mulatta: ultrastructure and histochemistry. Anat Embryol 1986; 174:167–178.

13. Leigh MW, Gambling TM, Carson JL, Collier AM, Wood RE, Boat TF. Postnatal development of tracheal surface epithelium and submucosal glands in the ferret. Exp Lung Res 1986; 10:153–169.

14. Balinsky BI. An Introduction to Embryology. Philadelphia: Saunders, 1963.

15. Tos M. Development of the mucous glands in the human main bronchus. Anat Anz Bd 1968; 123:376–389.

16. Jeffery PK, Reid L. Ultrastructure of airway epithelium and submucosal gland during development. In: Hodson WA, ed. The Development of the Lung. New York: Dekker, 1977:87–134.

17. Tatematsu M, Fukami H, Yamamoto M, Nakanishi H, Masui T, Kusakabe N, Sakakura T. Clonal analysis of glandular stomach carcinogenesis in C3H/HeN–BALB/c chimeric mice treated with N-methyl-N-nitrosourea. Cancer Lett 1994; 83: 37–42.

18. Tos M. Distribution and situation of the mucous glands in the main bronchus of human foetuses. Anat Anz Bd 1968; 123:481–495.

19. Evans MJ, Shami SG, Cabral-Anderson LJ, Dekker NP. Role of nonciliated cells in renewal of the bronchial epithelium of rats exposed to $NO_2$. Am J Pathol 1986; 123: 126–133.

20. Zhang X-M, McDowell EM. Vitamin A deficiency and inflammation: the pivotal role of secretory cells in the development of atrophic, hyperplastic and metaplastic change in the tracheal epithelium in vivo. Virchows Archiv B Cell Pathol 1992; 61: 375–387.

21. Randell SH, Shimuizu T, Bakewell W, Ramaekers FCS, Nettesheim P. Phenotypic marker expression during fetal and neonatal differentiation of rat tracheal epithelial cells. Am J Respir Cell Mol Biol 1993; 8:546–555.

22. Waseem N, Lane D. Monoclonal antibody analysis of the proliferating cellnuclear antigen (PCNA). Structural conservation and the detection of anucleolar form. J Cell Sci 1990; 96:121–129.

23. Ullrich A, Schlessinger J. Signal transduction by receptors with tyrosine kinase activity. Cell 1990; 61:203–212.

24. Rosen O, Herrera R, Olowe Y, Petruzelli L, Cobb M. Phosphorylation activates the insulin receptor tyrosine kinase. Proc Nat Acad Sci USA 1983; 80:3237–3240.

25. Solomon M, Glotzer M, Lee T, Philippe Kirschner M. Cyclin activation of p34cdc2. Cell 1990; 63:1013–1024.

26. King R, Jones M, Minoo P. Regulation of lung cell proliferation by polypeptide growth factors. Am J Physiol 1989; 1:L23–L38.
27. Lechner J, Haugen A, Autrup I, McClendon B, Trump F, Harris C. Clonal growth of epithelium from normal human bronchus. Cancer Res 1981; 41:2294–2304.
28. Lechner J, Laveck M. A serum-free method for culturing normal bronchial epithelial cells. J Tissue Cult Methods 1985; 9:43–48.
29. Thomassen D, Saffiotti U, Kaighn M. Clonal proliferation of rat tracheal epithelial cells in serum-free medium and their responses to hormones, growth factors and carcinogens. Carcinogenesis 1986; 7:2033–2039.
30. Wu R. In vitro differentiation of airway epithelial cells. In: Schiff, ed. In Vitro Models of Respiratory Epithelium. Boca Raton, FL: CRC Press, 1987:1–26.
31. Finch P, Rubin J, Miki T, Ron D, Aaronson S. Human KGF is FGF-related with properties of a paracrine effector of epithelial cell growth. Science 1989; 245:752–755.
32. Stahlman M, Orth D, Gray M. Immunocytochemical localization of epidermal growth factor in the developing human respiratory system and in acute and chronic lung disease in the neonate. Lab Invest 1989; 60:539–547.
33. Reponen P, Sahlberg C, Huhtala P, Hurskainen T, Thesleff I, Tryggvason K. Molecular cloning of murine 72-kDa type IV collagenase and its expression during mouse development. J Biol Chem 1992; 267:7856–7862.
34. Talhouk RS, Chin JR, Unemori EN, Werb Z, Bissell MJ. Proteinases of the mammary gland: developmental regulation in vivo and vectorial secretion in culture. Development 1991; 112:439–449.
35. Sheffield J, Graff D. Extracellular proteases in developing chick neural retina. Exp Eye Res 1991; 52:733–741.
36. Butler T, Zhu C, Mueller R, Fuller G, Lemaire W, Woessner J. Inhibition of ovulation in the perfused rat ovary by the synthetic collagenase inhibitor SC44463. Biol Reprod 1991; 4:1183–1188.
37. Grandahl-Hansen J, Ralfkiaer E, Kirkeby L, Kristenssen P, Lund L, Dano K. Localization of urokinase-type plasminogen activator in stromal cells in adenocarcinomas of the colon in humans. Am J Pathol 1991; 138:111–117.
38. Alexander CM, Werb A. Extracellular matrix degradation. In: Day ED, ed. Cell Biology of Extracellular Matrix. New York: Plenum Press, 1991:255–301.
39. Murphy G, Hembry R, Hughes C, Fosang A, Hardingham T. Role and regulation of metalloproteinases in connective tissue turnover. Biochem Soc Trans 1990; 18: 812–815.
40. Alexander CM, Werb Z. Proteinases and extracellular matrix remodeling. Curr Opin Cell Biol 1989; 1:974–982.
41. Tournier J-M, Polette M, Hinnrasky J, Beck J, Werb Z, Basbaum C. Expression of gelatinase A, a mediator of extracellular matrix remodeling, by tracheal gland cells in culture and in vivo. J Biol Chem 1994; 269:25454–25464.
42. Murphy G, Docherty AJP. The matrix metalloproteinases and their inhibitors. Am J Respir Cell Mol Biol 1992; 7:120–125.
43. Matrisian L. Metalloproteinases and their inhibitors in matrix remodeling. Trends Genet 1990; 6:121–125.

44. Docherty A, Lyons A, Smith B. Sequence of human tissue inhibitor of metallo-proteinases and its identity to erytroid-potentiating activity. Nature 1985; 318: 66–69.
45. Boone T, Johnson M, DeClerck Y, Langley K. cDNA cloning and expression of a metalloproteinase inhibitor related to tissue inhibitor of metalloproteinases. Proc Natl Acad Sci USA 1990; 87:2800–2804.
46. Saksela O, Rifkin DB. Cell-associated plasminogen activation: regulation and physiological functions. Ann Rev Cell Biol 1988; 4:93–126.
47. Larsson L, Skriver L, Nielson L, Grondahl-Hansen J, Kristensen P, Dano K. Distribution of urokinase-type plasminogen activator in the mouse. J Cell Biol 1984; 98: 894–903.
48. Hollas W, Balsi F, Boyd D. Role of the urokinase receptor in facilitating extracellular matrix invasion by cultured colon cancer. Cancer Res 1991; 51:3690–3695.
49. Grimaldi G, Di Fiore P, Locatelli E, Falco J, Blasi F. Modulation of urokinase plasminogen activator gene expression during the transition from quiescent to proliferative state in normal mouse cells. EMBO J 1986; 5:855–861.
50. Moscatelli D, Presta M, Rifkin D. Purification of a factor from human placenta that stimulates capillary endothelial cell protease production. Proc Natl Acad Sci (USA) 1986; 83:2091–2095.
51. Presta M, Moscatelli D, Joseph-Silverstein J, Rifkin D. Purification from a human hepatoma cell line of a basic fibroblast growth factor-like molecule that stimulates capillary endothelial cell plasminogen activator production, DNA synthesis and migration. Mol Cell Biol 1986; 6:4060–4066.
52. Stopelli M, Verdi P, Grimaldi G, Locatelli E, Blasi F. Increase in urokinase plasminogen activator mRNA synthesis in human carcinoma cells is a primary effect of the potent tumor promoter, phorbol myristate acetate. J Cell Biol 1986; 102:1235–1241.
53. Saksela O, Moscatelli D, Rifkin D. The opposing effects of basic fibroblast growth factor and transforming growth factor β on the regulation of plasminogen activator activity in capillary endothelial cells. J Cell Biol 1987; 105:957–963.
54. Berkenpas M, Quigley J. Transformation-dependent activation of urokinase-type plasminogen activator by a plasmin-dependent mechanism: involvement of cell surface membranes. Proc Natl Acad Sci USA 1991; 88:7768–7772.
55. Manchanda N, Schwartz B. Single chain urokinase: augmentation of enzymatic activity upon binding to monocytes. J Biol Chem 1991; 266:14580–14584.
56. Loskutoff D, Linders M, Keijer J, Veerman H, van Heerikhuizen H, Pannekoek H. Structure of the human plasminogen activator inhibitor gene: nonrandom distribution of introns. Biochemistry 1987; 26:3763–3768.
57. Kawano T, Mormoto K, Uemura Y. Partial purification and propertiew of urokinase inhibitor from human placenta. J Biochem 1970; 67:333–342.
58. Baker J, Low D, Simmer R, Cunningham D. Protease nexin: a cellular component that links thrombin and plasminogen activator and mediates their binding to cells. Cell 1980; 21:37–45.
59. DiPersio CM, Jackson DA, Zaret KS. The extracellular matrix coordinately modulates liver transcription factors and hepatocyte morphology. Mol Cell Biol 1991; 11:4405–4414.

60. Cutler LS. The role of extracellular matrix in the morphogenesis and differentiation of salivary glands. FASEB J 1990; 3:27–36.
61. Roskelley CD, Desprez PY, Bissell MJ. Extracellular matrix-dependent tissue-specific gene expression in mammary epithelial cells requires both physical and biochemical signal transduction. Proc Natl Acad Sci USA 1994; 91:12378–12382.
62. Flaumenhaft R, Rifkin D. Extracellular matrix regulation of growth factor an protease activity. Cell Biol 1991; 3:817–823.
63. Hall DE, Neugebauer KM, Reichardt LF. Embryonic neural retinal cell response to extracellular matrix proteins: Developmental changes and effects of the cell substratum attachment antibody (CSAT). J Cell Biol 1987; 104:623–634.
64. Kraemer PM. Perspectives in extracellular matrix research: the role of cell culture models. In Hawkes S, Wang, J, eds. Extracellular Matrix. New York: Academic Press, 1982:3–11.
65. Maresh GA, Timmons TM, Dunbar BS. Effects of extracellular matrix on the expression of specific ovarian proteins. Biol Reprod 1990; 43:965–976.
66. McGowan SE. Extracellular matrix and the regulation of lung development and repair. FASEB J 1992; 6:2895–2904.
67. Silberstein GB, Flanders KC, Roberts AB, Daniel CW. Regulation of mammary morphogenesis: Evidence for extracellular matrix-mediated inhibition of ductal budding by transforming growth factor-β1. Dev Biol 1992; 152:354–362.
68. Tournier J-M, Goldstein GR, Hall DE, Damsky CH, Basbaum CB. Extracellular matrix proteins regulate morphological and biochemical properties of tracheal gland serous cells through integrins. Am J Respir Cell Mol Biol 1992; 6:461–467.
69. Woodcock-Mitchell J, Rannels SR, Mitchell J, Rannels DE, Low RB. Modulation of keratin expression in type II pneumocytes by the extracellular matrix. Am Rev Respir Dis 1989; 139:343–351.
70. Jowett A, Vainio S, Ferguson M, Sharpe P, Thesleff I. Epithelial-mesenchymal interactions are required for msx 1 and msx 2 gene expression in the developing murine tooth. Development 1993; 117:461–470.
71. Liu J-K, DiPersio CM, Zaret KS. Extracellular signals that regulate liver transcription factors during hepatic differentiation in vitro. Mol Cell Biol 1991; 11:773–784.
72. Cooke PS, Uchima F-D A, Fujii DK, Bern HA, Cunha GR. Restoration of normal morphology and estrogen responsiveness in cultured vaginal and uterine epithelia transplanted with stroma. Proc Natl Acad Sci USA 1986; 83:2109–2113.
73. Cunha G, Alarid E, Turner T, Donjacour A, Boutin E, Foster B. Normal and abnormal development of the male urogenital tract: role of androgens, mesenchymal-epithelial interactions, and growth factors. J Androl 1992; 13:465–475.
74. Infeld MD, Brennan JA, Davis PB. Human fetal fibroblasts promote invasion of extracellular matrix by normal human tracheobronchial epithelial cells in vitro: a model of airway gland development. Am J Respir Cell Mol Biol 1993; 8:69–76.
75. Streuli C, Bailey N, Bissell M. Control of mammary epithelial differentiation: basement membrane induces tissue-specific gene expression in the absence of cell-cell interaction and morphological polarity. J Cell Biol 1991; 115:1383–1395.
76. Schmidhauser C, Bissell M, Meyers C, Casperson G. Proc Natl Acad Sci (USA) 1990; 87:9118–9122.

77. Schmidhauser C, Casperson G, Meyers C, Sanzo K, Bolton S, Bissell M. A novel transcriptional enhancer is involved in the prolactin- and extracellular matrix-dependent regulation of beta casein gene expression. Mol Biol Cell 1992; 3:699–709.

78. Lassar A, Munsterberg A. Wiring diagrams: regulatory circuits and the control of skeletal myogenesis. Curr Opin Cell Biol 1994; 6:432–442.

79. Crabtree G, Schibler, U, Scott M. Trascriptional regulatory mechanisms in liver and midgut morphogenesis of vertebrates and invertebrates. Vol 2, McKnight S, Yamamoto K, eds. Cold Spring Harbor, NY: Cold Spring Harbor Laboratory Press, 1994: 1063–1102.

80. Simmons D, Voss J, Ingraham H, Hollaway J, Broide R, Rosenfeld M, Swanson L. Pituitary cell phenotypes involve cell-specific Pit-1 mRNA translation and synergistic interactions with other classes of transcription factors. Genes Dev 1990; 4: 695–711.

81. Sassoon D. Myogenic regulatory factors: Dissecting their role and regulation during vertebrate embryogenesis. Dev Bio 1993; 156:11–23.

82. Ang S-L, Wierda A, Wong D, Stevens K, Cascio S, Rossant J, Zaret K. The formation and maintenance of the definitive endoderm lineage in the mouse: involvement of HNF3/forkhead proteins. Development 1993; 119:1301–1315.

83. Cheng T, Hanley T, Mudd J, Merlie J, Olson E. Mapping of myogenin transcription during embryogenesis using transgenes linked to the myogenin control region. J Cell Biol 1992. 119:1649–1656.

84. Thayer M, Tapscott S, Davis R, Wright W, Lassar A, Weintraub H. Positive autoregulation of the myogenic determination gene MyoD1. Cell 1989; 58(2):241–248.

85. Miner J, Wold B. Herculin, a fourth member of the MyoD family of myogenic regulatory genes. Proc Natl Acad Sci (USA) 1990; 87:1089–1093.

86. Taylor S, Jones P. Multiple new phenotypes induced in 10T1/2 and 3T3 cells treated with 5-azacytidine. Cell 1979; 63:23–32.

87. Konieczny S, Emerson C. Differentiation, not determination regulates muscle gene activation: transfection of troponin I genes into multipotential and muscle lineages of 10T½ cells. Mol Cell Biol 1985; 5:2423–2432.

88. Davis R, Weintraub H, Lassar A. Expression of a single transfected cDNA converts fibroblasts to myoblasts. Cell 1987; 51:987–1000.

89. Caraglia M, Pinto A, Correale P, Zagonal V, Genua G, Leardi A, Pepe S, Bianco A, Tagliaferri P. 5-Aza-2'-deoxycytidine induces growth inhibition and upregulation of epidermal growth factor receptor on human epithelial cancer cells. Ann Oncol 1994; 5:269–276.

90. Baik J, Chikhi N, Bulle F, Giuli G, Guellaen G, Siegrist S. Repetitive 5-azacytidine treatments of Fao cells induce a stable and strong expression of gamma-glutamyl transpeptidase. J Cell Physiol 1992; 153:408–416.

91. Endo T, Ishibashi Y, Shiokawa S, Fukumaki Y, Okano H. Differential induction of adult and fetal globin gene expression in the human CML cell subline KU-812F/33. J Biochem 1994; 115:540–544.

92. Visvader J, Adams J. Megakaryocytic differentiation induced in 416B myeloid cells by GATA-2 and GATA-3 transgenes or 5-azacytidine is tightly coupled to GATA-1 expression. Blood 1993; 82:1493–1501.

93. Kroll T, Peters B, Hustad C, Jones P, Killen P, Ruddon R. Expression of laminin chains during myogenic differentiation. J Biol Chem 1994; 269:9270–9277.

94. Mitchell P, Tjian R. Transcriptional regulation in mammalian cells by sequence-specific DNA binding proteins. Science 1989; 245:371–378.

95. Klockars M, Reitamo S. Tissue distribution of lysozyme in man. J Histochem Cytochem 1975; 23:932–940.

96. Klockars M, Osserman EF. Localization of lysozyme in normal rat tissues by an immunoperoxidase method. J Histochem Cytochem 1974; 22:139–146.

97. Mason D, Taylor C. The distribution of muramidase (lysozyme) in human tissues. J Clin Res 1975; 28:124–132.

98. Bowes D, Corrin B. Ultrastructural immunocytochemical localisation of lysozyme in human bronchial glands. Thorax 1977; 32:163–170.

99. Dohrman A, Tsuda T, Escudier E, Cardone M, Jany B, Gum J, Kim Y, Basbaum C. Distribution of lysozyme and mucin (MUC 2 and MUC 3) mRNA in human bronchus. Exp Lung Res 1994; 20:367–380.

100. Matthias P, Renkawitz R, Grez M, Schutz G. EMBO J 1982; 1(10):1207–1212.

101. Renkawitz GR, Schutz R, von der Ahe D, Beato M. Sequences in the promoter region of the chicken lysozyme gene required for steroid regulation and receptor binding. Cell 1984; 37:503–510.

102. Hecht A, Berkenstam A, Stromstedt P, Gustafsson J, Sippel A. A progesterone-responsive element maps to the far upstream steroid-dependent DNase hypersensitive site of chicken lysozyme chromatin. EMBO J 1988; 7:2063–2073.

103. Steiner C, Muller M, Baniahmad A, Renkawitz R. Lysozyme gene activity in chicken macrophages is controlled by positive and negative regulatory elements. Nucleic Acids Res 1987; 15:4163–4178.

104. Theisen M, Stief A, Sippel A. The lysozyme enhancer: cell-specific activation of the chicken lysozyme gene by a far upstream DNA element. EMBO J 1986; 5:719–724.

105. Baniahmad A, Muller M, Steiner C, Renkawitz R. Activity of two different silencer elements of the chicken lysozyme gene can be compensated by enhancer elements. EMBO J 1987; 6:2297–2303.

106. Irwin DM, Sidow A, White RT, Wilson AC. Multiple genes for ruminant lysozymes. In: Smith-Gill S, Sercarz BB, eds. The Immune Response to Structurally Defined Proteins: The Lysozyme Model. Guilderland, NY: Adenine Press, 1989:73–85.

107. Takeuchi K, Irwin D, Gallup M, Shinbrot E, Stewart C-B, Basbaum C. Multiple cDNA sequences encoding bovine tracheal lysozyme. J Biol Chem 1993; 268: 27440–27446.

108. Gendler SJ, Lancaster CA, Taylor-Papadimitriou J, Duhig T, Peat N, Burchell J, Pemberton K, Lalani EN, Wilson D. Molecular cloning and expression of human tumor-associated polymorphic epithelial mucin. J Biol Chem 1990; 265:15286–15293.

109. Porchet N, Van Cong N, Dufosse J, Audie JP, Guyonnet-Duperat V, Gross MS, Denis C, Degand P, Bernheim A, Aubert JP. Molecular cloning and chromosomal localization of a novel human tracheo-bronchial mucin cDNA containing tandemly repeated sequences of 48 base pairs. Biochem Biophys Res Commun 1991; 175:414–422.

110. Aubert J-P, Porchet N, Crepin M, Duterque-Coquillaud M, Vergnes G, Mazzuca M,

Debuire B, Petiprez D, Degand P. Evidence for different human tracheobronchial mucin peptides deduced from nucleotide cDNA sequences. Am J Respir Cell Mol Biol 1991; 5:178–185.

111. Gum JR, Byrd JC, Hicks JW, Toribara NW, Lamport DTA, Kim YS. Molecular cloning of human intestinal mucin cDNAs. J Biol Chem 1989; 264:6480–6487.

112. Toribara N, Roberton A, Ho S, Kuo W-L, Gum E, Hicks J, Gum J, Byrd J, Siddiki B, Kim Y. Human gastric mucin: identification of a unique species by expression cloning. J Biol Chem 1993; 268:5879–5885.

113. Gum JR, Hicks JW, Swallow DM, Lagace RL, Byrd JC, Lamport DTA, Siddiki B, Kim YS. Molecular cloning of cDNAs derived from a novel human intestinal mucin gene. Biochem Biophys Res Commun 1990; 171:407–415.

114. Meerzamam D, Charles P, Daskal E, Polymeropoulos M, Martin B, Rose M. Cloning and analysis of cDNA encoding a major airway glycoprotein, human tracheo-bronchial mucin (MUC 5). J Biol Chem 1984; 269:12932–12939.

115. Bobek L, Tsai H, Biesbrock A, Levine M. Molecular cloning, sequence, and speci-ficity of expression of the gene encoding the low molecular weight human salivary mucin (MUC 7). J Biol Chem 1993; 268:20563–20569.

116. Shankar V, Gilmore M, Elkins R, Sachdev G. A novel human airway mucin cDNA encodes a protein with unique tandem-repeat organization. Biochem J 1994; 300: 295–298.

117. Gendler S, Spicer A, Lalani EN, Duhig T, Peat N, Burchell J, Pemberton L, Boshell M, Taylor-Papadimitriou J. Structure and biology of a carcinoma-associated mucin, MUC 1. Am Rev Respir Dis 1991; 144:S42–S47.

118. Gum J, Hicks J, Toribara N, Siddiki B, Kim Y. Molecular cloning of human intestinal mucin (MUC 2) cDNA: identification of the amino terminus and overall sequence similarity to pre-pro-von Willebrand factor. J Biol Chem 1994; 269:2440–2446.

119. Ohmori H, Dohrman A, Gallup M, Kai H, Gum J, Kim Y, Basbaum C. Molecular cloning of the amino terminal region of a rat MUC 2 mucin gene homologue. J Biol Chem 1994; 269:17833–17840.

120. Jany B, Gallup M, Yan P, Gum J, Kim Y, Basbaum C. Human bronchus and intestine express the same mucin gene. J Clin Invest 1991; 87:77–82.

121. Doherty M, Liu J, Randell S, Carter C, Davis W, Nettesheim P, Ferriola P. Phenotype and differentiation potential of a novel rat tracheal epithelial cell line. Am J Respir Cell Mol Biol 1995; 12:385–395.

122. Kai H, Takeuchi K, Ohmori H, Gallup M, Basbaum C. PEA 3 motif contributes to tracheal gland serous cell-specific lysozyme transcription. J Cell Biochem 1996 (in press).

# 7

## Clara Cells

**CHARLES G. PLOPPER**

University of California
Davis School of Veterinary Medicine
Davis, California

## I.  Introduction—Defining a Clara cell

The epithelium of distal conducting airways generally consists of two epithelial populations: ciliated and nonciliated, or Clara, cells. The role of the nonciliated population in normal lung function and during lung development is not well understood. Studies oriented toward defining specific functions for the Clara cell population in the normal lung and establishing the developmental pattern for and regulation of Clara cell differentiation are complicated owing to the great inter-species heterogeneity in distribution and phenotypic expression of this cell population. Because of the heterogeneity of Clara cell phenotypic expression in the adult, developing a satisfactory working definition for this cell type is difficult. The early descriptions, especially those by Max Clara, were of the nonciliated epithelial cells lining the distal conducting airways at the junction with the gas exchange area (1). They were cuboidal cells which extended from the basement membrane to the lumen and had basal nuclei and apical secretory granules. Two species were studied: humans and rabbits. As described below, we now know that these cells differ markedly between the two species in a number of ultrastructural features, including: the abundance of smooth endoplasmic reticulum and apical secretory granules and the extent of the apical projection into the lumen. We also know that the distribution of cells with those characteristics differs throughout the airway tree, as does the organization of the microenvironment (terminal and respiratory, or transitional, bronchioles) in which they are found. For the purposes of this chapter, we have used the following definition for Clara cells: cuboidal to columnar (nonsquamous) epithelial cells which line the distal conducting airways, extend from the basal lamina to the lumen and lack cilia, long apical microvilli, and dense-cored neurosecretory granules. Epithelial cells in more proximal airways which have the same ultrastructural features as those in the distal airways of that species are also considered Clara cells.

This chapter takes a two-step approach to the developmental biology of Clara cells. The first is to summarize the aspects of the biology of this phenotype which are relevant to understanding Clara cell development, including; (1) the characteristics of the microenvironment in which Clara cells are found, (2) the phenotypic markers for the differentiated cell, (3) the functional significance of these markers, and (4) the role of the nonciliated cells in the kinetic activity of the bronchioles. Secondly, based on the phenotypic characteristics of this cell population in adults, the pattern of cytodifferentiation is evaluated for each of the phenotypic markers and the mechanisms regulating marker expression during development are discussed.

## II. Bronchiolar Microenvironment in Adults

In adult mammals, the principal location of Clara cells is the proximal, or central, portion of the pulmonary acinus. This is the zone of transition between the conducting airways and the gas-exchange area. The most distal of the conducting airways proximal to the pulmonary acinus are termed bronchioles. The microenvironment in which the bronchiolar epithelial cell population exists varies greatly from species to species in a number of factors, including: (1) relative position of the bronchiole within the airway tree, (2) extent of the transitional zone, and (3) interrelationship between connective tissue, vascular and epithelial elements of the gas-exchange area and those of the conducting airway. The term *transitional* bronchiole has been used as a descriptive term for the bronchiole where the most proximal gas-exchange unit, or alveolus, can be identified (2,3). The position of this transitional, or respiratory, bronchiole averages 14 generations of branching from the trachea in the lungs of humans (3) and from 9 to 22 generations in adult macaque monkeys (4), 8 to 25 (mean 15) in the rat (2), 12 to 26 (mean 18) in the rabbit (2), and 30 to 35 in the sheep (5).

The organization of the epithelial lining of the transitional bronchiole also varies markedly from species to species. In primates, the epithelial populations of the gas-exchange area, alveolar type I and II cells lining an alveolus, are surrounded by simple cuboidal or pseudostratified ciliated epithelial populations

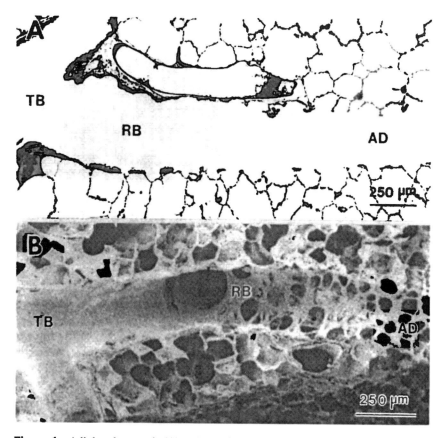

**Figure 1** A light microscopic (A) and scanning electron microscopic (B) comparison of the centriacinar region of a species with extensive respiratory bronchioles (cat). TB, terminal bronchiole; RB, respiratory bronchiole; AD, alveolar duct.

(4,6) (Fig. 1). This arrangement occurs over a variable number of generations of branching within the pulmonary acinus (7). The respiratory bronchiole is extensive (exceeding three generations) in humans, macaque monkeys, dogs, cats, and ferrets. In the rhesus monkey, and possibly in other primates including humans, the two epithelial populations, bronchiolar and alveolar, are distributed on opposite sides of the airway in relation to the position of the pulmonary arteriole (4). A pseudostratified population with ciliated cells lines numerous generations of respiratory bronchioles on the side adjacent to the pulmonary arteriole. The alveolarized areas are surrounded by a simple cuboidal bronchiolar epithelial population on the side opposite the arteriole. In the majority of mammalian species, the bronchiolar epithelium occupies the proximal portion of the transi-

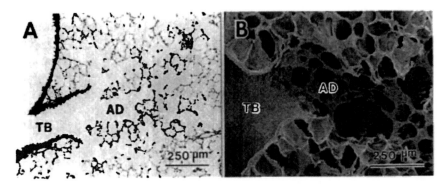

**Figure 2** A light microscopic and scanning electron microscopic comparison of the centriacinar region of species with short, or poorly developed, respiratory bronchioles (mouse, A; rat, B). TB, terminal bronchiole; AD, alveolar duct.

tional bronchiole and alveolar gas-exchange epithelium lines the distal portion (Fig. 2). This is the case for mice, hamsters, rats, guinea pigs, rabbits, pigs, sheep, cattle, and horses.

The composition of the peribronchiolar region associated with Clara cells includes the presence of smooth muscle adjacent to the basal lamina, and extensive collagen interspersed with elastin and few capillaries. Those capillaries that are present are not closely associated with the epithelial basal lamina. The principal vessel in the area is the pulmonary arteriole. In contrast, the alveolar portions of this transitional zone generally include a substantial capillary bed closely applied to the basal lamina of the alveolar epithelial populations. Although the matrix composition of the alveolar gas-exchange portions of the lung have been studied in some detail, the same is not true for the matrix associated with the bronchioles (8).

## III. Bronchiolar Morphogenesis

In fetal animals, in which the majority of epithelial cells are poorly differentiated or undifferentiated, the boundary between the epithelium lining presumptive distal conducting airways and that lining future gas-exchange regions is relatively easily defined in some species (9–11). The features include differences in epithelial configuration and modifications in the surrounding mesenchymally derived components. Most of these components, including smooth muscle and fibroblast-like cells, appear to mature somewhat more quickly then do the associated epithelium (12,13). The morphogenesis of the respiratory bronchiole during fetal lung development has been studied in detail in only one species—the rhesus monkey (12).

The respiratory bronchiole begins as a tube lined by glycogen-filled cuboidal cells intermixed with an occasional ciliated cell. Alveolarization begins in the most proximal aspect of the respiratory bronchiole; at approximately 60% gestation in the rhesus monkey and in humans. The alveolarization appears as a formation of outpocketings into surrounding extracellular matrix. The outpocketings, which are lined by cuboidal epithelium, occur only on the side of the potential respiratory bronchiole opposite the pulmonary arteriole. They begin at the same time that secondary septa are forming in the distal acinus. Outpocketing or alveolarization occurs over a very short period of time (5 days) in the rhesus monkey. As alveolarization progresses from proximal to distal in the potential respiratory bronchiole, the epithelial cells also differentiate. By 67% gestation, ciliated cells are confined to the epithelium adjacent to the pulmonary arteriole and the cyto-differentiation of the epithelial cells characteristic of alveoli is beginning in the outpocketings. Contacts between epithelium and underlying fibroblastic cells were observed for a very brief period in regions of respiratory bronchiole development. The epithelium of proximal generations of respiratory bronchiole differentiates earlier than more distal generations but much later than in the trachea.

## IV.  Phenotypic Markers for Differentiated Cells

### A.  Cellular Density in Bronchiolar Epithelium

The density of differentiated Clara cells in the epithelial populations of terminal and respiratory bronchioles in adult animals is species-specific. The absolute numerical density (as number of cells per square millimeter of basal lamina) has been determined morphometrically for six species: mouse (14), hamster (14), rat (Sprague Dawley [14] and Fisher 344 [15]), rabbit (16), cat (17), and bonnet monkey (18) (Table 1). The numerical density of the entire bronchiolar epithelial population is widely variable from species to species, as is the percentage of the population made up of Clara cells (Table 1). The rat and rabbit encompass the range in terms of percentage and density of the epithelial population for species with short transitional bronchioles (Table 1). In species with extensive respiratory bronchioles, Clara cells represent 90% or more of the cells throughout the transitional bronchiolar zone. In the cat, the numerical density for the entire epithelial population, as well as for the Clara cells, is somewhat larger than that for the other species (Table 1). The numerical density of the entire population and of Clara cells in macaques (e.g., bonnet monkey) is approximately half that of species with short transitional bronchioles and almost a third that of cats. The organization and numerical density of the cell populations in the adult human lung has not yet been clearly defined. However, qualitative studies indicate that the organization of these populations and the density of the cells within them are very similar to that of nonhuman primates (4).

**Table 1** Comparison of Numerical Density and Percentage of Clara Cells in the Bronchiolar Epithelial Population of Adults

| Species | Bronchiolar epithelium density (#/mm$^2$) | Clara cells | | References |
| | | Density[a] (#/mm$^2$) | % of cells | |
| --- | --- | --- | --- | --- |
| Mouse | 9759 ± 1700 | 8730 ± 1966 | 89.5 | 14 |
| Hamster | 14,238 ± 2794 | 8248 ± 2106 | 57.9 | 14 |
| Rat (Sprague-Dawley) | 18,813 ± 2722 | 14,028 ± 2918 | 82.2 | 14 |
| Rat (Fisher 344) | 17,070 ± 791 | 4336 ± 201 | 25.4 | 15, 114, 115 |
| Rabbit | 15,073 ± 706 | 9261 ± 434 | 61.44 | 16 |
| Cat | 19,532 ± 383 | 19,532 ± 383 | 100 | 17 |
| Bonnet Monkey | 9565 ± 304 | 8800 ± 280 | 92 | 18, 116 |

[a]Mean ± 1 standard deviation.

## B.  Cellular Ultrastructure

In adult animals, ultrastructural features are the most thoroughly characterized markers of differentiated Clara cells. There is considerable interspecies variability in these phenotypic characteristics (Fig. 3). The relative proportions of most of the cellular components of Clara cells vary considerably. In humans and other primates, Clara cells are characterized as low cuboidal cells with minimal apical projections bound to each other by junctional complexes on the luminal aspects of the basolateral membrane (Fig. 3). The distribution of organelles within the cytoplasm shows little polarization and includes small amounts (<10%) of granular (or rough) (GER) and agranular (or smooth) (AER) endoplasmic reticulum, mitochondria, and Golgi apparatus. The nucleus is approximately one third the total volume of the cell and is centrally located. The apical portion of the cytoplasm generally contains a small number of ovoid, electron-dense membrane-bound secretory granules. This structural composition has been defined for humans and three species of macaque monkeys (4,6,18,19). In contrast, the ultrastructure of the nonciliated cell in the majority of mammalian species is characterized by an extensive apical projection into the airway lumen, a polarized organization of organelles, and a predominance of one of two cellular cytoplasmic components (Fig. 3). In most species, there is an abundance of apical AER. Greater than 40% of the cytoplasmic volume is composed of AER in these species: mouse, hamster, rat, guinea pig, rabbit, pig, sheep, and horse (Fig. 3). GER is generally restricted to the basolateral portions of the cytoplasm surrounding the nucleus. Mitochondria are distributed throughout the cell but show significant interspecies variation in size and internal organization. Most Clara cells contain electron-dense, ovoid secretory granules in their apical cytoplasm, but in

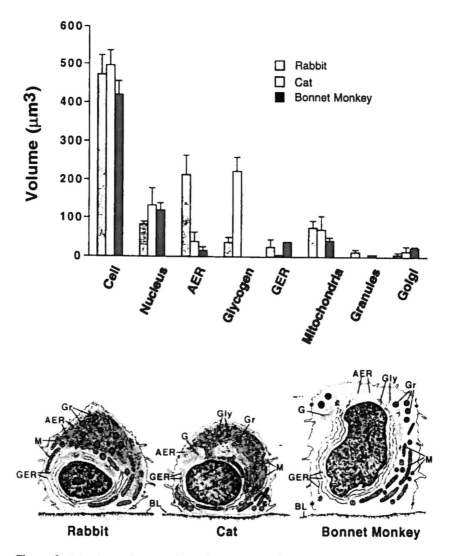

**Figure 3** Morphometric comparison of the volumes of cellular components in the Clara cells of three species (rabbit, cat, and bonnet monkey) with diagrammatic representations of their ultrastructural organization. N, nucleus; Gly, glycogen; AER, agranular endoplasmic reticulum; M, mitochondria; Gr, secretory granules; GER, granular endoplasmic reticulum; G, Golgi apparatus.

some species, such as guinea pig, these granules are of variable densities with the most dense portion in the center of the granule. In the dog, cat, and ferret, the predominant cytoplasmic constituent is glycogen, which is 40% of the cytoplasmic volume (Fig. 3). AER and GER are less than 10% of the cytoplasmic volume. Whether Clara cells of these species contain secretory granules and what they secrete is not clear. The lateral surfaces of Clara cells in all species have extensive cytoplasmic interdigitations. The apical projections found in many species appear to be due to a specific organization of microfilaments (20).

### C.  Cytochrome P450 Monooxygenases

Cytochrome P450 monooxygenases are a family of proteins whose expression is highly characteristic of Clara cells. Evidence from a number of different approaches has established that the Clara cell population is one of the primary sites in the lung for xenobiotic metabolism via the P450 system (6,21). This very active system metabolizes a wide variety of substrates. Although the gene superfamily is very large, only a limited number of isozymes have been identified in Clara cells of adult animals. Isozyme subfamily CYP2B, a form which is highly inducible by phenobarbital in the liver but expressed in very high levels in the lung in the steady state, has been identified in Clara cells of rats (22), mice (23–25), rabbits (26), hamsters (27), and rhesus monkeys (28). Two isozymes of the CYP4 family (CYP4B and 4A) have been identified in the Clara cells of rabbits, rats, mice, and hamsters. Isozyme CYP1A1, the polyaromatic hydrocarbon (PAH)–inducible form in the liver, is also inducible in some species but is found in the steady state in others. In rats, CYP1A1 is constitutively expressed within Clara cells and can be elevated in adult animals by a number of inducers, including 2,3,7,8-tetrachloro-dibenzo-p-dioxin (TCDD). CYP1A1 can also be induced in the rabbit (29) and the mouse (23,24). CYP1A1 is not detectable in the steady state in mice (23,25). An isozyme uniquely expressed in high amounts only in Clara cells of the mouse is CYP2F2 (25,28). Ultrastructural studies in rabbits have shown that P450 protein is associated with the plasma membrane as well as AER-rich zones (26). The NADPH-cytochrome P450 reductase has also been identified as most strongly expressed in Clara cells within the lung in mice, hamsters, rats, and rabbits (25,28,29,30) and in relatively low levels in Clara cells in the rhesus monkey. CYP2E, which is inducible by alcohol, acetone, and hyperoxia, has been identified in Clara cells of rats but has been little studied in other species. The function of these proteins has been substantiated by enzymatic activity studies using isolated Clara cells produced by enzymatic digestion or by microdissection of bronchioles (21,25,28,31). Isolation of free cells relies on protease digestion of lung tissue followed by enrichment for Clara cells by centrifugal elutriation, density gradient centrifugation, or immune panning. This approach has been applied to rabbits, rats, and mice. The yield of Clara cells varies widely from species to species.

Purity also varies from as low as 30–60% for rats to as high as 80–90% for mice and rabbits (21). One major drawback of protease digestion is degradation of the enzyme systems of interest, specifically cytochrome P450 monooxygenases. Factors which can reduce proteolysis include reduction in protease incubation time, decrease in protease concentration, degasing the lung tissue after mincing, and elimination of stirring of minced tissue. Another drawback of studies with isolated Clara cells is that the isolated cells come from throughout the airway tree and cannot be segregated based on specific microenvironments.

A spectrophotometric comparison of cytochrome P450 proteins in microsomal preparations from isolated rabbit Clara cells, alveolar type II cells, and pulmonary alveolar macrophages shows that the Clara cell has approximately four times the P450 activity of either of the other two cell types (21). Western blot analysis of rabbit Clara cells indicates that, per milligram protein, there is approximately the same amount of cytochrome P450 detectable protein in isolated Clara cells as in alveolar type II cells. The P450 level in Clara cells is approximately four times that in macrophages. The NADPH cytochrome P450 reductase is also approximately twice as high in isolated Clara cells as it is in alveolar type II cells. The following cytochrome P450–dependent monooxygenase metabolic activities have been evaluated in isolated Clara cells: 7-ethoxycoumarin (7EC) O-deethylation, coumarin hydroxylation, benzo(a)pyrene (B[a]P) hydroxylation, 7-ethoxyresorufin (7ERF) O-deethylation, naphthalene monooxygenase, and 2-acetylaminofluorene hydroxylation. Deethylation of 7EC was highest in Clara cells from mice as compared with rabbits or rats and twice as high in Clara cells as in alveolar type II cells. Coumarin hydroxylation is 10–20 times as high in isolated Clara cells as it is in alveolar type II cells for both rabbits and mice. B(a)P hydroxylation is twice as high in Clara cells as it is in alveolar type II cells in the rabbit and is very low in rat Clara cells. 7-ERF deethylation is mediated in rabbit lungs by pulmonary cytochrome P4501A1. The activities are very low, but detectable, in Clara cells, alveolar type II cells, and pulmonary alveolar macrophages isolated from rabbit lungs. Treatment with TCCD elevates these activities by about 20-fold. 2-Acetylaminofluorene is actively metabolized by Clara cells, alveolar type II cells, and pulmonary alveolar macrophages.

### D. Clara Cell Secretory Protein

In the earliest studies of differentiated Clara cells, it was suggested that their primary function was as the secretory cell for the distal conducting airways. The major biosynthetic products of Clara cells have now been recognized as at least three different groups of related proteins. Clara cells produce a group of secretory proteins ranging in size from less than 10 to 200 kDa (6,32). Antibodies to the low molecular weight secretory product produced by the rat cross react with mouse and hamster. There appear to be two antigenically distinct proteins produced in the rat with three molecular weights on SDS-PAGE: 12, 55, and 200 kDa. Antibodies from the smallest and the largest cross react with each other but not with the medium-sized protein (32). In the rabbit, there are four proteins of different molecular weights. The lowest molecular weight protein accounts for less than 5% of the cell and surfactant-free pulmonary alveolar lavage protein. Manabe et al. (33) has confirmed that the proteinaceous material obtained from lung lavage could be detected by a specific antiserum within Clara cells and in the airway surface lining of rats as well as mice. This antiserum, however, did not cross react with hamsters, guinea pigs, dogs, cats, monkeys, or humans. The protein with an apparent molecular weight of approximately 10 kDa, which is the unreduced form, and 5 kDa, the reduced form, constitutes as much as 40% of the secretory protein synthesized by cells isolated from rabbits (34,35). Using antibodies raised against the rat protein, the amino acid sequence has been determined for the human product (36). The primary transformation product is 7.3 kDa for both the rat and rabbit. The secretory protein in both cases is resistant to digestion with trypsin, but the primary translation product, which is approximately 1 kDa larger, is digestible (34). This suggests there is posttranslational modification of the protein prior to secretion. Further, it appears that in the rat this protein has approximately 60% homology with uteroglobin produced by rabbit uterus (34–36). The homology of the rabbit Clara cell protein to uteroglobin is even greater (37). The mRNA for the low molecular weight protein is also expressed in nonciliated cells lining both bronchioles and bronchi of human lung (38). The cellular distribution of the Clara cell secretory protein is predominantly in secretory granules with a lower concentration in the agranular and granular endoplasmic reticulum (39). Its presence in other cell populations within the lung is minimal.

### E. Other Enzymes and Secretory Products

A number of other enzyme systems, especially those involved in aspects of xenobiotic metabolism, have been identified in Clara cells, but they do not have the high levels of expression found for P450s and the Clara cell secretory protein. Enzymes involved in the second phase of xenobiotic metabolism have been measured in isolated Clara cells, including epoxide hydrolase and glutathione S-transferase (GST). The activity for these enzymes ranges anywhere from 2- to 20-fold that found in alveolar type II cells. Clara cells also appear to be the source of some pulmonary surfactant apoproteins (6,32,40–43). Although a number of previous studies had suggested similarities in proteinaceous antigens between Clara cells and alveolar type II cells, it now appears that the small molecular weight secretory protein is not the same as one of the surfactant apoproteins. Both Clara cells and type II cells in humans express mRNA for one of the smaller molecular weight apoproteins (surfactant apoprotein B), but only type II cells have mRNA for surfactant apoprotein A.

The Clara cell also appears to be one of the major sources of the anti-leukoproteases such as secretory leukocyte proteinase inhibitor (SLPI) found in the surface lining material of peripheral airways in humans (44–47). This protein has a molecular weight of approximately 15 kDa and has a strong inhibitory effect on neutrophil proteinases. It accounts for approximately 70% of the inhibiting capacity of bronchiolar lavage fluid in humans. It is present in Clara cells and in serous cells of tracheobronchial glands. It is now apparent that the Clara cell is a very metabolically active cell which is secreting at least one, and possibly more, protein with inhibitory effects on some proteinases and possibly plays a role in regulating pulmonary surfactant function. These proteins may bind certain classes of polychlorinated biphenyls (48).

Clara cells may also be a source of arachidonic acid metabolites (49,50). Clara cells take up large amounts of platelet-activating factor, which is thought to be remetabolized through the arachidonic acid cascade (50). In contrast, Clara cells do not metabolize prostaglandin $F_{2\alpha}$ ($PGF_{2\alpha}$) to the same extent as do alveolar type II cells (49). The Clara cell may prove to be the principal regulatory cell for cellular activity in the centriacinar zone. It takes up protein components of pulmonary alveolar surfactant, may synthesize some of them, produces protease inhibitors which are induced by disease processes, produces binding proteins for bronchiolar toxicants, and may also be a source of arachidonic acid metabolites.

## V. Role as the Bronchiolar Progenitor Cell

One of the primary functions of the Clara cell in distal bronchioles appears to be that of progenitor for replacement of itself and ciliated cells. The majority of the studies which have established this role have been ones which evaluated cell kinetics in an experimental injury situation (6). In the steady-state condition, the turnover of epithelial populations in the bronchiolar region of adult lungs is very low. In species in which terminal bronchioles (TBs) predominate, less than 1% of the epithelial cells incorporate tritiated thymidine in the steady state: rat, 0.2%; mouse, 0.3%. This is also true for species with extensive respiratory bronchioles (RBs): cat, 0.05% (TBs) and 0.076% (RBs); bonnet monkey, 0.1% (RBs); rhesus monkey, less than 0.1% (RBs). The index is approximately the same for postnatal animals nearing maturation: 1-month-old rat, 1.1%; young mouse, 0.75%. However, in response to injury to bronchiolar ciliated cells by $NO_2$, the labeling index of bronchiolar epithelium increases dramatically, as much as 10- to 20-fold (51). Over 90% of the cells taking up thymidine 1 hr after injection are nonciliated cells lacking both agranular endoplasmic reticulum and ovoid secretory granules. There is a shift in the percentage of labeled cells following injury, but no labeled ciliated cells are identified until two days following thymidine injection. Other studies using exposure to $NO_2$, $O_3$, or $O_2$ confirm that the majority of labeled bronchiolar cells following injury are nonciliated, and that ciliated cells represent a larger proportion of labeled cells at later time points. Studies in ozone-exposed macaques and diesel-exposed cats establish that the Clara cell is also the bronchiolar progenitor cell in species with extensive respiratory bronchioles. This is supported by repopulation studies in which preparations of Clara cells isolated from adult lungs (90–95% purity) repopulate denuded tracheas transplanted onto nude mice and form an epithelium composed of Clara cells and ciliated cells (52,53). Although the composition of the epithelium resembled that in rabbit bronchioles, the Clara cells in the transplants did not have secretory granules, suggesting they may not be completely differentiated.

Developmental studies in the rat and rabbit have shown that the predominant cell type prenatally is not ciliated and that ciliated cells increase in abundance postnatally (16,32,54–56). A study using the proliferating cell nuclear antigen, which is expressed in the late $G_1$ through the S phase of the cell cycle, suggests that in some strains of mice, mitotic activity may be much higher than indicated by autoradiographic studies (55). The pattern of proliferation and differentiation of ciliated and nonciliated cells was evaluated in the lungs of fetuses and offspring from time-mated New Zealand white rabbits beginning in late gestation (24 days) and terminating in adults at 25 weeks postnatal (56). Three categories of cells were distinguishable in terminal bronchioles: nonciliated cells with abundant glycogen and variable numbers of organelles; nonciliated cells with little glycogen, large numbers of polyribosomes, and variable numbers of basal bodies; and ciliated cells with cilia of varying height (Fig. 4). Both types of nonciliated cells combined were 100% of the epithelium in late fetal animals (24 and 27 days gestational age [DGA]), 85% of the population immediately before birth (30 DGA), and 75–81% of the total population in postnatal animals. Nonciliated cells with polyribosomes and basal bodies were 10–20% of the total nonciliated cell population in the perinatal period (24 DGA to 1 week postnatal [PN]) and were extremely rare in older animals. No ciliated cells were detectable in animals younger than 30 DGA. In a tritiated thymidine-uptake study conducted in the perinatal period (28 DGA), it was clear that the nonciliated cells were the predominant labeled cell 1 hr postinjection, comprising 98% of the labeled cells. The labeled cells contained large amounts of glycogen and no basal bodies. A small subpopulation of the remainder (2–3%) of the labeled cells consisted of nonciliated cells with basal bodies at all three time points evaluated. Twenty-four hours after injection, ciliated cells became 2% of the labeled population and increased to 7% by 2 days. It appears that the differentiation of ciliated cells, at least in the rabbit, occurs over a short period of time immediately before and after parturition, and that the majority of these ciliated cells differentiate from nonciliated cells via a transitional cell. The primary conversions are a loss of glycogen and production of polyribosomes followed by synthesis of basal bodies and then cilia. Kinetic studies suggest that the nonciliated bronchiolar cells which are highly undifferentiated in young animals serve as progenitors for increasing the population of nonciliated as well as ciliated cells (56). Clara cells appear in fetal human lungs by

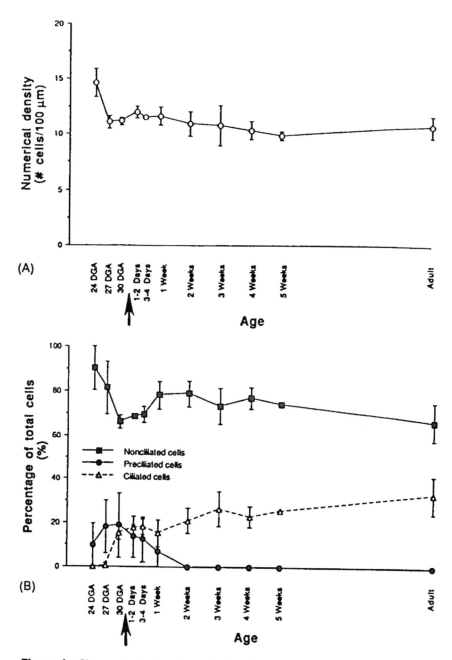

**Figure 4** Changes in the abundance of ciliated and nonciliated cells in terminal bronchioles of prenatal and postnatal rabbits. Birth is indicated by the arrows. (A) Numerical density of epithelium in terminal bronchioles of both pre-and postnatal animals presented as the number per 100 μm of basal lamina. (B) The relative proportion (%) of cells within the bronchiolar epithelium. Solid squares equal nonciliated cells; open triangles equal ciliated cells; solid circles equal nonciliated cells with polyribosomes.

15 weeks of gestation and comprise 24% of the epithelium by 24 weeks of gestation (57).

## VI. Patterns of Expression of Phenotypic Markers During Cytodifferentiation

### A. Cell Ultrastructure

The process of cytodifferentiation of the nonciliated cells of distal bronchioles entails substantial rearrangement, loss, and biogenesis of cellular organelles. Up to late fetal age, terminal bronchioles are lined by simple cuboidal to columnar epithelium composed of glycogen-filled nonciliated cells with few organelles. The shifts in cellular components with time for species in which the predominant cellular constituent in adults is AER, such as the mouse, hamster, rat, and rabbit, are summarized in Figure 5. The pattern is essentially similar for these species. What varies from species to species is the timing of these events. The first event is a dramatic loss in cytoplasmic glycogen. In rabbits, this drop is from approximately 70% of cytoplasmic volume to less than 10% cytoplasmic volume in adults. A similar substantial loss occurs in rats, hamsters, and mice. In the rabbit, this loss begins immediately prior to birth and continues for up to 4 weeks of postnatal age (58). A similar change occurs in the mouse (59). In the rat, the loss of cytoplasmic glycogen begins at birth and drops to adult levels within the first week of postnatal life (32). In the hamster, cytoplasmic glycogen is not detectable immediately after birth (60,61). Associated with the drop in cellular glycogen is a substantial biogenesis of membranous organelles, especially AER (Table 2). Smooth endoplasmic reticulum is not detected in nonciliated cells until immediately prior to birth in the rabbit (Fig. 6) (58). At birth, less than 20% of the cells contain greater than 10% AER. By 2 weeks, in almost 70% of the nonciliated cells AER occupies greater than 10% (up to 50%) of the cell volume. The adult configuration is reached at approximately 28 days PN in rabbits. In mice, the adult configuration of AER is reached at approximately 3 weeks PN (59). RER in prenatal animals is approximately twice as abundant in rabbit Clara cells as it is in rats (Fig. 6) (62). The drop in cellular abundance of GER occurs gradually in rabbits and is still double the adult configuration (2% of cell volume) at 4 weeks PN, but in the rat, the level decreases by 50% immediately postpartum and is at or near the adult configuration (<1%) by 10 days PN (62). The situation for the rat and the mouse appears similar to the rabbit, but for the hamster, GER is near the adult configuration immediately postpartum (60,61). Secretory granule appearance also varies by species. The earliest time at which secretory granules are detected in the Clara cells of rabbits and mice is within the first week of postnatal life, whereas in rats and hamsters, granules are abundant prenatally. In the rabbit as well as the mouse, granule abundance resembling adult levels occurs by 21 days

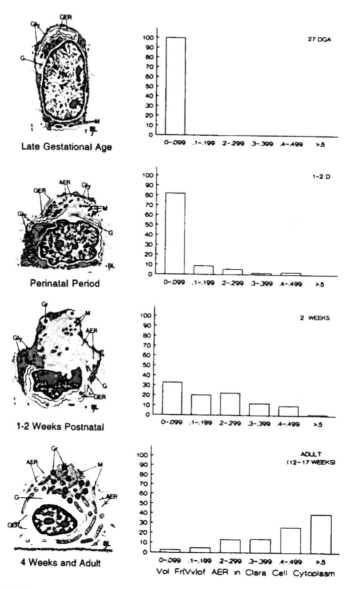

**Figure 5** Diagrammatic representations of changes in cellular composition of Clara cells during pre- and postnatal differentiation. The drawings correlate with the graphs of the percentage of Clara cell cytoplasm containing agranular endoplasmic reticulum (AER) as determined by morphometric measurements. The total number of cells counted is divided into groups based on the abundance (volume fraction) of endoplasmic reticulum.

**Table 2** Development of AER, P450 Reductase, and Monooxygenase Enzymes in Rabbit Lung

| Assay | | 27–28 DGA | 1–2 DPN | 7 DPN | 14 DPN | 20 DPN | Adult |
|---|---|---|---|---|---|---|---|
| | | | | % of adult value | | | |
| AER[a,b] | | 0.2 | 8.2 | 8.2 | 30.1 | 64.5 | 100 |
| P450 reductase | Immunohistochemistry[b,c] | ± | + | ++ | ++ | ++++ | ++++ |
| | Western blot | + | + | ++ | ++ | ++++ | ++++ |
| P450 isozyme 2B | Immunohistochemistry[b] | 0 | ± | + | ++ | ++++ | ++++ |
| | Western blot | 0 | 0 | ± | + | ++++ | ++++ |
| P450 isozyme 4B | Immunohistochemistry[b] | 0 | + | ++ | ++ | ++++ | ++++ |
| | Western blot | 0 | ± | + | ++ | +++ | ++++ |
| Microsomal P450[d] | | 0 | 10.8 | 20.9 | 44.5 | 56.0 | 100 |
| P450 activity | Ethoxyresorufin[e] | 0 | 6.5 | 11.7 | 14.9 | 59.3 | 100 |
| | Pentoxyresorufin[f] | 0 | | 8.1 | 29.9 | 51.8 | 100 |

[a] Average adult cell volume for AER is 43.9 ± 3.5%.
[b] Bronchiolar epithelium.
[c] Symbols indicate staining intensities in relation to adult (++++).
[d] Average adult level of microsomal P450 is 0.575 ± 0.238 nmol/mg of microsomal protein.
[e] Average adult ethoxyresorufin O-dealkylase activity is 47.99 ± 14.69 pmole/mg of protein/min.
[f] Average adult pentoxyresorufin O-dealkylase activity is 64.07 ± 64.51 pmol/mg of protein/min.

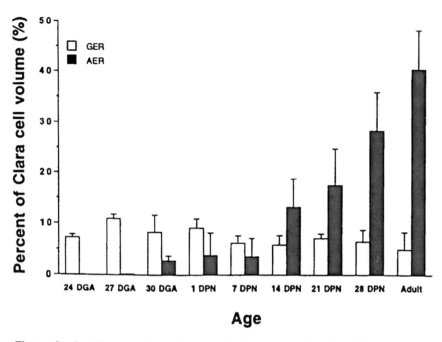

**Age**

**Figure 6** Graphic comparison of changes in the amount of rough (GER) and smooth (AER) endoplasmic reticulum in Clara cells of the rabbit during pre- and postnatal development. Data were determined morphometrically and are presented as a percent of total cell volume.

PN. In the rat, granule abundance reaches adult abundance by 7 days PN and is at adult configuration immediately postpartum in the hamster. The only species in which Clara cell differentiation has been fully characterized where the adult Clara cell population does not have an abundance of AER is the rhesus monkey (13). In that species, the loss of cytoplasmic glycogen and an increase, rather than a decrease, in GER occurs over a substantial period both prenatally and postnatally. Studies in humans suggest that developmental events for Clara cells are similar to those of the rhesus monkey but may extend longer than the 6 months to a year (postnatal) required for differentiation of all the nonciliated cells in terminal respiratory bronchioles of monkeys.

### B. Cytochrome P450 Monooxygenases

The expression of cytochrome P450 monooxygenases in Clara cells during their differentiation has been evaluated in only three species: rabbit, hamster, and rat (60,63,64). Protein for the NADPH P450 reductase and CYP2B is detected earliest, with the reductase being somewhat later than CYP2B in the rabbit. CYP4B is detected 2–3 days of age later (see Table 2). The initial distribution is in the most apical border of a small percentage of the nonciliated cell population. During the period of time in which the amount of detectable protein increases, the distribution changes in two ways. First, an immunologically detectable protein is found in an increasing proportion of the nonciliated cells as animals become older. Second, the distribution of detectable protein within an individual cell increases from the apex to the base with increasing age. The youngest ages at which intracellular protein can be detected immunohistochemically vary substantially within these three species. Protein becomes detectable in the hamster approximately 3–4 days prior to birth, and it reaches the distribution and intensity observed in the adult by 3 days PN. CYB4B is not detectable before 1 day PN, but it is at adult levels a short time thereafter. In the rabbit and the rat, the timing is somewhat different. NADPH reductase is found initially just prior to birth in the rabbit and CYP2B and CYP4B are not observed until after birth. All these proteins have an adult distribution and intensity by 28 days PN. In the rat, CYP2B, CYP4B, and reductase are detected in the first 2–3 days of postnatal life and are apparently at adult densities and distributions by 21 days PN. CYP1A1 is not detectable prenatally in rats but can be detected in increasing, but small, amounts until it reaches adult levels at approximately 21 days PN (64). Intracellular expression of protein precedes the appearance and increase in the abundance of AER by 2–4 days in each of these species. Activity for these proteins is first detected approximately 2–3 days after the protein is immunologically detectable within Clara cells. The activity studies have been done with whole lung homogenates and reflect potential activity from other cell populations as well as from Clara cells. Although both the AER abundance and antigenic protein intensity reach the adult configuration in approximately 3–4 weeks in rats and rabbits, the activity for these isozymes is still considerably below that for adults. This suggests that the functionality of these proteins continues to increase after the protein density and organelle composition have reached adult levels of expression. Table 2 summarizes the relationship between changes in AER abundance, expression of immunoreactive protein, and microsomal P450 activity for the rabbit. The timing for the rat is somewhat shifted to the left for postnatal time points and to the right for perinatal ones compared with the rabbit.

## C.  Clara Cell Secretory Protein

The pattern of expression of the Clara cell secretory protein is similar to that of the cytochrome P450 monooxygenase system in relation to the appearance of cellular organelles. Although there is substantial interspecies variability in the timing of expression, the general pattern is similar, at least for the four species studied in most detail: the rat, rabbit, hamster, and mouse (59,62,65–70). The protein appears earliest in the central or apical portion of a few cells per bronchiole, and the number of cells in which antigen can be detected increases with increasing age. In the hamster, the secretory protein antigen can be detected in a number of cells by the beginning of the last trimester of pregnancy and reaches the adult configuration in terms of density and number of cells labeled at about 3–4 days PN. In the rat, a small proportion of the cells are labeled prenatally, and the distribution observed in the adult is present at about 7 days of PN. This adult configuration occurs between 3 and 4 weeks in the rabbit, and the earliest detectable signal in the Clara cells is immediately prior to birth. The timing in the mouse and rat is similar to that in the rabbit. Immunoreactive protein has also been detected in late fetal humans, but when the distribution resembles adults has not been determined. Intracellular expression of the protein follows the changes in GER and is closely related to the first appearance and increase in the abundance of secretory granules. Western blotting of this protein indicates that it is present earlier in lung homogenate than its appearance in bronchiolar Clara cells suggests. This is due to the fact that secretory cells in proximal airways express the protein much earlier and in general are more differentiated in the perinatal period than are secretory cells of bronchioles. In the hamster the situation is the inverse, with the bronchioles differentiating in this respect prior to the bronchi.

### D. Surfactant-Associated Proteins

Expression of the surfactant-associated proteins in differentiating Clara cells during lung development is species specific. The pattern has been assessed for both mRNA and immunoreactive protein expression. mRNA expression leads expression of by a short, but variable, period of time. In the rabbit and rat (71–73), this pattern holds true for surfactant proteins A and B (SP-A and SP-B). In both species, the proteins are detected shortly prior to birth and are observed in differentiated cells within the first 2 weeks of postnatal life. The appearance of SP-A also occurs in Clara cells in the mouse immediately prior to birth (59). However, that study concluded that the protein is located in the Clara cell secretory granules but is not being synthesized by the Clara cell. Whether this is actually the case cannot be determined because of a lack of information regarding mRNA expression. SPA-A expression is predominately postnatal in all three species and occurs to a greater extent in alveolar type II cells than Clara cells. SP-C has not been detected in Clara cells; at least for the rat (71). SP-B is detected in a small number of Clara cells in late fetal and early postnatal humans, as well as in adults (74). SP-A has not been detected in the nonciliated cells of the respiratory bronchiole in the adult rhesus monkey. SP-B is detected by the 19th week in some humans, but not in others.

## VII.  Extracellular Matrix

The role which extracellular matrix components play in bronchiolar morphogenesis or in bronchiolar epithelial differentiation is poorly understood. A variety of extracellular matrix components appear to play a role in morphogenesis of the gas-exchange area, but it is unclear what their impact is on bronchiolar epithelial cells. Transforming growth factor—$\beta_1$, collagen I, collagen III, fibronectin, and glycosaminoglycans are abundant in fetal lungs and have been suggested to have a role in branching morphogenesis (75). Tenascin-C also has a pattern of distribution which varies during lung development and may be involved in branching morphogenesis (76). Neutralization of laminin by antilaminin antibodies markedly inhibits branching morphogenesis and significantly distorts the bronchial tree, as well as inhibiting overall growth rate (77). Fibronectin is found in high concentrations in the basal lamina surrounding distal bronchioles in the fetal lung (78,79). However, it is unclear whether changes in the density of any of these extracellular matrix or basal lamina components play a significant role in bronchiolar epithelial differentiation. Their distribution and time course postnatally have not been evaluated in detail during the period when bronchiolar epithelial cells are undergoing cytodifferentiation. Given the important role which extracellular matrix components play in the healing response to injury in a variety of organs, the particular role which extracellular matrix components play in cellular development in the lung needs more thorough exploration.

## VIII.  Regulation of Differentiation

Factors regulating Clara cell differentiation are not well understood. The postnatal nature of the majority of the cytodifferentiation process in most species suggests that it is independent of the hormones associated with pregnancy and parturition. The fact that the timing varies by as much as 2–3 weeks in different species would further suggest that the process may be under regulation of a variety of factors which act in different temporal sequences and with different levels of influence in different species. A number of mediators have been shown to stimulate cytodifferentiation of type II alveolar epithelial cells and produce architectural rearrangements of lung connective tissue elements to promote gas exchange, including corticosteroids, thyroid hormone, epidermal growth factor, and cyclic AMP (80). Whether all of these mediators influence Clara cell differentiation is not known. The best studied are the glucocorticoids, especially dexamethasone. Treatment in the perinatal period retards Clara cell differentiation as evidenced by an increase in cytoplasmic glycogen and minimal alterations in organelles in both rats and mice (81,82). Dexamethasone administered either prenatally or immediately postnatally elevates the SP-B mRNA levels in the lungs of rats of all ages, producing this elevation in both alveolar type II cells and Clara cells (83). Glucocorticoid administered to pregnant rabbits appears to have a stimulatory effect on the differentiation of secretory potential in fetal Clara cells by elevating the amount of the uteroglobin-like Clara cell secretory protein (84,85). Dexamethasone administered to pregnant rabbits also has a stimulatory effect on the pulmonary cytochrome P450 system in fetuses based on measurements of whole lung microsomes (86–88). Although glycogenolysis is retarded by dexamethasone treatment, glucagon, epinephrine, and 8-bromo-cAMP produce a rapid drop in Clara cell glycogen content (32).

One of the factors which appears to have the most impact on Clara cell differentiation is injury during the developmental period in which normal differentiation occurs. Normal differentiation is characterized by loss of glycogen and appearance of secretory granules and by differentiation of Clara cells into ciliated cells even in the absence of frank injury to either ciliated or Clara cells. Postnatal exposure to compounds which injure the respiratory system retard Clara cell differentiation. Hyperoxia during the early postnatal period inhibits differentiation (89,90). Injury by treatment with 4-ipomeanol impedes Clara cell differentiation even for a short term after treatment is discontinued (91). Not only are Clara cells in postnatal animals more susceptible to injury than are Clara cells in the adult, but the expression of the P450 system in the post-treatment period is markedly reduced. In the rat, exposure to cigarette smoke of either the pregnant mother or the newborn accelerates the appearance of one cytochrome P450 monooxygenase isozyme, CYP1A1, but not CYP2B (64). The increased P450 expression is primarily in the Clara cell population and is not found in either alveolar type II cells or in the vascular endothelium, which are both targets for inducers in adult animals. Other factors besides postnatal hyperoxia, including maternal undernutrition during the last 5 days of pregnancy, produce retardation of Clara cell differentiation, but these effects appear to be reversible with time (32,90,92,93).

There is considerable indirect evidence to suggest that a number of growth factors, inluding transforming growth factor-$\alpha$ (TGF-$\alpha$), epidermal growth factor (EGF), basic fibroblast growth factor (b-FGF), insulin-like growth factors, and platelet-derived growth factor, may play roles in regulating bronchiolar epithelial differentiation (94,95). The epidermal growth factor receptor (EGFR) has been detected in bronchiolar epithelium throughout pre- and postnatal lung development in the rat and prenatal development in the lamb (96,97). EGFR has also been detected in human lung at midgestation (98) and has been detected in human and rat fetal lung extracts (96,99). Both ligands of EGFR, as well as TGF-$\alpha$ and EGF, have been detected immunohistochemically in bronchiolar epithelium in a number of species. EGF is barely detectable in bronchiolar epithelium of fetal humans (first and second trimester) but is present in postnatal human lung (100). EGF has been reported in homogenates of lung from late fetal (21 days' gestational age) and adult rats (101), and immunoreactive protein has been detected in bronchiolar epithelium throughout fetal development in the rat and mouse (96,102). TGF-α has been detected in the bronchiolar epithelium of midgestational humans (103). It can be extracted, and mRNA can be detected in fetal rat lung homogenates (104). Late fetal (21 days' gestational age) and adult rat lung contains EGF (101). TGF-α is observed in bronchiolar epithelium of fetal rats (96). Platelet-derived growth factor receptor has also been detected in bronchiolar epithelium during most of the prenatal stages of lung development. Basic FGF and its receptor are found in bronchiolar epithelium during most of fetal rat lung development (107). Both the FGF receptor and the protein appear to colocalize in the epithelium and adjacent interstitial compartments. There is some suggestion that insulin-like growth factors are involved in aspects of epithelial development in bronchioles (108). These growth factors may play a role in autocrine regulation because both receptors and the proteins themselves appear within the bronchiolar epithelium. They also may play a paracrine role, because growth factor protein appears to be distributed to interstitial cell components, fibroblasts, and smooth muscle surrounding bronchiolar epithelium during various stages of lung development. At present, there is no direct evidence that any of these factors influence bronchiolar epithelial maturation. There is, however, evidence that EGF given in pharmacological doses alters branching morphogenesis in the mouse (109); enhances differentiation of alveolar type II cells in fetal rabbits, monkeys, and sheep (110–112); and alters the differentiation of tracheal epithelium in rhesus monkeys (113). Additional studies are needed to determine what role any of these growth factors or receptors may play in the differentiation of bronchiolar epithelium.

## References

1.  Clara M. Zur Histobiologie des Bronchalepithels. Ztschr Mikroskopi-anat Forsch 1937; 41:321–347.
2.  Rodriguez M, Bur S, Favre A, Weibel ER. Pulmonary acinus: geometry and morphometry of the peripheral airway system in rat and rabbit. Am J Anat 1987; 180: 143–155.
3.  Haefeli-Bleuer B, Weibel ER. Morphometry of the human pulmonary acinus. Anat Rec 1988; 220:401–414.
4.  Tyler NK, Plopper CG. Morphology of the distal conducting airways in rhesus monkey lungs. Anat Rec 1985; 211:295–303.
5.  Mariassy AT, Plopper CG. Tracheobronchial epithelium of the sheep. I. Quantitative light microscopic study of epithelial cell abundance, and distribution. Anat Rec 1983; 205:263–275.
6.  Plopper CG, Dungworth DL. Structure, function, cell injury and cell renewal of bronchiolar and alveolar epithelium. In: McDowell EM, ed. Lung Carcinomas. London: Churchill Livingstone, 1987:94–128.

7. Tyler WS. Comparative subgross anatomy of lungs: pleuras, interlobular septa, and distal airways. Am Rev Respir Dis 1983; 128:S32–S36.
8. Sannes PL. Basement membrane and extracellular matrix. In: Parent RA, ed. Comparative Biology of the Normal Lung. Boca Raton, FL: CRC Press, 1992:129–144.
9. ten Have-Opbroek AAW. The structural composition of the pulmonary acinus in the mouse. Anat Embryol 1986; 174:49–57.
10. ten Have-Opbroek AAW. Lung development in the mouse embryo. Exp Lung Res 1991; 17:111–130.
11. ten Have-Opbroek AAW, Otto-Verberne CJM, Dubbeldam JA, Dykman JH. The proximal border of the human respiratory unit, as shown by scanning and transmission electron microscopy and light microscopical cytochemistry. Anat Rec 1991; 229:339–354.
12. Tyler NK, Hyde DM, Hendrickx AG, Plopper CG. Morphogenesis of the respiratory bronchiole in rhesus monkey lungs. Am J Anat 1988; 182:215–223.
13. Tyler NK, Hyde DM, Hendrickx AG, Plopper CG. Cytodifferentiation of two epithelial populations of the respiratory bronchiole during fetal lung development in the rhesus monkey. Anat Rec 1989; 225:297–309.
14. Plopper CG, Macklin J, Nishio SJ, Hyde DM, Buckpitt AR. Relationship of cytochrome P450 activity to Clara cell cytotoxicity: III. Morphometric comparison of changes in the epithelial populations of terminal bronchioles and lobar bronchi in mice, hamsters, and rats after parenteral administration of naphthalene. Lab Invest 1992; 67:553–565.
15. Chang L-Y, Mercer RR, Stockstill BL, Miller FJ, Graham JA, Ospital JJ, Crapo JD. Effects of low levels of N02 on terminal bronchiolar cells and its relative toxicity compared to 03. Toxicol Appl Pharmacol 1988; 96:451–464.
16. Hyde DM, Plopper CG, Kass PH, Alley JL. Estimation of cell numbers and volumes of bronchiolar epithelium during rabbit lung maturation. Am J Anat 1983; 167:359–370.
17. Hyde DM, Plopper CG, Weir AJ, Murnane RD, Warren DL, Last JA. Peribronchiolar fibrosis in lungs of cats chronically exposed to diesel exhaust. Lab Invest 1985; 52:195–206.
18. Moffatt RK, Hyde DM, Plopper CG, Tyler WS, Putney LF. Ozone-induced adaptive and reactive cellular changes in respiratory bronchioles of bonnet monkeys. Exp Lung Res 1987; 12:57–74.
19. Plopper CG. Comparative morphologic features of broinchiolar epithelial cells: the Clara cell. Am Rev Respir Dis 1983; 128:S37–S41.
20. Sasaki J, Watanabe W, Nomura T, Wada T, Tanaka Y, Kanda S, Otsuka N. Presence of filaments in the nonciliated bronchiolar epithelial (Clara) cell of mammalian lung. Okajimas Folia Anat Jpn 1988; 65:155–170.
21. Devereux TR, Domin BA, Philpot RM. Xenobiotic metabolism by isolated pulmonary cells. Pharmacol Ther 1989; 41:243–256.
22. Baron J, Burke JP, Guengerich FP, Jakoby WB, Voigt JM. Sites for xenobiotic activation and detoxication within the respiratory tract: implications for chemically induced toxicity. Toxicol Appl Pharmacol 1988; 93:493–505.

23. Forkert PG, Vessey ML, Elce JS, Park SS, Gelboin HV, Cole SPC. Localization of phenobarbital- and 3-methylcholanthrene–inducible cytochromes P-450 in mouse lung with monoclonal antibodies. Res Commun Chem Pathol Pharmacol 1986; 53: 147–157.

24. Walker SR, Hale S, Malkinson AM, Mason RJ. Properties of isolated nonciliated bronchiolar cells from mouse lung. Exp Lung Res 1989; 15:553–573.

25. Chichester CH, Philpot RM, Weir AJ, Buckpitt AR, Plopper CG. Characterization of the cytochrome P-450 monooxygenase system in nonciliated bronchiolar epithelial (Clara) cells isolated from mouse lung. Am J Respir Cell Mol Biol 1991; 4:179–186.

26. Serabjit-Singh CJ, Nishio SJ, Philpot RM, Plopper CG. The distribution of cytochrome P-450 monooxygenase in cells of the rabbit lung: an ultrastructural immunocytochemical characterization. Mol Pharmacol 1988; 33:279–289.

27. Strum J, Ito T, Philpot R, DeSanti A, McDowell E. The immunocytochemical detection of cytochrome P-450 monooxygenase in the lungs of fetal, neonatal, and adult hamsters. Am J. Respir Cell Mol Biol 1990; 2:493–501.

28. Buckpitt A, Chang A, Weir A, Van Winkle L, Duan X, Philpot R, Plopper C. Relationship of cytochrome P450 activity to Clara cell cytotoxicity. IV. Metabolism of naphthalene and naphthalene oxide in microdissected airways from the mouse, rat, and hamster. Mol Pharmacol 1995; 47:74–81.

29. Overby LH, Nishio S, Weir A, Carver GT, Plopper CG, Philpot RM. Distribution of cytochrome P450 1A1 and NADPH-cytochrome P450 reductase in lungs of rabbits treated with 2,3,7,8-tetrachlorodibenzo-p-dioxin: ultrastructural immunolocalization and *in situ* hybridization. Mol Pharmacol 1992; 41:1039–1046.

30. Overby L, Nishio S, Lawton M, Plopper C, Philpot, R. Cellular localization of flavin-containing monooxygenase in rabbit lung. Exp Lung Res 1992; 18:131–144.

31. Plopper CG, Chang AM, Pang A, Buckpitt AR. Use of microdissected airways to define metabolism and cytotoxicity in murine bronchiolar epithelium. Exp Lung Res 1991; 17:197–212.

32. Massaro GD. Nonciliated Bronchiolar Epithelial (Clara) Cells. In: Massaro D, ed. Lung Cell Biology. New York: Dekker, 1989:81–114.

33. Manabe T, Ikeda H, Moriya T, Yamashita K. Immunohistochemical localization of the secretory products of rat Clara cells. Anat Rec 1987; 217:164–171.

34. Gupta RP, Patton SE, Jetten AM, Hook GER. Purification, characterization and proteinase-inhibitory activity of a Clara-cell secretory protein from the pulmonary extracellular lining of rabbits. Biochem J 1987; 248:337–344.

35. Singh G, Katyal SL, Brown WE, Phillips S, Kennedy AL, Anthony J. Amino-acid and CDNA nucleotide sequences of human Clara cell 10 kDa protein. Biochim Biophys Acta 1988; 950:329–337.

36. Gupta RP, Hook GER. In vitro translation of rabbit lung clara cell secretory protein mRNA. Biochem Biophys Res Commun 1988; 153:470–478.

37. Lopez de Haro MS, Alvarez L, Nieto A. Evidence for the identity of anti-proteinase pulmonary protein CCSP and uteroglobin. FEBS Lett 1988; 232:351–353.

38. Jensen SM, Jones JE, Pass H, Steinberg SM, Linnoila RI. Clara cell 10kDa protein mRNA in normal and atypical regions of human respiratory epithelium. Int J Cancer 1994; 58:629–637.

39. Patton SE, Gupta RP, Nishio SJ, Eddy M, Jetten AM, Plopper CG, Nettescheim P, Hook GER. Ultrastructural immunohistochemical localization of Clara cell secretory protein in pulmonary epithelium of rabbits. Environ Health Perspect 1991; 93: 225–232.
40. Miller YE, Walker SR, Spencer JS, Kubo RT, Mason RJ. Monoclonal antibodies specific for antigens expressed by rat type II alveolar epithelial and nonciliated bronchiolar cells. Exp Lung Res 1989; 15:635–649.
41. Suehiro T, Maeda K, Sueishi K. Immunohistochemical study of lung adenocarcinoma using monoclonal antibody for 60-kilodalton antigen in type II pneumocytes and nonciliated bronchiolar epithelial cells: comparison with two antisurfactant apoprotein antibodies. Am J Clin Pathol 1989; 92:150–158.
42. O'Reilly MA, Weaver TE, Pilot-Matias TJ, Sarin VK, Gazdar AF, Whitsett JA. In vitro translation, post-translational processing and secretion of pulmonary surfactant protein B precursors. Biochim Biophys Acta 1989; 1011:140–148.
43. Phelps D, Floros J. Localization of pulmonary surfactant proteins using immunohistochemistry and tissue in situ hybridization. Expl Lung Res 1991; 17:985–995.
44. De Water R, Willems LNA, van Muijen GNP, Franken C, Fransen JAM, Dijkman JH, Kramps JA. Ultrastructural localization of bronchial antileukoprotease in central and peripheral human airways by a gold-labeling technique using monoclonal antibodies. Am Rev Respir Dis 1986; 133:882–890.
45. Willems LNA, Kramps JA, Stijnen T, Sterk PJ, Weening JJ, Dijkman JH. Antileukoprotease-containing bronchiolar cells. Am Rev Respir Dis 1989; 139: 1244–1250.
46. Sallenave JM, Silva A. Marsden ME, Ryle AP. Secretion of mucus proteinase inhibitor and elafin by Clara cell and type II pneumocyte cell lines. Am J Respir Cell Mol Biol 1993; 8:126–133.
47. Sallenave JM, Shulmann J, Crossley J, Jordana M, Gauldie J. Regulation of secretory leukocyte proteinase inhibitor (SLPI) and elastase-specific inhibitor (ESI/elafin) in human airway epithelial cells by cytokines and neutrophilic enzymes. Am J Respir Cell Mol Biol 1994; 11:733–741.
48. Lund J, Devereux TR, Glaumann H, Gustafsson JA. Cellular and subcellular localization of a binding protein for polychlorinated biphenyls in rat lung. Drug Metab Dispos 1988; 16:590–599.
49. Devereux TR, Fouts JR, Eling TE. Metabolism of prostaglandin PG-F2alpha by freshly isolated alveolar type II cells from lungs of adult male or pregnant rabbits. Prostaglandins Leukotrienes Med 1987; 27:43–52.
50. Haroldsen PE, Voelkel NF, Henson JE, Henson PM, Murphy RC. Metabolism of platelet-activating factor in isolated perfused rat lung. J Clin Invest 1987; 79:1860–1867.
51. Evans MJ, Johnson LV, Stephens RJ, Freeman G. Renewal of the terminal bronchiolar epithelium in the rat following exposure to $NO_2$ or $O_3$. Lab Invest 1976; 35: 246–257.
52. Brody AR, Hook GER, Cameron GS, Jetten AM, Butterick CJ, Nettesheim P. The differentiation capacity of Clara cells isolated from the lungs of rabbits. Lab Invest 1987; 57:219–229.

53.  Hook GER, Brody AR, Cameron GS, Jetten AM, Gilmore LB, Nettesheim P. Repopulation of denuded tracheas by Clara Cells isolated from the lungs of rabbits. Exp Lung Res 1987; 12:311–329.

54.  Blanco A, Mendez A, Carrasco L, Bautista MJ, Sierra MA. Morphology and changes in Clara cells in the foetal bronchioles of Swiss mice. Histol Histopathol 1994; 9:251–258.

55.  Thaete LG, Ahnen DJ, Malkinson AM. Proliferating cell nuclear antigen (PCNA/Cyclin) immunocytochemistry as a labeling index in mouse lung tissues. Cell Tissue Res 1989; 256:167–173.

56.  Plopper CG, Nishio SJ, Alley JL, Kass P, Hyde DM. The role of the nonciliated bronchiolar epithelial (Clara) cell as the progenitor cell during bronchiolar epithelial differentiation in the perinatal rabbit lung. Am J Respir Cell Mol Biol 1992; 7: 606–613.

57.  Barth PJ, Wolf M, Ramaswamy A. Distribution and number of Clara cells in the normal and disturbed development of the human fetal lung. Pediatr Pathol 1994; 14: 637–651.

58.  Plopper CG, Alley JL, Serabjit-Singh CJ, Philpot RM. Cytodifferentiation of the nonciliated bronchiolar epithelial (Clara) cell during rabbit lung maturation: an ultrastructural and morphometric study. Am J Anat 1983; 167:329–357.

59.  ten Have-Opbroek AAW, De Vries ECP. Clara cell differentiation in the mouse: Ultrastructural morphology and cytochemistry for surfactant protein A and clara cell 10 kDa protein. Micros Res Tech 1993; 26:400–411.

60.  Strum JM, Ito T, Philpot RM, DeSanti AM, McDowell EM. The immunocytochemical detection of cytochrome P-450 monooxygenase in the lungs of fetal, neonatal, and adult hamsters. Am J Respir Cell Mol Biol 1990; 2:493–501.

61.  Ito T, Newkirk C, Strum JM, McDowell EM. Modulation of glycogen stores in epithelial cells during airway development in Syrian golden hamsters: a histochemical study comparing concanavalin A binding with the periodic acid-Schiff reaction. J Histochem Cytochem 1990; 38:691–697.

62.  Cardoso W, Stewart LG, Pinkerton KE, Ji C, Hook GER, Singh G, Katyal SL, Thurlbeck WM, Plopper CG. Secretory product expression during clara cell differentiation in the rabbit and rat. Am J Physiol 1993; 8:L543–L552.

63.  Plopper CG, Weir AJ, Morin D, Chang A, Philpot RM, Buckpitt AR. Postnatal changes in the expression and distribution of pulmonary cytochrome P450 mono-oxygenases during Clara cell differentiation in the rabbit. Mol Pharmacol 1993; 44:51–61.

64.  Ji CM, Plopper CG, Witschi HP, Pinkerton KE. Exposure to sidestream cigarette smoke alters bronchiolar epithelial cell differentiation in the postnatal rat lung. Am J Respir Cell Mol Biol 1994; 11:312–320.

65.  Strum JM, Singh G, Katyal SL, McDowell EM. Immunochemical localization of Clara cell protein by light and electron microscopy in conducting airways of fetal and neonatal hamster lung. Anat Rec 1990; 227:77–86.

66.  Nord M, Andersson O, Brönnegård M, Lund J. Rat lung polychlorinated biphenyl-binding protein: effect of glucocorticoids on the expression of the Clara cell-specific protein during fetal development. Arch Biochem Biophys 1992; 296:302–307.

67. Katyal SL, Singh G, Brown WE, Kennedy AL, Squeglia N, Wong-Chong ML. Clara cell secretory (10 kDaltons) protein: amino acid and CDNA nucleotide sequences, and developmental expression. Prog Respir Res 1990; 25:29–35.
68. Strum JM, Compton RS, Katyal SL, Singh G. The regulated expression of mRNA for Clara cell protein in the developing airways of the rat, as revealed by tissue *in situ* hybridization. Tissue Cell 1992; 24:461–471.
69. Singh G, Katyal SK. Secretory proteins of Clara cells and type II cells. In: Parent RA, ed. Comparative Biology of the Normal Lung. Boca Raton, FL: CRC Press, 1992:93–108.
70. Singh G, Katyal SL, Wong-Chong ML. A quantitative assay for a Clara cell-specific protein and its application in the study of development of pulmonary airways in the rat. Pediatr Res 1986; 20:802–805.
71. Kalina M, Mason R, Shannon JM. Surfactant protein C is expressed in alveolar type II cells but not in Clara cells of rat lung. Am J Respir Cell Mol Biol 1992; 6: 594–600.
72. Wohlford-Lenane CL, Snyder JM. Localization of surfactant-associated proteins SP-A and SP-B mRNA in rabbit fetal lung tissue by in situ hybridization. Am J Respir Cell Mol Biol 1992; 7:335–343.
73. Auten RL, Watkins RH, Shapiro DL, Horowitz S. Surfactant apoprotein A (SP-A) is synthesized in airway cells. Am J Respir Cell Mol Biol 1990; 3:491–496.
74. Stahlman MT, Gray ME, Whitsett JA. The ontogeny and distribution of surfactant protein B in human fetuses and newborns. J Histochem Cytochem 1992; 40:1471–1480.
75. Heine UI, Munoz EF, Flanders KC, Roberts AB, Sporn MB. Colocalization of TGF-beta 1 and collagen I and III, fibronectin and glycosaminoglycans during lung branching morphogenesis. Development 1990; 109:29–36.
76. Young SL, Chang LY, Erickson HP. Tenascin-C in rat lung: distribution, ontogeny and role in branching morphogenesis. Dev Biol 1994; 161:615–625.
77. Schuger L, O'Shea S, Rheinheimer J, Varani J. Laminin in lung development: effects of anti-laminin antibody in murine lung morphogenesis. Dev Biol 1990; 137:26–32.
78. Snyder JM, O'Brien JA, Rodgers HF. Localization and accumulation of fibronectin in rabbit fetal lung tissue. Differentiation 1987; 34:32–39.
79. Roman J, McDonald JA. Expression fibronectin, the integrin alpha5, and alpha-smooth muscle actin in heart and lung development. Am J Respir Cell Mol Biol 1992; 6:472–480.
80. Smith BT. Lung maturation in the fetal rat: acceleration by injection of fibroblast-pneumonocyte factor. Science 1979; 204:1094–1095.
81. Sepulveda J, Velasquez BJ. Study of the influence of NA-872 (Ambroxol) and dexamethasone on the differentiation of Clara cells in albino mice. Respiration 1982; 43:363–368.
82. Massaro D, Massaro G. Dexamethasone accelerates postnatal alveolar wall thinning and alters wall composition. Am J Physiol 1986; 251:R218–R224.
83. Phelps DS, Floros J. Dexamethasone in vivo raises surfactant protein B mRNA in alveolar and bronchiolar epithelium. Am J Physiol 1991; 260:L146–L152.
84. Fernandez-Renau D, Lombardero M, Nieto A. Glucocorticoid-dependent utero-

globin synthesis and uteroglobulin mRNA levels in rabbit lung explants cultured in vitro. Eur J Biochem 1984; 144:523–527.

85. Lombardero M, Nieto A. Glucocorticoid and developmental regulation of utero-globin synthesis in rabbit lung. Biochem J 1981; 200:487–494.

86. Devereux TR, Fouts JR. Effect of pregnancy or treatment with certain steroids on N, N-dimethylaniline demethylation and N-oxidation by rabbit liver or lung micro-somes. Drug Metab Dispos 1975; 3:254–258.

87. Devereux TR, Fouts JR. Effect of dexamethasone treatment on N, N-dimethylaniline demethylation and N-oxidation in pulmonary microsomes from pregnant and fetal rabbits. Biochem Pharmacol 1977; 27:1007–1008.

88. Fouts JR, Devereux TR. Developmental aspects of hepatic and extrahepatic drug-metabolizing enzyme systems: microsomal enzymes and components in rabbit liver and lung during the first month of life. J Pharmacol Exp Ther 1972; 183:458–468.

89. Massaro GD, Olivier J, Massaro D. Brief perinatal hypoxia impairs postnatal devel-opment of the bronchiolar epithelium. Am J Physiol 1989; 257:L80–L85.

90. Massaro GD, McCoy L, Massaro D. Development of bronchiolar epithelium: time course of response to oxygen and recovery. Am J Physiol 1988; 254:R755–R760.

91. Plopper CG, Weir AJ, Nishio SJ, Chang A, Voit M, Philpot RM, Buckpitt AR. Elevated susceptibility to 4-ipomeanol cytotoxicity in immature Clara cells of neonatal rabbits. J Pharmacol Exp Ther 1994; 269:867–880.

92. Massaro GD, McCoy L, Massaro D. Hyperoxia reversibly suppresses development of bronchiolar epithelium. Am J Physiol 1986; 251:R1045–R1050.

93. Massaro GD, McCoy L, Massaro D. Postnatal undernutrition slows development of bronchiolar epithelium in rats. 1988. Unpublished.

94. Jetten AM. Growth and differentiation factors in tracheobronchial epithelium. Am J Physiol Lung Cell Mol Physiol 1991; 260:L361–L373.

95. Kelley J. Cytokines of the lung. Am Rev Respir Dis 1990; 141:765–788.

96. Strandjord TP, Clark JG, Madtes DK. Expression of TGF-a, EGF, and EGF receptor in fetal rat lung. Am J Physiol Lung Cell Mol Physiol 1995; 11:L384–L389.

97. Johnson MD, Gray ME, Carpenter G, Pepinsky RB, Sundell H, Stahlman MT. Ontogeny of epidermal growth factor receptor/kinase and of lipocortin-1 in the ovine lung. Pediatr Res 1989; 25:535–541.

98. Johnson MD, Gray ME, Carpenter G, Pepinsky RB, Stahlman MT. Ontogeny of epidermal growth factor receptor and lipocortin-1 in fetal and neonatal human lungs. Hum Pathol 1990; 21:182–191.

99. Nexo E, Kryger-Baggesen N. The receptor for epidermal growth factor is present in human fetal kidney, liver and lung. Regul Pept 1989; 26:1–8.

100. Stahlman MT, Orth DN, Gray ME. Immunocytochemical localization of epidermal growth factor in the developing human respiratory system and in acute and chronic lung disease in the neonate. Lab Invest 1989; 60:539–547.

101. Raaberg L, Seier Poulsen S, Nexo E. Epidermal growth factor in the rat lung. Histochemistry 1991; 95:471–475.

102. Snead ML, Luo W, Oliver P, Nakamura M, Don-Wheeler G, Bessem C, Bell GI, Rall LB, Slavkin HC. Localization of epidermal growth factor precursor in tooth and lung during embryonic mouse development. Dev Biol 1989; 134:420–429.

103. Strandjord TP, Clark JG, Hodson WA, Schmidt RA, Madtes DK. Expression of transforming growth factor alpha in mid-gestation human fetal lung. Am J Respir Cell Mol Biol 1993; 8:266–272.
104. Kida K, Utsuyama M, Takizawa T, Thurlbeck WM. Changes in lung morphologic features and elasticity caused by streptozotocin-induced diabetes mellitus in growing rats. Am Rev Respir Dis 1983; 128:125–131.
105. Caniggia I, Liu J, Han R, Buch S, Funa K, Tanswell K, Post M. Fetal lung epithelial cells express receptors for platelet-derived growth factor. Am J Respir Cell Mol Biol 1993; 9:54–63.
106. Han RNN, Liu J, Tanswell K, Post M. Ontogeny of platelet-derived growth factor receptor in fetal rat lung. Micros Res Tech 1993; 26:381–388.
107. Han RNN, Liu J, Tanswell AK, Post M. Expression of basic fibroblast growth factor and receptor: immunolocalization studies in developing rat fetal lung. Pediatr Res 1992; 31:435–440.
108. Stiles AD, D'Ercole AJ. The insulin-like growth factors and the lung. Am J Respir Cell Mol Biol 1990; 3:93–100.
109. Warburton D, Seth R, Shum L, Horcher PG, Hall FL, Werb Z, Slavkin HC. Epigenetic role of epidermal growth factor expression and signalling in embryonic mouse lung morphogenesis. Dev Biol 1992; 149:123–133.
110. Catterton WZ, Escobedo MB, Sexson WR, Gray ME, Sundell HW, Stahlman MT. Effect of epidermal growth factor on lung maturation in fetal rabbits. Pediatr Res 1979; 13:104–108.
111. Plopper CG, St. George JA, Read LC, Nishio SJ, Weir AJ, Edwards L, Tarantal AF, Pinkerton KE, Merritt TA, Whitsett JA, George-Nascimento C, Styne D. Acceleration of alveolar type II cell differentiation in fetal rhesus monkey lung by administration of EGF. Lung Cell Mol Physiol 1992; 6:L313–L321.
112. Sundell HW, Gray ME, Serenius FS, Escobedo MB, Stahlman MT. Effects of epidermal growth factor on lung maturation in fetal lambs. Am J Pathol 1980; 100:707–726.
113. St. George JA, Read LC, Cranz DL, Tarantal AF, George-Nascimento C, Plopper CG. Effect of epidermal growth factor on the fetal development of the tracheobronchial secretory apparatus in rhesus monkey. Am J Respir Cell Mol Biol 1991; 4:95–101.
114. Young SL, Fram EK, Randell SH. Quantitative three-dimensional reconstruction and carbohydrate cytochemistry of rat nonciliated bronchiolar (clara) cells. Am Rev Respir Dis 1986; 133:899–907.
115. Barry BE, Mercer RR, Miller FJ, Crapo JD. Effects of inhalation of 0.25 ppm ozone on the terminal bronchioles of juvenile and adult rats. Exp Lung Res 1988; 14: 225–245.
116. Fujinaka LE, Hyde DM, Plopper CG, Tyler WS, Dungworth DL, Lollini LO. Respiratory bronchiolitis following long-term ozone exposure in bonnet monkeys: a morphometric study. Exp Lung Res 1985; 8:167–190.

# 8

## Growth and Differentiation of Tracheobronchial Epithelial Cells

**REEN WU**

California Regional Primate Research Center
and University of California at Davis
Davis, California

## I. Introduction

In a broad sense, airway diseases are a result related to a failure of airway epithelium to perform a homeostatic role in airway lumen. At least three features of the "epithelial failure" have been characterized. The first feature involves an uncontrolled cell proliferation in certain epithelial cell types that leads to bronchogenic neoplasm development. Four main histopathological types of lung cancer—adenocarcinoma, squamous cell carcinoma, small cell carcinoma, and large cell carcinoma—have been described (1–3). The cell type origins of these neoplasms are still poorly understood, even though some cancer cells in these lung tumors often retain many characteristics of normal airway epithelial cells; for instance, adenocarcinoma cells exhibit secretory features of mucous cell type, squamous carcinoma cells exhibit high tonofilament features resembling the basal cell type, and small cell carcinomas maintain some neuroendocrine characteristics. Reasons for this poor understanding are many. One problem is lack of a reproducible and predictable carcinogenesis model for manipulating both the initiation and the progression of bronchogenic tumors. The other reason is related to a plasticity of airway epithelium which can modify their intrinsic function (4). It is common to see a diverse histological appearance in the same neoplasm. This phenomenon has led to the interpretation that all cancer cell types and tumor types may derive from a common stem cell. Aberrations in the tracheobronchial epithelial stem cell could account for the heterogeneity and diversity in lung cancers. Clearly, identification of the stem cell population in tracheobronchial epithelium and elucidation of the pathway of cell differentiation and its regulation in these stem cells will lead us to a better understanding of neoplastic development in the lung (5).

The second feature related to epithelial failure is a change in cell differentiated function. The normal tracheobronchial lining is a well-differentiated mucociliary epithelium typified by the presence of basal, ciliated, and a variety of secretory cells (mucous secretory, serous, Clara, and neuroendocrine cells) (6). Under usual circumstances, the airway epithelium represents the first line of defense against noxious stimuli from inhalation. To exert the defense mechanism, the secretory cells in the epithelium are the principal cell type responsible for the secretion and maintenance of a viscoelastic mucous blanket to cover the epithelial cell surface. This mucous blanket serves as a protective layer that traps or modifies the inhalants. The complexes are then removed from the airway lumen through the coordinately ciliary escalation. It appears that the coordination between the mucous rheology and ciliary activity is an important factor in determining the efficiency of mucociliary clearance. Thus, it is possible that an alteration of mucous rheology, such as in the case of cystic fibrosis, could impair the mucociliary transport. It is also possible that a hypermucous secretion that occurs in the airway at the wrong place, such as in the bronchiolar region, or at the wrong time, such as during the disease stage, could jeopardize the clearance of ciliary escalation. As a consequence, the excess mucus and trapped molecules become the media that support the proliferation of various infectious agents. These infectious agents are capable of further damaging airway epithelium, and they cause epithelial cells to call on the migration of additional inflammatory cells in the airway lumen to initiate a vicious inflammatory cycle, which then leads to the change in the differentiation of airway epithelium. Indeed, a hypermucous secretion is a clinical hallmark that is frequently associated with various infectious airway diseases. By contrast, a reduced mucous secretion or a change of differentiated function from mucociliary to squamous by chemical or mechanical injury (7–10) would also impair this first line of defense, causing more damage in the epithelium. Clearly, epithelium repair of injury and restoration to an active and coordinately normal mucociliary function are essential to the homeostasis of the respiratory system (11).

The third feature of epithelial failure is the inability to prevent further migration of the inflammatory system into the airway lumen. Epithelial cells are known to produce both chemoattractants (12,13) and inhibitors (12) for inflammatory cell migration. Normally, airway epithelium has the instinct to call on the migration of inflammatory cells when it is under stress or damaged. However, these inflammatory cells also carry a battery of enzymes and mediators that are able to modify the extracellular matrix and the epithelial cell properties. These modifications, a good intention of the defense mechanism by the inflammatory cells, could produce a permanent scar in the epithelium. The size of the scar depends on how fast epithelial cells repair the injury and return to a differentiated state of mucociliary epithelium. The failure of the epithelial cells to repair the scar and the failure to prevent further influx of the inflammatory cells in the lumen by epithelial cells are the major symptoms associated with various airway diseases, such as asthma, cystic fibrosis, and bronchitis.

Aberrant cell proliferation and differentiation in tracheobronchial epithelium are clearly not only the cause but also the consequence of airway diseases. To develop a strategy that not only combats the cause but also the consequence requires a better understanding of the fundamental process that regulates the life cycle of tracheobronchial epithelium. Such an elucidation is the key to developing an effective strategy that can modulate airway disease at different stages of injury and repair. Progress has been made both in vivo and in vitro in understanding the biology of tracheobronchial epithelial cells. However, more work needs to be done. The purpose of this chapter is to review recent findings regarding the life cycle and functions of bronchial epithelial cells with a special focus on adult human and nonhuman primate species.

## II. Growth Regulation in Tracheobronchial Epithelium

### A. Progenitor Cell Type

Tracheobronchial epithelium, like many epithelia, is continually renewing itself. To identify the progenitor cell types that are involved in the self renewal in vivo, the traditional approach is to carry out mitotic index and nuclear labeling studies. For the nuclear labeling study, the incorporation of [³H]thymidine or bromdeoxy-uridine is used. Using these approaches, most of the data suggest that less than 1% of the epithelial cell population is involved in cell proliferation (14–18). Both basal and secretory cell types are capable of incorporating these nucleotide precursors and mitosis, whereas ciliated cells are considered to be terminally differentiated and incapable of division (19). In fact, it is only under exceptional circumstances that the ciliated cells of isolated hamster trachea are capable of synthesizing DNA, as evidenced by the incorporation of [³H]thymidine (20). Since differentiation and proliferation are normally inversely related, based on this view a number of investigators (21,22) suggest that it is the basal cell type that serves as the stem cells or the progenitor cell type that is involved in normal maintenance as well as in the regeneration and redifferentiation of bronchial epithelium after injury. However, this view is inconsistent with the data obtained from the developmental study and the injury/repair results. In the developing tracheas of a number of animal species, including human and nonhuman primates, basal cells are derived from an undifferentiated columnar epithelium (23). The appearance of the basal cell type in the tracheal surface lining layer appears after the appearance of ciliated and nonciliated secretory cell types (24). Furthermore, in the growing intrapulmonary airways (25,26), the basal cell type is not found in the smallest airway (23). In the injury models, such as the mechanical and toxic gases exposure model, hyperproliferation is seen in the secretory cell type, not in the basal cell type (4,8,18,27). These results point out that it is less likely for the basal cell type to serve as a progenitor cell type that initiates the growth of airway epithelium and the repair of epithelial damage (23).

New experiments in the repopulation of epithelial cells on denuded tracheal grafts have been used to assess the "progenitor" nature of various bronchial epithelial cell types. Denuded tracheal grafts are generally produced by removing the lining epithelial layer by repeated freezing and thawing of tracheal grafts, a technique developed several years ago by Nettesheim and his colleagues (28). Using this technique, combined with the cell separation technique, Hook and his colleagues have demonstrated the repopulation of a mucociliary epithelium in the denuded tracheal graft by enriched basal cell population from the rabbit and rat (29,30). These experiments clearly demonstrate the polypotent nature of the basal cell type. However, there are several deficiencies in these experiments. First of all, the definition of basal cell type is based on the ultrastructural picture and the immunohistochemical stain. However, it is well known that secretory cells lose their differentiated features on cell isolation and culturing in vitro. The degranulated secretory cells may resemble the basal cell type, and the morphological tools used in these studies cannot satisfactorily distinguish the basal one from the degranulated secretory cell type in dissociated and isolated cell preparations. Furthermore, for the preparations in these studies, the purity of basal cell type population is only 90%. Johnson et al. (31) used flow cytometry to isolate basal cells. They found that basal cells from rat trachea had a colony-forming efficiency of 0.6%, whereas secretory cells and unsorted cells had efficiencies of 3.4 and 2.6%, respectively. From these results, the investigators concluded that basal cells had less proliferative activity than secretory cells. It is therefore difficult to conclude from these tracheal graft repopulation studies that basal cell type is the progenitor cell type responsible for the initiation of airway epithelial cell growth and the repair response to injury.

Recently, the use of the molecular expression technique has allowed researchers to tag a proliferative cell population in vitro and then repopulate these tagged cells into denuded rat trachea, which were implanted subcutaneously into athymic mice. This approach will allow the analysis of the dynamics of cell turnover, lineage, and differentiation pattern. Wilson and his colleagues (32,33) used the retroviral system to tag cultured cells with an expression of various reporter genes (e.g., β-galactosidase) and used these cells to repopulate a denuded tracheal graft. By following the clusters of transgene-expressing cells in the newly repopulated tracheal graft, it was found that these retroviral tagged cells had the capacity to generate different sizes of cluster cells and a variety of differentiated cell types. A substantial number of clones showed transgene expression in basal as well as differentiated columnar cells, which supports the existence of a cell type within the tracheobronchial epithelium that is capable of extensive self-renewal and pluripotent development. Further characterization of these potential stem cells will be an important task to further advance our knowledge of the pathogenesis of various airway diseases.

## B. Growth of Tracheobronchial Epithelial Cells in Culture

To elucidate growth factors and mechanisms involved in growth regulation, airway epithelium is best studied in vitro. A number of primary epithelial cell culture systems for human airway tissues has been developed (34–39). These include the 3T3 feeder layer system (34,35), explant outgrowth system (34,35), dissociated cell culture system (36–38), and the newly developed brush system (39) from clinic patients. The basic principle behind the success in growing airway epithelial cells is based on the development of serum-free hormone-supplemented medium. The development of the hormone/growth factor supplements is based on the growth study showing that deleting one of these growth supplements would decrease the growth (cell number) in these primary tracheobronchial epithelial cultures. An example of such a study is shown in Figure 1 which demonstrated the optimal growth of human tracheobronchial epithelial (TBE) cells on various substrata is dependent on the supplement of these seven factors. Primary epithelial cells grown under these conditions, especially at low calcium (0.1 mM) level and on a plastic cell culture surface or a culture surface coated with a very small amount of collagen, can be passaged several times. Passage of primary cultures grown on collagen gel substratum or on a culture surface coated with thick collagen is difficult even though these types of substratum help epithelial cell differentiation in culture.

Despite the success in growing primary bronchial epithelial cells in culture and the development of a technique to passage them and maintain them in culture, few studies have focused on the origin of these cultured cells. In our laboratory, we have previously observed that both beating cilia and mucous-secreting granules can be found in the first 72 hr of primary culture of dissociated rat tracheal epithelial cells (40). However, these differentiated features are rapidly lost in culture, and as a result, most cultured cells did not exhibit any differentiated features. Interestingly, more than 90% of cultured cells are engaged in DNA synthesis within 48 hr after plating. This study demonstrated that airway epithelial cells, like many other epithelial cell types, are capable of cell proliferation despite their differentiated features. In the airway in vivo injury model, the adjacent

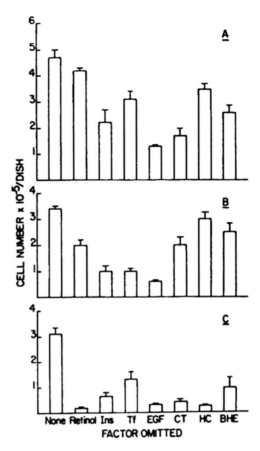

**Figure 1**   Effects of minus one factor on the growth of primary human tracheobronchial epithelial (TBE) cells in culture. Human TBE cells were isolated as previously described and were plated on various culture surfaces in the complete medium supplemented with the seven growth factors or in the minus one factor medium as indicated. The seven growth factor supplements are vitamin A (A, retinol, 0.1 μM), insulin (Ins, 5 μg/ml), transferrin (Tf, 5 μg/ml), epidermal growth factor (EGF, 10 ng/ml), hydrocortisone (HC, 1 μM), cholera toxin (CT, 10 ng/ml), and bovine hypothalamus extract (BHE, 15 μg/ml). The cell seeding density was $2 \times 10^5$ cells/dish and cell counting was carried out after 7 days of incubation. Similar results were obtained independently from three different monkey airway tissues. (A) Plastic culture surface; (B) collagen coated surface; (C) collagen gel substratum. Collage coated surface was prepared by treating plastic culture surface with 30 μg/cm² of type I collagen and air-dried overnight. Collagen gel substratum was prepared according to the procedure in previously published (38).

epithelial cells with mucous granules are able to transform into a different type of secretory cells, such as those containing small mucous granules or no granule as an intermediate undifferentiated cell type to engage in DNA synthesis (17,18). A similar transformation between differentiated features and cell proliferation has recently been demonstrated in vitro by Randall and his colleagues (41). In their study, markers for basal and differentiated cell types have been developed. Using the cell separation technique, they are able to enrich the basal and mucous cell types in the preparations. They have observed that when basal cells are plated on a culture dish, the cultured cells eventually develop the markers for both basal and mucous cell types. Similarly, the mucous cell type after plating in culture can develop both the basal and mucous cell types. These results strengthen the notion that various TBE cells are able to differentiate and proliferate if the conditions to stimulate their growth and differentiation exist. These results also support the notion as described above that there are heterogeneous progenitor cell types which have different life spans and differentiated properties.

## C. Ability of Epithelial Cells to Secrete Growth Factor

It was observed many years ago that mechanical or toxic injury (7–9,17,18) and vitamin A deficiency were able to induce hyperplasia and squamous cell metaplasia in tracheobronchial epithelia (22,42–45). These conditions increase dramatically the mitotic rate of TBE cells. A similar step of hyperplasia and squamous cell metaplasia has been implicated in the development of bronchogenic cancer. However, the nature of the hyperplasia is not known. For mechanical and toxic injury, it is reasonable to assume that the influx of inflammatory cells and the growth factors to the lumen through underlying basal lamina may be partly responsible for the initiation of cell proliferation. However, in the case of vitamin A–deficiency induced hyperplasia, the influx does not occur unless an infection develops. Therefore, the initiation of cell proliferation is related to the intrinsic property of epithelial cells in response to vitamin A deficiency.

To elucidate the mechanism of the hyperplasia phenomenon, we and workers at several other laboratories have examined the effects of vitamin A on the primary tracheobronchial epithelial cultures. In the serum-free hormone-supplemented medium, we have observed that vitamin A and its synthetic derivatives (retinoids) stimulate growth in tracheobronchial epithelial cells (46,47). When cells are plated on an uncoated plastic culture surface, the stimulatory effect is small; 20–60% of the overall growth in a 7-day assay. However, on the collagen gel substratum, retinoid is absolutely essential for the continuous growth and proliferation of monkey and human TBE cells. Interestingly, retinoid treatment alters the responsiveness of TBE cells to epidermal growth factor (EGF). As shown in Figure 2, depriving one growth factor from the complete medium reduced the growth of primary TBE cells. Among these studies, insulin and

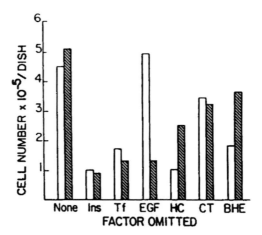

**Figure 2** Effects of vitamin A on the response of human tracheobronchial epithelial (TBE) cells to various growth factor supplements. Human TBE cells were isolated and plated on culture dishes in the complete medium supplemented with six growth factor supplements or in the minus one of these growth factor supplements medium as described in Figure 1. Retinol (shaded bars) was added to the culture medium at 0.1 μM one day after the plating. The control cultures (open bars) have no retinol added. Cell number was determined after 7 days in culture. Note: The response of human TBE cells to EGF-dependent growth stimulation is affected by the presence or absence of retinol. Experiments have been carried out independently in separate three human airway tissues with similar results.

transferrin are the two most important factors. However, when retinoid is added to the culture system, an additional requirement for EGF is seen. The simplest way to interpret this result is that TBE cells under the vitamin A–sufficient condition require EGF for their growth, whereas in the vitamin A–deficient medium, EGF is not needed. There are several explanations for this phenomenon. However, we favor the explanation that epithelial cells are capable of secreting EGF-like growth factor(s) in the vitamin A–deficient condition, whereas this secretion is inhibited by vitamin A. To further elaborate this mechanism, we have demonstrated that both human and monkey tracheobronchial epithelial cells in primary cultures in the absence of vitamin A supplement are capable of secreting growth-stimulating activity (46). This growth-stimulating activity can replace the EGF requirement and downregulate the EGF receptor after incubation. In a study using the neutralizing anti-transforming growth factor-α (anti–TGF-α) antibody, the growth-stimulating activity is inhibited, suggesting that TGF-α–like activity is involved. Nettesheim and his colleague have also demonstrated that TGF-α is secreted by primary rat tracheal epithelial cells and several transformed TBE cell lines (48,49).

Because it is difficult to translate the cell culture data to the in vivo situation, especially in the development of a vitamin A–deficient animal model, we used the organ culture system to achieve a vitamin A–deficient stage. As shown in Figure 3, a vitamin A–deficient squamous cell metaplasia can be achieved in the organ culture system. In contrast, a mucociliary epithelium is continuously maintained if the culture medium is supplemented with vitamin A (47). Using the cRNA probe in the in situ hybridization, we observed that the TGF-α message level is elevated in the squamous epithelium, whereas the level is reduced in the presence of vitamin A. These results support the notion that tracheobronchial epithelial cells are capable of producing autocrine/paracrine growth factor(s), and this production may be regulated by vitamin A.

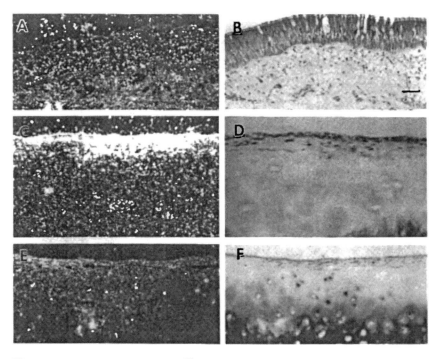

**Figure 3**  In situ hybridization of $^{35}$S-cRNA of TGF-α in paraffin sections of human tracheobronchial tissues. Airway tissues were maintained as organ cultures in the presence of vitamin A (A,B) or in its absence (C–E). (A,C,E) Darkfield micrography of hybridization; (B,D,F) bright field micrography. Sense (E,F) and antisense (A–D) cRNA probes were generated as described before and were used for the hybridization. Note: TGF-α message in tracheobronchial epithelium is elevated in the organ culture without the vitamin A supplement. Bar=10 μm

In addition to the presence of stimulatory factor, vitamin A can also regulate the production of growth inhibitor. In a recent study, it was shown that the expression of TGF-β is elevated by the vitamin A treatment (C.B. Robinson and R. Wu, unpublished data). TGF-β is generally a growth inhibitor for various epithelial cell types, including the transformed cell types (50). However, the potential role of this autocrine/paracrine secretion of TGF-β in TBE cell culture is still uncertain (49,50). This is because more than 90% of TGF-β secreted in culture is in a latent form, which requires activation in order to be active.

### D.  A Hypothesis of Paracrine/Autocrine Growth Regulation in Airway Epithelium

In summary, tracheobronchial epithelium has limited cell proliferation under normal conditions. However, hyperplasia of airway epithelium can be induced by injuries related to vitamin A deficiency, carcinogens, and mechanical treatments. We have observed an imbalance of growth supplements in the local airway environment after vitamin A deficiency (Fig. 4). This type of imbalance is different from the one induced by carcinogens or mechanical injury. This difference is

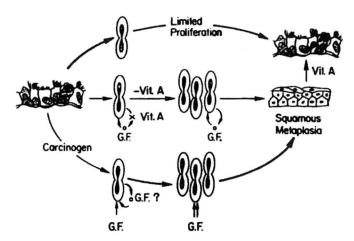

**Figure 4**   A hypothesis based on autocrine/paracrine growth regulation for airway epithelial cells during vitamin A deficiency and carcinogen treatment. Under the normal condition, the mucociliary epithelium has limited proliferation activity, and a differentiated mucociliary epithelium is continuously maintained. During the vitamin A deficiency (-Vit. A), epithelial cells secrete growth factors (as indicated by G.F.) to promote cell proliferation, resulting in the formation of squamous metaplasia. This secretion is inhibited by vitamin A. A similar mechanism is proposed for the carcinogen-exposed airway epithelium in which growth factors are either secreted by epithelial cells or obtained from the basal lamina.

consistent with the morphological analysis which shows in the keratinized epithelia induced by vitamin A deficiency that the basement membrane is still intact, whereas it is fragmented in airways after carcinogen treatment (9,51). It is possible that the carcinogen-induced squamous cell metaplasia is influenced by the influx of various exogenous growth factors and hormones through the under layer tissue. In this situation, the recovery of the lesion may depend on the repair-completion of the basement membrane. This notion is also consistent with the reports that carcinogen-induced metaplastic lesions are greatly enhanced when vitamin A is depleted (52,53).

## III. Regulation of Mucociliary Differentiation

### A. In Vivo Studies of the Plasticity of Airway Epithelium

Depending on species, at least eight different epithelial cell types have been morphologically delineated in airway surface epithelium (9,54–56) Based on their functions, these epithelial cell types can be roughly divided into three groups. One is the basal cell type, which is proposed by Evans and his colleagues as an anchoraged cell type (23), especially in airways with a large diameter. Ciliated cell type is present throughout the entire airway epithelium and is responsible for ciliary beating. The secretory cell type, although heterogeneous, is responsible for the secretion of vasoelastic mucus. As described above, based on the kinetics of the [3H]thymidine pulse and chase experiments, it is generally accepted that both basal and nonciliated columnar cells contribute significantly to steady-state turnover. The chase experiment also supports the notion that these proliferative cell types after DNA synthesis are able to differentiate into various cell types seen in the mucociliary epithelium. It is often seen that the progeny of dividing cells follow a differentiation pathway different from that of the original cell. A similar pattern of cell division and differentiation is also seen in airway injury in which more columnar cells are recruited to proliferate and then to differentiate. However, there is evidence to support the idea that the differentiation pattern is greatly influenced by the environment. Under normal conditions, differentiation is fixed by the environment, which varies little from the previous one. Therefore, under normal conditions, the cells differentiate to mucociliary epithelium, whereas under injury conditions, the influx of inflammatory cells through their secretion is able to modulate the surrounding tissue architecture and may significantly influence the pathway of cell differentiation. Depending on the injury model, both mucous cell metaplasia and squamous cell metaplasia are seen. However, compared with the in vitro experiments, relatively few experiments have been carried out in vivo to elucidate the nature of the regulation of mucociliary differentiation. Reasons for fewer experiments in vivo are many, but the major problem is that it is difficult to carry out mechanistic experiments in vivo. A majority of in vivo experiments are descriptive. The straightforward information reveals the plasticity of airway epithelial cell properties (4). Other studies have revealed that aberrant cell differentiation results in the phenomena of hypermucous secretion (57,58) and squamous cell differentiation (5).

### B.  Hypermucous Secretion—Mucous Cell Metaplasia

Hypermucous secretion is one of the major hallmarks clinically associated with the airway disease of infection. These diseases include cystic fibrosis, asthma, and bronchitis. In many of these diseases, an initial infection or damage by toxic gas, such as $SO_2$, causes an irritation of epithelial cells, which then call on the migration of inflammatory cells. It is still unclear how the persistent presence of inflammatory cells and infectious microorganisms in the airway lumen can influence the differentiation of TBE cells toward a hyper-mucous secretion stage. Recently, Basbaum and her colleagues have demonstrated in vitro that treatment of bronchial epithelial cells with lipopolysaccharides stimulates the expression of several human apomucin genes, such as MUC-2 and MUC-5, in cultured airway epithelial cells (C.B. Basbaum, personal communication). This result is consistent with the notion that a persistent presence of bacterial product influences the transformation of airway epithelial cells to express various mucous cell markers.

### C.  In Vitro Studies of Mucociliary Cell Differentiation

Tracheobronchial epithelial cells, like many other epithelial cells, tend to lose their differentiated functions when cultured in vitro. However, the loss of differentiated functions—at least in the primary tracheobronchial epithelial culture—is transient. Evidence of transient dedifferentiation comes from two experiments. One is the repopulation study in which cultured cells are replated on denuded tracheal grafts which are carried by immune-deficient mice (28). It was observed more than 14 years ago that undifferentiated rabbit tracheal epithelial cells maintained long-term in culture are able to repopulate on denuded rat tracheal grafts and form a new mucociliary epithelium (59,60). This result suggests that epithelial cells, despite dedifferentiation in culture, are able to maintain their intrinsic differentiated potential which is eventually expressed if an appropriate environment is provided. Because of this encouraging result, subsequent developments in optimizing hormonal requirements and the utilization of vitamin A supplement and collagen gel substratum (36,61) for epithelial cultures further enhance the differentiated nature of cultured tracheobronchial epithelial cells. We were the first to demonstrate new ciliogenesis in primary hamster tracheal epithelial cultures based on the semiquantitative determination of ciliated population (62). Subsequently, we were able to demonstrate that mucous cell differentiation also occurs in hamster tracheal cultures (63). We, as well as Kim's laboratory, have demonstrated that the large molecular weight of secretory glycoproteins by cultured hamster tracheal epithelial cells are O-glycosidic linked to protein (63,64). Based on the amino acid and carbohydrate composition analyses of the in vitro secretory products as compared with the in vivo mucin products purified from sputum and epithelial cell layer, we concluded that cultured hamster tracheal epithelial cells are able to secrete authentic mucin (65). Similar results have since been demonstrated in both human (38) and guinea pig (66) tracheobronchial epithelial cultures. These developments further strengthen the notion that a mucociliary epithelium can be achieved in culture if the culture condition is properly developed.

In 1986, we developed a Whitcutt's chamber to grow airway epithelial cells between air and a liquid medium interface (67). The development of this chamber is based on the physiological consideration that airway epithelial cells in vivo are usually located between air and a liquid interface. This notion is quite different from the traditional tissue culture technique which tends to culture cells under a medium-immersed condition. Using this chamber, we observed columnarized formation of cultured epithelial cells and further development of mucociliary differentiation in culture (68,69). We as well as others (70,71) have recently applied the biphasic culture systems to both human and monkey tracheobronchial epithelial cells and have observed the formation of a fully differentiated epithelial cell layer with prominent features of ciliary beating (Fig. 5) and mucous-secreting granules (Fig. 6). However, in contrast to airway epithelial cells derived from rodents, mucociliary differentiation of human and monkey cultures occurs at a much later time (at least 21 days after plating). We have observed that one of the major problems associated with such a long-term biphasic culture is the drying out on the apical side of cultured epithelial cell layers despite 100% humidity in the incubator. To avoid such a problem, a trace amount of culture medium is added on the apical side of the culture. We have observed that the addition of 0.05 ml of culture medium on top of an approximately 5-cm$^2$ surface of a monkey tracheobronchial epithelial culture was able to maintain the culture more than 2 months without any deterioration. As shown in Figure 5, scanning electron microscopy has demonstrated extensive ciliary features on the culture surface, and transmission electron micrography (data not shown; cf. Fig. 6) has demonstrated the formation of abundant mucous-secreting granules and the columnarized features with two- to four-cell layer. Interestingly, the "basal" cell layer is compressed and resembles the in vivo basal cell type with such features as prominent tonofilament structure and high nucleus/cytoplasm ratio. In contrast, if excessive medium (e.g., 0.5 ml) was added on the apical side of the culture, a condition similar to the traditional immersed culture system, both the compact and columnarized features are reduced. Furthermore, the extent of mucociliary differentiation in such a culture is qualitatively decreased.

In summary, there are at least three stages of development of the airway epithelial cell culture system. First, the development of serum-free hormone-supplemented medium allows a continuous cultivation of various tracheo-

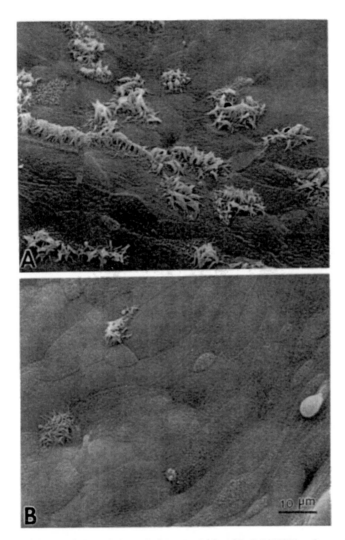

**Figure 5**  Ciliogenesis in monkey tracheobronchial epithelial (TBE) cultures. Monkey
TBE cells were plated in the biphasic culture chambers (25 mm diameter) with variable
amounts of culture medium (from 0 to 1 ml) on the apical side of epithelial layer. After 21–
28 days of incubation, chambers were fixed for scanning electron microscopic analysis.
Without the culture medium, there is a dryness of epithelial layer observed (data not
shown). The presence of 0.05 ml medium on the apical side of epithelial layer is sufficient to
prevent this problem (A). Increased medium overlayer volume (e.g., B at 0.5 ml) reduces
the ciliated cell population as evidenced by the scanning electron micrograph.

bronchial epithelial cells in culture. Successful completion of this stage allows the second stage of development to incorporate critical factors, such as vitamin A and the collagen gel substratum, for airway epithelial cell differentiation. In the third stage of development, a physiology-relevant culture condition is developed. The development of a biphasic culture system for bronchial epithelial cells is a major advance in the in vitro model to study airway epithelial cell physiology and injury and repair. Application of the biphasic culture system to ozone exposure has recently been demonstrated (72,73).

## IV. Role of Vitamin A in Airway Mucociliary Cell Differentiation

### A. Effects of Vitamin A Deficiency and Supplement

Tracheobronchial epithelium is one of the vitamin A–targeted tissues (42–45). The epithelium requires vitamin A for the preservation and induction of the expression of differentiated functions. Keratinizing squamous metaplasia of normal mucociliary epithelium is the primary lesion that occurs in the vitamin A-deficient state. The normal, columnar, mucociliary epithelium becomes underlaid with the new, stratified, squamous, keratinizing epithelium; distinctive keratohyaline granules can usually be seen before the development of sheets of keratin. Accompanying these morphological changes is a reduction in the synthesis of mucous glycoproteins. Both in vivo and in vitro organ culture studies have shown that the administration of vitamin A or its synthetic derivatives (retinoids) can reverse this phenomenon. At the other extreme, excess vitamin A can even convert stratified skin epithelium in chick embryos to an epithelium containing mucous-secreting granules (74). Thus, it appears that the controls for mucous cell differentiation and squamous metaplasia are inversely linked by vitamin A.

The cell type responsive to vitamin A regulation of squamous cell differentiation and mucous cell differentiation in airway epithelium has not been identified. There are at least two possibilities. One possibility is that both mucous and squamous cells are derived from different cell types and both of them are competing for the same growth environment. The presence of vitamin A alters the growth environment, which favors the proliferation of mucous progenitor cells, whereas the absence of vitamin A favors the proliferation of the progenitor cell type of squamous cell epithelium. McDowell and her colleagues have demonstrated that vitamin A treatment enhances the proliferation of small mucous-granular cell type in primary hamster tracheal epithelial cultures (75–77). However, it has not been demonstrated that vitamin A deficiency leads to enhanced squamous cell proliferation. In a separate study, vitamin A was shown to enhance DNA synthesis of basal cells of keratinocyte cultures (78). In addition, there is no evidence that

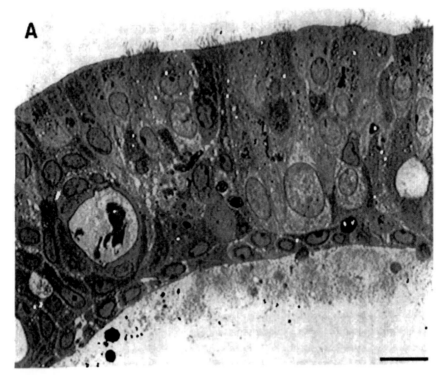

**Figure 6** Light microscopic cross section of monkey tracheobronchial cultures maintained in the biphasic culture chambers. Experiments were carried out as described in Figure 5. Chambers were fixed and ultra-thin sections were prepared and stained with toluidine blue. As described in Figure 5, the apical side of epithelial layer contained the medium volume of 0.05 and 0.5 ml, respectively, for (A and B). Bar=10μm

vitamin A inhibits squamous cell proliferation. The other possibility is that both mucous and squamous cells are derived from the same cell type, and vitamin A stimulates this uncommitted cell type to express mucous cell phenotypes. There is some evidence to support this explanation. It is not unusual to observe cells with the differentiated features of both mucous cell type (i.e., secretory granules) and squamous cell type (i.e., tonofilaments). Furthermore, it is known from the in vivo injury-repair study that degranulated mucous cells (or an intermediate cell type) are capable of incorporating [³H]thymidine and then differentiating into squamous cell type. In vitro, we have observed that a similar phenomenon exists in primary tracheobronchial epithelial cultures immediately after plating. These results support the notion that the progenitor cell types of mucous and squamous epithelia are

B

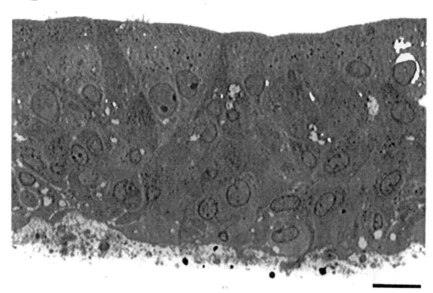

related and the differential expression of these phenotypes is regulated by vitamin A.

### B. Cellular Basis of Vitamin A–Dependent Mucous Cell Differentiation in Culture

To elucidate the role of vitamin A in cell differentiation, we use the in vitro cell culture system to address this question. We have observed that vitamin A is very important for human and monkey tracheobronchial epithelial cells to express mucous differentiated functions. As shown in Figure 7, the presence of vitamin A is essential for a continuous maintenance of the integrity of airway epithelium cultured on collagen gel substratum. In the absence of vitamin A supplements, the epithelium deteriorates within 1–2 weeks, whereas a multiple cell layer of epithelium can be maintained long term in the vitamin A–supplemented condition. We have observed that the expression of mucous differentiated cell types in culture depends on vitamin A. To further trace the origin of the mucous cell type in culture, we carried out kinetics studies with pulse and chase of [³H]thymidine labeling. Data for this cytokinetic study are currently in preparation for a publication, and Figure 8 best describes the conclusion of this study. According to the cell kinetics, we observed that a majority of the mucous cell type in culture is derived

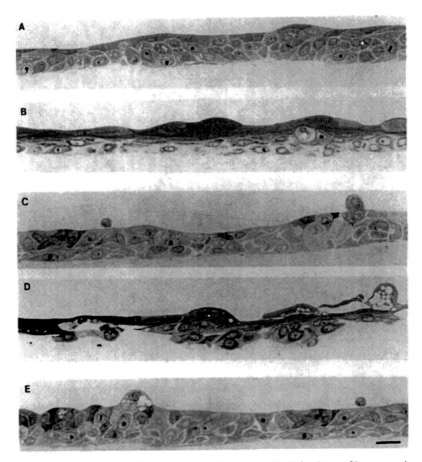

**Figure 7** Morphologies of cross-sections of airway epithelial cultures. Human tracheo-bronchial epithelial cells were maintained in the serum-free hormone-supplemented medium with vitamin A (A,C,E) and without (B,D) on collagen gel substratum. Cultures were harvested 1 (A,B), 2 (C,D), or 4 (E) weeks after plating and fixed for methacrylate embedding. Vertical sections of the blocks were prepared and stained with toluidine blue. Note: Vitamin A is required by human epithelial cells to maintain the integrity of epithelium in culture. Bar = 2 μm.

from a process of cell differentiation independent from cell proliferation. A mucous cell population capable of DNA synthesis in culture is rare, occurring only during the early period of primary culture. Within 4 to 6 days, a majority of the new mucous cell population is developed from a replicative nonmucous cell type after DNA synthesis has ceased. Vitamin A and its derivatives apparently

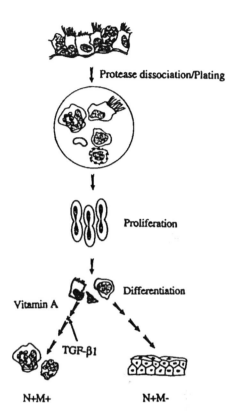

**Figure 8** A cellular model of vitamin A–dependent mucous cell differentiation in primary cultures of airway epithelial cells. Most of cells labeled with [³H]thymidine (indicated as N+) have no mucous cell function (indicated as N+M-). However, after DNA synthesis, some of these nonmucous cells (indicated as N+M-) are able to differentiate into mucous cell type (indicated as N+M+). This DNA replication-independent mucous cell differentiation is dependent on vitamin A treatment but is inhibited by TGF-β1.

play an essential role in this transformation. Interestingly, this transformation is inhibited by TGF-β1.

## C. Molecular Basis of Mucous Cell Differentiation

It is still unclear how vitamin A regulates these differential functions. At the biochemical level, one of the major differences between squamous and mucous cell differentiation is the production of the mucous glycoprotein mucin. Understanding the biochemical mechanism(s) of vitamin A control of mucin synthesis will significantly increase our understanding of the cellular processes related to airway mucociliary cell differentiation. Recent data establish that vitamin A regulates cell differentiation at the transcriptional level. There is a wealth of information about the transcriptional roles of retinoids, especially the active form, retinoic acid (RA). Retinol is biologically active, but its affinity for nuclear retinoid receptors is approximately 1% of that exhibited by all-*trans*–retinoic acid. Three major classes of nuclear binding proteins or retinoic acid receptors (RAR) have been characterized and are termed $\alpha$, $\beta$, and $\gamma$, respectively (79–84). These receptors are members of a superfamily of nuclear receptors, which includes the receptors for steroid and thyroid hormones and for vitamin $D_3$. The RARs are 50,000-d DNA binding proteins that contain six domains, designated A–F from amino to carboxyl termini, respectively. The C region contains two zinc fingers that interact with DNA response elements; namely, retinoic acid response elements (RAREs). The response element contains a sequence that is usually composed of two tandemly arranged half-site sequences, (Pu)G(G/T)TCA (opposite strand: TGA[C/A]C[Py]) separated by a spacer which is from one to five nucleotides long (85). The RA binding portion of the RAR lies within domain E, and this region, along with the C region, is highly conserved among these three types of RARs (86). The A and F regions are not conserved among the RARs but are highly conserved among species. The RARs can dimerize with other DNA binding proteins such as the retinoid X receptors (RXRs) (87). Dimerization between RAR and RXR increases the stability of the receptor-DNA complex and greatly enhances the transcriptional activity. Three types of RXRs, $\alpha$, $\beta$, and $\gamma$, have been described. Although RXR binds all-*trans*–RA, the affinity is 40-fold less than the affinity with their natural ligand 9-*cis*-RA. RXR homodimers can also bind to RXREs in the presence of ligand (87). Recently, evidence has shown that RXR is capable of forming heterodimers with various steroid receptors such as GR, TR, and VDR. In addition, RAR can also influence the activity of other transcriptional factors such as AP-2 and AP-1. This information shows that these RARs and RXRs are among the most dynamic transcriptional factors involved in various transcriptional regulation activities (88).

To further elucidate the nature of vitamin A–dependent mucous cell differentiation in culture, we carried out an RNA microinjection study. The purpose of this study is to determine whether change of cell differentiation occurs at the genetic level. RNA was isolated from primary human and monkey tracheobronchial epithelial cultures which were plated on collagen gel substratum and maintained in the medium with or without vitamin A. RNA at 10–100 μg/ml were microinjected into cells. After 4–6 hr of incubation, cells were fixed and immunostained with mucin-specific monoclonal antibodies, 17B1 and 17Q2 (89,90). The epitope of both antibodies has been localized on the mucous-secreting granules of both human and monkey airway epithelium by the immunogold electron microscopic technique (J.A. St. George and C.G. Plopper, unpublished data). As shown in Figure 9, the host cells, which are derived from an immortalized human

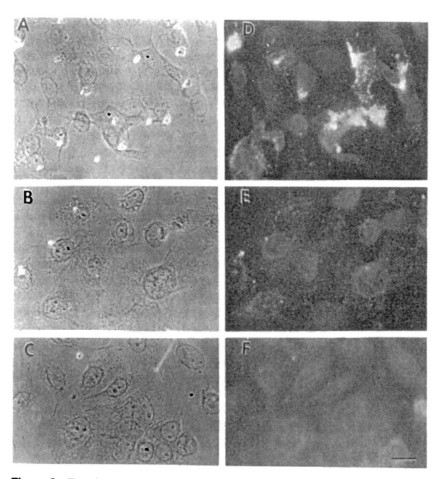

**Figure 9** Transformation of nonmucous cells to mucous cell type by RNA microinjection. BEAS-2B cell line grew in culture expressed no mucous cell function as indicated by a negative immunofluorescent stain with antimucin–specific antibody (C, F). When BEAS-2B cells were microinjected with RNA isolated from primary airway epithelial cultures which expressed mucociliary differentiation, the injected cells (A, as shown by the presence of holes in the injected cell) became positive to antimucin antibody staining (D). In contrast, when BEAS-2B cells were microinjected with RNA isolated from undifferentiated cultures, the injected cells (B, as shown by the presence of holes in the cells) were still negative to antimucin antibody staining (E). (A–C) Phase contrast micrographs; (D–F) Fluorescent micrographs. Bar: 10 μm.

bronchial epithelial cell line, BEAS-2B, have no fluorescent stain with these antibodies. After microinjection with RNA from collagen gel primary culture maintained in vitamin A–supplemented medium, injected cells are able to express mucin-like synthesis and have positive fluorescent stain from reacting with these antibodies. However, the microinjection with RNA derived from the vitamin A–deficient culture has less or no fluorescent stain. These results suggest that the change in differentiation between the vitamin A–supplemented and vitamin A–absent cultures takes place at the genetic level. To further elucidate the nature of this change, molecular cloning of these genes will be essential. One potential difference at the genetic level is the change in the expression of the mucin core protein genes, MUC genes.

Airway mucous that covers the surface of conducting airways is the first line of lung defense against airborne pollutants and microorganisms. The mucous gel layer relies on mucous glycoproteins (mucins) for its viscoelastic properties and hence its ability to effectively clear foreign particles from airways. Mucin glycoproteins are large, highly glycosylated macromolecules (91,92). Carbohydrate, which makes up 80–90% of airway mucins by weight, is the major determinant of the gelation and bacteria binding (93) properties of mucins. Mucin carbohydrates are extremely heterogeneous with respect to size, structure, and acidic properties (94). Differences in carbohydrate chains, composition, and structures have been demonstrated among different airway diseases. The cause of the difference among carbohydrate chains in different diseases is not known.

Mucins constitute a family of glycoproteins whose members exhibit similar characteristics in their protein backbones and their O-glycosidic oligosaccharide chains (95,96). Over the last several years, at least seven human MUC genes have been isolated and characterized (95–97). The complete primary structures have been elucidated only for MUC1 (98,99), MUC7 (97), and recently MUC2 (100,101). Both MUC1 (102) and MUC2 (103–106) are known to be expressed in airway epithelial cells. We have recently demonstrated that the expression of the MUC2 gene in both human and monkey TBE cultures is downregulated by vitamin A at the transcriptional level (106). MUC4, a human tracheobronchial mucin gene, is expressed in both airways and intestine (107). The MUC5 cDNA has recently been cloned from the library derived from human lung (108,109). MUC6 is not expressed in airways (96). It is not yet known whether MUC3 and MUC7 are expressed in respiratory tract epithelium.

The major approach in cloning MUC genes is based on the development of antibodies specific to deglycosylated mucin core protein (apomucin) (110). These antibodies are then used as immunoprobes for screening a λgt11 cDNA library derived from lung or airways. This approach has been successful in the cloning of MUC2, MUC4, and MUC5 from a human respiratory tract cDNA library. Putative apomucin is prepared from highly deglycosylated mucin by either the enzymatic approach or by chemicals such as HF and TFMS. Because of the complexity of mucin and the likely contaminants of nonmucin in the preparation, the contribution of these MUC gene products to airway mucin remains to be elucidated. Based on the amino acid sequence information of isolated tryptic peptide derived from mucin preparation, Rose and her colleagues were able to use degenerated oligonucleotide primer to clone MUC5 cDNA (109). Both the antibody and the degenerated oligomer approaches yielded the same clone, suggesting the contribution of MUC5 gene product to airway mucin. However, the contribution of other MUC genes to airway mucin remains to be explained. We have recently observed that MUC2 gene expression in primary TBE cultures is inhibited by vitamin A at the transcriptional level (106). Similarly, MUC2 gene product is not abundant in normal, uninjured airway tissues. However, the MUC2 message is abundant in airways from patients with ceptic fibrosis (CF) and bronchitis or tissues from animals exposed to $SO_2$ (103–105). Taken together, these data suggest that the expression of the MUC2 gene is not consistent with normal mucous cell differentiation. Clearly, at this moment, we do not have any conclusive candidate among MUC gene products to serve as the core protein of major airway mucin.

## V. Summary and Future Studies

Tracheobronchial epithelial cells play a critical factor in the maintenance of the homeostasis of the airway lumen. Epithelial injury and alteration of mucociliary function are the main initiation events and causes associated with various airway diseases. Much has been learned about the structure and functions of tracheobronchial epithelial cells. However, we still do not know how to maintain the integrity and facilitate the injury-repair mechanism of the epithelium. This chapter has examined two areas of research. One is to focus on the control of the life cycle in tracheobronchial epithelium. Progress has been made in tracing the cell lineage and the progenitor-progeny relationship in various airway epithelial cell types in vivo. Recent progress in combining the molecular gene transfer technique and the tracheal graft repopulation approach should yield new information regarding the cell lineage of various airway epithelial cell types. The development of the biphasic culture system for in vitro mucociliary differentiation should provide a model system by which the mechanism and hypothesis of cell differentiation can be approached and tested. The other focus is on the control of mucociliary differentiation. Studying this requires the understanding of the plasticity of airway epithelial cell differentiation. Squamous cell metaplasia is frequently expressed in this nonkeratinized epithelium. Jetten (5,49) has provided an elegant review on this subject. Using the RNA microinjection approach, we have demonstrated that the expression of differentiated function is regulated at the genetic level. Although mucin genes have been isolated, it is still unclear which one is the authentic airway mucin gene. The elevation of MUC2 gene expression in various airway disease tissues is interesting. Further study focusing on the regulation of the MUC2 gene is important to the understanding of aberrant hypermucous secretion in various airway diseases. Here, we showed the important role vitamin A plays in the regulation of epithelial cell growth and differentiation. We demonstrated that a potential autocrine/paracrine growth regulation mechanism is involved in the regulation of airway epithelium prior to bronchogenic cancer development. Furthermore, vitamin A is absolutely essential for mucociliary cell differentiation. This effect occurs again at the genetic level. The isolation and characterization of differentiation genes will further advance our understanding of the molecular basis of mucociliary cell differentiation.

## Acknowledgments

The author gratefully acknowledges the many scientific contributions and valuable discussions by C.G. Plopper, D.M. Carlson, T. Huang, G. An, C. B. Robinson, M. J. Chang, and Y.H. Zhao. I also gratefully acknowledge the editing work of G. Konas on this manuscript prior to its submission. The work described in the author's laboratory was supported by grants from NIH, American Cancer Society, and the California Tobacco-Related Disease Research Program.

## References

1. McDowell EM, Harris CC, Trump BF. Histogenesis and morphogenesis of bronchial neoplasms. In: Shimosato Y, Melamed MR, Nettesheim P, eds. Morphogenesis of Lung Cancer. Vol. II. Boca Raton, FL, CRC Press, 1982:1–37.
2. Melamed MR, Zaman MB. Pathogenesis of epidermoid carcinoma of lung. In: Shimosato Y, Melamed MR, Nettesheim P, eds. Morphogenesis of Lung Cancer. Vol. II. Boca Raton, FL, CRC Press, 1982:37–65.
3. World Health Organization, Histological typing of lung tumors. 2nd ed. Am J Clin Pathol 1982; 77:123–136.
4. Basbaum C, Jany B. Plasticity in the airway epithelium. Am J Physiol (Lung Cell Mol Physiol) 1990; 259:L38–L46.
5. Jetten AM. Proliferation and differentiation in normal and neoplastic tracheobronchial epithelial cells. In: Bernal SD, Hesketh PJ, eds. Lung Cancer and Differentiation: Implications for Diagnosis and Treatment. New York: Dekker, 1993:3–43.
6. Harkema JR, Mariassy A, St. George J, Hyde DM, Plopper CG. Epithelial cells of the conducting airways, a species comparison. In: Farmer SG, Hay DWP, eds. The Airway Epithelium: Physiology, Pathology, and Pharmacology. New York: Dekker, 1991:3–39.
7. Klein-Szanto AJP, Topping DC, Heckman CA, Nettesheim P. Ultrastructural characteristics of carcinogen-induced dysplastic change in tracheal epithelium. Am J Pathol 1980; 98:83–100.

8. Keenan KP, Wilson TS, McDowell EM. Regeneration of hamster tracheal epithelium after mechanical injury. IV Histochemical, immunocytochemical and ultrastructural studies. Virchows Arch Cell Pathol 1983; 43:213–240.

9. Woodworth CD, Mossman BT, Craighead JE. Squamous metaplasia of the respiratory tract: possible pathogenic role in asbestos-associated bronchogenic carcinoma. Lab Invest 1983; 48:578–584.

10. Keenan KP, Saffiotti U, Stinson SF, Riggs CW, McDowell EM. Morphological and cytokinetic responses of hamster airways to intralaryngeal or intratracheal cannulation with instillation of saline or ferric oxide particles in saline. Cancer Res 1989; 49:1521–1527.

11. Boucher RC, van Scott MR, Willumsen N, Stutts MJ. Epithelial injury: mechanisms and cell biology of airway epithelial injury. Am Rev Respir Dis 1989; 138: S41–S44.

12. Widdicombe JH. Physiology of airway epithelia. In: Farmer SG, Hay DWP, eds. The Airway Epithelium: Physiology, Pathology, and Pharmacology. Vol. 55. New York: Dekker, 1991:41–64.

13. Massion P, Inoue H, Richman-Eisenstat J, Grunberger D, Jorens PG, Houssel B, Wiener-Kronish JP, Nadel J. Novel Pseudomonas product stimulates interleukin-8 production in airway epithelial cells in vitro. J Clin Invest 1994; 93:26–32.

14. Lane BP, Gordon RE. Regeneration of rat tracheal epithelium after mechanical injury. I. The relationship between mitotic activity and cellular differentiation. Proc Soc Exp Biol Med 1974; 145:1139–1144.

15. Boren HG, Paradise LJ. Cytokinetics of lung. In: Harris CC, ed. Pathogenesis and Therapy of Lung Cancer. Vol. 10. New York: Dekker, 1978:369–418.

16. Donnelly HM, Haack DG, Heird CS. Tracheal epithelium: Cell kinetics and differentiation in normal rat tissue. Cell Tissue Kinet 1982; 15:119–130.

17. Keenan KP, Combs JW, McDowell EM. Regeneration of hamster tracheal epithelium after mechanical injury. Virchows Arch Cell Pathol 1982; 41:215–229.

18. Evans MJ, Shami SG. Lung cell kinetics. In: Massaro D, ed. Lung Cell Biology. Vol. 41. New York: Dekker, 1989:1–31.

19. McDowell EM, Trump BF. Conceptual review: histogenesis of preneoplastic and neoplastic lesions in tracheobronchial epithelium. Surv Synth Pathol Res 1984; 2:235–279.

20. Rutten AJL, Beems RB, Wilmer JWGM, Feron VJ. Ciliated cells in vitamin A–deprived culture hamster tracheal epithelium to divide. In Vitro Cell Dev Biol 24:931–935.

21. Jeffery PK, Ayers M, Rogers D. The mechanisms and control of bronchial mucous cell hyperplasia. In: Chantler, EN, Elder JB, Elstein M, eds. Mucous in Health and Disease II. New York: Plenum Press, 1982:399–409.

22. Chopra DP. Squamous metaplasia in organ culture of vitamin A-deficient hamster trachea: cytokinetic and ultrastructural alterations. J Natl Cancer Inst 1982; 69: 895–905.

23. Evans MJ, Moller PC. Biology of airway basal cells. Exp. Lung Res. 1991; 17: 513–531.

24. Plopper CG, St. George J, Pinkerton RE, Tyler N, Mariassey A, Wilson D, Wu R, Hyde DM, Evans MJ. Tracheobronchial epithelium in vivo: composition, differentiation and response to hormones. In: Thomassen DG, Nettesheim P, eds. Biology,

Toxicology and Carcinogenesis of Respiratory Epithelium. New York: Hemisphere, 1990:6–23.

25. Hislop A, Muir DCF, Jacobsen M, Simon G, Reid L. Postnatal growth and function of the pre-acinar airways. Thorax 1972; 27:265–274.

26. Burrington JD. Tracheal growth and healing. J Thorac Cadiovasc Surg 1978; 76:453–458.

27. Johnson NF, Hubbs AF. Epithelial progenitor cells in the rat trachea. Am J Respir Cell Mol Biol 1990; 3:579–585.

28. Terzaghi M, Nettesheim P, Williams ML. Repopulation of denuded tracheal grafts with normal, preneoplastic, and neoplastic epithelial cell population. Cancer Res 1978; 38:4546–4553.

29. Inayama Y, Hook GER, Brody AR, Cameron G, Jetten AM, Gilmore LB, Gray T, Nettesheim P. The differentiation potential of tracheal basal cells. Lab Invest 1988; 58:706–717.

30. Inayama Y, Hook GER, Brody AR, Jetten AM, Gray T, Nettesheim P. In vitro and in vivo growth and differentiation of clones of tracheal basal cells. Am J Pathol 1989; 134:539–550.

31. Johnson NF, Hubbs AF, Thomassen DG. Epithelial progenitor cells in the rat respiratory tract. In: Thomassen DG, Nettesheim P, eds. Biology, Toxicology and Carcinogenesis of Respiratory Epithelium. Washington, DC: Hemisphere, 1990: 88–98.

32. Engelhardt JF, Allen E, Wilson JM. Reconstitution of tracheal grafts with a genetically modified epithelium. Proc Natl Acad Sci USA 1991; 88:11192–11196.

33. Zepeda MI, Chinoy MR, Wilson JM. Characterization of stem cells in human airway capable of reconstituting a fully differentiated bronchial epithelium. Somatic Cell Mol Genet 1995; 21:61–73.

34. Lechner JF, Haugen A, Autrup H, McClendon IA, Trump BF, Harris CC. Clonal growth of epithelial from normal human bronchous. Cancer Res. 41:2294–2304.

35. Lechner JF, Stoner GD, Yoakum GH, Willey JC, Grafstrom RC, Mastui T, LaVeck MA, Harris CC. In vitro carcinogenesis studies with human tracheobronchial tissues and cells. In: Schiff LJ, ed. In Vitro Models of Respiratory Epithelium. Boca Raton, FL: CRC Press, 1986:143–159.

36. Wu R. In vitro differentiation of airway epithelial cells. In: Schiff LJ, ed. In Vitro Models of Respiratory Epithelium. Boca Raton, FL: CRC Press, 1986:1–26.

37. Wu R, Yankaskas J, Cheng E, Knowles MR, Boucher R. Growth and differentiation of human nasal epithelial cells in culture: serum-free, hormone supplemented medium and proteoglycan synthesis. Am Rev Respir Dis 1985; 132:311–320.

38. Wu R, Martin WR, St. George JA, Plopper CG, Kurland G, Last JA, Cross CE, McDonald RJ, Boucher R. Expression of mucin synthesis and secretion in human tracheobronchial epithelial cells grown in culture. Am J Respir Cell Mol Biol 1990; 3:467–478.

39. De Jong PM, van Sterkenburg MAJA, Kempenaar JA, Dijkman JH, Ponec M. Serial culturing of human bronchial epithelial cells derived from biopsies. In Vitro Cell Dev Biol 1993; 29A:379–387.

40. Chang LY, Wu R, Nettesheim P. Morphological changes in rat tracheal cell cultures

during the adaptive and early growth phase in primary cell culture. J Cell Sci 1985; 74:283–301.

41. Randall SH. Progenitor-progeny relationships in airway epithelium. Chest 1992; 101:llS–16S.

42. Wolbach SB, Howe PR. Tissue changes following deprivation of fat-soluble A vitamin. J Exp Med 1926; 42:753–781.

43. Wong YC, Buck RC. An electronic microscopic study of metaplasia of the rat tracheal epithelium in vitamin A deficiency. Lab Invest 1971; 24:55–66.

44. Harris CC, Silverman T, Jackson F, Boren HG. Proliferation of tracheal epithelial cells in normal and vitamin A-deficient Syrian golden hamsters. J Natl Cancer Inst 1973; 51:1059–1062.

45. Sporn MI, Clamon GH, Dunlop NJ, Newton DL, Smith JM, Saffiotti U. Activity of vitamin A analogues in cell cultures of mouse epidermis and organ cultures of hamster trachea. Nature 1975; 253:47–49.

46. Miller L, Wu R. Inhibition of epidermal growth factor-like growth factor secretion in tracheobronchial epithelial cells by vitamin A. Cancer Res 1993; 53:2527–2533.

47. Miller L, Zhao YH, Wu R. Down regulation of TGF-α gene expression by vitamin A in conducting airway epithelium. J Clin Invest 1996. In press.

48. Ferriola PC, Walker C, Robertson AT, Earp HS, Rusnak DW, Nettesheim P. Altered growth factor dependence and transforming growth factor gene expression in transformed rat tracheal epithelial cells. Mol Carcinogen 1990; 2:336–344.

49. Jetten AM. Growth and differentiation factors in tracheobronchial epithelium. Am J Physiol (Lung Cell Mol. Physiol. 4) 1991; 260:L361–L373.

50. Wakefield LM, Smith DM, Masui T, Harris CC, Sporn MB. Distribution and modulation of the cellular receptor for transforming growth factor-beta. J Cell Biol 1987; 105:965–975.

51. Becci PJ, McDowell EM, Trump BF. The respiratory epithelium IV. Histogenesis of epidermoid metaplasia and carcinoma in situ in the hamster. J Natl Cancer Inst 1978; 61:577–586.

52. Crocker TT, Sanders LL. Influence of vitamin A and 3,7 dimethyl 2,6-octadienal (citral) on the effect of benzo(a)oyrene hamster trachea in organ culture. Cancer Res 1970; 30:1312–1318.

53. Genta VM, Kaufman DG, Harris CC, Smith JM, Sporn MD, Saffiotti U. Vitamin A-deficiency enhances binding of benzopyrene to tracheal epithelial DNA. Nature 1974; 247:48–49.

54. Jeffery PK, Reid L. New observations of rat airway epithelium: A quantitative electron microscopic study. J Anat 1975; 120:295–320.

55. Breeze RG, Wheeldon EB. The cells of the pulmonary airways. State of the art. Am. Rev. Respir. Dis. 1977; 116:705–777.

56. Jeffery PK. Morphology of airway surface epithelial cells and glands. Am Rev Respir Dis 1983; 128:S14–S20.

57. St. George JA, Plopper CG, Wang S. Development of the airway secretory apparatus. Patterns of mucous cell differentiation. In: Takishima T, Shimura S, eds. Airway Secretion. Physiological Bases for the Control of Mucous Hypersecretion. Vol. 72. New York: Dekker, 1994:123–147.

58. Jeffery PK. Microscopic structure of airway secretory cells. Variation in hypersecretory disease and effects of drugs. In: Takishima T, Shimura S, eds. Airway Secretion. Physiological Bases for the Control of Mucous Hypersecretion. Vol. 72. New York: Dekker, 1994:149–215.

59. Wu R, Smith D. Continuous multiplication of rabbit tracheal epithelial cells in a defined hormone-supplemented medium. In Vitro 1982; 18:800–812.

60. Wu R, Groelke JW, Chang LY, Porter ME, Smith D, Nettesheim P. Effects of hormones on the multiplication and differentiation of tracheal epithelial cells in culture. In: Sirbasku D, Sato GH, Pardee A, eds. Growth of Cells in Hormonally Defined Media. Cold Spring Harbor, NY: Cold Spring Harbor Laboratory, 1982:641–656.

61. Robinson CB, Wu R. Culture of conducting airway epithelial cells in serum-free medium. J Tissue Cult Method 1991; 13:95–102.

62. Lee TC, Wu R, Brody AR, Barrett JC, Nettesheim P. Growth and differentiation of hamster tracheal epithelial cells in culture. Exp Lung Res 1983; 6:27–45.

63. Wu R, Nolan E, Turner C. Expression of tracheal differentiated functions in a serum-free hormone-supplemented medium. J Cell Physiol 1985; 125:167–181.

64. Kim KC, Rearick JI, Nettesheim P, Jetten AM. Biochemical characterization of mucin secreted by hamster tracheal epithelial cells in primary culture. J Biol Chem 1985; 260:4021–4027.

65. Wu R, Plopper CG, Cheng PW. Mucin-like glycoprotein secreted by cultured hamster tracheal epithelial cells: Biochemical and immunological characterization. Biochem J 1991; 277:713–718.

66. Adler KB, Cheng PW, Kim KC. Characterization of guinea pig tracheal epithelial cells maintained in biphasic organotypic culture: cellular composition and biochemical analysis of released glycoconjugates. Am J Respir Cell Mol Biol 1990; 2: 145–154.

67. Wu R, Sato GH, Whitcutt JM. Developing differentiated epithelial cell cultures: airway epithelial cells. Fundam Appl Toxicol 1986; 6:680–689.

68. Adler KB, Schwarz JE, Whitcutt MJ, Wu R. A new chamber system for maintaining differentiated guinea pig respiratory epithelial cells between air and liquid phases. Biotechniques 1987; 5:462–465.

69. Whitcutt MJ, Adler KB, Wu R. A biphasic chamber system for maintaining polarity of differentiation of cultured respiratory tract epithelial cells. In Vitro Cell Dev Biol 1988; 24:420–428.

70. de Jong PM, van Strekenburg MAJA, Hesseling SC, Kempenaar JA, Mulder AA, Mommaas AM, Dijkman JH, Ponec M. Ciliogenesis in human bronchial epithelial cells cultured at the air-liquid interface. Am J Respir Cell Mol Biol 1994; 10: 271–277.

71. Gray TE, Guzman K, Davis CW, Abdullah LH, Nettesheim P. Mucociliary differentiation of serially passaged normal human tracheobronchial epithelial cells. Am J Respir Cell Mol Biol 1996; 14:104–112.

72. Tarkington BK, Wu R, Sun WM, Nikula J, Wilson DW, Last JA. In vitro exposure of tracheobronchial epithelial cells and of tracheal explants to ozone. Toxicology 1994; 88:51–68.

73. Sun WM, Wu R, Last JA. Coordinated expression of 45kd protein synthesis and ozone toxicity in human bronchial epithelial cell line. Am J Respir Cell Mol Biol 1994; 10:673–682.
74. Fell HB, Mellanby E. Metaplasia produced in cultures of chick ectoderm by high vitamin A. J Physiol 1953; 119:470–488.
75. McDowell EM, Ben T, Coleman B, Chang S, Newkirk C, De Luca LM. Effects of retinoic acid on the growth and morphology of hamster tracheal epithelial cells in primary culture. Virchows Archiv B Cell Pathol 1987; 54:38–51.
76. De Luca LM, McDowell EM. Effects of vitamin A status on hamster tracheal epithelium in vivo and in vitro. Food Nutr Bull 1989; 11:20–24.
77. McDowell EM, DeSanti AM, Newkirk C, Strum JM. Effects of vitamin A-deficiency and inflammation on the conducting airway epithelium of Syrian golden hamsters. Virchows Archiv B. Cell Pathol. 1990; 59:231–242.
78. Kopan R, Fuchs E. The use of retinoic acid to probe the relation between hyperproliferation-associated keratins and cell proliferation in normal and malignant epidermal cells. J Cell Biol 1989; 109:209–307.
79. Petkovich M, Brand N, Krust A, Chambon P. A human retinoic acid receptor which belongs to the family of nuclear receptors. Nature 1987; 330:444–450.
80. Giguere V, Ong ES, Segui P, Evans RM. Identification of a receptor for the morphogen retinoic acid. Nature 1987; 330:620–629.
81. Brand N, Petkovich M, Krust A, Chambon P, de The HD, Marchio A, Tiollais P, Dejean A. Identification of a second human retinoic acid receptor. Nature 1988; 332:850–853.
82. Benbrook D, Lernhardt E, Pfahl M. A new retinoic acid receptor identified from a hepatocellular carcinoma. Nature 1988; 333:669–672.
83. Krust A, Kastner PH, Petkovich M, Zelent A, Chambon P. A third human retinoic acid receptor, hRAR-γ. Proc Natl Acad Sci USA 1989; 86:5310–5314.
84. Zelent A, Krust A, Petkovich M, Kastner PH, Chambon P. Cloning of murine α and β retinoic acid receptors and a novel receptor γ predominantly expressed in skin. Nature 1989; 339:714–717.
85. Mader S, Pierre L, Chen JY, Chambon P. Multiple parameters control the selectivity of nuclear receptors for their response elements. J Biol Chem 1993; 268:591–600.
86. De Luca LM. Retinoids and their receptors in differentiation, embryogenesis, and neoplasia. FASEB J 1991; 5:2924–2933.
87. Allenby G, Bocquel MT, Saunders M, et al. Retinoic acid receptors and retinoid X receptors: Interactions with endogenous retinoic acids. Proc Natl Acad Sci USA 1993; 90:30–34.
88. Mangelsdorf DJ, Evans RM. The RXR heterodimers and orphan receptors. Cell 1995; 83:841–850.
89. St. George JA, Cranz DL, Zicker S, Etchison JR, Dungworth DL, Plopper CG. An immunohistochemical characterization of rhesus monkey respiratory secretions using monoclonal antibodies. Am Rev Respir Dis 1985; 132:556–563.
90. Lin H, Carlson DM, St. George JA, Plopper CG, Wu R. An ELISA method for the quantitation of tracheal mucins from human and nonhuman primates. Am J Respir Cell Mol Biol 1989; 1:41–48.

91.  Wu R, Carlson DM. Structure and synthesis of mucins. In: Crystal RG, West JB, eds. The Lung: Scientific Foundations. New York: Raven Press, 1991:183–188.

92.  Boat TF, Cheng PW, Leigh MW. Biochemistry of mucous. In: Takishima T, Shimura S, eds. Airway Secretion. Physiological Bases for the Control of Mucous Hypersecretion. Vol. 72. New York: Dekker, 1994:217–282.

93.  Ramphal R, Carnoy C, Fierre S, Michelski J, Houdret N, Lamblin G, Strecker G, Roussel P. Pseudomonas aeruginosa recognizes carbohydrate chains containing type 1 (Gal β3 GlcNAc) or type 2 (Gal β4 GlcNAc) disaccharide units. Infect Immun 1991; 59:700–704.

94.  Schachter H. Enzymes associated with glycosylation. Curr Opin Structure Biol 1993; 1:755–765.

95.  Gum JR. Mucin genes and the proteins they encode: structure, diversity, and regulation. Am J Respir Cell Mol Biol 1992; 7:557–564.

96.  Rose MC. Mucins: structure, function, and role in pulmonary diseases. Am J Physiol (Lung Cell Mol. Physiol.) 1992; 263:L413–L429.

97.  Bobek LA, Tsai H, Biesbrock AR, Levine MJ. J Biol Chem 1993; 268:20563–20569.

98.  Gendler SJ, Lancaster CA, Taylor-Papadimitriou J, Duhig T, Peat N, Burchell J, Pemberton L, Lalani E, Wilson D. Molecular cloning and expression of human tumor-associated polymorphic epithelial mucin. J Biol Chem 1990; 265:15286–15293.

99.  Lan MS, Batra SK, Qi W, Metzgar RS, Hollingsworth MA. Cloning and sequencing of a human pancreatic tumor mucin cDNA. J Biol Chem 1990; 265:15294–15299.

100. Gum JR, Hicks JW, Toribara NW, Siddiki B, Kim YS. Molecular cloning of human intestinal mucin (MUC2) cDNA: Identification of the amino terminus and overall sequence similarity to prepro-von Willebrand factor. J Biol Chem 1994; 269:2440–2446.

101. Ohmori H, Dohrman AF, Gallup M, Tsuda T, Kai H, Gum JR, Kim YS, Basbaum CB. Molecular cloning of the amino-terminal region of a rat MUC2 mucin gene homologue: Evidence for expression in both intestine and airway. J Biol Chem 1994; 269:17833–17840.

102. Hollingsworth MA, Batra D, Qu WN, Yankaskas JR. Am J Resp Cell Mol Biol 1992; 6:516–520.

103. Jany BH, Gallup MW, Tsuda T, Basbaum CB. Mucin gene expression in rat airways following infection and irritation. Biochem Biophys Res Commun 1991; 181:1–8.

104. Jany BH, Gallup MW, Yan P, Gum JR, Kim YS, Basbaum CB. Human bronchus and intestine express the same mucin gene. J Clin Invest 1991; 87:77–82.

105. Gerard C, Eddy RL, Shows TB. The core polypeptide of cystic fibrosis tracheal mucin contains a tandem repeat structure. Evidence for a common mucin in airway and gastrointestinal tissue. J Clin Invest 1990; 86:1921–1927.

106. An G, Luo G, Wu R. Expression of MUC2 gene is down-regulated by vitamin A at the transcriptional level in vitro in tracheobronchial epithelial cells. Am J Resp Cell Mol Biol 1994; 10:546–551.

107. Porchet N, Nguyen VC, Dufosse J, Audie JP, Guyonnet-Duperat V, Gross MS, Denis C, Degamd P, Bernheim A, Aubert JP. Molecular cloning and chromosomal localiza-

tion of a novel human tracheo-bronchial mucin cDNA containing tandemly repeated sequences of 48 base pairs. Biochem Biophys Res Commun 1991; 175:414–422.

108. Aubert JP, Porchet N, Crepin M, Duterque-Coquillaud M, Vergnes G, Mazzuca M, Debuire B, Pettprez D, Degand P. Evidence for different human tracheobronchial mucin peptides deduced from nucleotide cDNA sequences. Am J Resp Cell Mol Biol 1991; 5:175–185.

109. Meerzaman D, Charles P, Daskal E, Polymeropoulos MH, Martin BM, Rose MC. Cloning and analysis of cDNA encoding a major airway glycoprotein, human tracheobronchial mucin (MUC5). J Biol Chem 1994; 269:12932–12939.

110. Thornton DJ, Howard M, Devine PL, Sheehan JK. Methods for separation and deglycosylation of mucin subunits. Anal Biochem 1995; 227:162–167.

# 9

# Development of Innervation in the Lung

**RICHARD D. DEY**

West Virginia University
Morgantown, West Virginia

**KUEN-SHAN HUNG**

University of Kansas Medical Center
Kansas City, Kansas

## I. Introduction

The nerve supply to the lung follows the classic organization of sensory, sympathetic, and parasympathetic systems. Most ganglionic cells and the supporting Schwann cells are derived from the neural crest in the embryo. In the human, by the 6th week of embryonic life, the essential anatomical features of the autonomic nervous system are established. These primitive nerves form a plexus into which the lung bud grows as it emerges from the embryonic foregut. Continued migration of neuroblasts and growth of nerve fibers establish the connections of nerve fibers with their targets in the lung. During the time since the development of the nervous system in the lung was last reviewed in the Lung Biology Series (1), much progress has been made on the understanding of the adult lung innervation. However, there have been relatively few investigations on the nervous system in the developing lung. This chapter presents the current concepts of the development of the innervation of the human and animal lungs, emphasizing the studies that have been undertaken since 1977. There are still many fundamental questions which cannot be answered, but hopefully, this chapter will stimulate others to undertake the important task of further studies.

## II. Embryonic Precursors of the Pulmonary Nervous System

### A. Origin of the Pulmonary Plexus

Although the embryonic precursor cells that give rise to the epithelium and glands, cartilage, and connective tissues are present as primary components of the foregut, the cells that form the pulmonary nervous system arrive at the foregut through cell migration and directed growth of axonal processes. Based on studies in chick embryos, the nervous system is established around the foregut prior to the initiation of the laryngotracheal diverticulum and lung buds. Using anti-neurofilament antibodies (NFP) to demonstrate nerve cell projections, Kuratani and Tanaka (2) showed that a neuronal arborization forms along the embryonic foregut. The arborization receives contributions from both vagal and sympathetic nerve trunks and accompanies the lung buds as they grow, forming the pulmonary plexus on the trachea and airways (Fig. 1). The arborization around the esophagus begins to separate bilaterally into dorsal and ventral plexuses. The ventral plexus migrates around the esophagus, eventually fusing in the midline forming the plexus located on the dorsal surface of the trachealis muscle. With further growth of the respiratory diverticulum and the development of the lung bud, the plexus begins to form two distinct vagal branches: a rostral branch corresponding to the recurrent laryngeal nerve and a caudal branch going to each lung bud forming the pulmonary vagal branches. These branches contain both preganglionic parasympathetic axons growing from neurons in the brain stem and sensory fibers originating from vagal sensory ganglia (jugular and nodose). These nerve bundles may be expected to contain sympathetic postganglionic fibers, since the original arborization included sympathetic branches. Other sympathetic nerves may form separately from the sympathetic trunk and fuse with the tracheal and pulmonary plexuses.

The cholinergic, postganglionic parasympathetic neurons in the airways and the intrinsic airway neurons that contribute to the nonadrenergic/noncholinergic innervation are all believed to originate from neural crest cells that migrated to the embryonic foregut prior to the formation of the lung buds (3) (Table 1). Although there have been no studies that directly evaluated neural crest contributions to the lung, several studies have examined the arrival and fate of neural crest cells in the embryonic foregut. The parallel development of the gut tube and lung should allow reliable extrapolation of at least the general principles involved in the formation of the pulmonary plexus.

### B. Neural Crest

The neural crest forms from ectoderm as a transitory structure during the formation of the neural tube (4) (Fig. 2A). As the dorsal neural plate forms and begins to invaginate to form the neural tube, some cells separate from the neural fold,

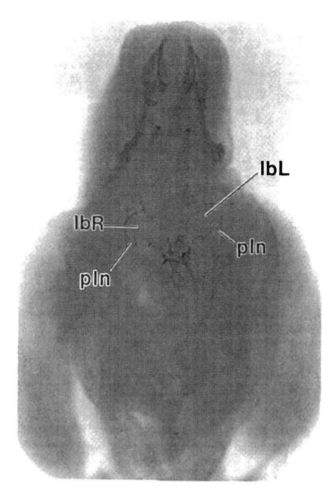

**Figure 1** Stage 25 chick embryo stained with anti-NFP antibody. The embryo has been sectioned in a transverse plane to show the initial innervation of lung buds (lbR and lbL) by the vagus nerve. Lung innervation begins as the intestinal arborization which surrounds the embryonic foregut. The respiratory diverticulum emerges from the foregut, and the lung buds grow into a region of the arborization identified as the precursors of the pulmonary nerve branch (pln). (4×) (From ref. 2.)

**Table 1**  Chronology of Neuronal Development in the Lung

| Species | Neural crest cell migration | Respiratory diverticulum | First identifiable NCBs or fibers (NSE, neural morphology) | Appearance of cholinergic proprieties | Appearance of peptidergic or adrenergic proprieties |
|---|---|---|---|---|---|
| | | | Glandular stage | | Canalicular stage |
| Chick | 1.5 days (63) | 2.5 days (63) | 8 days (23) | ND | 12 days (23) |
| Mouse | 8 days (64) | 9.5 days (64) | 15 days[a] (41) | 15 days (41) | 15–19 days (41) |
| Rat | ND | ND | 13 days (40) | 13 days (40) | 18–20 days (39,40) |
| Rabbit | ND | ND | 17 days (42) | 19–21 days (42) | 25 days (42) |
| Human | 21 days (65) | 22 days (65) | 6–7 weeks (24) | 12 weeks (24) | 16–20 weeks (24) |

ND, not determined; NCB, nerve cell body; NSE, neuron-specific enolase.
[a]Earliest fetal age studied.

migrate laterally to form the neural crest, and assume locations near the somites. As soon as they aggregate into neural crest, they begin to migrate through the surrounding tissues and give rise to diverse structures, including neurons and supporting cells of sensory and autonomic ganglia, melanocytes in the skin, and certain musculature and skeletal structures in the head (Fig. 2B). The definitive experimental approach proving that neurons of the gut originated from neural crest were performed in the 1970s and early 1980s. The now classic experiments developed by Le Douarin and colleagues consisted of replacing neural crest tissues in chick embryos with transplants of quail neural crest tissue (5,6). After suitable developmental periods, the migrating quail neural crest cells can be distinguished from chick-derived cells by the staining pattern of nuclear heterochromatin. Although studies prior to these had indicated that the neural crest generally contributed to the enteric nervous system, the precise segmental origin remained elusive. Le Douarin and colleagues showed that the enteric nervous system in the foregut and midgut originated from neural crest cells associated with somites 1–7. Airway neurons undoubtedly originate from these same levels.

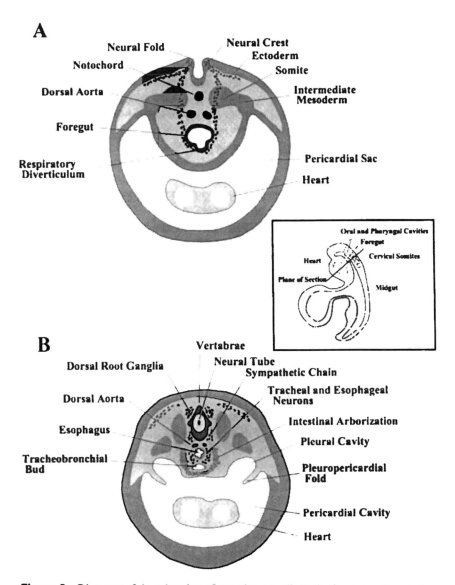

**Figure 2** Diagrams of the migration of neural crest cells to the foregut and respiratory diverticulum in transverse sections at the level of the cervical somites (see inset) of the human fetus. (A) On day 21, cells begin migrating in ventral medial and dorsal lateral directions from the neural crest located near the edges of the neural fold. The neural crest cells travel through somitic mesoderm toward the embryonic foregut. On day 22, a small evagination forms in the ventral wall of the embryonic foregut and develops as the respiratory diverticulum. (B) By day 28, collections of neural crest cells are distributed along the dorsal surface of the tracheobronchial buds and ventrolateral to the esophagus. A network of vagosympathetic fibers around the foregut (intestinal arborization) has formed by this stage. Other groups of neural crest cells are forming the sympathetic chain, dorsal root ganglia, and melanocytes of the dermis. Pleuropericardial folds grow from the lateral body wall eventually create separate pleural and pericardial cavities.

### C. Autonomic Ganglia

It is now generally accepted that postganglionic neurons of both the sympathetic and parasympathetic nervous systems originate from neural crest (4,7). In addition, all sensory neurons of the dorsal root ganglia and most neurons of the jugular ganglia originate from neural crest. Neurons in the nodose ganglion, however, develop from ectodermal placodes, which are condensations of ectoderm that form in association with the branchial arches. The distinction of embryological origin of sensory neurons may be relevant to the lung. Substance P (SP)–containing cells of the jugular ganglion originate from neural crest cells, whereas the SP-containing neurons in the nodose ganglion are derived from the ectodermal placodes (8,9). These findings suggest that precursors of the C-fiber afferent neurons responsible for neurogenic inflammatory responses in the airways (10,11) may originate from either neural crest or ectodermal placodes.

### D. Guidance of Axonal Growth by Target Tissues

Another aspect of early neuronal development relevant to lung embryology is the question of how growing axons find appropriate targets. The process of axonal growth includes both the connection of preganglionic axon terminals to postganglionic nerve cells and the growth of postganglionic axons to target structures in the airways. Much of the current information suggests that molecules encountered in the interstitial environment play essential roles in guiding axons to target cells. Normal axonal growth is strongly influenced by adherence molecules, growth factors, and extracellular matrix proteins (12). In the lung, the local mesodermal composition probably serves to guide the growth of axons to appropriate targets such as airway smooth muscle, glands, epithelium, and blood vessels.

Preganglionic innervation of postganglionic neurons probably occurs shortly after neural crest cells arrive at their final location. During sympathetic ganglion development in the rat, neural crest cells arrive in thoracic and then cervical regions as early as embryonic day (ED) 12, forming the stellate and superior ganglia (13). At about the same time, preganglionic axons emerge from the thoracic spinal cord through the ventral rami and begin to travel toward and even into the sympathetic chain. Connections with the ganglia are not established until ED 13 or 14 (14). These findings demonstrate that neural crest cells forming autonomic ganglia migrate to a location and are subsequently innervated by growing preganglionic fibers.

### E. Multipotent Neural Crest Cells

Neural crest cells are multipotent prior to their arrival at a final destination. Using the quail chick chimera model, Le Douarin and colleagues transplanted quail neural crest cells from somite levels 1–5, normally destined for enteric ganglia, into somite levels 18–24 in chicks, levels which normally form the adrenal medulla (3). The transplanted cells readily formed normal adrenal medulla cells, supporting the hypothesis that neural crest cells are multipotent and are determined in large part by the environment through which they migrate. Furthermore, even cells that have already migrated to target organs, like the gastrointestinal (GI) tract, will form adrenal medulla when transplanted into younger chicks and allowed to migrate a second time from the appropriate level. The influence of environment in determining the fate of neural crest cells is probably true in mammals as well. By injecting neural crest cells at different locations along their migratory path, it has been shown that determination of neural crest cells does not occur until the cells are near or in the final target (15).

### F.  Formation of Ganglia

Neural crest cells arrive at the gut about ED 2.5 in the chick and continue to divide until about ED 10.5 (16). During this time, a network of nerve fibers and neurons grows in conjunction with gut tube. Groups of cell bodies coalesce forming ganglia. The ganglia continue to be connected by strands of the network, thus forming the myenteric plexus. Epstein and colleagues noted that neuronal cell precursors were formed in the gut wall prior to the time these cells were connected to the vagus nerve (17). This further supports the hypothesis that preganglionic innervation of postganglionic neurons occurs after neural crest cells have arrived at their targets.

### G.  Neurotransmitter Expression

Early neural crest cells demonstrate features of nerve cells including neurite extensions and changing from fusiform to spherical shape. In the mouse gut, phenotypic expression of small molecular weight neurotransmitters like acetylcholine (ACh) and 5-hydroxytryptamine (5-HT) occurs at approximately ED 9, whereas expression of neuropeptides seems to lag behind (18). In the avian gut, vasoactive intestinal peptide (VIP) and SP appear near ED 14 even though the precursor cells of peptidergic neurons are present by ED 11 (19). It has been suggested that either the precursor of peptidergic neurons are programmed to differentiate later than cholinergic and 5-HT–containing neurons or that the microenvironment of the maturing host tissue induces continued development and expression of peptidergic phenotypes.

The factors that regulate phenotypic expression have been investigated in elegant studies by Landis and colleagues during the past 15 years (20). They have shown that chemical signals released by the target tissues determine phenotypic expression in sympathetic neurons. When cultured with salivary glands, normally innervated by adrenergic nerves, sympathetic neurons continue to express norepinephrine (NE). However, when the same neurons are cultured with sweat glands, a target that normally received cholinergic sympathetic innervation, the sympathetic neurons express ACh. Soluble molecules capable of inducing cholinergic phenotype in sympathetic neurons include ciliary neurotrophic factor (CNF) and cholinergic differentiating factor (21,22). These molecules are synthesized and released by targets as a mechanism of regulating neurotransmitter expression. Recent studies have shown that the release of CNF by sweat glands is mediated through adrenoceptors in the acinar cell membranes that are activated by the release of NE from approaching sympathetic fibers (20). Thus, these studies suggest that phenotypic expression of neurotransmitters by neurons is strongly influenced by molecules released from the targets that are being innervated.

It is difficult precisely to describe the sequence and timing of neurotransmitter expression in pulmonary neurons, because so few studies have been conducted. In chick embryos, neuropeptide expression lags behind the formation of new airways by several days. Salvi and Renda (23) have shown that VIP-, SP- and galanin-containing nerve cells in chicks appear at approximately ED 12, whereas primary bronchi begin to develop at ED 5. Peptide expression in the foregut also precedes that in the lung. Fontaine-Perus and colleagues showed that VIP and SP neurons are first visible in the esophagus at ED 9, and they appear throughout the entire intestine by ED 12 (19). These findings suggest that maturation of the local environment may be important in the timing of phenotypic expression in pulmonary neurons. In human fetuses, staining of neurons by neuron-specific enolase (NSE) is first seen at 8 weeks of gestation (24). This suggests that the neural crest–derived precursors are beginning to mature at this time. However, expression of cholinergic neurons, identified as acetylcholinesterase (AChE)–positive neurons, is delayed until 10–12 weeks. The expression of adrenergic and peptidergic phenotypes is reportedly delayed until 20 weeks, although our studies suggest that VIP and SP are present by 16 weeks (Figs. 3–5). Ghatei and colleagues (25) showed that VIP extracted from fetal lungs was detectable during the canalicular stage of lung development, and it did not change markedly during the caniculur stage but decreased during the terminal sac stage. These findings probably reflect the fact that VIP is primarily found in airway walls and large vessels. The increasing proportion of parenchymal lung mass during the terminal sac stage dilutes neuropeptides localized in the airways.

With these limited studies, it seems appropriate to conclude that neuronal precursors are present at the time the lung buds form around 5 weeks of gestation. However, phenotypic expression of known pulmonary neurotransmitters and neuropeptides is delayed until the airways are quite well developed during the late canalicular and pseudoglandular stages. Studies so far have not attempted to correlate airway maturity and neurotransmitter expression. But the maturation of innervated targets like smooth muscle, glands, and blood vessels may be important determinants in the induction and specification of neurotransmitter phenotypic expression.

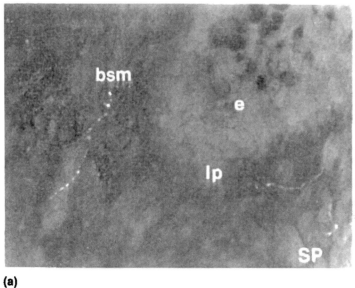

**(a)**

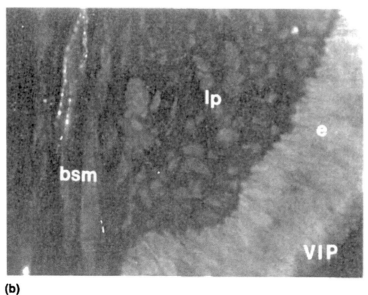

**(b)**

**Figure 3** Localization of (a) VIP- and (b) SP-like immunoreactivity in nerve fibers associated with bronchial smooth muscle (bsm) from a 16-week human fetus. The airway epithelium (e) and lamina propria (lp) are also present. (580×)

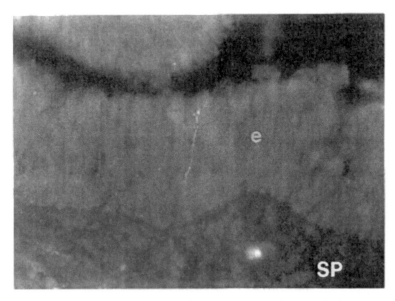

**Figure 4** A SP-immunoreactivity nerve fiber located in the airway epithelium (e) of a 16-week human fetus. Epithelial SP-containing fiber represents sensory C-fibers characterized in adult airways. (580×)

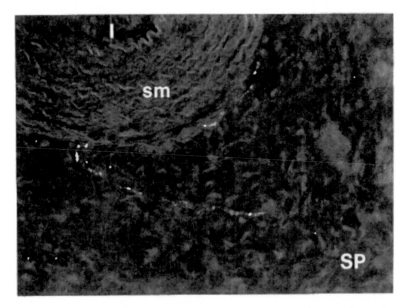

**Figure 5** SP-containing nerve fibers located near the outer edge of the smooth muscle layer (sm) of a pulmonary artery in the lung of a 16-week week human fetus. Autofluorescent elastic fibers are seen in the wall of the blood vessel and close to the vessel lumen (1). (580×)

## III. Development of Lung Innervation

### A. Innervation in the Human Fetal and Neonatal Lung

Using a series of fetal lung specimens of gestational age from 7, 10, 12, 14, and 16 weeks and 5, 6, 8, and 10 months and lungs from 8-month-old infants, it has been determined that neuroblasts and nerve fibers are already present in the primary bronchial region at 7 weeks of gestation (1). After that, there is a progressive growth of nerve tissue that follows the chronological development of the tracheobronchial tree, pulmonary arteries, and veins (26,27). Since the nervous tissue eventually reaches its target structures in different airway divisions of the lung, its distribution in development will be described based on its association with target structures. The observations are based on the specimens which are stained with routine histological staining methods (1) and other staining techniques specific for nervous tissue, including methylene blue (28,29), silver impregnation (27), cholinesterase enzyme histochemistry (26), and immunohistochemistry of neuronal markers (24).

### Trachea

Ganglion cells at 7 weeks of gestation appear in the extrachondrial tissue of the trachea. As growth proceeds, they form segmental ganglia and develop fibers, which penetrate the tissues between the tracheal cartilages and encircle the trachea to form a posterior plexus. Intrachondrial plexuses gradually develop and by 4 months show dense interplexus communications. Fibers extend to the tracheal muscle forming a primary muscle plexus with a fine network. Fibers from the extra- and intrachondrial plexuses also supply the glands, submucosa, and epithelial layer. At the bifurcation of the trachea, the extrachondrial plexus divides and is uniformly distributed about the right and left primary bronchi.

### Bronchus and Bronchiole

Poorly defined neuroblasts already migrate to the hilar region of the lung at 7 weeks of gestation (1). At this time period, the extrachondrial nerve plexuses surrounding the main bronchus extend only to the second order of bronchi, but at 4 months, they are present in all but the smallest bronchi. The intrachondrial plexus is relatively poorly formed at 12 weeks but are well developed in the main bronchi at 4 months. Neuroblasts and nerves show positive immunoreactivity for neuron-specific enolase (NSE) at 8 weeks, for acetylcholinesterase at 10–12 weeks, and for dopamine-β-hydroxylase and VIP at 20 weeks (24). At 20 weeks, NSE-positive nerves increase in density and distribution and extend from the adventitia between the cartilage plates to innervate the airway smooth muscle, seromucous glands, blood vessels, and the respiratory epithelium (24). At 4 months, cholinesterase-positive nerves supply the smooth muscle and mucous gland (26). Toward the distal parts of the bronchial tree, the extra- and intrachondrial plexuses are mixed into a single plexus, and weakly staining fibers extend as far as the bronchioles. Beginning myelination is present at 4 months. Developing ganglia along with extra- and intrachondrial plexuses are preferentially located at bronchial bifurcations, although they may also be seen in the adventitial tissue throughout the bronchi.

At 5 months of gestation, there is further development of nerve tissue in the walls of the bronchi. Immature ganglia are present in the extrachondrial tissue of the major bronchi. Most of the nerve cells are small, oval, and hyperchromic (Figs. 6–9). Other large multipolar cells give rise to axons that divide and terminate on developing smooth muscle. Occasional fibers terminating between smooth muscle cells may be sensory in nature. At 6 and 8 months, nerve fibers entering the lung from the hilum are well developed. Axonal processes of the ganglionic cells are more extensive. At 8 months, the nerve cells contain fibrils and are generally multipolar, sending branches to the submucosal nerve plexus. Nerve fibers from this plexus terminate on smooth muscle and in the intercellular spaces in the epithelium.

The ganglion cells and ganglia are readily recognized in embryonic lungs in the early stages of development and throughout the prenatal period. As the lung grows, however, they are observed progressively less frequently, and they are seldom seen in histological sections of the adult lungs. In random sections of bronchi, at 9–12 weeks of gestation, about 87% of the bronchi have ganglionic cells in their wall; at 23–28 weeks, about 78%; at 38–40 weeks, about 9%; and at 3 months to 18 years of postnatal age, about 8% (1). The decline in the number of ganglionic cells found associated with the airways is undoubtedly due to the fact that the fast growth of lung parenchyma dilutes the presence of slow-growing nervous tissue.

In fetal lungs at term and in the neonate, innervation of bronchi with cartilages and mucous glands is profuse and rather complete. NSE-positive nerves extend as far as bronchioles (24). The ganglion cells are mostly multipolar in shape. Extra- and intrachondrial ganglia communicate and receive and give off fibers to the intrabronchial nerves. The thick fibers (presumably sensory) of the bronchial nerves terminate in the perichondrium, smooth muscle, lamina propria, and bronchial epithelium. The fine fibers (presumably motor) from the ganglia terminate on smooth muscle of the bronchi and blood vessels and on mucous glands. The fine fibers can be followed as far as the respiratory bronchioles. The bronchial arteries are surrounded by a fine beaded nerve plexus. Fibers from this plexus form a major supply to the bronchial mucous glands, which is very apparent in the lungs of a child of 8 months (26–29).

The study of the nerve tissue in well-prepared lungs of an 8-month-old child, reported in 1933, is widely accepted as that present in the adult (29). Nerve trunks entering the lung at the hilum come from the pulmonary plexus. The bronchial plexus divides into extra- and intrachondrial plexuses. The extrachondrial plexus contains both myelinated and unmyelinated nerve fibers, which branch and anastomose. Clusters of ganglion cells lie in and along nerve trunks as

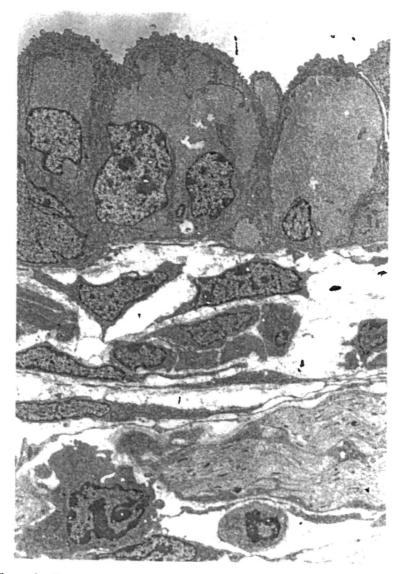

**Figure 6** Electron micrograph showing a developing bronchus. Epithelial cells with a typically high content of glycogen are on the top. Developing smooth muscle cells are under the epithelium, and a large nerve bundle occupies the lower right field. 18-day mouse fetus. (4480×)

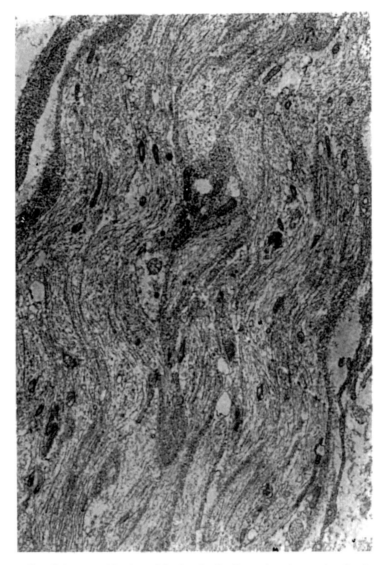

**Figure 7**   Higher magnification of the longitudinally sectioned nerve bundle shown in Figure 1. Note that it consists of unmyelinated axons only. Thin and dark Schwann cell cytoplasm covers the surface of the nerve bundle and extends into the bundle to cover some individual axons. 18-day mouse fetus. (16,800×)

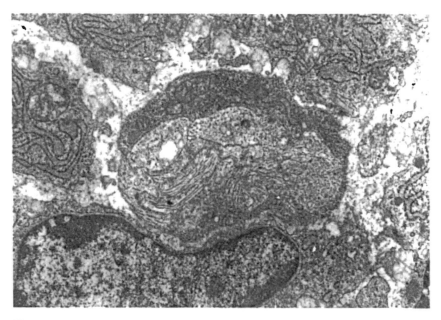

**Figure 8**  A cross-sectioned nerve bundle. Its surface is covered by the dark cytoplasm of Schwann cell. All axons are unmyelinated. 18-day mouse fetus. (16,800×)

far as the smaller bronchi. These cells are positive for acetylcholinesterase (26). The ganglion cells are multipolar and surrounded by capsules. Some cells are surrounded by pericellular preganglionic fibers. The ganglion cells have unmyelinated axons and send fibers to the intrachondrial plexus, which in turn sends fibers to mucous glands and airway smooth muscle as far distal as the alveolar ducts. Clusters of ganglion cells send fibers that form pericellular baskets about mucous glands. Such fibers to the muscle and mucous glands are motor and belong to the vagus element. Afferent endings are found in walls of bronchi as far as the alveolar ducts and terminate on the bronchial smooth muscle bands (29).

### Intraepithelial Nerves and Innervation of Neuroepithelial Bodies

The presence of intraepithelial nerves in the prenatal lungs has been described in early studies. Although poorly developed, these nerves in the bronchus of 6-month and older fetuses have been reported (27,28). These are unbranched fibers which penetrate the developing ciliated epithelium from the lamina propria. Although these fibers may be seen associated with different cell types in the epithelium, they often make contact with neuroendocrine cells and neuroepithelial bodies (NEBs) in the bronchi and bronchioles. The neuroendocrine cells are nonciliated and are

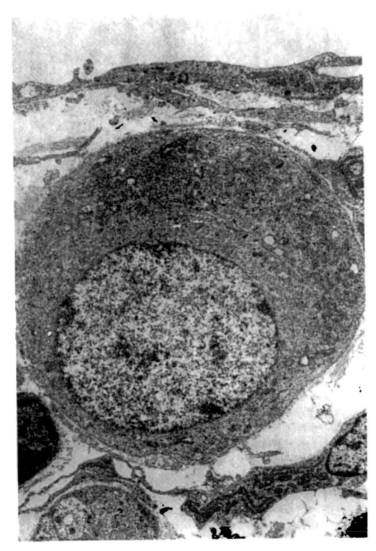

**Figure 9**   A developing ganglionic cell. The nucleus is lightly stained, and the cytoplasm has mitochondria, free ribosomes, Golgi apparatus, as well as typically high contents of rough endoplasmic reticulum. A thin sheath of cytoplasm from the satellite cell covers part of the neuron. Axons and dendrites from this cell are not shown at this sectioning level. 18-day mouse fetus. (8,190×)

characterized by cytoplasmic granules containing neuropeptides and other neural or endocrine markers. Clusters of these specialized cells organize into corpuscular structures called NEBs. Using NSE as a marker, precursor cells are first seen at 8 weeks of gestation while the lung is still at the beginning of the pseudoglandular stage (24,30). These cells differentiate early in embryonic life and are more often seen in fetal and neonatal lung sections. Light and electron microscopy has revealed both motor and sensory nerves in direct contact with these cells in human lungs (31–34), but more detailed observations of the innervation of these cells are derived from the study of animal lungs (see below).

### Alveolar Ducts and Alveoli

By the 6th month, the alveolar ducts and alveoli begin to develop, and small nerve branches from the bronchioles extend into the alveolar ducts surrounded by the alveoli (27). Nerve fibers in the alveolar ducts in the lungs of an 8 month old child has already been reported in 1933 (29). The existence of unmyelinated axons in the gas exchange region of the lung has been confirmed with electron microscopy in the adult human, and their ultrastructural appearance generally indicates sensory function (35,36). Additional types of nerves associated with the alveolar walls are seen in animal lungs (see below).

### Pulmonary Vessels

At 10 weeks of gestation, the major extrapulmonary arteries and veins are well supplied with nerves. The major extra- and intrapulmonary vessels are well supplied from 10 weeks onward, with arteries exhibiting a more profuse innervation as fetal growth occurs and as the vessel walls become larger and more distinct. The fibers are spiral and lie in the tunica adventitia and do not enter the tunica media. At 4 months, still no nerve fibers are seen entering the muscular coat. Occasional ganglia are present at bifurcations of vessels in the hilar region. Small ganglia in the perivascular tissue between arteries and veins are present. Although the adventitia of major extrapulmonary arteries and veins contain many more nerves than intrapulmonary vessels, nerve supply to intrapulmonary vessels increases with age.

At term and in the neonate, the pulmonary arteries contain a few large and many fine nerve fibers in the adventitia. The fine fibers form plexuses about the vessels and extend to as far as the arterioles. They also intermingle freely with fibers derived from the peribronchial nerves but do not extend into the alveolar walls. Nerves also accompany the pulmonary veins. A few fibers end in the adventitia and media, but most pass into the intimal layer forming a network under the endothelium.

A set of nerves originating in perivenous ganglia accompanies the veins in the septal tissue and course spirally along the vessels. These nerves give off fine fibers to the venous walls as far as the smaller venules. Their arrangement suggests they are motor in function. A second set of nerves ends in the walls of the subseptal alveoli (26–29,37).

The periarterial plexus in the lungs of the 8-month child is made up of large nerve trunks about the base of the pulmonary artery and its branches. The nerves diminish in size with the arteries to single fibers about the smaller arterioles. Some fibers branch into the lung parenchyma. In the parenchyma, nerve fibers follow the course of capillaries in the alveolar ducts and air sacs and end in relation to the capillary walls (29).

The small arterial nerve plexus in close proximity with terminal bronchioles appears to receive fibers from and send fibers to bronchial plexus. These interminglings probably have no functional significance. From the periarterial plexus, nerve fibers end on smooth muscle of the pulmonary and bronchial arteries. Afferent nerve endings (sensory type) are present in the arterial walls, in the adventitia of the pulmonary artery, and in the perichondrium of bronchial cartilages on the side toward the bronchial lumen (29).

## B.  Development of Lung Innervation in Animals

Since the last review of the topic (1), reports on the development of pulmonary innervation in experimental animals, including the rat (38–40), mouse (41), and rabbit (42), have been published. Because of the possible species variation, the development of the nervous system in these animals will be described separately.

### Rat

Fetal, perinatal, and adult rat lungs are processed for acetylcholinesterase histochemistry to study nerve development (40,43). At day 13 of gestation, acetylcholinesterase-positive neuroblasts are seen in the mesenchyme surrounding the trachea for the first time. At day 17, the myoblasts condense to form recognizable smooth muscle around the bronchi, and neuroblasts outside the smooth muscle differentiate into more mature ganglion cells characterized by clear nuclei with multiple nucleoli. Smaller acetylcholinesterase-positive neuroblasts are also seen in the submucosa (40). Neuroblasts in isolated lungs from day 12 fetuses prepared for culture develop similarly as those in vivo (43). On day 18, acetylcholinesterase-positive NEBs begin to appear, and distal neuroblasts further differentiate and assume paramuscular and submucosal positions. Neither neuroblasts, ganglion cells, nor nerve fibers could be demonstrated by these techniques distal to the third branching point from the trachea in the embryonic, perinatal, and adult lungs (40,43). Using calcitonin gene–related peptide (CGRP) as a marker (39), airway endocrine cells become positive for CGRP at day 17, and nerve fibers in the trachea, stem bronchi, and proximal intrapulmonary airways become positive at day 18 while the lung is at the pseudoglandular stage of development. By days 19 (canalicular stage) and 20 (terminal sac stage), additional tiny varicose fibers are also seen among smooth muscle and around blood vessels present in the adventitia of the major airways. The fine network below and within the epithelium lining of the trachea and stem bronchi is first detected by day 1 after birth (39). Other investigators have reported that in the rat, cholinergic nerves are not found until 5 days after birth, but intrapulmonary adrenergic nerves supplying bronchial arteries are seen in 20-day-old fetuses (38).

### Mouse

The nerve supply to the tracheas and lungs of mouse fetuses at 15–21 days of gestation and postnatal mice of 2, 5, 9, and 18 days old were studied with silver impregnation, cholinesterase histochemistry, and glyoxylic acid technique for histofluorescence of catecholamines (41) as well as electron microscopy. The silver impregnation technique provides good demonstration of the general distribution of the nervous tissue. The growth of the nervous tissue is already well established in 15–day fetuses, which is the earliest fetal age studied. In these fetuses, the nerve bundles accompany the tracheas, bronchi, and large bronchioles, and the developing autonomic ganglia are located in the hilum of the lungs, and a few single nerve fibers extend into the connective tissue area between the developing air passages. In fetuses 18 days and older and in postnatal mice, in addition to these ganglia and nerve bundles, single nerve fibers are located close to the developing smooth muscle of the airways of various sizes and in the walls of the pulmonary veins. Single fibers also penetrate the epithelial lining of the bronchi and bronchioles and innervate the NEBs, and other fibers following the terminal bronchioles may extend into the alveolar walls.

In 15-day-old fetuses, cholinesterase activity is associated with nerve bundles running along the tracheas. Beginning at day 18, the cholinergic nerves are located near the tracheal, bronchial, and bronchiolar smooth muscle as well as the cardiac muscle of the pulmonary veins. These nerves are more prominent in fullterm fetuses and young postnatal mice. At 15 days of fetal age, fluorescent adrenergic nerves are located in connective tissue surrounding tracheas and in the hilum. In 18-day and older fetuses and in young postnatal mice, fluorescent nerves follow the tracheas, bronchi, bronchioles, and pulmonary veins; some of these nerves are near the muscle layer of the airways.

Transmission electron microscopy of proximal airways from 18-day fetuses shows that the airway wall consists of the epithelium with differentiating epithelial cells, the underlying immature smooth muscle, and nerve bundle in peribronchial connective tissue (Fig. 6). The nerve bundle is formed by unmyelinated axons partially surrounded by Schwann cells (Figs. 7 and 8). The ganglionic cell can be identified by its light-staining nucleus, large amount of cytoplasm, and basal lamina (Fig. 9). The cell may appear singly, is small in comparison with mature neurons, and has an abundance of cell organelles (Fig. 9).

### Rabbit

Studies on the development of nervous tissue in the fetal rabbit lungs have been conducted using neurohistological techniques, including silver impregnation, cholinesterase histochemistry, and glyoxylic acid–induced monoamine histofluorescence (42). Nerve fibers and primitive ganglionic cells enter the developing lungs by day 17; some fibers closely follow the bronchi, but others are surrounded by mesenchymal tissues. Close contact of nerve fibers with bronchial smooth muscle is found at day 21, which coincides with the first detection of acetylcholinesterase and epinephrine (adrenaline) in the nerve fibers. At day 25, single nerve fibers and nerve bundles can be seen in the developing alveolar walls and in or near the pleura. At day 25, nerve fibers accompany pulmonary arteries but not pulmonary veins; these fibers were positive for epinephrine but negative for acetylcholinesterase. Acetylcholinesterase-positive neurons begin to appear at day 27, and this enzyme reactivity is very strong by 31 days (term fetus). At 31 days, extensive adrenergic nerve plexuses with a characteristic beaded appearance are seen in the walls of the proximal bronchi and in the tunica adventitia and tunica media of the pulmonary arteries.

These observations indicate that in the rabbit fetuses, the nervous tissue is present in the lungs during the glandular stage of development (17–23 days of gestation), and differentiation of the adrenergic and cholinergic nerves occurs during the late glandular stage (42). This pattern of development in the nervous system of the lung in relation to the stages of lung development is in general agreement with that reported in the rat and mouse (Table 1).

It is interesting to point out that nerve fibers reach the developing alveolar wall as early as 25 days of gestation in rabbits. These nerves in the lungs of adult guinea pig, rat, hamster, cat, and dog are shown to be immunoreactive for tachykinin, protein gene product 9.5, and calcitonin gene-related peptide and are thought to have sensory function (44).

In the rabbit fetuses, endocrine cells and NEBs are argyrophilic acetylcholinesterase-positive and contain serotonin detected with glyoxylic acid–induced histofluorescence. They are seen at 19–21 days of gestation while the lung is still in glandular stage of development (42). Such an early differentiation of NEBs also occurs in humans and other animals (30). In the rabbit, these cells receive a nerve supply at day 21 of gestation; and some of these nerves become positive for epinephrine at day 25. Light and electron microscopy and denervation studies have characterized these nerves as sensory, adrenergic, cholinergic, and nonadrenergic and noncholinergic (NANC, or peptidergic) (30,31,45,46). In the lungs of the adult rabbit, hamster, and rat, these nerves are positive for NSE, substance P, calcitonin gene-related peptide, and protein gene peptide 9.5 (45). Using electron microscopy, axons with small clear vesicles (about 40 nm in diameter) are identified as cholinergic; axons with small dense core vesicles (40–80 nm in diameter) are adrenergic; and NANC terminals usually have larger dense vesicles 80–225 nm in diameter) (30,45).

### C. Denervation of the Lung: Fetal, Neonatal, and Adult

Unilateral vagotomy and sympathectomy during the first 3 weeks after birth in the rat and rabbit do not change dry lung weight, lung volume, and the size of subpleural alveoli in the rat, and they also do not change lung mechanical properties (static and dynamic lung compliances, lung resistance, frequency dependence of compliance) in the rabbit (47). Follow-up studies also indicate that these procedures do not modify growth, ventilation, metabolism, and lung and heart macroscopic development, nor does it interfere with the changes of these variables induced by chronic hypoxia or hyperoxia (48). Hence, it has been suggested that lung innervation does not have an important role in the postnatal development of the lung even in conditions of altered oxygen supply (47,48). In contrast, bilateral vagotomy has been shown to alter the ultrastructure of the type II pneumocytes in the adult rat (49) and in the fetal lamb (50) and to cause respiratory distress in the adult rabbit (51). Additionally, chemical sympathectomy in neonatal rats causes alterations in lamellar bodies in the type II pneumocytes (52) and also prevents the development of normal β-adrenergic receptors (53). Furthermore, sympathetic stimulation reduces cytoplasmic lamellar bodies in the type II pneumocytes in the cat owing to increased exocytosis (54). On the other hand, bilateral vagotomy also has been shown to alter the ultrastructure of the type II pneumocytes in the adult rat (49) and in the fetal lamb (50) and to cause respiratory distress in the adult rabbit (51). Electron microscopy has identified axons terminating directly on the type II pneumocytes (55). These experiments point to the importance of a nerve supply in lung development and function. Because of the important role of surfactant in normal respiration, the possible neural control of surfactant secretion deserves further studies.

## IV. Summary

Studies in animals have indicated that the precursors of the nervous tissue destined for the lung are associated with the foregut before the appearance of the lung bud. As the lung bud is formed, the nervous tissue is incorporated into the developing lung and innervates various components of the air passages: epithelium, smooth muscle, glands, and blood vessels. In the fetus, histochemical and immunocytochemical techniques show an orderly expression of neurotransmitters as the lung develops. It should be noted that changes in airway innervation may also occur during postnatal growth (56). Although a lot is known about the functions of different types of nerves and ganglionic cells in the adult lung, the functions of the nerve tissue in the fetal lung await further study.

Our review regarding the basic principles regulating the interactions between the nervous system and the target tissues is based on work performed mostly in the gastrointestinal tract. There is a need for studies on the influence of target tissues on the developing nerves in the lung because of the complexity of the lung structures with various target cells at different airway levels.

Recent studies have also discovered nitric oxide synthase–containing neurons in the adult lung (57–59). The development of NO-producing nerves and their significance in the developing and growing lung need further study. Additionally, the lung is also an obvious site of neuroimmune interaction because of the bronchus-associated lymphoid tissue and the active secretion of immunoglobulin by airway epithelium. There are recent reports on this relationship in the adult lung (60–62). This too is an important area which warrants investigation in future studies on lung development.

### Acknowledgments

The authors thank Dr. Shigeru Kuratani for providing the original photograph used for Figure 1. We also thank Jeff Altemus for preparing the diagrams in Figure 2 and Sandy Baker for preparing Table 1.

### References

1. Loosli CG, Hung K-S. Development of pulmonary innervation. In: Hodson WA, ed. Development Of The Lung. New York: Dekker, 1977:269–306.
2. Kuratani S, Tanaka S. Peripheral development of the avian vagus nerve with special reference to the morphological innervation of heart and lung. Anat Embryol 1990; 182:435–445.
3. Le Douarin NM, Teillet M-A. The migration of neural crest cells to the wall of the digestive tract in avian embryo. J Embryol Exp Morphol 1973; 30:31–48.
4. Jacobson M. Developmental Neurobiology. New York: Plenum Press, 1991.
5. Le Douarin NM, Smith J, Teillet M-A, LeLievre CS, Ziller C. The neural crest and its developmental analysis in avian embryo chimaeras. TINS 1980; 3:39–42.
6. Le Douarin NM. The ontogeny of the neural crest in avian embryo chimaeras. Nature 1980; 286:663–668.
7. Purves D, Lichtman JW. Principles of Neural Development. Massachusetts: Sinauer, 1985.
8. Ayer-Le Leivre CS, Le Douarin NM. The early development of cranial sensory ganglia and the potentialities of their component cells studied in quail-chick chimeras. Dev Biol 1982; 94:291–310.
9. Fontaine-Perus J, Chanconie M, Le Douarin NM. Embryonic origin of substance P

containing neurons in cranial and spinal sensory ganglia of the avian embryo. Dev Biol 1985; 107:227–238.

10. Barnes PJ. Asthma as an axon reflex. Lancet 1986; 1:242–245.
11. Lundberg JM, Saria A, Brodin E, Rosell S, Folkers K. A substance P antagonist inhibits vagally induced increase in vascular permeability and bronchial smooth muscle contraction in the guinea pig. Proc Natl Acad Sci USA 1983; 80:1120–1124.
12. Chamak B, Pronchiantz A. Influence of extracellular matrix proteins on the expression of neuronal polarity. Development 1989; 106:483–491.
13. Rubin E. Development of the rat superior cervial ganglion: ganglion cell maturation. J Neurosci 1985; 5:673–684.
14. Rubin E. Development of the rat superior cervical ganglion: ingrowth of preganglionic axons. J Neurosci 1985; 5:685–696.
15. Bronner-Fraser M, Fraser SE. Cell lineage analysis of the avian neural crest. Development 1991; 2:17–22.
16. Epstein ML, Poulsen KT, Thiboldeaux R. Formation of ganglia in the gut of the chick embryo. J Comp Neurol 1991; 307:189–199.
17. Epstein ML, Saffrey MJ, Poulsen KT. Development and birthdates of vasoactive intestinal peptide immunoreactive neurons in the chick proventriculus. J Comp Neurol 1992; 321:83–92.
18. Rothman TP, Nilaver G, Gershon MD. Colonization of the developing murine enteric nervous system and subsequent phenotypic expression by the precursors of peptidergic neurons. J Comp Neurol 1984; 225:13–23.
19. Fontaine-Perus J, Chanconie M, Polak JM, Le Douarin NM. Origin and development of VIP and substance P containing neurons in the embryonic avian gut. Histochemistry 1981; 71:313–323.
20. Schotzinger R, Xinghuan Y, Landis S. Target determination of neurotransmitter phenotype in sympathetic neurons. J Neurobiol 1994; 25:620–639.
21. Symes AJ, Rao MS, Lewis SE, Landis SC, Hyman SE, Fink JS. Ciliary neurotrophic factor coordinately activates transcription of neuropeptide genes in a neuroblastoma cell line. Proc Natl Acad Sci USA 1993; 90:572–576.
22. Sun Y, Rao MS, Zigmond RE, Landis SC. Regulation of vasoactive intestinal peptide expression in sympathetic neurons in culture and after axotomy: the role of cholinergic differentiation factor/leukemia inhibitory factor. J Neurobiol 1994; 25:415–430.
23. Salvi E, Renda T. An immunohistochemical study on neurons and paraneurons of the pre- and post-natal chicken lung. Arch Histol Cytol 1992; 125:135.
24. Sheppard MN, Marangoss PJ, Bloom SR, Polak JM. Neuron specific enolase: a marker for the early development of nerves and endocrine cells in the human lung. Life Sci 1984; 34:265–271.
25. Ghatei MA, Sheppard MN, O'Shaughnessy DJ, et al. Regulatory peptides in the mammalian respiratory tract. Endocrinology 1982; 111:1248–1254.
26. Taylor IM, Smith RB. Intrinsic innervation of the human fetal lung between the 35 and 140 mm crown-rump length stages. Biol Neonate 1971; 18:193–202.
27. Mizukoshi T. Histological studies on the innervation of lung of human embryo. Tohoku J Exp Med 1953; 58:223–233.
28. Spencer H, Leof D. The innervation of the human lung. J Anat 1964; 98:599–609.
29. Larsell O, Dow RS. The innervation of the human lung. Am J Anat 1933; 52:125–145.

30. Sorokin SP, Hoyt RF, Jr. Neuroepithelial bodies and solitary small-granule cells. In: Massaro D, ed. Lung Cell Biology. New York: Dekker, 1989:191–344.

31. Hung K-S. Histology, ultrastructure and development of pulmonary endocrine cells. In: Becker KL, Gazdar AF, eds. The Endocrine Lung In Health And Disease. Vol. 1. Philadelphia: Sanders, 1984:162–192.

32. Lauweryns JM, Peuskens JC, Cokelaere M. Argyrophile, fluorescent and granulated (peptide and amine producing?) AFG cells in human infant bronchial epithelium. Light and electron microscopic studies. Life Sci 1970; 9:1417–1429.

33. Lauweryns JM, Peuskens JC. Neuro-epithelial bodies (neuroreceptors or secretory organs?) in human infant bronchial and bronchiolar epithelium. Anat Rec 1972; 172:471–482.

34. Stahlman MT, Gray ME. Ontogeny of neuroendocrine cells in human fetal lung. I. An electron microscopic study. Lab Invest 1984; 51:449–463.

35. Fox B, Bull TB, Guz A. Innervation of alveolar walls in the human lung: an electron microscopic study. J Anat 1980; 131:683–692.

36. Hertweck MS, Hung K-S. Ultrastructural evidence for the innervation of human pulmonary alveoli. Experientia 1980; 36:112.

37. Pessacq TP. The innervation of the lung of new born children. Acta Anat 1971; 79: 93–101.

38. El-Bermani A-WI, Bloomquist EI. Acetycholinesterase- and norepinephrine-containing nerves in developing rat lung. J Embryol Exp Morphol 1978; 48:177–183.

39. Cadieux A, Springall DR, Mulderry PK, et al. Occurrence, distribution and ontogeny of CGRP immunoreactivity in the rat lower respiratory tract: effect of capsaicin treatment and surgical denervations. Neuroscience 1986; 19:605–627.

40. Morikawa Y, Donahoe PK, Hendren WH. Cholinergic nerve development in fetal lung. Dev Biol 1978; 6:541–546.

41. Hung K-S. Innervation of the pre- and postnatal mouse tracheas and lungs (abstr). Anat Rec 1978; 190:427.

42. Hung K-S. Innervation of rabbit fetal lungs. Am J Anat 1980; 159:73–83.

43. Morikawa Y, Donahoe PK, Hendren WH. Cholinergic nerve development of fetal lung in vitro. J Pediatr Surg 1978; 13:653–661.

44. Nohr D, Weihe E. Tachykinin-, calcitonin gene–related peptide-, and protein gene product 9.5-immunoreactive nerve fibers in alveolar walls of mammals. Neurosci Lett 1991; 134:17–20.

45. Adriaensen D, Scheuermann DW. Neuroendocrine cells and nerves of the lung. Anat Rec 1993; 236:70–85.

46. Scheuermann DW. Morphology and cytochemistry of the endocrine epithelial system in the lung. Int Rev Cytol 1987; 106:35–88.

47. Mortola JP, Saetta M, Bartlett D, Jr. Postnatal development of the lung following denervation. Respir Physiol 1987; 67:137–145.

48. Dotta A, Mortola JP. Postnatal development of the denervated lung in normoxia, hypoxia, or hyperoxia. J Appl Physiol 1992; 73:1461–1466.

49. Goldenberg VE, Buckingham S, Sommers SC. Pulmonary alveolar lesions in vagotomized rats. Lab Invest 1967; 16:693–705.

50. Alcorn D, Adamson TM, Maloney JE, Robinson PM. Morphological effects of

chronic bilateral phrenectomy or vagotomy in the fetal lamb lung. J Anat 1980; 130:683–695.

51. Berry D, Ikegami M, Jobe A. Respiratory distress and surfactant inhibition following vagotomy in rabbits. J Appl Physiol 1986; 61:1741–1748.

52. de Camara D, Moss GS, Das Gupta TK. Alterations in pulmonary surfactant following sympathectomy. Surg Forum 1976; 27:182–184.

53. Slotkin TA, Lau C, Kavlock RJ, et al. Trophic control of lung development by sympathetic neurons: effects of neonatal sympathectomy with 6-hydroxydopamine. J Dev Physiol 1988; 100:577–590.

54. Crittenden DJ, Alexander LA, Beckman DL. Sympathetic nerve influence on alveolar type II cell ultrastructure. Life Sci 1994; 55:1229–1235.

55. Hung K-S, Hertweck MS, Hardy JD, Loosli CG. Innervation of pulmonary alveoli of the mouse lung: an electron microscopic study. Am J Anat 1972; 135:477–495.

56. Hislop AA, Wharton J, Allen KM, Polak JM, Haworth SG. Immunohistochemical localization of peptide-containing nerves in human airways: age-related changes. Am J Respir Cell Mol Biol 1990; 3:191–198.

57. Díaz de Rada O, Villaro AC, Montuenga LM, Martínez A, Springall DR, Polak JM. Nitric oxide synthase-immunoreactive neurons in human and porcine respiratory tract. Neurosci Lett 1993; 162:121–124.

58. Fischer A, Mundel P, Mayer B, Preissler U, Philippin B, Kummer W. Nitric oxide synthase in guinea pig lower airway innervation. Neurosci Lett 1993; 149:157–160.

59. Dey RD, Mayer B, Said SI. Colocalization of vasoactive intestinal peptide and nitric oxide synthase in neurons of the ferret trachea. Neuroscience 1993; 54:839–843.

60. Nilsson G, Alving K, Ahlstedt S, Hokfelt T, Lundberg JM. Peptidergic innervation of rat lymphoid tissue and lung: relation to mast cells and sensitivity to capsaicin and immunization. Cell Tissue Res 1990; 262:125–133.

61. Inoue N, Magari S, Sakanaka M. Distribution of peptidergic nerve fibers in rat bronchus-associated lymphoid tissue: Light microscopic observations. Lymphology 1990; 23:155–160.

62. Nohr D, Weihe E. The neuroimmune link in the bronchus-associated lymphoid tissue (BALT) of cat and rat: peptides and neural markers. Brain Behav Immun 1991; 5: 84–101.

63. Patten BM. Early Embryology Of The Chick. New York: McGraw-Hill, 1971.

64. Rugh R. The Mouse: Its Reproduction And Development. Minneapolis: Burgess, 1968.

65. Larsen WJ. Human Embryology. New York: Churchill Livingstone, 1993.

# 10

# Development of Airway Smooth Muscle

**PAUL B. McCRAY, JR.**

University of Iowa College of Medicine
Iowa City, Iowa

**KENNETH T. NAKAMURA**

Kapiolani Medical Center
John A. Burns School of Medicine
Honolulu, Hawaii

## I. Introduction

The development of airway smooth muscle in the fetal lung is intimately linked with the formation of the tracheobronchial tree. In the human, the lung begins around the 4th week of gestation as a ventral outgrowth of foregut endoderm which becomes invested in splanchnic mesoderm. As the airways form by dichotomous branching, a complex process involving epithelial-mesenchymal interactions, smooth muscle cells first become visible as a condensation of the mesenchyme near the basement membrane along the epithelial tubules. In humans, this is evident by 6–8 weeks of gestation (1,2). As development progresses, the smooth muscle cell investment around the airways extends from its origins in the trachea, mainstem, and lobar bronchi to the segmental bronchi, terminal and respiratory bronchioles, and alveolar ducts (1,3). Early in gestation, the airway smooth muscle becomes innervated and responsive to contractile and relaxing stimuli (4,5).

The postnatal functions of airway smooth muscle, including protective responses and the regulation of airflow within the lung, and its role in lung diseases, are well documented. An intriguing question is why airway smooth muscle is functionally expressed from such an early developmental time point. In this chapter, we review the developmental biology of smooth muscle expression in the fetal lung, discuss the physiology of airway smooth muscle in the fetus and newborn, and outline how alterations of normal development may lead to clinical lung disease in infants.

## II.  Developmental Biology of Airway Smooth Muscle

### A.  Myogenesis

Understanding of the genes regulating skeletal muscle myogenesis has progressed tremendously in the last decade. However, similar detailed knowledge of the regulation of airway smooth muscle development is lacking. Nonetheless, a brief discussion of skeletal muscle myogenesis may serve as a useful framework for conceptualizing muscle development in general.

The embryonic precursors of mammalian skeletal muscle originate as myoblasts in the mesodermal somites (6,7). Before skeletal muscle fibers or contractile proteins are expressed, mammalian myogenic cells express genes of the *MyoD*, myogenin, *Myf-5*, and MRF4/herculin/*Myf-6* families. This family of genes has proven to be a major group of regulatory genes controlling the expression of the skeletal muscle cell phenotype. Expression of *MyoD* genes in a variety of cultured nonmuscle cells confers a skeletal muscle phenotype (8). Members of these gene families code for nuclear proteins which may bind to the consensus sequence CANNTG in the promoter and enhancer regions of several muscle genes. The proteins share a common helix-loop-helix (HLH) domain and may form homodimers or heterodimers with themselves and other family members. Binding of these proteins can produce either positive or negative regulatory effects on the transcription of muscle genes and thus influence the muscle cell phenotype (6). Myogenic factors may be phosphorylated, allowing a way for growth factors or second messengers to regulate their function (6). Furthermore, growth factors and other cell-specific transcription factors also influence the expression of myogenic genes.

Known members of the *MyoD* and myogenin families are not expressed in airway smooth muscle. Whether the tissue-specific regulation of smooth muscle gene expression in the fetal lung involves a similar family of genes or novel transcription factors remains to be determined. This is an important area of research in smooth muscle biology.

### B.  Ontogeny of Smooth Muscle Cell Protein Expression

Airway smooth muscle cells arise from pluripotent mesodermal cells that become myoblasts under the appropriate signals. The smooth muscle investment surrounding the epithelial tubules develops as a condensation of mesodermal cells while branching morphogenesis occurs. Interactions between the epithelial and mesenchymal cells and their respective extracellular matrices and regulatory factors are critical to this process (9,10). The extracellular matrix and its associated growth factors play an important role in the development and differentiation of the smooth muscle phenotype in vascular smooth muscle (11). Limited information is available regarding the role of such factors in airway smooth muscle differentiation and development, but growth factors and cytokines are likely to act as important autocrine or paracrine signals. Transforming growth factor-$\beta$ (TGF-$\beta$) increased $\alpha$ smooth muscle actin expression in cultured adult rat pulmonary mesenchymal cell lines (12). Heparin and TGF-$\beta$1 have also been observed to induce $\alpha$ smooth muscle actin expression in cultured rat and human fibroblasts (13). These observations suggest that similar factors may influence the differentiation and maturation of the smooth muscle phenotype in fetal airway smooth muscle.

The expression of desmin and $\alpha$ smooth muscle actin genes in the cells along the developing airways is one of the earliest signs of smooth muscle cell differentiation in the lung mesenchyme (14). In a study of developing rat lung, Mitchell and colleagues used antibodies to contractile and cytoskeletal proteins to examine the differentiation and tissue distribution of smooth muscle and fibroblastic cells (14). Smooth muscle cell differentiation from the mesenchyme followed epithelial tubule branching. They observed that the condensation of cells along the epithelial tubules of the pseudoglandular stage lung expressed the intermediate filament protein desmin (Fig. 1). This appeared to replace vimentin as differentiation occurred, a pattern that was maintained as development progressed.

$\alpha$ Smooth muscle actin is the actin isoform characteristically expressed by airway smooth muscle cells. The expression of the actin multigene family members has been shown to be developmentally regulated in a fashion that is both temporally and tissue specific (15,16). Mitchell et al. found that $\alpha$ smooth muscle actin staining along the length of branching tubules was prominent, whereas it was absent from the epithelia and mesenchyme of the pseudoglandular stage rat lung (see Fig. 1) (14). Similar findings were noted in day 11 fetal mouse lung (17) and first-trimester human fetal lung (2,4). The expression of the matrix protein fibronectin and its receptor follows a similar pattern during branching morphogenesis (17,18). $\alpha$ Smooth muscle actin and the fibronectin receptor marker a5 were coexpressed in the parabronchial cells. These observations suggest that fibronectin may influence the differentiation and migration pattern of mesenchymal cells toward a smooth muscle cell phenotype (17). Interestingly, $\alpha$ smooth muscle actin staining was also prominent in the clefts of branch points of the pseudoglandular stage (14).

Booth and colleagues localized the expression of several smooth muscle–associated proteins in fetal pig trachealis muscle using immunocytochemistry (19). Myosin, caldesmon, and filamin were all abundantly expressed in animals as small as 7 g (~30% of gestation). Two-dimensional gel electrophoresis of proteins

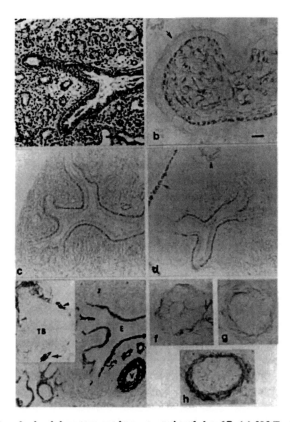

**Figure 1** Pseudoglandular stage rat lung, gestational day 17. (a) H&E stained section. (b) Diffuse antivimentin reactivity (DAB) product (black) is seen in mesenchyme, especially at the borders of epithelial tubes. Epithelial cells themselves (arrow) are negative. Endothelial lining of blood vessels shows discrete staining (arrowhead). (c) Desmin staining of thin cell layer around epithelial tree. (d) Smooth muscle myosin reactivity around epithelial tube. Note prominent staining of smooth muscle around large "airway" tube (arrow) and weaker reactivity of the companion blood vessel (arrowhead). (e) Prominent anti–smooth muscle α-actin staining is seen at the margins of the epithelial (E) and blood vessel (V) tubes. The insert shows the distal extension of α-actin reactivity (arrowheads) to the sides of a terminal bulb (TB). Also note reactive cell (arrow) in the notch where epithelial tube bifurcation is beginning. (f) Anti–smooth muscle myosin, (g) antidesmin, and (h) anti–α-actin reactivity around similar epithelial tubes in the peripheral lung. Bar in panel a equals 50 μm and applies to panels a, c, d, and e. Bar in panel b equals 10 μm and applies to panels b, f, g, h, and inset in panel e. (From ref. 14.)

from the trachea and bronchi of early-gestation fetuses demonstrated that actin, tropomyosin, and calponin were expressed in the fetal pig (20).

Myosin proteins form essential components of the contractile apparatus in muscle and are coded for by members of a related multigene family (21). In skeletal and cardiac muscle, myosin isoform expression is developmentally regulated and correlates with functional properties (22). Thus, myosin isoform expression also serves as a marker of muscle cell differentiation. Specific myosin heavy chain isomers are expressed in airway smooth muscle and the expression of myosin isoforms in developing airway smooth muscle has been examined in several species. In the developing rat lung, a polyclonal antibody recognizing multiple myosin isoforms stained muscle cells surrounding lobar, segmental, and subsegmental airways (12). This contrasted with the pattern obtained with specific antisera against two myosin heavy chain isoforms (SM1 and SM2) expressed in airway smooth muscle. SM1 immunoreactivity was present only along larger developing airways, whereas SM2 immunoreactivity was absent from fetal lung (12). In the adult rat lung, both heavy chain isomers were easily detected along the length of the airways. These findings in the rat suggest that there may be myosin isoforms unique to the developing lung that are currently unknown.

The expression of two myosin heavy chain isomers (204 and 200 kDa) has also been studied during development in the pig using densitometric quantitation of Western blots from different regions of the airways (23). Overall, the myosin content of airway tissues increased throughout maturation from fetal to adult time points. The myosin content of the trachea was greater than the peripheral airways at all developmental ages and increased fivefold by adulthood. The ratio of myosin heavy chains (204 to 200 kDa) was greatest in the fetus and declined with maturation. The ability of airways to develop stress in response to pharmacological interventions was normalized to myosin content. Suckling airways developed the greatest stress in response to carbachol or histamine, whereas isolated tracheal fiber bundles from fetal and suckling pigs demonstrated greater sensitivity to $Ca^{2+}$ (23). These findings raise the issue of whether the changes in myosin heavy chain isoforms that occur with maturation are responsible for the differences in the physiological properties of airway smooth muscle.

The distribution of myosin heavy chain isoforms in newborn and adult human airways was studied using immunochemistry by Mohammad et al. (24). The 204- and 200-kDa isoforms were identified in newborn and adult tracheas and bronchi in a ratio of 0.69:1.0 (MHC1/MHC2), a ratio that was remarkably constant between newborn and adult. In addition, a putative third myosin heavy chain isoform was found in bronchi and parenchyma which was unique to humans (24). The observation that the ratio of the heavy chain isoforms did not change between infancy and adulthood suggests that the myosin components of the contractile apparatus may be mature by the early postnatal period in humans.

These studies clearly document that the protein components of the airway smooth muscle contractile machinery are expressed from early in fetal life in several species. Together these results would suggest that all elements are in place for airway smooth muscle to exhibit contractility during fetal life.

## III. Physiology

During the first half of the 19th century, the contractile abilities of airway smooth muscle were not well established. In 1840, the seminal work of Charles J. B. Williams clearly documented airway smooth muscle contractility and several important regulatory mechanisms in vivo, including contraction in response to electrical and irritant stimuli and inhibition by anticholinergic agents. These original observations have been reviewed in tribute to one of the most important contributors to the knowledge of airway pathophysiology (25).

### A. Spontaneous Contractility of Fetal Airway Smooth Muscle

A surprising aspect of airway smooth muscle development is the observation that spontaneous contractility and pharmacological responsiveness occur early in fetal life. Lewis first reported fetal airway and air sac smooth muscle contractility in chick embryos and cultured chick lung and noted that contractions were temperature dependent, had a frequency of ~2/min, and occurred without histological evidence of innervation (26). Spontaneous contractility of fetal airway smooth muscle was also described by Schopper, who observed similar findings in chick and guinea pig embryos and cultured guinea pig lung tissue (27,28). Sollman and Gilbert also described spontaneous contractility of airway smooth muscle in preparations from puppies and mid gestation human fetal lung and reported the pharmacological responses to adrenergic and cholinergic stimuli and other agents (29). Sorokin observed contractions of fetal airway smooth muscle which were present after 2–3 days in culture in cultured rat lungs and speculated that the distention of the distal lung units produced by such contractions might influence the development of the respiratory portion of the lungs (30). Furthermore, spontaneous electrical slow-wave activity accompanied by mechanical evidence of contractions has been described in isolated adult human tracheal smooth muscle (31,32) and guinea pig airway smooth muscle (33). The reports of similar spontaneous airway smooth muscle contractility in several species, including embryos, cultured fetal lung explants, and isolated adult smooth muscle preparations, support the notion that these contractions occur in vivo.

Studies of early first-trimester human lung tissue and cultured lung tissue explants documented that human fetal airway smooth muscle is also spontaneously contractile (4). When observed using videomicroscopy, fetal airway smooth muscle contractions produced visible movement of intraluminal fluid and distention of the distal ends of epithelial tubules, suggesting that the contractions produced significant changes in intraluminal pressure (Fig. 2). The interval be-

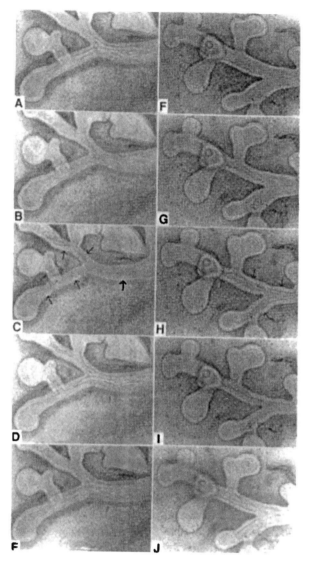

**Figure 2** Photomicrographs of cycle of smooth muscle contractions in two representative cultured first-trimester human fetal lung explants. Each series of photos (A–E; F–J) shows one cycle of airway smooth muscle contraction. Note progressive change in diameter of airway lumen (arrows) as contraction proceeds. Bar equals 100 μm. (From ref. 4.)

tween contractions was regular and ranged from 8–135 sec (mean $\pm$ SE = 54 $\pm$ 5 sec). Spontaneous fetal airway smooth muscle contractility was not inhibited by tetrodotoxin or atropine, implying a myogenic rather than a neurogenic origin of the contractility. The cholinergic agonists acetylcholine and carbachol increased human fetal airway smooth muscle contractility, and contractile activity was inhibited by the calcium channel blockers $CdCl_2$ and nifedipine, suggesting that fetal airway smooth muscle contractions are accompanied by an influx of extracellular $Ca^{2+}$. Isoproterenol caused dilation of the contractile regions of the epithelial tubules and cessation of contractions. Lemakalim, an activator of smooth muscle ATP-sensitive $K^+$ channels, also stopped contractions and caused relaxation of fetal airway smooth muscle (4).

Detailed studies of airways from 40- to 45-day gestation fetal pigs (term = 115 days) has further characterized the functional properties of airway smooth muscle in early fetal mammalian lungs (5). The bronchial tree was dissected free from the parenchyma and narrowing of the airways recorded in real time with videomicroscopy. Spontaneous narrowing and relaxation was noted to occur throughout the bronchial tree in these specimens. Bronchoconstriction occurred in response to acetylcholine, histamine, substance P, and depolarizing concentrations of $K^+$. Interestingly, small airways showed greater narrowing in response to acetylcholine than medium- or large-diameter airways. The $\beta$-agonist isoproterenol induced relaxation of constricted fetal airways. Electrical field stimulation also produced marked narrowing of the fetal airways, a response that was inhibited by atropine. Using immunohistochemical techniques, nerve trunks could be demonstrated coursing from the carina to bronchioles of 75–155 $\mu$m external diameter (Fig. 3) (5). Neurofilament staining does not detect all nerves. Recent immunolocalization experiments by Everett and colleagues (34) using an antisynaptic vesicle antibody reveals a dense innervation to all airways with an abundance of varicosities in the nerves of fetal pigs (first trimester) and fetal rabbits (near term). A plexus of fine nerves was distributed over the smooth muscle surface of the bronchial wall with an abundance of prominent varicosities 1–3 $\mu$m in diameter and 3–10 $\mu$m apart which were distributed both over and in the smooth muscle layer. Antineurofilament stained a much smaller population of nerves. This is consistent which the presence of functional cholinergic nerves and pharmacological responsiveness qualitatively similar to adult airway smooth muscle early in development (5).

The contractile force of tracheal smooth muscle from fetal pigs in response to acetylcholine, $K^+$ depolarizing solution, and electrical field stimulation (EFS) was measured by Booth et al. (19). Trachealis muscle from animals as small as 9 g body weight contracted in response to agonists and to EFS. Isometric force corrected for cross-sectional area of smooth muscle was the same from 17- to 600-g fetuses. When the force in response to EFS was normalized to the maximal

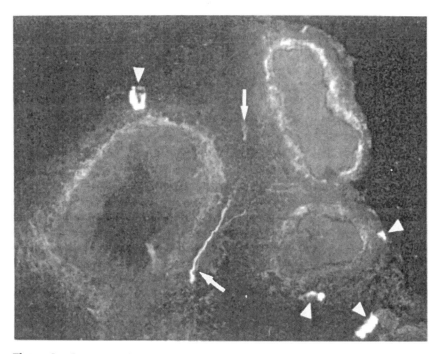

**Figure 3** Cryostat sections of three branches of an airway from a fetal pig bronchial tree that have been stained concurrently for nerve trunks (arrowheads) and fiber bundles (arrows) with the 68-kDa neurofilament antibody (FITC conjugate) and for smooth muscle using smooth muscle myosin (rhodamine red conjugate). The FITC nerve staining is shown, but some of the intense rhodamine red signal has passed through the FITC filter showing the smooth muscle. Overexposure during photography has enabled the mucosal layer and the mesenchymal matrix to be seen in the background but causing the nerve trunks to be slightly blurred. (Scale bar equals 100 μm). FITC, fluorescein isothiocyanate. (From ref. 5.)

response to acetylcholine, 11- to 300-g fetuses all had similar responses. EFS induced contractions were inhibited by atropine and tetrodotoxin (19).

It is not certain what purpose the contractile activity of the fetal airway smooth muscle serves, but clearly this tissue is functional very early in fetal life. One speculation is that it may play a role in lung development by signals transduced via phasic changes in the intraluminal pressure. Several physical factors have been implicated in lung development (35), including fluid secretion by the pulmonary epithelium (36–38), the maintenance of a positive intraluminal pressure by the fetal glottis and upper airways (39,40), patency of the fetal airways

(41,42), adequate intrathoracic and amniotic fluid volumes (43,44), and fetal breathing movements (35). Spontaneous fetal airway smooth muscle contractions result in mechanical distortion or stretching of the fetal pulmonary epithelium and mesenchyme (4,5). Wirtz and Dobbs reported that a single mechanical stretch of alveolar type II cells stimulated release of surfactant and a sustained increase in intracellular calcium and hypothesized that phasic distention of the alveolar epithelium is a mechanical signal for surfactant release mediated through calcium-induced exocytosis (45). Similarly, in the heart, it has been shown that stretch induces increases in myocyte total RNA and protein synthesis, and it also causes induction of several genes, resulting in myocyte hypertrophy (46,47). Perhaps similar mechanisms exist in the fetal lung where changes in intraluminal pressure produce a mechanical signal resulting in the release of growth factors or regulation of gene expression. Two studies show that pulsatile mechanical stretching of fetal rat lung organotypic cultures stimulates prostacyclin production and increases cAMP production, whereas also increasing lung cell growth as measured by thymidine incorporation (48,49). Further study of this hypothesis in the developing lung may provide new insights into how physical forces influence lung development.

### B.  Developmental Physiology of Airway Smooth Muscle Contractility

*Ontogeny of Airway Smooth Muscle Contractility*

The functional capabilities of airway smooth muscle during ontogeny have only recently begun to attract the interest of smooth muscle physiologists (50). In vivo studies of airway smooth muscle contraction comparing the newborn and adult suggest that the newborn possesses a reduced capability to narrow airway diameter relative to the adult, although potential weaknesses regarding interpretations of data obtained on the basis of in vivo measurements have been discussed (50).

In contrast to conclusions based on in vivo studies, in vitro investigations suggest airway smooth muscle from neonatal or young animals has an enhanced capability to generate isometric force compared with the adult (23,51–54). Comparisons of maximal isometric force generated in vitro by neonatal and adult tissue may be influenced by the maturational status of the species at birth, since the majority of previous studies were conducted in precocial species (pig, sheep, guinea pig) with a fairly wide range of postnatal age as opposed to altricial species such as the dog. In the isolated trachea from the newborn dog, reduced isometric force generation is seen relative to the adult (50). A comparison between immature and adult tissues among several species is shown in Figure 4. In addition, comparisons of maximal isometric force between animals of different ages require normalization, and the choice of the normalization factor may be critical to the interpretation of results. Although a traditional basis for comparing tissues has

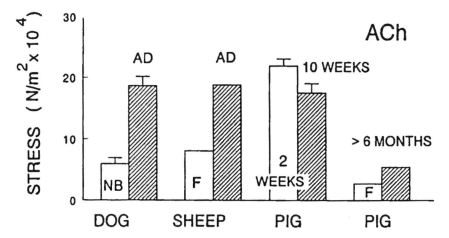

**Figure 4** Comparison of maximal values of stress in response to acetylcholine between fetal (F), newborn (NB), or suckling (2 weeks) animals of several species to those obtained in the adult (AD). Note that on the basis of tissue stress, values are generally lower in the newborn than the adult. Data for the dog are from Fisher et al. (1992) (50) and those of Mitchell et al. (1987), sheep from Panitch et al. (1989) (56), suckling pig from Murphy et al. (1989) (69), and the fetal pig from Sparrow and Mitchell (1990) (23). (From ref. 50.)

been to divide force by cross-sectional area of the tissue to yield stress (Fig. 4), this procedure assumes that there is a similar contribution of contractile and noncontractile components of the tissues being compared which may not be valid in developmental studies (51). In fact, evidence supporting the notion that noncontractile components of the airway are indeed different during development is presented below.

More recently, morphological and biochemical methods of normalization have been employed. Sparrow and Mitchell (23) were the first to normalize force on the basis of smooth muscle contractile protein content during development. Based on this normalization scheme, the very small tissue stress present in fetal trachea relative to the adult reflected the paucity of myosin heavy chain and smooth muscle present and not "less effective" airway smooth muscle (Fig. 5) (23).

Murphy et al. (52) studied the relationship of airway morphometry, the content of myosin heavy chain and isoform stoichiometry, and the distribution of bronchoconstrictor responses in the airways of maturing swine between 2 and 10 weeks of age. In this comprehensive investigation, the investigators concluded that force of airway smooth muscle contraction normalized to tissue weight, smooth muscle content, and/or tissue myosin content decreases systematically in the major resistance airways of swine during maturation. Decreased contractile

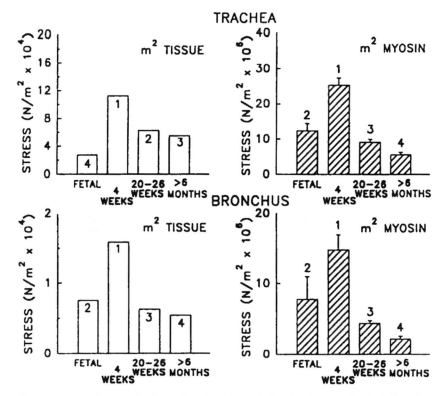

**Figure 5** Comparison of values of maximal force during development in the pig based on tissue cross-sectional area ($m^2$ tissue) and myosin heavy chain cross-sectional area ($m^2$ myosin) normalizations. Note that myosin normalization for tracheal smooth muscle alters the rank order of the maximal force from largest (1) to smallest (4) and tends to reduce the relative difference between groups. In bronchial tissue, the rank order is not altered by myosin normalization, but the relative difference between bronchial and tracheal stress is reduced by myosin normalization. (Data from Sparrow and Mitchell (1990) (23). (From ref. 50.)

response with maturation is receptor independent and is not related to the changes in the nonmuscular tissues of the airway. Because smooth muscle content remains comparable and nonmuscle to muscle ratio is not altered, changes in contractile response cannot be related to differences in relative smooth muscle cross-sectional area occurring with maturation. They further conclude that myosin isoforms associated with smooth muscle contraction do not differ substantially during maturation but that total tissue content of functional myosin within each airway generation is diminished.

Unlike adult human airways, studies of airway responsiveness in human neonates have been lacking. However, a recent detailed study of human neonatal bronchi shows that mechanisms controlling airway tone in adults are functional in the neonate (55). These investigators found the rank of maximal contractile force to be carbachol > histamine > KCl > neurokinin A (NKA), with sensitivities ($EC_{50}$) NKA < carbachol < histamine < KCl. In addition, these human neonatal sensitivities to the cholinergic agonist carbachol and to histamine are similar with those of the lamb (56), guinea pig (57), and pig (23), as well as having similar slopes of the concentration response curves to newborn guinea pigs (57).

### Neural Regulation of Airway Smooth Muscle During Development

The postnatal human airways are richly innervated by the autonomical nervous system, including well-documented cholinergic and but sparse adrenergic inputs. There are also nonadrenergic noncholinergic nerves in which peptides such as vasoactive intestinal peptide and substance P serve as neurotransmitters (58,59). The development of lung innervation and neuropeptides in the lung development are the subjects of other chapters in this volume to which the reader is referred for an analysis of these topics. Unfortunately, there is little detailed information regarding the development of innervation in the early human lung.

Two aspects of the development of pulmonary innervation deserve specific attention in view of fetal airway smooth muscle spontaneous contractility. The first is that the innervation of the lung is established prenatally (1). In the chick model, innervation of the airways appears to follow lung branching morphogenesis (60). Evidence suggests that these fibers are present in early gestation and could therefore influence the contractility of fetal airway smooth muscle (1,5,60). Sparrow and colleagues have documented that electrical field stimulation of fetal airway smooth muscle induces contractile responses early in gestation, suggesting that the cholinergic innervation is functional (5,19). The second is the finding that neuroendocrine cells expressing peptides, including bombesin and calcitonin gene–related peptide, are present in the lung during the first trimester in the human (61–63). In addition to its mitogenic effects on lung cells, bombesin is a potent bronchoconstrictor and could conceivably influence smooth muscle contractility in the fetus (64,65).

Vagal control of pulmonary resistance has been demonstrated in premature lambs (0.87% gestation) as well as in term lambs (66), piglets (67), puppies, and kittens (68). Isolated airway contractile response of young postnatal swine to parasympathetic nerve stimulation is greater than in older swine (69), which is at least in part related to reduced acetylcholinesterase activity in immature animals (70). In addition, functional nonadrenergic noncholinergic inhibitory (iNANC) nerves have been demonstrated in approximately 2-week-old newborn guinea pigs (71) and newborn cats (72). With the recent discovery that NO is a mediator in iNANC (73), it is expected that additional work in this area will be forthcoming.

Other neuromodulators of airway function during the postnatal period have been investigated (74,75). Tanaka and Grunstein (74), demonstrated that the neurokinin substance P (SP), a potent bronchoconstrictor identified in airway nerves, has a significantly enhanced neuromedulatory effect on acetylcholine release during postnatal development. Studies in piglets between <4 days to 10 weeks of age found a progressive increase in in situ tracheal tension to intravenous infusions of SP with a weaker response to neurokinin A (NKA) during postnatal maturation (75). Studies in anesthetized 2-week-old and adult guinea pigs found that the young animals required larger doses of SP and NKA than adults to cause significant airflow obstruction (76). Similar to these animal studies, results in human airway demonstrate an increase in force generation induced by NKA with maturation (55).

### Maturation of Intracellular Messengers

Schramm et al. (77) investigated the maturational changes in the binding characteristics of the Ins (1,4,5)P3 receptor and the modulation of Ins(1,4,5)P3 binding by $Ca^{2+}$ in rabbit tracheal smooth muscle in vitro. Under basal conditions, both the Ins(1,4,5)P3 receptor affinity and density do not change with postnatal age, but $Ca^{2+}$ exerts an inhibitory effect on binding in adult tracheal smooth muscle, whereas it is potentiated in immature tracheal smooth muscle. This suggests that $Ca^{2+}$-dependent potentiation of binding in immature rabbit airway smooth muscle may contribute, at least in part, to the increased airway reactivity observed in newborns.

### Effect of Relaxants

The bronchodilator effects of β-adrenoceptor–mediated agonists and their mechanisms of action via stimulation of cAMP have been well described (58,78). The original subdivision of β-adrenoceptors was based on the finding that the relative potency of a series of catecholamines causing bronchodilatation in the guinea pig differed from that causing cardiac stimulation in the rabbit (79,80). Since then, tracheal smooth muscle, particularly from the guinea pig, has been extensively employed to investigate airway smooth muscle responses to catecholamines (81), as well as other receptor- and nonreceptor-dependent stimulants of airway smooth muscle tone (51,82–85).

Ontogeny of β-Adrenoceptor Function

The ontogeny of β-adrenergic receptors in the developing lung has been extensively studied (86,87). Binding assays demonstrated that β-receptor density progressively increases as gestation advances and continues postnatally in the rabbit and rat (86). Localization studies have shown that β-receptors are present on vascular and airway smooth muscle in addition to the alveolar epithelia of the fetal and postnatal lung (86). The maturation of β-receptor expression in the lung is also under hormonal regulation and is precociously accelerated by glucocorticoids (86). The coupling of the β-receptor to adenylate cyclase and the generation of cAMP also undergoes changes with maturation. The levels of adenylate cyclase activity of lung cell membranes decreases with maturation while the response to β-agonist stimulation increases (86).

The majority of β-adrenoceptors in airway smooth muscle are the $\beta_2$ subtype (88). It has been demonstrated that β-adrenoceptor responsiveness and sensitivity in airway smooth muscle decreases with age (51,82,89,90). Evidence that ontogenic modification may occur at the receptor level has been provided (89), since forskolin, a direct stimulator of adenylate cyclase, did not show any modified effect as a function of age in rats. Several important pharmacological characteristics described for β-adrenoceptor function in airway smooth muscle may have clinical correlates: (1) airway smooth muscle is relatively more sensitive to β-adrenoceptor–mediated relaxation when contracted by inflammatory mediators such as histamine compared with contraction by muscarinic agents (88,91); (2) as bronchoconstriction becomes more intense, the bronchodilator efficacy of these agonists declines (88); (3) downregulation of lung β-adrenoceptors occurs in a guinea pig model of asthma (88), suggesting that hyperresponsive airways may be less sensitive to β-adrenoceptor–mediated agonists.

In elucidating mechanisms of airway smooth muscle relaxation, the considerable progress made in identifying the molecular basis for receptor/G-protein coupling and other regulatory processes leading to both activation and downregulation of the adenylate cyclase/cAMP system has been thoroughly reviewed by Schramm and Grunstein (78). However, there remains a sizable gap in our knowledge of the developmental aspects of airway smooth muscle second-messenger pathways.

### Other Agents

Agents acting via nonadrenergic mechanisms are also known to produce airway relaxation and may have potential therapeutic value. Drugs that stimulate increases in intracellular cGMP such as sodium nitroprusside and atrial natriuretic factor can relax airway smooth muscle (92–94). Preliminary studies have begun to determine the ontogenic pattern of cGMP-mediated airway relaxation (95). In addition, the recent interest in nitric oxide (96) has focused investigators' efforts in determining the role of nitric oxide in airway function (73,97).

Furosemide, a potent loop diuretic, has also been found to decrease airway hyperresponsiveness when inhaled in adults (98–101) and children (102) and to relax fetal and newborn airway tissue in vitro (103). In airways, in addition to having a direct, nonepithelial–dependent relaxant effect (103), furosemide appears to act via modulation of nonadrenergic, noncholinergic nerve activity (104,105). Thus, it is conceivable that the clinical benefit of systemically administered furosemide in improving pulmonary function in infants with chronic lung disease might be related in part to alterations in airway tone (106).

### Effect of the Airway Epithelium

The influence of airway epithelium in modulating airway responsiveness in adults has been the subject of intense investigation (107–109). However, the effect of epithelium removal has only been recently investigated in fetal and newborn guinea pigs (53) and pigs (110). In both studies, no evidence for an epithelial derived relaxing factor could be demonstrated. On the other hand, Panitch and co-workers (111) found agonist-selective modulation by the epithelium in preterm sheep. In addition, the magnitude of epithelial-dependent effects may be different during pathological conditions as the development of bronchiolar epithelium is attenuated during hyperoxic exposure (112). Epithelium-derived prostaglandin(s) also contributes to observed increases in maximal airway contractility in hyperoxic exposed immature rats (113). Finally, epithelial damage from mechanical ventilation may alter smooth muscle responsiveness in premature newborns (111).

### Influence of Structural Support of Airways on Smooth Muscle Function

Raeburn et al. (85) have found reduced smooth muscle reactivity to histamine and KCl in airway preparations devoid of cartilage. This finding, coupled with their observation that basal $^{45}Ca^{2+}$ uptake in guinea pig isolated trachealis muscle is reduced if cartilage is removed (114), has led to the suggestion that airway cartilage may supply $Ca^{2+}$ to the muscle for contraction. In addition, cartilage may be important in providing necessary structural support for airway smooth muscle contraction and underlying airway tone. Moreover, the importance of tracheal smooth muscle tone in maintaining normal newborn respiratory physiology has recently been emphasized (115,116). The immature airway is more compliant than adult airways and is less able to resist deformational changes with barotrauma (117). In preterm lambs, both tracheal rings as well as the cartilage alone are more compliant compared with adult sheep (118) and parallel developmental differences observed in tracheal pressure-flow characteristics (119). Detailed anatomical investigations during the third-trimester of gestation in sheep demonstrate progressive increases in tracheal ring and changes in the compositional characteristics of tracheal cartilage occur with maturation and provide evidence to explain why greater stiffness of the trachea is seen in older animals (120). These results have been extended to human infants, in whom the propensity toward airway collapse decreases with advancing gestational age (121). Finally, since preterm infants tend to increase extrathoracic airway (ETA) stability with increasing postnatal age rather than with postconceptional age, Duara et al. (121) suggests that extrauterine factors not yet determined promote ETA stability in otherwise healthy premature infants.

## IV. Relevance to Disease in the Premature and Newborn Infant

The main clinical manifestation of diseases affecting airway smooth muscle in infancy is airway obstruction. Premature and term newborns are predisposed to develop airway obstruction for several reasons, with the primary ones being anatomical. The diameter of a peripheral airway in an infant is approximately half that of a corresponding airway in an adult (122,123). Since resistance to airflow is inversely related to the airway radius to the fourth power, any narrowing of the airway lumen in an infant will be more likely to result in symptoms. In addition, the chest wall and cartilaginous support of the airways are more compliant in infants than in older children and adults. Furthermore, medical interventions used to treat lung disease in newborns (e.g., mechanical ventilation and supplemental oxygen) may injure the airways and contribute to airway obstruction (124). Premature infants also have increased bronchial smooth muscle for their postconceptual age and mechanical ventilation appears to further increase the smooth muscle area in the airway (125). Finally, asthma usually has its onset in childhood, often in infancy. These topics are discussed in detail below.

### A. Oxygen Toxicity

Studies examining the effects of hyperoxia on the newborn's lungs have concentrated on damage to the lung parenchyma and vasculature, with less consideration of functional changes that may also be occurring in the airways. Szarek (126) reported increased bronchial responsiveness to 5-hydroxytryptamine in hyperoxia-exposed adult rats. In young animals, Hershenson et al. (127) observed that chronic exposure to hyperoxia ($>95\%$ $O_2$ for 8 days) caused airway muscarinic hyperresponsiveness in the developing Sprague-Dawley rat in vivo. In these animals, increased airway thickening correlated with airway hyperresponsiveness, suggesting that airway remodeling may be responsible in part for the hyperresponsiveness. In addition, epithelial removal and treatment with indomethacin attenuated the hyperresponsiveness (113). Further work from this group found that remodeling and hyperresponsiveness are reversible (128). Newborn guinea pigs exposed to 85% $O_2$ for 48 hr were found to have increased airway smooth muscle contractility in vitro (57). Finally, preliminary data (129) suggest that relaxation responses may also be impaired after hyperoxic exposure.

However, a better understanding of the relationship between hyperoxic airway injury and prematurity is necessary since premature infants are much more likely to be exposed to high $O_2$ concentrations for prolonged periods. Recently, Sosenko and Frank found that preterm guinea pigs were less susceptible to hyperoxic-induced lung damage (130). In contrast, Kelly and co-workers (131) reported that preterm guinea pigs were more susceptible than term guinea pigs to lung injury after hyperoxic exposure. The guinea pig, with the capacity for premature survivability, may serve as a useful model to study effects of various interventions on immature lung function without the confounding presence of surfactant deficiency (130–132). However, further investigations are necessary using this or other species (133) specifically to determine the effect of hyperoxia on airway responsiveness in premature animals.

## B. Bronchopulmonary Dysplasia

The most common neonatal lung disease, neonatal respiratory distress syndrome (RDS), occurs less frequently in females (134), but in both males and females may be complicated by a form of unresolved lung injury referred to as bronchopulmonary dysplasia (BPD). In certain populations, BPD may occur in up to 68% of surviving very low birth weight infants (124). Further, treatment of RDS is believed to be partially responsible for the emergence of BPD by mechanisms such as oxygen toxicity and barotrauma. Exposure of the lung to increased concentrations of inspired oxygen is associated with adverse respiratory effects (127,135,136) and probably plays an important role as a complicating or intensifying factor in preventing normal growth and recovery of acute lung injury (124). RDS and BPD are the subjects of a chapter in this volume to which the reader is referred for a more detailed discussion.

BPD is characterized in part by increased airway hyperreactivity (137–141) and bronchodilators are frequently employed in the management of this condition (142). On postmortem examination, the lungs of infants with BPD commonly demonstrate tracheal muscle hyperplasia and bronchiolar smooth muscle hypertrophy (143,144). Neonates with BPD often show clinical improvement with bronchodilator therapy (142), and common stimuli, such as airway cooling, produce bronchoconstriction (145), a finding previously demonstrated in animals (146). Moreover, bronchodilators may improve pulmonary function in neonates with BPD (138–141). However, it is also known that airway smooth muscle sensitivity to the relaxant effects of β-adrenergic agonists depends importantly on the specific contractile agonist used to induce tone (58), suggesting that the pathophysiology of airway constriction is important in determining pharmacological therapy in induced relaxation. For example, airway smooth muscle is relatively sensitive to relaxant effects of β-adrenergic agonists when contracted by inflammatory mediators, such as histamine, compared with effects observed when contracted by muscarinic agonists (58). Since the inflammatory process has been implicated in the development of airway reactivity in BPD, one may speculate that β-adrenergic agonists may be of greater benefit if hyperresponsiveness is mediated by histamine rather than acetylcholine. Furthermore, this provides a rationale for the use of steroids to treat the chronic lung disease associated with BPD (147,148). In addition, increased muscarinic activation of airway smooth muscle in neonates with BPD (149) suggests that combining bronchodilator therapies with different mechanisms of action may enhance improvements in pulmonary function.

In contrast, large-airway collapse may also contribute to airway obstruction in BPD patients (150–152), and bronchodilators may worsen airway obstruction owing to large airway collapse (151). In addition, neonates with BPD are prone to episodes of acute hypoxemia which increase airway constriction (153,154). However, hypoxia causes reversible reductions in active tension of in vitro tracheal smooth muscle preparations (155–158). It is unclear whether these differences observed with in vivo and in vitro studies are related to the methodology used or to age-dependent effects, since hypoxic bronchodilation has been observed in adult patients (159). In any case, abnormal airway smooth muscle tone appears to play an essential role in the symptoms of BPD and consequently the importance of optimal tracheal smooth muscle tone on neonatal airway mechanics has been emphasized (115,116). Conversely, increases in tracheal smooth muscle tone may enhance airway rigidity and provide a protective mechanism against compression of the intrathoracic airway (115,116,151). Thus, the magnitude and sensitivity of contractile and relaxant responses to various stimuli may be important in determining pharmacological therapy to optimize airway smooth muscle tone in BPD.

Tracheobronchial pathology, including epithelial injury, has been reported in many conditions affecting the sick newborn, including BPD (124), asthma (58,107), assisted ventilation (160), virus-induced airway disease (161), and following nursing procedures such as endotracheal suctioning (162). Thus, it is important to understand the role of airway smooth muscle in postnatal lung growth and how alterations in airway smooth muscle in a sick neonate may contribute to the development of BPD (163).

### C. Development of Reversible Airway Obstruction in Early Childhood

The American Thoracic Society defines asthma as, "a disease characterized by an increased responsiveness of the trachea and bronchi to various stimuli and manifested by widespread narrowing of the airways that changes in severity either spontaneously or as a result of therapy." Asthma is a variable disease with complex pathology involving the airway lumen, epithelium, and submucosal glands in addition to airway smooth muscle. Multiple factors may contribute to bronchial smooth muscle hyperreactivity, including inflammation, alterations in the neural control of the airways, and smooth muscle hypertrophy (164). However, there is no conclusive evidence that a primary defect in airway smooth muscle causes asthma.

Several factors may contribute to the development of clinical asthma symptoms in infants and young children. Well-documented predisposing factors include heredity and prematurity, environmental factors such as air pollution and parental smoking, atopy, respiratory infections, and socioeconomic factors (165–172). A thorough review of these topics is beyond the scope of this chapter; however, the relationship between respiratory infections and asthma symptoms in infancy and childhood deserves particular comment.

Respiratory pathogens are the most common trigger of lower airway obstruction in infants and children, which is a pattern that contrasts with that of adults with asthma (172,173). Common agents include respiratory syncytial virus (RSV), parainfluenza, adenovirus, and rhinovirus (161,173–175). In a comprehensive, primary care–based study, Denny and colleagues reported that 30% of children with lower respiratory infections developed associated wheezing (174). Wheezing with respiratory infection was most likely to occur in children under the age of 2 years (174). The pathogens isolated from children with wheezing–associated respiratory infections varied with the child's age. RSV was the most commonly recovered virus in children less than 5 years old (174).

Viral infections may contribute to small airway obstruction by several mechanisms, including increased thickness of the airway wall, increased luminal contents, and airway smooth muscle contraction (161,173). Several lines of evidence point to inflammation as key factor in virus-induced bronchospasm in children. Welliver and colleagues found that children infected with RSV or parainfluenza who developed bronchiolitis or croup syndromes were more likely to secrete specific IgE antibodies in their nasal secretions (176–178). Infants with bronchiolitis and higher RSV IgE titers also had increased levels of histamine in nasal secretions and lower arterial oxygen concentrations (176). Interestingly, the infants who continued to have detectable levels of RSV IgE antibodies months after an episode of bronchiolitis had an increased incidence of recurrent wheezing episodes compared with those with no detectable antibodies (178). These findings, although correlative rather than causative, raise the interesting speculation that the development of virus-specific immunity and subsequent reexposure to the virus leads to the release of mediators and inflammation. These conditions may contribute to epithelial injury, airway obstruction, and airway hyperreactivity. There is also convincing evidence that infants may manifest bronchial hyperreactivity with bronchoprovocation maneuvers such as methacholine and histamine challenge or inhalation of cold, dry air (179). This suggests that nonspecific airway reactivity is present in some infants and may predate any lung injury or infection.

The incidence of reactive airway disease in cystic fibrosis (CF) is significantly increased over the general population and recalcitrant wheezing may occur in CF infants (180). Patients with CF commonly present in infancy or early childhood with respiratory symptoms from airway inflammation and infection and small airways obstruction. Furthermore, pulmonary inflammation and altered lung function may occur in infancy before the onset of clinical symptoms of respiratory disease or bacterial colonization (181–184). In two preliminary reports, pro-inflammatory cytokines were detected in the bronchoalveolar lavage fluid of CF infants and children in the absence of viral or bacterial infection (181,182). Thus, airway inflammation from a variety of causes may lead to airway obstruction, bronchospasm, and increased airway hyperreactivity in infants and children.

Respiratory infections also contribute to airway obstruction by increasing the luminal contents through alterations in mucociliary clearance, sloughing of epithelia, and alterations in mucous secretion (161). Viral infections can also cause airway smooth muscle contraction through several mechanisms, including exposure of irritant receptors, damage to the epithelium, inhibition of NANC bronchodilatory peptides, or induction of β-adrenergic hyporesponsiveness (161).

Whether there is a causal relationship between episodes of wheezing in children with respiratory infections and the development of recurrent asthma symptoms is controversial. Several investigators have presented evidence that children hospitalized with bronchiolitis have an increased incidence of airway hyperreactivity and recurrent asthma (185–187). Alternatively, Samet and co-workers found no conclusive evidence that respiratory infections in childhood altered normal lung development or predisposed children to recurrent episodes of wheezing (188). A prospective study by Martinez et al. studied the relationship between lung function before the first respiratory infection in infancy and later episodes of lower respiratory tract disease symptoms in the first year of life (189). They observed a significantly increased incidence of wheezing illnesses in infants whose values for total respiratory system conductance (the inverse of resistance) were in the lowest third. These findings from a large longitudinal study suggest that infants with preexisting lower values for respiratory conductance are at an increased risk for wheezing lower respiratory tract illness (189). In a follow-up to this study with longitudinal data from birth to age 6 years (190), Martinez et al. found that children with recurrent wheezing from early in life to age 6 years were more likely to have mothers with a history of asthma, persistently elevated serum IgE levels, and normal lung function in the first year of life but diminished lung function at age 6 years. In contrast, children with wheezing before age 3 years but not at age 6 years were more likely to have mothers who smoked, have normal IgE levels, and exhibit diminished lung function before age 1 year which persisted at 6 years.

## V. Areas for Future Research

Several areas for future investigation can be suggested. In order to understand the biology of smooth muscle development in the airways the transcription factors and genes regulating airway smooth muscle expression must be identified. Further investigations into the possible relationship between fetal airway smooth muscle contractility and normal lung development of the lung are needed. The ontogeny of the innervation of the human lung needs to be better defined. Emphasis on the genetic determinants of airway reactivity are needed to understand the pathophysiology of developmental airway disorders (191). Along these lines, animal models with genetically hyperresponsive airways have been described (192) and genetic manipulations to decrease lung injury in immature animals have been reported (193). Gene targeting techniques may be very useful in creating animals models to study the regulation of smooth muscle development (194).

## Acknowledgments

We thank Drs. John T. Fisher and Malcolm Sparrow for reviewing the chapter and offering critical commentary and for their willingness to share data. This work was supported in part by the NIH: HL-02767, the Roy J. Carver Foundation, the Children's Miracle Network Telethon (P.B.M.) and by NIH: HL-45220 (K.J.N.).

## References

1. Loosli CG, Hung K-S. Development of pulmonary innervation. In: Lenfant C, Hodson WA, eds. Development of the Lung. New York, N.Y.: Dekker, 1977: 269–306.
2. Leslie K, Mitchell J, Woodcock-Mitchell J, Low RB. Alpha smooth muscle actin expression in developing and adult human lung. Differentiation 1990; 44:143–149.
3. Langston C, Kida K, Reed M, Thurlbeck WM. Human lung growth in late gestation and in the neonate. Am Rev Respir Dis 1984; 129:607–613.
4. McCray PB, Jr. Spontaneous contractility of human fetal airway smooth muscle. Am J Respir Cell Mol Biol 1993; 8:573–580.
5. Sparrow MP, Warwick SP, Mitchell HW. Foetal airway motor tone in prenatal lung development of the pig. Eur Respir J 1994; 7:1416–1424.
6. Buckingham M. Molecular biology of muscle development. Cell 1994; 78:15–21. 7.
7. Stockdale FE. Myogenic cell lineages. Dev Biol 1992; 154:284–298.
8. Olson EN. MyoD family: a paradigm for development? Genes Dev 1990; 4:2104–2111.
9. Hirai Y, Takebe K, Takashina M, Kobayashi S, Takeichi M. Epimorphin: A mesenchymal protein essential for epithelial morphogenesis. Cell 1992; 69:471–481.
10. Minoo P, King RJ. Epithelial-mesenchymal interactions in lung development. Annu Rev Physiol 1994; 56:13–45.
11. Herman IM. Controlling the expression of smooth muscle contractile protein isoforms: a role for the extracellular matrix? Am J Respir Cell Mol Biol 1993; 9:3–4.
12. Woodcock-Mitchell J, White S, Stirewalt W, Periasamy M, Mitchell J, Low RB. Myosin isoform expression in developing and remodeling rat lung. Am J Respir Cell Mol Biol 1993; 8:617–625.

13. Desmouliere A, Geinoz A, Gabbiani F, Gabbiani G. Transforming growth factor b-1 induces a-smooth muscle actin expression in granulation tissue myofibroblasts and in quiescent and growing cultured fibroblasts. J Cell Biol 1993; 122:103–111.

14. Mitchell J, Reynolds S, O'Leslie K, Low RB, Woodcock-Mitchell J. Smooth muscle cell markers in developing rat lung. Am J Respir Cell Mol Biol 1990; 3:515–523.

15. Sawtell N, Lessard J. Cellular distribution of smooth muscle actins during mammalian embryogenesis: expression of the α-vascular but not the g-enteric isoform in differentiating striated myocytes. J Cell Biol 1989; 109(No. 6, Pt. 1):2929–2937.

16. McHugh KM, Crawford K, Lessard JL. A comprehensive analysis of the developmental and tissue-specific expresion of the isoactin multigene family in the rat. Dev Biol 1991; 148:442–458.

17. Roman J, McDonald JA. Expression of fibronectin, the integrin α5, and α smooth muscle actin in heart and lung development. Am J Respir Cell Mol Biol 1992; 6: 472–480.

18. Snyder JM, O'Brien JA, Rodgers HF. Localization and accumulation of fibronectin in rabbit fetal lung tissue. Differentiation 1987; 34:32–39.

19. Booth RJ, Sparrow MP, Mitchell HW. Early maturation of force production in pig tracheal smooth muscle during fetal development. Am J Respir Cell Mol Biol 1992; 7:590–597.

20. Gimona M, Sparrow MP, Strasser P, Herzog M, Small JV. Calponin and SM 22 isoforms in avian and mammalian smooth muscle. Eur J Biochem 1992; 205:1067–1075.

21. Emerson CP, Jr., Bernstein SI. Molecular genetics of myosin. Ann Rev Biochem 1987; 56:695–726.

22. Sweeney HL, Kushmerick MJ, Mabuchi K, Gergely J, Sreter FA. Velocity of shortening and myosin isozymes in two types of rabbit fast-twitch muscle fibers. Am J Physiol 1986; 251:C431–C434.

23. Sparrow MP, Mitchell HW. Contraction of smooth muscle of pig airway tissues from before birth to maturity. J Appl Physiol 1990; 68:468–477.

24. Mohammad MA, Sparrow MP. The distribution of heavy-chain isoforms of myosin in airways smooth muscle from adult and neonate humans. Biochem J 1989; 260: 421–426.

25. Lotvall J. Contractility of lungs and air-tubes: experiments performed in 1840 by Charles J.B. Williams. Eur Respir J 1994; 7:592–595.

26. Lewis MR. Spontaneous rhythmical contraction of the muscles of the bronchial tubes and air sacs of the chick embryo. Am J Physiol 1924; 68:385–388.

27. Schopper W. Embryonales und erwachsenes Lungengewebe vom Meerschweinchen und Huhn in der Kultur mit Zeitrafferbeobachtungen an Flimmerepithel, sog. Alveolarphagocyten und von Kontraktionen der Bronchialmuskulatur. Virchows Arch Pathol Anat Physiol 1935; 295:623–644.

28. Schopper W. Uber das Verhalten des Lungengewebes in der Gewebekultur (Filmdemonstration). Arch Exp Zellforsch 1937; 19:326–328.

29. Sollmann T, Gilbert AJ. Microscopic observations of bronchiolar reactions. J Pharmacol Exp Ther 1937; 61:272–285.

30. Sorokin S. A study of development in organ cultures of mammalian lungs. Dev Biol 1961; 3:60–83.

31. Davis C, Kannan MS, Jones TR, Daniel EE. Control of human airway smooth muscle: in vitro studies. J Appl Physiol 1982; 53:1080–1087.

32. Honda K, Tomita T. Electrical activity in isolated human tracheal muscle. Jpn J Physiol 1987; 37:333–336.

33. Small RC. Electrical slow waves and tone of guinea-pig isolated trachealis muscle: effects of drugs and temperature changes. Br J Pharmacol 1982; 77:45–54.

34. Weichselbaum M, Everett AW, Sparrow MP. Mapping the innervation of the bronchial tree in fetal and postnatal pig lung using antibodies to PGP 9.5 and SV2. Am J Respir Cell Moll Biol 1996; 15.

35. Kitterman JA. Physical factors and fetal lung growth. In: Johnston BM, Gluckman PD, eds. Reproductive and Perinatal Medicine (III). Respiratory Control and Lung Development in the Fetus and Newborn. Ithaca, NY: Perinatology Press, 1986: 64–85.

36. Alcorn D, Adamson TM, Lambert TF, Maloney JE, Ritchie BC, Robinison PM. Morphological effects of chronic tracheal ligation and drainage in the fetal lamb lung. J Anat 1977; 123:649–660.

37. Fewell JE, Hislop AA, Kitterman JA, Johnson P. Effect of tracheostomy on lung development in fetal lambs. J Appl Physiol 1983; 55:1103–1108.

38. McCray PB, Jr., Bettencourt JD, Bastacky J. Developing bronchopulmonary epithelium of the human fetus secretes fluid. Am J Physiol 1992; 262:L270–L279.

39. Vilos GA, Liggins GC. Intrathoracic pressures in fetal sheep. J Dev Physiol 1982; 4:247–256.

40. Harding R, Bocking AD, Sigger JN. Influence of upper respiratory tract on liquid flow to and from fetal lungs. J Appl Physiol 1986; 61:68–74.

41. Potter EL, Bohlender GP. Intrauterine respiration in relation to development of the fetal lung. Am J Obstet Gynecol 1941; 42:14–22.

42. Griscom NT, Harris GBC, Wohl MEB, Vawter GF, Eraklis AJ. Fluid-filled lung due to airway obstruction in the newborn. Pediatrics 1969; 43:383–390.

43. Harrison MR, Jester JA, Ross NA. Correction of congenital diaphragmatic hernia in utero. I. The model: intrathoracic balloon produces fatal pulmonary hypoplasia. Surgery 1980; 88:174–182.

44. Potter EL. Bilateral renal agenesis. J Pediatr 1946; 29:68–76.

45. Wirtz HR, Dobbs LG. Calcium mobilization and exocytosis after one mechanical stretch of lung epithelial cells. Science 1990; 250:1266–1269.

46. Sadoshima J-I, Jahn L, Takahashi T, Kulik TJ, Izumo S. Molecular characterization of the stretch-induced adaptation of cultured cardiac cells. J Biol Chem 1992; 267: 10551–10560.

47. Komuro I, Katoh Y, Kaida Y, et al. Mechanical loading stimulates cell hypertrophy and specific gene expression in cultured rat cardiac myocytes. J Biol Chem 1991; 266:1265–1268.

48. Skinner SJM, Somervell CE, Olson DM. The effects of mechanical stretching on fetal rat lung cell prostacyclin production. Prostaglandins 1992; 43:413–433.

49. Liu M, Skinner SJM, Xu J, Han RNN, Tanswell AK, Post M. Stimulation of fetal rat lung cell proliferation in vitro by mechanical stretch. Am J Physiol 1992; 263:L376–L383.

50. Fisher JT. Airway smooth muscle contraction at birth: in vivo versus in vitro comparisons to the adult. Can J Physiol Pharmacol 1992; 70:590–596.

51. Duncan PG, Douglas JS. Age-related changes in guinea pig respiratory tissues: considerations for assessment of bronchodilators. Eur J Pharmacol 1985; 108:39–48.

52. Murphy TM, Mitchell RW, Halayko A, et al. Effect of maturational changes in myosin content and morphometry on airway smooth muscle contraction. Am J Physiol 1991; 260:L471–L480.

53. Southgate WM, Pichoff BE, Stevens EL, Balaraman V, Uyehara CFT, Nakamura KT. Ontogeny of epithelial modulation of airway smooth muscle function in the guinea pig. Pediatr Pulmonol 1993; 15:105–110.

54. Pichoff BE, Uyehara CFT, Nakamura KT. Effect of calcium agonists, BAY K 8644 and CGP 28392, on guinea pig airway smooth muscle function during development. J Pharmacol Exp Ther 1993; 265:524–528.

55. Fayon M, Ben-Jebria A, Elleau C, et al. Human airway smooth muscle responsiveness in neonatal lung specimens. Am J Physiol 1994; 267:L180–L186.

56. Panitch HB, Allen JL, Ryan JP, Wolfson MR, Shaffer TH. A comparison of preterm and adult airway smooth muscle mechanics. J Appl Physiol 1989; 66:1760–1765.

57. Uyehara CFT, Pichoff BE, Sim HH, Nakamura KT. Hyperoxic exposure enhances airway reactivity of newborn guinea pigs. J Appl Physiol 1993; 74:2649–2654.

58. Leff AR. Endogenous regulation of bronchomotor tone. Am Rev Respir Dis 1988; 137:1198–1216.

59. Barnes PJ. Neural control of human airways in health and disease. Am Rev Respir Dis 1986; 134:1289–1314.

60. Kuratani S, Tanaka S. Peripheral development of the avian vagus nerve with special reference to the morphological innervation of heart and lung. Anat Embryol 1990; 182:435–445.

61. Stahlman MT, Kasselberg AG, Orth DN, Gray ME. Ontogeny of neuroendocrine cells in human fetal lung: II. An immunohistochemical study. Lab Invest 1985; 52:52–60.

62. Sheppard MN, Marangos PJ, Bloom SR, Polak JM. Neuron specific enolase: a marker for the early development of nerves and endocrine cells in the human lung. Life Sci 1984; 34:265–271.

63. Sunday ME, Kaplan LM, Motoyama E, Chin WW, Spindel ER. Gastrin-releasing peptide (mammalian bombesin) gene expression in health and disease. Lab Invest 1988; 59:5–24.

64. Said SI. Influence of neuropeptides on airway smooth muscle. Am Rev Respir Dis 1987; 136:S52–S58.

65. Impicciatore M, Bertaccini G. The bronchoconstrictor action of the tetradecapeptide bombesin in the guinea-pig. J Pharm Pharmacol 1973; 25:872–875.

66. Perez Fontan JJ, Kinlock LP. Control of bronchomotor tone during perinatal development in sheep. J Appl Physiol 1993; 75:1486–1496.

67. Perez Fontan JJ, Ray AO. Vagal control of central and peripheral pulmonary resistance in developing piglets. J Appl Physiol 1991; 70:1617–1626.

68. Fisher JT, Brundage KL, Waldron MA, Connelly BJ. Vagal cholinergic innervation of the airways in newborn cat and dog. J Appl Physiol 1990; 69:1525–1531.

69. Murphy TM, Mitchell RW, Blake JS, et al. Expression of airway contractile properties and acetylcholinesterase activity in swine. J Appl Physiol 1989; 67:174–180.

70. Mitchell RW, Murphy TM, Kelly E, Leff AR. Maturation of acetylcholinesterase expression in tracheal smooth muscle contraction. Am J Physiol 1990; 259:L130–L135.

71. Clerici C, MacQuin-Mavier I, Harf A. Nonadrenergic bronchodilation in adult and young guinea pigs. J Appl Physiol 1989; 67:1764–1769.

72. Waldron MA, Connelly BJ, Fisher JT. Nonadrenergic inhibitory innervation to the airways of the newborn cat. J Appl Physiol 1989; 66:1995–2000.

73. Gaston B, Drazen JM, Loscalzo J, Stamler JS. The biology of nitrogen oxides in the airways. Am J Respir Crit Care Med 1994; 149:538–551.

74. Tanaka DT, Grunstein MM. Maturation of neuromodulatory effect of substance P in rabbit airways. J Clin Invest 1990; 85:345–350.

75. Haxhiu-Poskurica B, Haxhiu MA, Kumar GK, Miller MJ, Martin RJ. Tracheal smooth muscle responses to substance P and neurokinin A in the piglet. J Appl Physiol 1992; 72:1090–1095.

76. Tokuyama K, Yokoyama T, Morikawa A, Mochizuki H, Kuroume T, Barnes PJ. Attenuation of tachykinin-induced airflow obstruction and microvascular leakage in immature airways. Br J Pharmacol 1993; 108:23–29.

77. Schramm CM, Chuang ST, Grunstein MM. Maturation of inositol 1,4,5-trisphosphate receptor binding in rabbit tracheal smooth muscle. Am J Physiol 1992; 263:L501–L505.

78. Schramm CM, Grunstein MM. Assessment of signal transduction mechanisms regulating airway smooth muscle contractility. Am J Physiol 1992; 262:L119–L139.

79. Lands AM, Arnold A, McAuliff JP, Luduena FP, Brown TG. Differentiation of receptor systems activated by sympathomimetic amines. Nature 1967; 214:597–598.

80. Lands AM, Luduena FP, Buzzo HJ. Differentiation of receptors responsive to isoproterenol. Life Sci 1967; 6:2241–2249.

81. Bulbring E, Tomita T. Catecholamine action on smooth muscle. Pharmacol Rev 1987; 39:49–96.

82. Brink C, Duncan PG, Midzenski M, Douglas JS. Response and sensitivity of female guinea-pig respiratory tissues to agonists during ontogenesis. J Pharmacol Exp Ther 1980; 215:426–433.

83. Mansour S, Daniel EE. Responsiveness of isolated tracheal smooth muscle from normal and sensitized guinea pigs. Can J Physiol Pharmacol 1987; 65:1942–1950.

84. Orehek J, Douglas JS, Bouhuys A. Contractile responses of the guinea-pig trachea in vitro: modification by prostaglandin synthesis-inhibiting drugs. J Pharmacol Exp Ther 1975; 194:554–564.

85. Raeburn D, Hay DWP, Farmer SG, Fedan JS. Influence of cartilage on reactivity and on the effectiveness of verapamil in guinea pig isolated airway smooth muscle. J Pharmacol Exp Ther 1987; 242:450–454.

86. Ballard PL. Hormones and Lung Maturation. Berlin, Heidelberg: Springer-Verlag, 1986:236–277.

87. Schell DN, Durham D, Murphree SS, Muntz KH, Shaul PW. Ontogeny of β-adrenergic receptors in pulmonary arterial smooth muscle, bronchial smooth muscle, and alveolar lining cells in the rat. Am J Respir Cell Mol Biol 1992; 7:317–324.

88. Townley RG, Agrawal DK. Adrenergic and chlinergic receptors and airway responsiveness. In: Agrawal DK, Townley RG, eds. Airway Smooth Muscle: Modulation of Receptors and Response. Boca Raton, FL: CRC Press, 1990:229–257.

89. Frossard N, Landry Y. Physiological approach of beta receptor coupling to adenylate cyclase in rat airways: ontogenical modification and functional antagonism. J Pharmacol Exp Ther 1985; 233:168–175.

90. Aberg G, Adler G, Ericsson E. The effect of age on betaβ-adrenoceptor activity in tracheal smooth muscle. Br J Pharmacol 1973; 47:181–182.

91. Madison JM, Brown JK. Differential inhibitory effects of forskolin, isoproterenol, and dibutyryl cyclic adenosine monophosphate on phosphoinositide hydrolysis in canine tracheal smooth muscle. J Clin Invest 1988; 82:1462–1465.

92. Ishii K, Murad F. ANP relaxes bovine tracheal smooth muscle and increases cGMP. Am J Physiol 1989; 256:C495–C500.

93. O'Donnell M, Garippa R, Welton AF. Relaxant activity of atriopeptins in isolated guinea pig airway and vascular smooth muscle. Peptides 1985; 6:597–601.

94. Watanabe H, Takagi K, Satake T. Relaxant effects of atrial natriuretic polypeptide on guinea pig tracheal smooth muscle. Prog Biochem Pharmacol 1988; 23:136–141.

95. Balaraman V, Kullama LK, Fujiwara N, Sato AK, Nakamura KT. Mechanisms of cGMP dependent relaxation to sodium nitroprusside and atriopeptin III in aorta of fetal and adult guinea pigs. Pediatr Res 1990; 27:56A.

96. Moncada S, Palmer RMJ, Higgs EA. Nitric oxide: Physiology, pathophysiology and pharmacology. Pharmacol Rev 1991; 43:109–142.

97. Dupuy PM, Shore SA, Drazen JM, Frostell C, Hill WA, Zapol WM. Bronchodilator action of inhaled nitric oxide in guinea pigs. J Clin Invest 1992; 90:421–428.

98. Bianco S, Vaghi A, Robuschi M, Pasargiklian M. Prevention of exercise-induced bronchoconstriction by inhaled frusemide. Lancet 1988; 2:252–255.

99. Bianco S, Pieroni MG, Refini RM, Rottoli L, Sestini P. Protective effect of inhaled furosemide on allergen-induced early and late asthmatic reactions. N Engl J Med 1989; 321:1069–1073.

100. Nichol GM, Alton EWFW, Nix A, Geddes DM, Chung KF, Barnes PJ. Effect of inhaled furosemide on metabisulfite- and methacholine-induced bronchoconstriction and nasal potential difference in asthmatic subjects. Am Rev Respir Dis 1990; 142:576–580.

101. Moscato G, Dellabianca A, Falagiani P, Mistrello G, Rossi G, Rampulla C. Inhaled furosemide prevents both the bronchoconstriction and the increase in neutrophil chemotactic activity induced by ultrasonic "fog" of distilled water in asthmatics. Am Rev Respir Dis 1991; 143:561–566.

102. Chin T, Franchi L, Nussbaum E. Reversal of bronchial obstruction in children with mild stable asthma by aerosolized furosemide. Pediatr Pulmonol 1994; 18:93–98.

103. Stevens EL, Uyehara CFT, Southgate WM, Nakamura KT. Furosemide differentially relaxes airway and vascular smooth muscle in fetal, newborn, and adult guinea pigs. Am Rev Respir Dis 1992; 146:1192–1197.

104. Elwood W, Lotvall JO, Barnes PJ, Chung KF. Loop diuretics inhibit cholinergic and noncholinergic nerves in guinea-pig airways. Am Rev Respir Dis 1991; 143:1340–1344.

105. Verleden GM, Pype JL, Demedts MG. Furosemide and bumetanide, but not nedocromil sodium, modulate nonadrenergic relaxation in guinea pig trachea in vitro. Am J Respir Crit Care Med 1994; 149:138–144.

106. Rush MG, Engelhardt B, Parker RA, Hazinski TA. Double-blind, placebo-controlled trial of alternate-day furosemide therapy in infants with chronic bronchopulmonary dysplasia. J Pediatr 1990; 117:112–118.

107. Fedan JS, Hay DWP, Farmer SG, Raeburn D. Epithelial cells: Modulation of airway smooth muscle reactivity. In: Barnes P, ed. Asthma: Basic Mechanisms and Clinical Management. Academic Press, 1988:143–162.

108. Goldie RG, Fernandes LB, Rigby PJ, Paterson JW. Epithelial dysfunction and airway hyperreactivity in asthma. In: Armour CL, Black JL, eds. Mechanisms in asthma: Pharmacology, Physiology, and Management. New York: Liss, 1988: 317–329.

109. Stuart-Smith K, Vanhoutte PM. Epithelium-derived relaxing factor. In: Agrawal DK, Townley RG, eds. Airway Smooth Muscle: Modulation of Receptors and Response. Boca Raton, FL: CRC Press, 1990:129–146.

110. Fisher JT, Gray PR, Mitchell HW, Sparrow MP. Epithelial modulation of neonatal and fetal porcine bronchial contractile responses. Am J Respir Crit Care Med 1994; 149:1304–1310.

111. Panitch HB, Wolfson MR, Shaffer TH. Epithelial modulation of preterm airway smooth muscle contraction. J Appl Physiol 1993; 74:1437–1443.

112. Massaro GD, McCoy L, Massaro D. Development of bronchiolar epithelium: time course of response to oxygen and recovery. Am J Physiol 1988; 254:R755–R760.

113. Hershenson MB, Wylam ME, Punjabi N, et al. Exposure of immature rats to hyperoxia increases tracheal smooth muscle stress generation in vitro. J Appl Physiol 1994; 76:743–749.

114. Raeburn D, Rodger IW. Lack of effect of leukotriene D4 on Ca-uptake in airway smooth muscle. Br J Pharmacol 1984; 83:499–504.

115. Bhutani VK, Koslo RJ, Shaffer TH. The effect of tracheal smooth muscle tone on neonatal airway collapsibility. Pediatr Res 1986; 20:492–495.

116. Koslo RJ, Bhutani VK, Shaffer TH. The role of tracheal smooth muscle contraction on neonatal tracheal mechanics. Pediatr Res 1986; 20:1216–1220.

117. Panitch HB, Allen JL, Ryan JP, Wolfson MR, Shaffer TH. A comparison of preterm and adult airway smooth muscle mechanics. J Appl Physiol 1989; 66:1760–1765.

118. Penn RB, Wolfson MR, Shaffer TH. Developmental differences in tracheal cartilage mechanics. Pediatr Res 1989; 26:429–433.

119. Penn RB, Wolfson MR, Shaffer TH. Effect of tracheal smooth muscle tone on collapsibility of immature airways. J Appl Physiol 1988; 65:863–869.

120. Deoras KS, Wolfson MR, Searls RL, Hilfer SR, Shaffer TH. Developmental changes in tracheal structure. Pediatr Res 1991; 30:170–175.

121. Duara S, Neto GS, Claure N, Gerhardt T, Bancalari E. Effect of maturation on the extrathoracic airway stability of infants. J Appl Physiol 1992; 73:2368–2372.

122. Whittenborg MH, Gyepes MT, Crocker D. Tracheal dynamics in infants with respiratory distress, stridor and collapsing trachea. Radiology 1967; 88:653–662.

123. Engel S. Lung Structure. Springfield, IL: Thomas, 1962.

124. O'Brodovich HM, Mellins RB. Bronchopulmonary dysplasia: unresolved neonatal acute lung injury. Am Rev Respir Dis 1985; 132:694–709.

125. Hislop AA, Haworth SG. Airway size and structure in the normal fetal and infant lung and the effect of premature delivery and artificial ventilation. Am Rev Respir Dis 1989; 140:1717–1726.

126. Szarek JL. In vivo exposure to hyperoxia increases airway responsiveness in rats. Am Rev Respir Dis 1989; 140:942–947.

127. Hershenson MB, Aghili S, Punjabi N, et al. Hyperoxia-induced airway hyperresponsiveness and remodeling in immature rats. Am J Physiol 1992; 262:L263–L269.

128. Hershenson MB, Abe MK, Kelleher MD, et al. Recovery of airway structure and function after hyperoxic exposure in immature rats. Am J Respir Crit Care Med 1994; 149:1663–1669.

129. Marinkovich GA, Pichoff BE, Iwamotto LM, Nakamura KT. Acute oxygen injury attenuates the relaxing effects of "loop" diuretics, furosemide and ethacrynic acid, on large airways of newborn guinea pigs. Clin Res 1993; 41:30A.

130. Sosenko IRS, Frank L. Guinea pig lung development: antioxidant enzymes and premature survival in high $O_2$. Am J Physiol 1987; 252:R693–R698.

131. Kelly FJ, Town GI, Phillips GJ, Holgate ST, Roche WR, Postle AD. The pre-term guinea-pig: a model for the study of neonatal lung disease. Clin Sci 1991; 81: 439–446.

132. Sosenko IRS, Frank L. Lung development in the fetal guinea pig: surfactant, morphology, and premature viability. Pediatr Res 1987; 21:427–431.

133. Chen Y, Whitney PL, Frank L. Comparative responses of premature *versus* full-term newborn rats to prolonged hyperoxia. Pediatr Res 1994; 35:233–237.

134. Bone CR, Higgins MW, Hurd SS, Reynolds HY. Research needs and opportunities related to respiratory health of women. Am Rev Respir Dis 1992; 146:528–535.

135. Frank L, Bucher JR, Roberts RJ. Oxygen toxicity in neonatal and adult animals of various species. J Appl Physiol 1978; 45:699–704.

136. Shaffer SG, O'Neill D, Bradt SK, Thibeault DW. Chronic vascular pulmonary dysplasia associated with neonatal hyperoxia exposure in the rat. Pediatr Res 1987; 21:14–20.

137. Motoyama EK, Fort MD, Klesh KW, Mutich RL, Guthrie RD. Early onset of airway reactivity in premature infants with bronchopulmonary dysplasia. Am Rev Respir Dis 1987; 136:50–57.

138. Kao LC, Warburton D, Platzker ACG, Keens TG. Effect of isoproterenol inhalation on airway resistancein chronic bronchopulmonary dysplasia. Pediatrics 1984; 73: 509–514.

139. Smyth JA, Tabachnik E, Duncan WJ, Reilly BJ, Levison H. Pulmonary function and bronchial hyperreactivity in long-term survivors of bronchopulmonary dysplasia. Pediatrics 1981; 68:336–340.

140. Sosulski R, Abbasi S, Bhutani VK, Fox WW. Physiologic effects of terbutaline on pulmonary function of infants with bronchopulmonary dysplasia. Pediatr Pulmonol 1986; 2:269–273.

141. Wilkie RA, Bryan MH. Effect of bronchodilators on airway resistance in ventilator-dependent neonates with chronic lung disease. J Pediatr 1987; 111:278–282.

142. Roberts RJ. Pharmacologic approaches to the prevention and treatment of bronchopulmonary dysplasia. Respir Care 1986; 31:581–590.

143. Margraf LR, Tomashefski JF,Jr., Bruce MC, Dahms BB. Morphometric analysis of the lung in bronchopulmonary dysplasia. Am Rev Respir Dis 1991; 143:391–400.

144. Stocker JT. Pathologic features of lung-standing "healed" bronchopulmonary dysplasia: a study of 28 3-40 month-old infants. Hum Pathol 1986; 17:943–961.

145. Greenspan JS, DeGiulio PA, Bhutani VK. Airway reactivity as determined by a cold air challenge in infants with bronchopulmonary dysplasia. J Pediatr 1989; 114: 452–454.

146. Bratton DL, Tanaka DT, Grunstein MM. Effects of temperature on cholinergic contractility of rabbit airway smooth muscle. J Appl Physiol 1987; 63:1933–1941.

147. Cummings JJ, D'Eugenio DB, Gross SJ. A controlled trial of dexamethasone in preterm infants at high risk for bronchopulmonary dysplasia. N Engl J Med 1989; 320:1505–1510.

148. Avery GB, Fletcher AB, Kaplan M, Brudno DS. Controlled trial of dexamethasone in respirator-dependent infants with bronchopulmonary dysplasia. Pediatrics 1985; 75:106–111.

149. Brundage KL, Mohsini KG, Froese AB, Fisher JT. Bronchodilator response to ipratropium bromide in infants with bronchopulmonary dysplasia. Am Rev Respir Dis 1990; 142:1137–1142.

150. McCoy KS, Bagwell CE, Wagner M, Sallent J, O'Keefe M, Kosch PC. Spirometric and endoscopic evaluation of airway collapse in infants with bronchopulmonary dysplasia. Pediatr Pulmonol 1992; 14:23–27.

151. McCubbin M, Frey EE, Tribby R, Smith WL. Large airway collapse in bronchopulmonary dysplasia. J Pediatr 1989; 114:304–307.

152. Sotomayor JL, Godinez RI, Borden S, Wilmott RW. Large-airway collapse due to acquired tracheobronchomalacia in infancy. Am J Dis Child 1986; 140:367–371.

153. Teague WG, Pian MS, Heldt GP, Tooley WH. An acute reduction in the fraction of inspired oxygen increased airway constriction in infants with chronic lung disease. Am Rev Respir Dis 1988; 137:861–865.

154. Tay-Uyboco JS, Kwiatkowski K, Cates DB, Kavanagh L, Rigatto H. Hypoxic airway constriction in infants of very low birth weight recovering from moderate to severe bronchopulmonary dysplasia. J Pediatr 1989; 115:456–459.

155. Stephens NL, Meyers JL, Cherniack RM. Oxygen, carbon dioxide, $H^+$ ion and bronchial length-tension relationships. J Appl Physiol 1968; 25:376–383.

156. Stephens NL, Kroeger E. Effect of hypoxia on airway smooth muscle mechanics and physiology. J Appl Physiol 1970; 28:630–635.

157. Stephens NL, Chui BS. Mechanical properties of tracheal smooth muscle and effects of $O_2$, $CO_2$, and pH. Am J Physiol 1970; 219:1001–1008.

158. Fernandes LB, Stuart-Smith K, Croxton TL, Hirshman CA. Role of $CA^{2+}$ entry in the modulation of airway tone by hypoxia. Am J Physiol 1993; 264:L284–L289.

159. Dinh L, Maltais F, Series F. Influence of progressive and of transient hypoxia on upper airway resistance in normal humans. Am Rev Respir Dis 1991; 143:1312–1316.

160. Polak MJ, Donnelly WH, Bucciarelli RL. Comparison of airway pathologic lesions after high-frequency jet or conventional ventilation. Am J Dis Child 1989; 143: 228–232.

161. Smith JJ, Lemen RJ, Taussig LM. Mechanisms of viral-induced lower airway obstruction. Pediatr Infect Dis J 1987; 6:837–842.

162. Bailey C, Kattwinkel J, Teja K, Buckley T. Shallow versus deep endotracheal suctioning in young rabbits: pathologic effects on the tracheobronchial wall. Pediatrics 1988; 82:746–751.

163. Motoyama EK, Brody JS, Colten HR, Warshaw JB. Postnatal lung development in health and disease. Am Rev Respir Dis 1988; 137:742–746.

164. Busse WW, Reed CE. Asthma: Definition and pathogenesis. In: Middleton E Jr, Reed CE, Ellis EF, Adenson NF Jr, Yunginger JW, Busse WW, eds. Allergy Principles and Practice. St. Louis: Mosby-Year Book, 1993:1173–1201.

165. Weitzman M, Gortmaker S, Sobol A. Racial, social, and environmental risks for childhood asthma. Am J Dis Child 1990; 144:1189–1194.

166. Weitzman M, Gortmaker SL, Sobol AM, Perrin JM. Recent trends in the prevalence and severity of childhood asthma. JAMA 1992; 268:2673–2677.

167. Taylor WR, Newacheck PW. Impact of childhood asthma on health. Pediatrics 1992; 90:657–662.

168. Young S, LeSouef PN, Geelhoed GC, et al. The influence of a family history of asthma and parental smoking on airway responsiveness in early infancy. N Engl J Med 1991; 324:1168–1174.

169. Clifford RD, Pugsley A, Radford M, Holgate ST. Symptoms, atopy, and bronchial response to methacholine in parents with asthma and their children. Arch Dis Child 1987; 62:66–73.

170. Sibbald B, Horn MEC, Gregg I. A family study of genetic basis of asthma and wheezy bronchitis. Arch Dis Child 1980; 55:354–357.

171. Horwood LJ, Fergusson DM, Hons BA, Shannon FT. Social and familial factors in the development of early childhood asthma. Pediatrics 1985; 75:859–868.

172. Ellis EF. Asthma in infancy and childhood. In: Middleton E Jr, Reed CE, Ellis EF, Adkinson NF Jr, Yunginger JW, Busse WW, eds. Allergy Priniciples and Practice. St. Louis: Mosby-Year Book, 1993:1225–1262.

173. Busse WW. Respiratory infections: Their role in airway responsiveness and the pathogenesis of asthma. J Allergy Clin Immunol 1990; 85:671–683.

174. Henderson FW, Clyde WA,Jr., Collier AM, et al. The etiology and epidemiologic spectrum of bronchiolitis in pediatric practice. J Pediatr 1979; 95:183–190.

175. McIntosh K, Ellis EF, Hoffman LS, Lybass GT, Eller JJ, Fulginiti VA. The association of viral and bacterial respiratory infections with exacerbations of wheezing in young asthmatic children. J Pediatr 1973; 82:578.

176. Welliver RC, Wong DT, Sun M. The development of respiratory syncytial virus specific IgE and the release of histamine in nasopharyngeal secretions after infection. N Engl J Med 1981; 305:841.

177. Welliver RC, Wong DT, Middleton E,Jr.. Role of parainfluenza virus-specific IgE in pathogenesis of croup and wheezing subsequent to infection. J Pediatr 1979; 94:370.

178. Welliver RC, Sun M, Rinaldo D. Predictive value of respiratory syncytial virus-specific IgE responses for recurrent wheezing following bronchiolitis. J Pediatr 1986; 109:776.

179. Morgan WJ, Geller DE, Tepper RS, Taussig LM. Partial expiratory flow-volume curves in infants and young children. Pediatr Pulmonol 1988; 5:232–243.

180. Kerem E, Reisman J, Corey M, Bentur L, Canny G, Levison H. Wheezing in infants with cystic fibrosis: clinical course, pulmonary function, and survival analysis. Pediatrics 1992; 90:703–706.

181. Balough K, McCubbin M, Weinberger M, Smits W, Ahrens R, Fick R. The relationship between infection and inflammation in the early stages of lung disease from cystic fibrosis. Pediatr Pulmonol 1995; 20:63–70.

182. Khan TZ, Wagener JS, Bost T, Martinez J, Accurso FJ, Riches DWH. Early pulmonary inflammation in infants with cystic fibrosis. Am J Respir Crit Care Med 1995; 151:1075–1082.

183. Ackerman V, Montgomery G, Eigen H, Tepper RS. Assessment of airway responsiveness in infants with cystic fibrosis. Am Rev Respir Dis 1991; 144:344–346.

184. Hiatt P, Eigen H, Yu P, Tepper RS. Bronchodilator responsiveness in infants and young children with cystic fibrosis. Am Rev Respir Dis 1988; 137:119–122.

185. Zweiman B, Schoenwetter WF, Pappano JE. Patterns of allergic respiratory disease in children with a past history of bronchiolitis. J Allergy 1971; 48:283.

186. Gurwitz D, Mindorff C, Levison H. Increased incidence of bronchial reactivity in children with a history of bronchiolitis. J Pediatr 1981; 98:551–555.

187. Rooney JC, Williams HE. The relationship between proven viral bronchiolitis and subsequent wheezing. J Pediatr 1971; 79:744–747.

188. Samet JM, Tager IB, Speizer FE. The relationship between respiratory illness in childhood and chronic airflow obstruction in adulthood. Am Rev Respir Dis 1983; 127:508.

189. Martinez FD, Morgan WJ, Wright AL. Diminished lung function as a predisposing factor for wheezing respiratory illness in infants. N Engl J Med 1988; 319:1112.

190. Martinez FD, Wright AL, Taussig LM, et al. Asthma and wheezing in the first six years of life. N Engl J Med 1995; 332:133–138.

191. Wanner A, Abraham WM, Douglas JS, Drazen JM, Richerson HB, Sri Ram J. Models of airway hyperresponsiveness. Am Rev Respir Dis 1990; 141:253–257.

192. Levitt RC, Mitzner W, Kleeberger SR. A genetic approach to the study of lung physiology: Understanding biological variability in airway responsiveness. Am J Physiol 1990; 258:L157–L164.

193. Wispe JR, Warner BB, Clark JC, et al. Human Mn-superoxide dismutase in pulmonary epithelial cells of transgenic mice confers protection from oxygen injury. J Biol Chem 1992; 267:23937–23941.

194. Ho Y. Transgenic models for the study of lung biology and disease. Am J Physiol 1994; 266:L319–L352.

# 11

## Laminin in Lung Development

**LUCIA SCHUGER**

Wayne State University School of Medicine
Detroit, Michigan

## I. Introduction

Laminins are essential components of basement membranes and are widely expressed in the animal kingdom. This family of glycoproteins consists of trimeric isoforms linked together by disulfide bonds. Laminins play important roles in cell adhesion, proliferation, and differentiation. These biological activities are mediated by several functional domains and for some of them structure-function correlations have been established. Increasing evidence indicates that laminin is involved in numerous and important morphogenic events taking place during development. This chapter discusses the role of laminin in mouse lung organogenesis. Some of the studies presented herein represent our effort to understand how relatively simple cell behaviors result in a complex lung tissue structure. We are aware that our knowledge covers only a small part of the whole, and we believe that additional laminin-related mechanisms contributing to lung development will be elucidated in the incoming years.

## II. Molecular Structure of Laminin

Laminins are composed of three polypeptide chains originally referred to as A (400 kDa), B1 (200 kDa), and B2 (220 kDa) chains, when have been recently renamed $\alpha$, $\beta$, and $\gamma$, respectively, followed by an arabic numeral to identify the isoform (1). The first laminin identified, from the Engelbreth-Holm-Shwarin (EHS) tumor (2), is now referred as laminin-I with the chain composition $\alpha1\beta1\gamma1$. The genes for these chains have been cloned and sequenced (3–5) and are referred as LAMA1, LAMB1, and LAMC1, respectively. Electron microscopy of EHS laminin reveals a cruciform structure with three short arms and one long arm (6). The three similar short arms (domains III–VI) are contributed by the N-terminal regions of the $\alpha1$, $\beta1$ and, $\gamma1$ chains whereas the long arm (domains I, II) is formed by the three chains associated over a considerable length (Fig. 1). Structural elements characteristic of the short arms are multiple EGF-like repeats of about 60 residues each. These repeats are terminated or interrupted by seven globular domains of about 200 residues. The N-terminal globules are homologous. Several internal globules correspond to large loops inserted into an EGF-like repeat. At the center of the cross, all three chains are linked by three disulfide bonds. The sequences then continue for about 600 residues in the $\alpha$-helical domains I and II. The $\beta1$ and $\gamma1$ chains terminate at domain I and are connected by a disulfide bridge. The $\alpha1$ chain continues for about 1000 residues, which are folded into five homologous 150- to 180-residue G motifs (see Fig. 1). Although most biochemical and structural work was performed with the EHS laminin, this laminin is not a tumor-specific variant but is widely distributed as a major glycoprotein in basement membranes of the mouse, and closely related laminins have been found in other species.

Crucial evidence for the existence of isoforms of laminin chains different from those found in the EHS tumor came from CDNA sequencing (7–9) as well as from biosynthetic and biochemical data indicating different assembly forms and different tissue distributions (1,10,11). At present, eight different laminin chains and seven different heterotrimeric assembly forms have been identified (Table 1) (1). They include the $\alpha1$, $\alpha2$, and $\alpha3$ chains; the $\beta1$, $\beta2$, and $\beta3$ chains; and the $\gamma1$ and $\gamma2$ chains. Only heterotrimeric assembly forms including one of each of the three classes of chains have been identified. As shown, by electron microscopy and in part by sequence analysis, laminin-2, laminin-3, and laminin-4 have a very similar domain structure. The $\alpha3$, $\beta3$, and $\gamma2$ chains, however, have a number of deletions in the short arms but apparently maintain a long $\alpha$-helical domain and, in

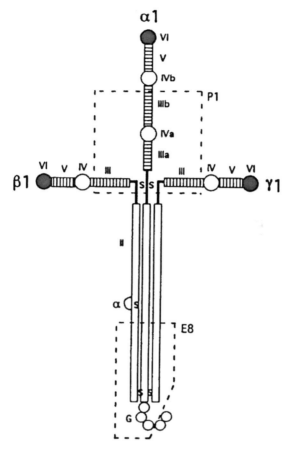

**Figure 1** Structural model of laminin-1. The three chains α1, β1, and γ1 are linked by disulfide bonds. Designation of sequence regions by roman numerals and G1–5 is according to Sasaki and Yamada (4). The positions of two functionally active proteolytic fragments (E8 and P1) are depicted. EGF-like repeats are indicated by lined boxes. Equal hatching of the globular domains represents homology. Open boxes mark α-helical domains. The C-terminal globular domains G1–5 are represented by small circles.

**Table 1**   New Nomenclaature for Established
Heterotrimeric Assembly Forms of Laminins[a]

| New name | Chain composition | Previous name |
|---|---|---|
| Laminin-1 | $\alpha1\beta1\gamma1$ | EHS laminin |
| Laminin-2 | $\alpha2\beta1\gamma1$ | Merosin |
| Laminin-3 | $\alpha1\beta2\gamma1$ | s-Laminin |
| Laminin-4 | $\alpha2\beta2\gamma1$ | s-Merosin |
| Laminin 5 | $\alpha3\beta3\gamma2$ | Kalinin/nicein |
| Laminin-6[b] | $\alpha3\beta1\gamma1$ | k-Laminin |
| Laminin-7[b] | $\alpha3\beta2\gamma1$ | ks-Laminin |

[a]According to Buergson et al. (1).
[b]The identity of the $\alpha3$ chain with that of laminin-5 has not
yet been completely established.

$\alpha3$, a G domain. This pattern strongly suggests that the $\alpha$-helical domain is essential for chain assembly and is thus a hallmark of laminin structure.

### III.   Biosynthesis and Glycosylation

Laminin chains are assembled in the rough endoplasmic reticulum (12,13) and then glycosylated within the Golgi apparatus prior to secretion (13,14). Variant chains are produced in the same organism or by the same cells (15,16). Although noncoordinated synthesis (17–19) and differences in the steady-state levels of mRNA (20,21) for each of the laminin chains have been observed, there is increasing evidence that only certain chain combinations are possible (22). Several investigators (13,15) found that laminins are secreted into the medium only after addition of the $\alpha$ chain.

Seventy-four potential N-glycosylation sites in laminin-1 are unevenly distributed between chains and are concentrated in the long arm. Forty possible acceptor sites are occupied by a variety of oligosaccharides (23–25). Glycosylation has been estimated in 25–30% (w/w) (25,26). A functional role for glycosylation of laminin was reported in tumor cell adhesion, cell spreading, neurite outgrowth (26–29), and integrin-laminin interaction (30). Glycosylation apparently does not influence chain assembly (31), heparin binding, and stability against proteases (32).

### IV.   Functions of Laminin

Laminins are large macromolecules with many structural domains; therefore it is not surprising that many if not all of the laminin functions are assigned to individual laminin domains. The evidence for such a site-function correlation has been provided by studying the biological activity of laminin proteolytic fragments, synthetic peptides reproducing laminin sequences, and site-specific antibodies. Laminin interacts with extracellular matrix and with cells. In vivo, these two types of interactions are closely related for laminin acts on cells as part of a supramolecular organization, which in turn is dependent on cellular interactions.

### A. Assembly Functions: Interaction with Other Extracellular Matrix Molecules

Because of their multidomain structure, laminins provide many interaction sites for other extracellular matrix/basement membrane–related constituents. In vitro, laminin can self-assemble into oligomers and large networks in the presence of $Ca^{2+}$ (33). This property of laminin has recently been attributed to the three VI globular domains at the N-termini of the short arms (34). $Ca^{2+}$ binding sites have been identified by these studies at the short arm structures (34,35). Laminin self-assembly into a polymer is considered to be fundamental to the supramolecular organization of basement membranes in vivo.

Laminin-1 interacts with entactin/nidogen with a high affinity ($K_d$ 1 nM) (36). This interaction is not calcium dependent (37). Electron microscopy showed that entactin binds to laminin at one of the short arms in a 1:1 stoichiometry. The entactin binding site was recently assigned to the fourth EGF-like repeat of domain III in the $\gamma$1 chain (38). Entactin also binds to type IV collagen, the other major component of basement membranes besides laminin, and therefore it has been proposed to link between the laminin and collagen type IV networks (36). Direct interactions between collagen IV and laminin do take place also (33).

Heparan sulfate proteoglycans (HSPGs) are additional important constituents of basement membranes. Laminin may interact with the heparan sulfate chains of proteoglycans via several heparin binding sites, one of them located in the G domain of the $\alpha$1 chain (39,40) and the other two in the inner and outer globular regions of the $\beta$1 chains (40,41). Through these sites, laminin may bind to the HSPG present on the cell surface (42,43).

Based on extensive studies, Yurchenco and Cheng (34) proposed a three-arm interaction model for the in vitro polymerization of laminin into a network similar to those found in basement membranes. In this model, the central nucleus of laminin polymerization is formed by the joining of an $\alpha$ short arm to both a $\beta$ short arm and a $\gamma$ short arm. Laminin monomers could thus bind to each other in a plantar array. The three-arm interaction model further suggests that the more flexible long arm of each monomer would be free to interact with cells or heparin/heparan sulfates out of the plane of the polymer. Since some cells preferentially recognize the end of long arms, these arms would be free to interact with them. It should be noted however that laminins that possess a truncated α chain (laminin-7) and laminins that lack the outer globular regions, such as laminin-5, would be unlikely to polymerize by this model mechanism.

### B. Interactions with Cellular Receptors

Cell binding to laminin occurs via a variety of cellular receptors, including integrins and nonintegrins receptors (44). At least six different integrins have been identified which bind to different laminins. Among them, the α6β1 integrin seems to be the major receptor for laminin-1 (45) and promotes cell adhesion and spreading by binding to the G region of the α chain (46). A similar specificity was found for the α7β1 integrin, which shows a more restricted expression in cells and tissues (44). Recent studies with recombinant fragments demonstrated that full activity of the binding site in the G domain requires stabilization by a portion of the long arm coiled coil (47).

Murine laminin-1 fragment P1 (see Fig. 1) is also a strongly cell-adhesive substrate (46) owing to exposure of a cryptic RCID site. However, this RGD is not conserved in the human laminin α chain, which possesses another RGD site in the G domain, the latter seems not to be recognized by RGD-dependent integrins (48). Whether such cryptic cell binding sites of laminin become functional during tissue remodeling and invasion remains to be shown.

Among the nonintegrin laminin binding proteins, a 67-kDa cell surface protein appears to be a high-affinity receptor (49–51) which is expressed in increased levels in many malignant tumors (52). The dystrophin-dystroglycan complex is another nonintegrin laminin receptor and connects laminin to the actin filaments of muscle cells (53).

### C. Major Biological Activities

The most critical and generalized function of laminin is to mediate cell adhesion (54). This function is accomplished by its interaction with cell receptors and surface "glycocalix," on one hand, and with itself and other extracellular matrix molecules on the other. Besides this fundamental function, laminin has been shown to possess mitogenic activity, which is localized in areas of EGF-like repeats and is independent of cell attachment (55). Chemotaxis, tumor metastasis induction (56), and triggering of various intracellular signal transduction pathways (57) are additional functions mediated by this molecule. The binding of cells to laminin has dramatic effects on cell phenotype (58); however, this effect is more permissive than instructive. In other words, laminin is required for the expression and maintenance of the full phenotype, but there is no evidence that laminin actually directs the process of cell differentiation toward one lineage or another. Laminin is known to play a role in the development of the peripheral nervous system (59–61), the kidney (62–64), and the lung (65–72).

## V. Laminin Expression in the Mouse Developing Lung

Laminins are expressed in the mouse embryo as early as the two-cell stage and subsequently are present in all newly formed basement membranes (18,31). In the developing lung, mRNA for all three laminin-1 chains is widely detected in epithelial and mesenchymal cells, and the steady-state levels gradually increase from early organogenesis onward (68,73). A predominance of β1 chain mRNA is observed through development and is maintained in the adult lung. Predominance of a particular chain mRNA is also found in other organs. Thus the liver and heart are characterized by an abundance of γ chains (20), whereas the lung and kidney express mainly β chains (20,63,64,74).

Lung epithelial and mesenchymal cell monocultures synthesize laminin α1 and β1/γ1 polypeptide chains as shown by sodium dodecyl sulfate polyacryl-amide gel electrophoresis and enzyme linked immunosorbent assays (68). A similar epithelial and mesenchymal dual origin of laminin was demonstrated in other developing tissues (75), suggesting that laminin is produced by cells at both sides of the basement membrane. This concept departs from the original belief that the basement membrane is wholly a product of epithelial cells. It is, however, unclear whether mesenchymal laminin is completely targeted to the basement membrane or if some laminin remains in the mesenchyme and serves local functions there. The latter possibility is supported by the immunodetection of laminin in the mesenchymal extracellular matrix using certain site-specific antilaminin antibodies (66).

## VI. Laminin Role in the Mouse Developing Lung

### A. Laminin in Lung Branching Morphogenesis

Evidence for a laminin role in lung branching morphogenesis derives from functional studies employing blocking antibodies, proteolytic fragments, and synthetic peptides. In an initial study (65), we determined whether exposure of lung explants to antibodies against major basement membrane constituents could affect in vitro morphogenesis. For these experiments, right lower lobes of lungs removed from day 12 embryos were placed in filter membrane assemblies. The explants were then cultured at the liquid-air interface for several days in the presence of antibodies to laminin, thrombospondin, entactin/nidogen, or preimmune serum, laminin-neutralized antilaminin antibody, or medium alone. Branching development was monitored daily. An initial concern regarding this experimental approach was whether antibodies could penetrate the lung explants. However, antibody localization studies (65) demonstrated that all the antibodies penetrated the explants and localized at the basement membrane site. Only the antilaminin antibody produced alterations in lung morphogenesis. These alterations consisted of a decrease in explant size, a marked inhibition of branching morphogenesis, and a distortion of the bronchial tree. The severity of these abnormalities was directly proportional to the concentration of the antibody in the culture medium (Table 2).

Additional functional studies employing site-specific monoclonal antibodies to laminin (termed AL-1, AL-2, AL-3, AL-4, and AL-5) (76,77) (Fig. 2) strongly suggest that the activity of laminin in the lung is localized to distinct domains. These laminin sites are the α chain at the center of the cross and the globular segments of the β and or γ chain(s) (domains IV, V, VI) blocked by antibodies AL-1 and AL-5, respectively (67). As in the previous study, explants exposed to each of these antibodies are smaller than controls and present a decrease in the total number of mitotic figures. Those explants exposed to antibody AL-5 exhibit severe alterations in the pattern of branching, a rather uncommon finding in the explants exposed to antibody AL-1, suggesting that the two are blocking different laminin functions (Fig. 3).

It should be noted that the epitopes for antibodies AL-1, AL-2, and AL-3 partially overlap; however, only AL-1 inhibits branching activity. This difference in effect may reflect differences in antibodies' affinity for a common epitope or alternatively; it may point to a relatively small epitope blocked only by antibody AL-1. If activity is dependent on a few amino acids, then blocking of this pinpoint sequence must occur to obtain an effect. Studies using synthetic peptides support this hypothesis.

Based on these observations, we have proposed that the α chain at the cross intersection and the globular domains of β/γ chains (domains IV, V, and VI) are

**Table 2**  Effects of Various Treatments on Branching Morphogenesis

| Treatment | N-Terminal buds | Inhibition/total[a] |
|---|---|---|
| None | 65 ± 15 | 0/18 |
| Normal rabbit serum | | |
| 1:10 dilution | 60 ± 10 | 2/16 |
| Antilaminin | | |
| 1:10 dilution | 30 ± 6 | 14/14 |
| 1:50 dilution | 34 ± 8 | 3/4 |
| Laminin-neutralized antilaminin | 62 ± 15 | 0/3 |
| Antithrombospondin | | |
| 100 μg/ml | 70 ± 18 | 0/3 |
| 500 μg/ml | 68 ± 12 | 0/3 |

Data are expressed as mean ± standard deviation.
[a]Number of experiments in which an inhibition of branching was observed/total number of experiments.

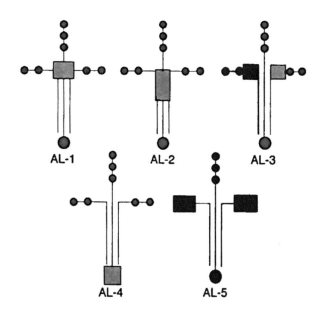

**Figure 2** Diagrammatic model of the monoclonal antibody binding sites on laminin (76,77). AL-1 to AL-5, were generated against murine EHS laminin by immunization of male LOU/MNCr rats. All of the monoclonal antibodies are of the IgG class except AL-5, which is an IgM. The preparation, purification, and characterization of these antibodies have been previously described (76,77). Each monoclonal antibody reacted with laminin by solid-phase radioimmunoassay and immunoprecipitation, and did not cross react with type IV collagen, thrombospondin, or fibronectin in an enzyme-linked immunosorbent assay. The regions on laminin to which each antibody binds were determined by immunoblotting in combination with rotary shadowing and electron microscopy. Monoclonal antibody AL-1 recognizes the α chain in immunoblots and binds to the cross region of laminin. Monoclonal antibody AL-2 recognizes α and β/γ chains and binds to the long arm of the molecule near the cross region. Monoclonal antibody AL-3 recognizes β/γ chains and binds to the inner rod segment of these chains. Monoclonal antibody AL-4 recognizes α chain and binds to the carboxyl end of the α chain. Monoclonal antibody AL-5 binds to the globular segments of the lateral short arms.

selectively involved in controlling morphogenesis. However, the previous studies did not address the question of how this control is exerted.

## B.  Laminin in Organotypic Pattern Formation

The role of laminin in establishing and maintaining tissue structure is supported by the ability of the glycoprotein to promote epithelial and mesenchymal cell sorting into different compartments when these cells are cocultured in an organotypic

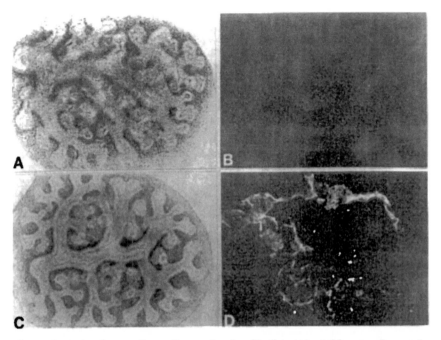

**Figure 3**   Left column: effects of monoclonal antibodies on branching morphogenesis.
Lung organ cultures were established on day 0 and incubated for 2 days in the presence of
100 μg/ml of normal rat IgG (A), antibody AL-3 (C), antibody AL-1 (E), or antibody AL-5
(G). Normal branching morphogenesis occurred in the explants exposed to IgG (A) and
AL-3 (C). Inhibition in branching activity is evident in the cultures exposed to AL-1 (E) and
AL-5 (G). Right column: Assessment of antibody penetration into the explant during organ
culture treatment. No immunoglobulin is bound to the tissue when explants are cultured in
the presence of normal rat IgG (B). When explants are cultured in the presence of AL-3 (D)
or AL-1 (F), the antibodies penetrate the tissue and bind to the basement membrane. AL-5
reacts with clusters of cells close to the basement membrane (H). Scale bars 100 μm.

system. Organotypic pattern formation is an in vitro phenomenon that results from
the ability of mixed cell populations from a certain organ to reaggregate in culture
and mimic their tissue of origin. Although this a pure in vitro phenomenon, it is the
result of normal cell behaviors occurring during embryogenesis. Cell movement/
motility, aggregation, sorting into epithelial and mesenchymal compartments, and
eventual polarization take place in this unique experimental system. Morphogenic
cell-cell and cell-matrix interactions can then be promoted, blocked, or manipulated to elucidate the mechanisms that govern them.

    Embryonic lung cells (early organogenesis, days 11–12 of gestation) reag-
gregate organotypically only if plated on basement membrane extracts rich in

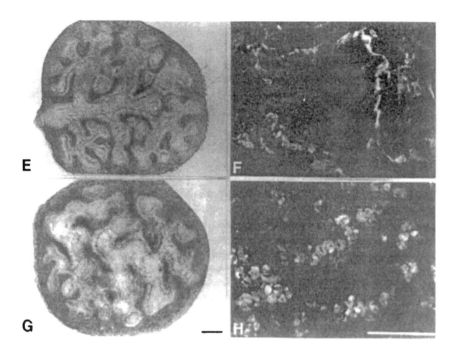

laminin such as Matrigel (Fig. 4) or on pure laminin gels (66). This effect is abolished by antilaminin antibodies in a dose-dependent manner. In contrast, epithelial and mesenchymal cells obtained from fetal lungs (late organogenesis, days 15–16 of gestation) which produce approximately 10-fold more laminin than embryonic cells rearrange in organotypic patterns spontaneously. Spontaneous rearrangement is blocked by antilaminin but not by antifibronectin antibodies (68). These observations suggest a direct correlation between laminin synthesis and the ability of the cells to establish and maintain a normal tissue structure.

Cell sorting requires an obligatory step of cell-cell recognition in which a cell identifies another as similar or different and, based on this information, establishes the proper relationship with it. Whether the effect of laminin in cell-cell recognition is indirect by facilitating cell motion or adhesion and thereby enhancing effective cell-cell contact or whether the molecule has a more direct role in this process is unclear. An attractive hypothesis is that epithelial cells recognize certain laminin domains, whereas mesenchymal cells interact with others. Laminin could then promote cell sorting as well as preserve epithelial-mesenchymal boundaries in the organ by adopting a critical orientation between the two cell types or within the basement membrane. This orientation could be such that it allows exposure of the proper domains at each side of the basement membrane. The histologically observed proximity of the laminin long arm to the

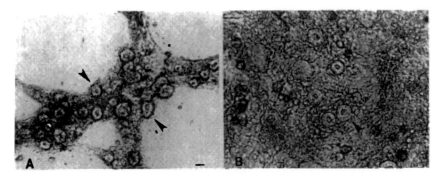

**Figure 4** Embryonic lungs dissociated into single-cell suspensions and plated on Matrigel. Phase-contrast images of cultures grown for 2 days on a gel (A) or film (B) of Matrigel. Both show organotypic cell rearrangement, characterized by the presence of multiple epithelial cysts (arrowed) with central lumen, surrounded by mesenchymal cells. Note that cultures grown on a gel (A) acquire a tri-dimensional configuration in which the epithelial component is embedded in a meshwork of mesenchymal cells, whereas cultures grown on a film (B) are flat and cover the entire dish surface. (C,D) Sections from organotypic cultures after 1 and 3 days in culture respectively. (C) A section cut perpendicular to the culture dish surface. Two small epithelial cysts are clearly distinguished from the surrounding mesenchymal cells. The mesenchymal cells are intermixed with Matrigel, which surrounds the entire structure (arrowed). (D) After 3 days in culture, the epithelial component exhibits substantial development. There is clear polarization of the epithelium with nuclei located basally; polarization of the mesenchymal cells nearest to the cysts is suggested by their alignment parallel to the base of the cysts. (E,F) Electron microscopic views of an organotypic culture after 3 days. The cyst epithelium is fully polarized. It is composed of low columnar cells with a basal nucleus and microvilli at the apical border. (F) A higher magnification micrograph of the interface between epithelium (e) and mesenchyme (m). A basal lamina–like structure is present between the two. Scale bars: A–D 50 μm, E 10 μm, F 1 μm.

plasma membrane of cells facing the basement membrane (78,79) fits with this notion.

## VII.  Basic Morphogenic Cell Behaviors Modulated by Laminin

Morphogenesis is the result of a limited number of basic cell behaviors taking place in a coordinated fashion. These include cell movement/motility, aggregation, sorting into epithelial and mesenchymal compartments, and polarization. In order to understand the role of laminin in lung branching morphogenesis, it is

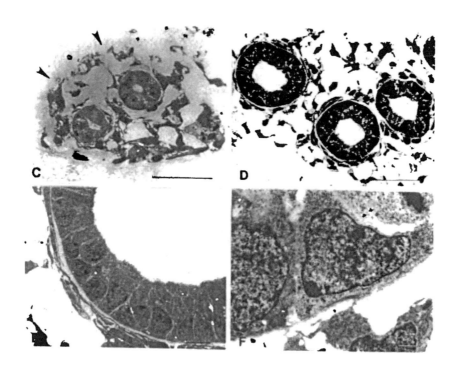

necessary to understand the function of laminin in these cell-cell and cell-matrix interactions.

## A.  Laminin In Lung Cell Attachment

Attachment of epithelial and mesenchymal lung cells is mediated by several laminin sites. One has been identified around the cross region of the α chain (70–72). Another cell attachment site has been recently located in the G region of the same chain (69). A third adhesion site seems to be present in the inner globular region of the β1 chain (71). All of these three sites are not specific for the lung but have been reported as major adhesion domains for a variety of cells other than those originated in the developing lung (46,69,76,80–83).

In the developing lung, the adhesion domain in the cross region of the a chain has been localized by a site-specific monoclonal antibody (monoclonal antibody AL-1). This antibody blocks the attachment of both epithelial and mesenchymal cell populations to each other, to the major basement membrane constituents laminin and type IV collagen, and to a basement membrane extract (Matrigel) (72). Since both epithelial and mesenchymal cells from the developing lung synthesize laminin (68), the inhibition of cell attachment to type IV collagen suggests that both cell types interact with type IV collagen through their own laminin. In support of this possibility, when the extracellular matrix production is decreased by exposing the cells to cycloheximide, monoclonal antibody AL-1 no longer blocks cell attachment to type IV collagen (Fig. 5) but still blocks attachment to laminin. Furthermore, early embryonic mesenchymal cells (day 11), which synthesize approximately 10-fold less laminin than day 15–16 cells, are not significantly affected in their attachment to type IV collagen by this antibody (unpublished observation).

The recent study by Matters and Laurie (69) showed that the carboxyterminal fragment E8 (see Fig. 1) blocked lung epithelial cell attachment and alveolar

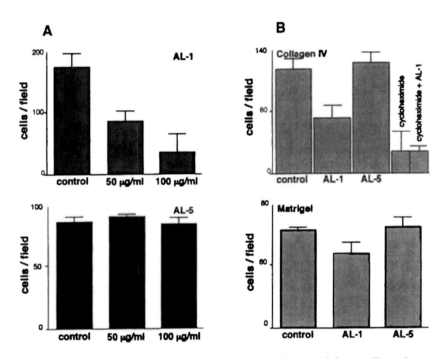

**Figure 5**  Effects of site-specific monoclonal antibodies to laminin on cell attachment. Mixed cell populations from fetal lungs were preincubated with the antibodies or control immunoglobulins and plated on laminin (A), type IV collagen, or Matrigel (B). Since the antibodies do not affect a particular cell population (epithelial or mesenchymal), the results are expressed as the total number of cells/field. Monoclonal antibody AL-1 has an inhibitory effect on both epithelial and mesenchymal cell populations ($P$ <.001 for 100 μg /ml antibody on laminin, and $P$ <.05 for the same concentration of antibody on type IV collagen). The effect of AL-1 on cell attachment to type IV collagen disappears by blocking protein synthesis with cycloheximide. Antibody AL-5 does not affect attachment to any of the substrata studied.

formation. The active site in the E8 fragment was further pinned down to the sequence SINNNR within the GI domain, which is conserved in a variety of animal species. The divalent cation dependence of this binding site raises the possibility that an integrin surface receptor may mediate cell interaction with this site. A likely candidate in such a case would be integrin α6β1, which has been shown to bind laminin fragment E8 (48).

The third laminin site with cell adhesive properties for lung epithelial and mesenchymal cells is located in the inner globular region of laminin β1 chain. It is represented by a 20 amino acid–long sequence (RYVVLPRPVCFEKGM-NYTVR) and has been referred as F-9 (41). This site also binds heparin, and our recent studies suggest that it is mainly involved in mediating cell attachment to HSPG via cell surface laminin, as presented below.

### B. Laminin in Epithelial Cell Proliferation

Although the effect of monoclonal antibody AL-1 on cell attachment is similar for both cell types epithelial and mesenchymal, this antibody selectively inhibits proliferation of epithelial cells (Fig. 6). This finding supports our previous studies

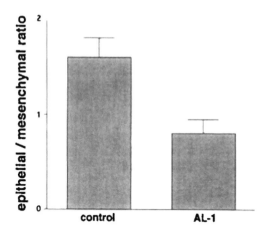

**Figure 6** Effect of monoclonal antibody AL-1 on epithelial and mesenchymal cell proliferation after 72 hr in coculture. Epithelial-mesenchymal cocultures were exposed to 100 μg/ml of monoclonal antibody AL-1 or control immunoglobulin for 72 hr. At the end of the culture period, the cocultures were fixed, immunostained with antikeratin antibodies, and the surfaces covered by either epithelial or mesenchymal cells were determined using the image analysis program Optimas 5.1. The ratio between the surface covered by epithelial cells and the surface covered by mesenchymal cells was then determined. The cocultures exposed to AL-1 have lower epithelial/mesenchymal ratios than those exposed to similar concentrations of IgG. The difference is statistically significant ($P < .01$).

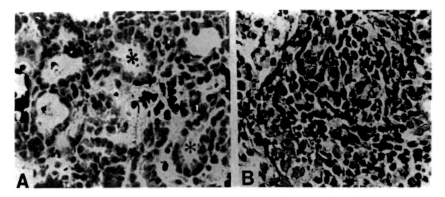

**Figure 7**  Effect of monoclonal antibodies AL-1 and AL-5 on epithelial cell polarization. (A,B) Cocultures of epithelial and mesenchymal cells isolated from fetal lungs. Cocultures exposed to AL-1 (A) present a normal organotypic formation. The general architectural pattern mimics that of the fetal lung (the cells sorted into epithelial and mesenchymal compartments, the clusters of epithelial cell polarized and created a central lumen, the mesenchymal cells rearranged surrounding them). Epithelial polarization is represented by a basal nucleus and apical cytoplasm. Cocultures exposed to monoclonal antibody AL-5 (B) do not show organotypic rearrangement. In these cocultures, the cells aggregate in pattern-less, large, solid masses. (C) An attached cell coculture exposed to AL-1 and stained with antitkeratin antibodies. The epithelial cells form a round tridimensional cystic structure, although the lumen is not visible because of the immunostaining. An electron microscopic view of one of these cysts discloses clear signs of epithelial polarization towards a central lumen (E). Compare to (D) representing an attached coculture exposed to AL-5 and stained with antikeratin. The cells arrange in flat, irregular clusters and their nuclei adopt a central (unpolarized) position. Scale bar = 10 μm, and 0.5 μM in E.

showing that the number of mitoses in AL-1–treated lung explants in organ culture is decreased in the epithelial but not in the mesenchymal compartment (67).

The preferential attachment of epithelial cells to laminin substrates (72) and the inhibition of epithelial cell adhesion and proliferation by monoclonal antibody AL-1 suggest that these cells are highly dependent on laminin for growth. Mesenchymal cells, however, are likely to rely on additional extracellular matrix constituents, such as type IV collagen, on which they attach in higher numbers than on laminin (72). The comparatively minor role of laminin in mesenchymal cell behavior is also suggested by their ability to proliferate in the presence of monoclonal antibody AL-1. Since AL-1 inhibits mesenchymal cell attachment, such proliferation can not occur unless the cells are able to overcome this inhibition by utilizing other extracellular matrix constituents. Another explanation for the difference in the proliferative response between epithelial and mesenchymal

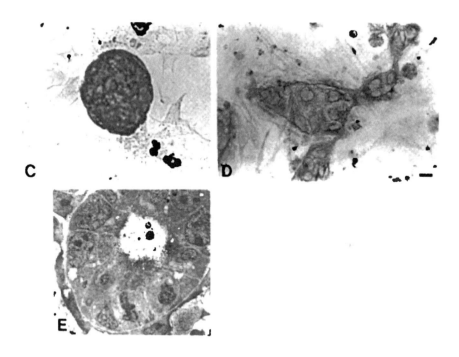

cells may be due to a higher epithelial cell sensitivity to the mitogenic activity localized in the cross region of laminin α chain (55,84). The stimulatory effect of the cross region of laminin has been attributed to EGF-like repeats (55) present in this segment (5) and is independent of cell attachment.

### C.   Laminin in Epithelial Cell Polarization and Lumen Formation

Previous studies demonstrated that cocultures of epithelial and mesenchymal cells from fetal organs can rearrange mimicking the organ of origin. We found that the degree and complexity of organotypic rearrangement of immature lung cells depends in part on the concentration of laminin in their environment (66,68). Additional studies using site-specific antibodies suggest that one of the mechanisms by which laminin induces organotypic pattern formation is by facilitating epithelial cell polarization. Induction of polarization seems to be mediated by the globular regions of the β and/or γ chains, because it is blocked by antibody AL-5 (Fig. 7). Although antibody AL-5 inhibits polarization, it does not affect cell sorting into epithelial and mesenchymal compartments. Since cell sorting involves homotypic cell recognition, the ability of the cells to sort in the presence of AL-5 suggests a selective effect of the α/γ chain(s) globular regions on epithelial-

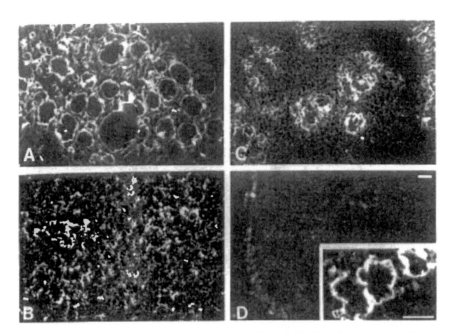

**Figure 8** Effect of monoclonal antibodies AL-1 and AL-5 on basement membrane formation. Immunohistochemical studies on suspension cocultures exposed to AL-1 disclose a linear pattern of laminin deposition along the epithelial-mesenchymal junction (A). This pattern is absent in cocultures exposed to AL-5, which present instead a diffuse, granular deposition of laminin in the extracellular space (B), or an irregular accumulation of laminin, probably around clusters of epithelial cells (C). In contrast to laminin, a linear deposition of type IV collagen is seen surrounding the irregular, unpolarized epithelial clusters in cocultures exposed to AL-5 (D, insert). (D) Control in which the primary antibody was omitted during the immunostaining procedure. (E,F) Additional sections from the same cocultures shown in (A–D) were stained with antikeratin antibodies. (E) Section from the coculture exposed to AL-1. Organotypic rearrangement indicated by epithelial cell clusters with smooth, round contours, and central lumen is seen. (F) Section from a coculture exposed to AL-5; note the irregular shape of the epithelial cell clusters and the absence of lumen. Scale bars = 20 μm.

mesenchymal interaction and not on interactions between homotypic cells. The effect of laminin on cell polarization has not been yet assigned to an specific amino acid sequence, and it may be possible that this process requires the full laminin region in its native configuration.

### D. Laminin in Basement Membrane Assembly

Several reports indicate that a basement membrane or a basement membrane–like structure is formed at the epithelial-mesenchymal interface of organotypic cocul-

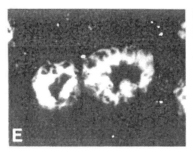
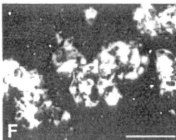

tures (66,85). Similar to a regular basement membrane, this structure is rich in laminin and type IV collagen. In comparison to this, cocultures exposed to antibody AL-5 disclose an almost complete absence of laminin deposition at the basement membrane site (Fig. 8). Since laminin is the major noncollagenous component of basement membranes, the lack of laminin represents a major and severe structural alteration.

Laminin self-assembles in vitro into a polymer by a reversible process dependent on the participation of the globular domains of the short arms (86). Type IV collagen forms an independent meshwork that binds to laminin (80,87) directly and indirectly through entactin/nidogen (36). Based on these studies, we propose that blockage of the globular region of laminin β and/or γ chain(s) prevents laminin assembly, and that the absence of a laminin polymer in the epithelial-mesenchymal interface precludes the establishment and maintenance of a polarized epithelium. In the lung organ cultures exposed to AL-5, this lack of proper laminin polymerization resulted in severe alterations in the pattern of branching instead of fewer branches as was seen when blocking the cross region of the α chain with antibody AL-1 (67).

A recent paper by Ekblom et al. (88) suggests that not only the proper assembly of laminin is important for the establishment of a normal basement membrane but also the correct link between laminin and entactin/nidogen. These investigators found that blocking antibodies to the laminin binding site of entactin/nidogen prevent the formation of a basement membrane in the developing kidney and lung which in turn results in severe alterations in organogenesis.

### E.   Laminin–Heparan Sulfate Proteoglycan Interaction

Laminin has at least three heparin binding sites; one in the G domain (39,40) and the other two in the outer and inner globular regions of the β chain (40,41). In the inner globular region, the binding site is centered in a 20 amino acid–long sequence (RYVVLPRPVCFEKGMNYTVR). This site, which has been termed F-9, binds to HSPG from the EHS tumor, to epithelial and mesenchymal lung cells (89), and to several other cell types (41). Incubation of early embryonic lung cells (days 11–12 of gestation) with the synthetic peptide F-9 triggers organotypic arrangement similar to that induced by basement membrane extracts or laminin gels. F-9–mediated organotypic rearrangement is inhibited by heparin, suggesting that HSPG produced by the lung cells plays a key role in this phenomenon. These studies indicate that HSPG may be involved in the events leading to organotypic rearrangement, such a cell-cell recognition and epithelial polarization. Laminin-HSPG interaction may be important in maintaining epithelial-mesenchymal structure when and where laminin levels are relatively low, such as in early lung morphogenesis or at the tips of the developing bronchial buds.

## VIII.  Laminin in Lung Cell Differentiation

Laminin has been shown to play a major role in the maintenance of the differentiated cell phenotype (58), including adult alveolar lung cells. In these cells, the production of surfactant (90) lung-specific apoprotein (91) and certain keratins (92) is stimulated by basement membrane extracts rich in laminin. Although laminin-coated dishes had a significant lesser effect on type II cells, this was probably related to the fact that laminin achieves its optimal biological activity if presented to cells as a gel. The possible role of laminin in embryonic and fetal lung cell differentiation remains unknown, perhaps because the lack of specific markers of differentiation for lung immature cells has discouraged research in this field.

## IX.  Summary and Conclusions

At least four laminin domains are involved in lung development and serve different roles during morphogenesis. By the mediation of these active sites, laminin stimulates epithelial and mesenchymal cell attachment, selective proliferation of epithelial cells, and establishment of a polarized epithelium. The latter is possible owing to the capability of laminin for self-assembly leading to an appropriate basement membrane network. Although the combinatory effect of these domains results in normal lung tissue structure and branching morphogenesis, different developmental abnormalities of the lung may result from alterations in each of these active sites.

At present, there is little information on which cellular receptors are involved in laminin interactions with embryonic and fetal lung cells. In part, this is due to the limited availability of probes for rodent extracellular matrix receptors. However, since most developmental lung research is carried out on rodents, several laboratories are currently developing such probes and we should soon have suitable reagents. Ultimately, understanding the specific receptors involved and the signal transduction pathways evoked by these receptors should provide important clues for the understanding of lung morphogenesis and how it is modulated by laminin.

## Acknowledgments

This work has been supported by NIH grants HL48730-01, American Lung Association grant RG/058N and a grant from The Council for Tobacco Research.

## References

1. Burgeson RE, Chiquet M, Deutzmann R, Ekblom P, Engel J, Kleinmann H, Martin GR, Meneguzzi G, Paulsson M, Sanes J, Timpl R, Tryggvason K, Yamada Y, Yurchenco PD. A new nomenclature for the laminins. Matrix Biol Chem 1988; 263: 16536–16544.
2. Timpl GR. Laminin-A glycoprotein from basement membranes. J Biol Chem 1979; 254:9933–9937.
3. Sasaki M, Kato S, Kohno K, Martin GR, Yamada Y. Sequence of the cDNA encoding the laminin β1 chain reveals a multidomain protein containing cysteine-rich repeats. Proc Natl Acad Sci USA 1987; 84:935–939.
4. Sasaki M, Yamada Y. The laminin β2 chain has a multidomain structure homologous to the β1 chain. J Biol Chem 1987; 262:17111–17117.
5. Sasaki M, Kleinmann HK, Huber H, Deutzmann R, Yamada Y. Laminin, a multi domain protein. The A chain has a unique globular domain and homology with the basement membrane proteoglycan and the laminin β chains. J Biol 1994; 14: 209–211.
6. Engel J, Odermatt E, Engel A, Madri JA, Furthmay H, Rohde H, Timpl R. Shapes, domain organizations and flexibility of laminin and fibronectin, two multifunctional proteins of the extracellular matrix. J Mol Biol 1981; 150:97–120.
7. Hunter DD, Shah V, Merlie JP, Sanes JR. A laminin-like adhesive protein concentrated in the synaptic cleft of the neuromuscular junction. Nature 1989; 338:229–234.
8. Ehrig K, Leivo I, Argraves WS, Ruoslahti E, Engvall E. Merosin, a tissue-specifric basement membrane protein, is a laminin-like protein. Proc Natl Acad Sci USA 1990; 87:3264–3268.
9. Kallunki P, Sainio K, Eddy R, Byers M, Kallunki T, Sariola H, Beck K, Hirvonen H, Shows TB, Tryggvason K. A truncated laminin chain homologous to the β2 chain: structure, spatial expression, and chromosomal assignment. J Cell Biol 1992; 119: 679–693.
10. Martin GR, Timpl R. Laminin and other basement membrane components. Ann Rev Cell Biol 1987; 3:57–85.
11. Paulsson M, Saladin K, Engvall E. Structure of laminin variants. The 300-kDa chains of murine and bovine heart laminin are related to the human placenta merosin heavy chain and replace the A chain in some laminin variants. J Biol Chem 1991; 266: 17545–17551.

12. Cooper AR, Kurkinen M, Taylor A, Hogan BLM. Studies on the biosynthesis of laminin by murine parietal endodermal cells. Eur J Biochem 1981; 119:189–197.

13. Peters BP, Hartle RJ, Krzesicki RF, Kroll TG, Perini F, Balun JE, Goldstein IJ, Ruddon RW. The biosynthesis, processing and secretion of laminin by human chorio-carcinoma cells. J Biol Chem 1985; 260:14732–14742.

14. Morita A, Sugimoto E, Kitagawa Y. Post-translational assembly and glycosylation of laminin subunits in parietal endoderm-like F9 cells. Biochem J 1985; 229:259–264.

15. Tokida Y, Aratani Y, Morita, A, Kitagawa Y. Production of two variants laminin forms by endothelial cells and shift of their relative levels by angiostatic steroids. J Biol Chem 1990; 265:18123–18129.

16. Greein TL, Hunter DD, Merlie JP, Sanes JR. Synthesis and assembly of the synaptic cleft protein S-laminin by cultured cells. J Biol Chem 1992; 267:2014–2022.

17. Kuhl U, Timpl R, von der Mark K. Synthesis of type IV collagen and laminin in cultures of skeletal muscle and their assembly on the surface of myotubules. Dev Biol 1982; 93:344–354.

18. Cooper AR, MacQueen HA. Subunits of laminin are differentially synthesized in mouse eggs and early embryos. Dev Biol 1983; 96:467–471.

19. Rao CN, Brinker JM, Kefalides NA. Changes in the subunit composition of laminin during the increased tumorigenesis of mouse A9 cells. Connect Tissue Res 1991; 25: 321–329.

20. Kleinmann HK, Ebihara I, Killen PD, Sasaki M, Cannon FB, Yamada Y, Martin GR. Genes for basement membrane proteins are coordinately expressed in differentiating F9 cells but not in normal adult murine tissues. Dev Biol 1987; 122:373–378.

21. Olsen D, Nagayoshi T, Fazio M, Peltonen J, Jaalola S, Sanborn D, Sasaki T, Kuivaniemi H, Chu ML, Deutzmann R, Timpl R, Uitto J. Human Laminin: cloning and sequence analysis of cDNAs encoding A, β1 and β2 chains, and expression of the corresponding genes in human skin and cultured cells. Lab Invest 1989; 60:772–782.

22. Engel J, Hunter I, Schulhers T, Beck K, Dixon TW, Parry DA. Assembly of laminin isoforms by triple- and double-stranded coiled-coil structures. Biochem Soc Trans 1991; 19:839–844.

23. Arumugham RG, Hsieh TCY, Tanzer ML, Laine RA. Structure of aspargine-linked oligosaccharides of the extracellular matrix component laminin. Biochim Biophys Acta 1986; 883:112–126.

24. Fujiwara S, Shinkai H, Deutzmann R, Paulsson M, Timpl R. Structure and distribu-tion of N-linked oligosaccharide chains on various domains of mouse tumor laminin. Biochem J 1988; 252:453–461.

25. Knibbs RN, Perini F, Goldstein I. Structure of the major concanavalin A reactive oligosaccharides of the extracellular matrix component laminin. J Biochem 1989; 28:6379–6392.

26. Chandrasekaran S, Dean JW, Griniger MS, Tanzer ML. Laminin carbohydrates are implicated in cell signalling J Cell Biochem 1991; 46:115–124.

27. Dennis JW, Waller CA, Schirrmacher V. Identification of aspargine-linked oligosac-charides involved in tumor cell adhesion to laminin and type IV collagen. J Cell Biol 1984; 99:1416–1423.

28. Bouzon M, Dussert C, Lissitzkyl JC, Martin PM. Spreading of B16 F1 cells on

laminin and its proteolytic fragments P1 and E8: involvement of laminin carbohydrate chains. Exp Cell Res 1990; 190:47–54.

29. Dean JW, Chandraserkaran S, Tanker ML. A biological role for the carbohydrate moieties of laminin. J Biol Chem 1990; 265:12553–12556.

30. Chammas R, Veiga SS, Line S, Potocnjak P, Brentani RR. Asn-linked oligosaccharide-dependent interaction between laminin and gp 120/140. An $\alpha6\beta1$ integrin. J Biol Chem 1991; 266:3349–3355.

31. Wu TC, Wan YJ, Chung AE, Damajonov I. Immunohistochemical localization of entactin and laminin in mouse embryos and fetuses. Dev Biol 1983; 100:496–505.

32. Howe CC. Functional role of laminin carbohydrate. Mol Cell Biol 1984; 4:1–7.

33. Yurchenco PD, Schittny JC. Molecular architecture of basement membranes. FASEB J 1990; 4:1577–1590.

34. Yurchenko PD, Cheng Y-S. Self-assembly and calcium binding sites in laminin: a three arm interaction model. J Biol Chem 1993; 268:17286–17299.

35. Paulsson M. The role of $Ca^{2+}$ binding in the self-aggregation of laminin-nidogen complexes. J Biol Chem 1988; 263:5425–5430.

36. Fox JW, Mayer R, Nischt R, Aumailley M, Reinhardt D, Wiedemann H, Mann K, Timpl R, Krieg T, Engel J, Chu M-L. Recombinant nidogen consists of three globular domains and mediates binding of laminin to collagen type IV. EMBO J 1991; 10: 3137–3146.

37. Paulsson M, Aumailley M, Deutzmann R, Timpl R, Beck K, Engel J. Laminin-nidogen complex. Extraction with chelating agents and structural characterization. Eur J Biochem 1987; 166:11–19.

38. Mayer U, Nischt R, Poschl E, Mann K, Fukuda K, Gerl M, Yamada Y, Timpl R. A single EGF-like motif of laminin is responsible for high affinity nidogen binding. EMBO J 1993; 12:1879–1885.

39. Ott VE, Odermatt E, Engel J, Furthmayr H, Timpl R. Protease resistance and conformation of laminin. Eur J Biochem 1982; 123:63–72.

40. Kouzi-Koliakos K, Koliakos GG, Tsilibary EC, Furcht LT, Charonis AS. Mapping of three major heparin binding sites on laminin and identification of a novel heparin-binding site on the B1 chain. J Biol Chem 1989; 264:17971–17978.

41. Charonis AS, Skubitz APN, Koliakos GG, Reger LA, Dege J, Vogel AM, Wohlueter R, Furcht LT. A novel synthetic peptide from the B1 chain of laminin with heparin-binding and cell adhesion-promoting activities. J Cell Biol 1988; 107:1253–1260.

42. Saunders S, Jalkanen M, O'Farrell S, Bernfield M. Molecular cloning of syndecan, an integral membrane proteoglycan. J Cell Biol 1989; 108:1547–1556.

43. Kjellen L, Lindahl U. Proteoglycans: structure and interactions. Annu Rev Biochem 1991; 60:443–475.

44. Kramer RH, Cheng YF, Clyman RI. Human vascular endothelial cells use $\beta1$ and $\beta3$ integrin receptor complexes to attach to laminin. J Cell Biol 1990; 110:1233–1243.

45. Sonnenberg A, Linders CJT, Modderman PW, Damsky CH, Aumailley M, Timpl R. Integrin recognition of different cell-binding fragments of laminin (P1, E3, E8) and evidence that $\alpha6\beta1$ but not $\alpha6\beta4$ functions as a major receptor for fragment E8. J Cell Biol 1990; 110:2145–2155.

46. Aumailley M, Nurcombe V, Edgar D, Paulsson M, Timpl R. The cellular interactions

of laminin fragments. Cell adhesion correlates with two fragment–specific high affinity binding sites. J Biol Chem 1987; 262:11532–11538.

47.  Sung U, O'Rear JJ, Yurchenco PD. Cell and heparin binding in the distal long arm of laminin: identification of active and cryptic sites with recombinant and hybrid glyco-protein. J Cell Biol 1993; 123:1255–1268.

48.  Aumailley M, Gerl M, Sonnenberg A, Deutzmann R, Timpl R. Identification of of the Arg-Gly-Asp sequence in laminin A chain as a latent cell-binding site being exposed in fragment P1. FEBS Lett 1990; 262:359–366.

49.  Malinoff H, Wicha MS. Isolation of a cell surface receptor protein laminin from murine fibrosarcoma cells. J Cell Biol 1983; 96:1475–1480.

50.  Lesot H, Kuhl U, von der Mark K. Isolation of a laminin binding protein from muscle cell membranes, EMBO J 1983; 2:861–869.

51.  Clement B, Segui-Real B, Savagner P, Kleinman HK, Yamada Y. Hepatocyte attach-ment to laminin is mediated through multiple receptors. 1990; 110:185–192.

52.  Cioce V, Castronovo V, Shmookler BM, Garbisa S, Grigioni WF, Liotta LA, Sobel ME. Increased expression of the laminin receptor in human colon cancer. J Natl Cancer Inst 1991; 83:29–36.

53.  Evaristi JM, Campbell KP. A role for the dystrophin-glycoprotein complex as a transmembrane linker between Laminin and actin. J Cell Biol 1993; 4:809–823.

54.  Beck K, Hunter I, Engel J. Structure and function of laminin: anatomy of a multi-domain glycoprotein. FASEB J 1990; 4:148–160.

55.  Panayotou G, End P, Aumailley M, Timpl R, Engel J. Domains of laminin with growth-factor activity. Cell 1989; 56:93–101.

56.  Kanemoto T, Reich R, Royce L, Greatorex D, Adler SH, Shiraishi N, Martin GR, Yamada Y, Kleinman H. Identification of an amino acid sequence from the laminin A chain that stimulates metastasis and collagenase IV production. Proc Natl Acad Sci, USA 1990; 87:2279–2283.

57.  Hynes RO. Integrins: versatilty, modulation and signalling in cell adhesion. Cell 1992; 69:11–25.

58.  Kleinman HK, Kibbey MC, Schnaper HW, Hadley MA, Dym M, Grant DS. Role of basement membrane in differentiation. In: Rohrbach DH, Timpl R, eds. Molecular and Cellular Aspects of Basement Membranes. San Diego: Academic Press, 1993: 309–326.

59.  Edgar D, Timpl R, Theonen H. The heparin-binding domain of laminin is responsible for the effects on neurite outgrowth and neuronal survival. EMBO J 1984; 3:1463–1468.

60.  Hunter DD, Cashman N, Morris-Valero R. An LRE (leucine-arginine-glutamate)–dependent mechanism for adhesion of neurons to S-laminin. J Neurosci 1991; 11:3960–3971.

61.  Skubitz AP, Letouneau PC, Wayner E, Furcht LT. Synthetic peptides from the carboxy-terminal globular domain of the A chain of laminin: their ability to promote cell adhesion and neurite outgrowth and interact with heparin and $\beta 1$ integrin subunit. J Cell Biol 1991; 115:1137–1148.

62.  Klein G, Langegger M, Timpl R, Ekblom P. Role of laminin A chain in the develop-ment of epithelial cell polarity. Cell 1988; 55:331–341.

63. Ekblom M, Klein G, Mugraver G, Fecker L, Deutzmann R, Timpl R, Ekblom P. Transient and locally restricted expression of laminin A chain mRNA by developing epithelial cells during kidney organogenesis. Cell 1990; 60:337–346.

64. Klein G, Ekblom M, Fecker L, Timpl R, Ekblom P. Differential expression of laminin A and B chains during development of embryonic mouse organs. Development 1990; 110:823–837.

65. Schuger L, O'Shea S, Rheinheimer J, Varani J. Laminin in lung development: effects of anti-laminin antibody in murine lung morphogenesis. Dev Biol 1990; 137:26–32.

66. Schuger L, O'Shea S, Nelson BB, Varani J. Organotypic arrangement of mouse embryonic lung cells on a basement membrane extract: involvement of laminin. Development 1990; 110:1091–1099.

67. Schuger L, Skubitz APN, O'Shea KS, Chang JF, Varani J. Identification of laminin domains involved in epithelial branching morphogenesis: effects of anti-laminin monoclonal antibodies on mouse embryonic lung development. Dev Biol 1991; 146: 531–541.

68. Schuger L, Varani J, Killen PD, Skubitz APN, Gilbride K. Laminin expression in the mouse lung increases with development and stimulates spontaneous organotypic rearrangement of mixed lung cells. Dev Dyn 1992; 195:43–54.

69. Matter ML, Laurie GW. A novel laminin E8 cell adhesion site required for lung alveolar formation *in vitro*. J Cell Biol 1994; 124:1083–1090.

70. Schuger L, Skubitz A, Gilbride K. The globular region of laminin B chain(s) is critical for epithelial cell polarization in the developing lung. Mol Biol Cell 1993; 4:377a.

71. Santora K, Skubitz APN, Gilbride K, Schuger L. Cell adhesion is promoted by different laminin sites during murine lung organogenesis. FASEB J 1993; 7:A834.

72. Schuger L, Skubitz APN, Morenas A, Gilbride K. Two separate domains of laminin promote lung organogenesis by different mechanisms of action. Dev Biol 1995; 169: 520–532.

73. Thomas T, Dziadek M. Expression of collagen alpha 1 (IV), laminin and nidogen genes in the embryonic mouse lung: implications for branching morphogenesis. Mech Dev 1994; 45:193–201.

74. Laurie GW, Horikoshi S, Killen PD, Segui-Real B, Yamada Y. In situ hybridization reveals temporal and spatial changes in cellular expression of mRNA for a laminin receptor, laminin, and basement membrane (type IV) collagen in the developing kidney. J Cell Biol 1989; 109:1352–1362.

75. Simon-Assmann P, Bouziges F, Arnold C, Haffen K, Kedinger M. Epithelial-mesenchymal interactions in the production of basement membrane components in the gut. Development 1988; 102:339–347.

76. Skubitz APN, Charonis AS, Tsilibary EC, Furcht LT. Localization of a tumor cell adhesion domain of laminin by a monoclonal antibody. Exp Cell Res 1987; 173: 349–360.

77. Skubitz APN, McCarthy JB, Charonis AS, Furcht LT. Localization of three distinct heparin-binding domains by monoclonal antibodies. J Biol Chem 1988; 263:4861–4868.

78. Schittny JC, Timpl R, Engel J. High resolution immuno electron microscopic localization of funtional domains of laminin, of nidogen, of heparan sulfate proteoglycan in

epithelial basment membrane of mouse cornea reveals different topological orientations J Cell Biol 1989; 107:1599–1610.

79. Abrahamson DR, Irwin MH, St. John PL, Perry EW, Accavitti MA, Heck LW, Couchman JR. Molecular orientation of laminin within basement membranes. J Cell Biol 1989; 109:3477–3491.

80. Terranova VP, Rao CN, Kalebic T. Laminin receptor on human breast carcinoma cells. Proc Natl Acad Sci USA 1983; 80:444–451.

81. Graf J, Iwamoto Y, Sasaki M, Martin GR, Kleinman HK, Robey F, Yamada Y. Identification of an amino acid sequence of laminin mediating cell attachment, chemotaxis, and receptor binding. Cell 1987; 48:989–996.

82. Kleinman HK, Graf J, Iwamoto Y, Sasaki M, Schasteen CS, Yamada Y, Martin GR, Robey FA. Identification of a second active site in laminin for promotion of cell adhesion and migration and inhibition of in vivo melanoma lung colonization. Arch Biochem Biophys 1989; 272:39–45.

83. Tashiro K, Sephel GC, Weeks B, Sasaki M, Martin GR, Kleinman HK, Yamada Y. A synthetic peptide containing the IKVAV sequence from the A chain of laminin mediate cell attachment, migration and neuritic outgrowth. J Biol Chem 1989; 264:16174–16182.

84. Terranova VP, Aumailley M, Sultan LH, Martin GR, Kleinman H. Regulation of cell attachment and cell number by fibronectin and laminin. J Cell Physiol 1986; 127:473–479.

85. McAteer JA, Dougherty GS, Gardner KD, Evan AP. Polarized epithelial cysts *in vitro*. A review of cell and explant culture systems that exhibit epithelial cyst formation. Scanning Electron Microsc 1988; 3:1739–1763.

86. Yurchenco PD, Cheng YS, Colognato H. Laminin forms an independent network in basement membranes. J Cell Biol 1992; 117:1119–1133.

87. Laurie GW, Bing JT, Kleinman HK, Hassell JR, Aumailley M, Martin GR, Feldmann RJ. Localization of binding sites for laminin, heparan sulfate proteoglycan and fibronectin on basement membrane (type IV) collagen. J Mol Biol 1986; 189: 205–216.

88. Ekblom P, Ekblom M, Fecker L, Klein G, Zhang H-Y, Kadoya Y, Chu M-L, Mayer U, Timpl R. Role of mesenchymal nidogen for epithelial morphogenesis in vitro. Development 1994; 120:2003–2014.

89. Schuger L, Skubitz APN, Gilbride K. Interaction between a site in the outer globular region of laminin β1 chain and heparan sulfate proteoglycan in early mouse lung development. Submitted to Dev Biol.

90. Rannels SR, Yarnell JA, Stinson Fisher C, Fabisiak JP, Rannels E. Role of laminin in maintainance of type II pneumocyte morphology and function. Am J Physiol 1987; 253(Cell Physiol 22):C835–C845.

91. Shannon JM, Emrie J, Fisher JH, Kuroki Y, Jennings SD, Mason R. Effect of a reconstituted basement membrane on expression of surfactant apoproteins in cultured adult rat alveolar type II cells. Am J Respir Cell Mol Biol 1990; 2:183–192.

92. Woodcock-Mitchell J, Rannels SR, Mitchell J, Rannels DE, Low RB. Modulation of keratin expression in type II pneumocytes by the extracellular matrix. Am Rev Respir Dis 1989; 139:343–351.

# 12

# Collagens and Elastic Fiber Proteins in Lung Development

**EDMOND C. CROUCH,
ROBERT P. MECHAM,
and ROSA M. DAVILA**

Washington University School of Medicine
St. Louis, Missouri

**AKIHIKO NOGUCHI**

Cardinal Glennon Children's Hospital
St. Louis University Medical Center
St. Louis, Missouri

## I. Introduction

The orderly deposition and remodeling of fibrous and elastic matrices and basement membranes is essential for the structural development of the conducting airways, pulmonary blood vessels, alveoli, and pleura. In addition to their important structural roles, matrix macromolecules participate in regulating critical aspects of pulmonary morphogenesis, including airway branching and epithelial differentiation. Although the number of matrix proteins that contribute to lung structure is quite large, this chapter focuses on two major classes of lung matrix macromolecules—the collagens and elastic fiber proteins—and examines their roles in human lung development.

The importance of collagen and elastic fibers for the mechanical and gas-exchange properties of the postnatal lung is emphasized by the effects of abnormal collagen deposition in diffuse pulmonary fibrosis and of extensive elastic fiber degradation in emphysema. It should not be surprising that fetal lung growth and development are characterized by increases in collagenous and elastic lung matrix and by alterations in the numbers and spatial relationships of collagen- and elastin-producing cells. However, remarkably little is still known about the organization of collagens, elastin, and microfibrillar proteins within various anatomical compartments and subcompartments of the lung. Even less is known about the cellular and extracellular mechanisms that regulate the local deposition and turnover of these components during lung development. Accordingly, this chapter provides a brief overview of the fetal lung matrix and reviews important structural features of the known pulmonary collagens and components of the elastic fiber. We also review recent data relating to the production and extracellular turnover of these proteins, and examine their probable participation in specific aspects of lung development.

## II.  Matrix Alterations in Lung Development

The intrauterine development of the lung can be divided into two phases comprising at least three overlapping stages: glandular/pseudoglandular, canalicular, and terminal sac/alveolar. The first phase establishes the general structural organization of air-conducting system, whereas the second phase leads to the formation of the gas-exchange tissues. Both phases are characterized by conspicuous alterations in the amount, spatial organization, and composition of extracellular matrix.

### A.  Early Phase

Lung development and maturation proceed from proximal to distal. The lung bud forms at 4–5 weeks' gestation as an outpouching of endoderm of the foregut into the supporting mesenchyme. This outpouching gives rise to two endodermal rudiments that subsequently undergo progressive branching. The embryonic mesenchyme, which surrounds the rudiments, is highly hydrated and rich in hyaluronic acid and proteoglycans. However, it also contains small numbers of interspersed fibrils comprising various collagens and various noncollagenous glycoproteins. From the earliest stages of lung morphogenesis, the epithelial compartment is at least partly surrounded by a basement membrane that contains type IV collagen as well as basement membrane glycoproteins and proteoglycans. No elastic fibers are identified within the mesenchyme or in association with the primitive airways.

The adult pattern of conducting airways and arteries is established by approximately 16 weeks' gestation. In addition, branching of the pulmonary arteries closely follows the pattern of airway branching both temporally and spatially. By 16 weeks' gestation, connective tissue subcompartments can also be identified within each of the major pulmonary compartments. The large airways show a continuous subepithelial basement membrane, submucosal matrix, smooth muscle layer, perichondrium, and cartilage. The pleural compartment can be identified with mesothelial cells supported by a basement membrane and loose fibrous matrix. The arteries show identifiable medial and adventitial layers containing elastic lamellae.

## B. Late Phase

Subsequent fetal lung development and maturation are characterized by the peripheral multiplication of noncartilagenous airways and the formation of alveolar sacs as well as the continued growth and maturation of the previously formed parenchymal elements. These events are accompanied by a peripheral extension of the microvasculature, and progressive thinning and remodeling of the interstitial matrix. At birth, the pulmonary blood vessels undergo marked remodeling as they adapt to systemic pressures. Alveolar multiplication with associated matrix and microvascular remodeling is very rapid during the neonatal period but continues through childhood and into adolescence.

## C. Collagen and Elastic Fiber Deposition

As indicated above, collagenous fibers are present in comparatively small numbers during the pseudoglandular phase. However, subsequently an increasingly large proportion of the interstitium is occupied by collagenous fibrils and fibers which are often concentrated initially subjacent to the epithelial basement membrane.

Elastic fibers are first detected by histological staining at 3 months of gestation in the walls of the trachea and main stem bronchi, the pleura, and the pulmonary artery (1). A marked increase in elastogenesis occurs during the last trimester of gestation as the respiratory region of the lung differentiates. Elastic fibers are identified with the appearance of alveolar septal primordial cells (2,3) and in association with smooth muscle cells at bifurcations in the late glandular stage (4). At the beginning of the alveolar phase, elastic fiber bundles are confined largely to areas immediately surrounding the mouths of the alveoli but expand into the alveolar wall during the neonatal and adolescent phase of life (1,5,6). Concentrations of elastic fibers are also found where two alveolar septa meet in a tent-like configuration.

Although there are significant species differences in the timing of these events relative to total gestation, there appears to be a good correlation between alterations in the expression of collagen and elastic fiber proteins and specific morphogenetic events. For example, the correlation of elastin expression with changes in the spatial distribution of elastic fibers is essentially the same for all mammalian species. Thus, in the rat, secondary septal development in the air sac starts postnatally and is essentially complete within the first 2 weeks of life. In the human, this stage begins in the last trimester of gestation and continues into adolescence. This correlation is consistent with the important roles of collagen and elastin and matrix-producing cells in pulmonary morphogenesis as well as in determining the mechanical properties of the tissue.

## III. Collagens

The collagens are a diverse family of matrix proteins characterized by one or more triple helical domains (7). Structural differences within the collagen or noncollagenous domains of the various collagen types result in differences in molecular aggregation, fiber formation, and intermolecular cross linking that influence matrix organization and the mechanical properties of the tissue. Such differences also result in collagen type–dependent differences in the ability to interact with degradative enzymes. Finally, differences in collagen structure may influence interactions with specific cellular receptors and thereby influence matrix assembly and turnover as well as the phenotype of associated cells.

Although collagens account for >60% of the total matrix protein and 15–20% of the dry weight of the normal adult human lung (8), the relative proportion of collagen and noncollagenous molecules changes dramatically during development. For example, collagens account for ±1.5% of the dry weight of the late second-trimester fetal human lung (8).

There are at least 12 types of matrix collagen in the lung, each consisting of one or more genetically different collagen chains or splicing variants (Table 1). However, the contribution of individual collagen types must vary considerably during the course of lung development. Because the structural features of these molecules have been extensively reviewed (7,9), only those features of probable relevance to lung development will be presented in this chapter. It should be appreciated that there are no published studies that have examined the absolute or relative amounts of collagen or of specific collagen types in mammalian lungs as a function of developmental age, and very little is known about the distribution of expression of specific collagen transcripts.

### A. Collagens: Classified by Supramolecular Organization

The various matrix collagens can be classified based on their predominant pattern of supramolecular organization (10). The major classes include fibrillar collagens that participate in quarter-staggered fibers or fibrils, fibril-associated collagens with interrupted triple helical domains, sheet-forming collagens, and beaded filament–forming collagens (Table 2). Another more recently described group consists of collagens characterized by multiple triple helical domains with intervening noncollagenous sequences; this includes types XV and XVIII collagen (11).

Pulmonary collagens fall into at least three of the above classes, including collagens that form quarter-stagger fibers and those that form sheets or micro-

**Table 1** Pulmonary Collagens

| Type | Chains[a] | Predominant form(s) |
|------|-----------|---------------------|
| I | α1,α2 | $[\alpha 1(I)]_{\alpha 2} \gg [\alpha 1]_3$ |
| II | α1 | $[\alpha 1(II)]_3$ |
| III | α1 | $[\alpha 1(III)]_3$ |
| IV | α1,α2,α3,α4,α5,α6 | $[\alpha 1(IV)]_2 \alpha 2 >, [\alpha 3(IV)]_2 \alpha 4?, [\alpha 5(IV)]_2, \alpha 6?$ |
| V | α1,α2,α3 | $[\alpha 1(V)]_2 \alpha 2, [\alpha 1, \alpha 2, \alpha 3]?$ |
| VI | α1,α2,α3 | $[\alpha 1, \alpha 2, \alpha 3]$ |
| VII | α1 | $[\alpha 1(VII)]_3$ |
| VIII | α1,α2 | |
| IX? | α1,α2,α3,α1' | $[\alpha 1, \alpha 2, \alpha 3]$ |
| XI | α1,α2,α3 | ? |
| XIII[b] | α1,? | ? |
| XVIII[c] | α1,? | ? |

[a]Present in lung of at least some species based on biochemical, immunohistochemical, and/or nucleic acid hybridization assays.
[b]Ref. 11.
[c]Ref. 133.
[d]Ref. 134.

fibrils. Several of the collagens are probably restricted to the same anatomical structures or compartments in developing and mature lung. For example, type II collagen appears restricted to cartilage. However, some collagens, such as type IV collagen, show age-dependent differences in site-specific accumulation.

### Collagens Forming Quarter-Stagger Fibers and Fibrils

Types I and III Collagen

Types I and II collagen are virtually ubiquitous in the mature lung and are extensively codistributed at the light microscopic level (12–15). However, they

**Table 2** Classification of Lung Collagens by Their Patterns of Supramolecular Organization

| | |
|---|---|
| Quarter-stagger fibers/fibrils | Types I, III, and V |
| | Types II and XI |
| | Type VII |
| Sheet-forming collagens | Type IV |
| Microfibril | Type VI and VIII |
| | Type IV ? |

are also widely distributed in the fetal lung (16), and are components of mesenchymal fibrils observed during early lung development.

Together, types I and III collagen account for the majority of total peripheral lung collagen and are present in a ratio of approximately 2:1 in the adult lung of most mammalian species. Although type III collagen is typically enriched in fetal tissues, the proportions of these collagens in specific areas of the lung have not been determined. Types I and III collagen are primarily synthesized by embryonic mesenchyme and interstitial connective tissue cells and are deposited in the matrix as fibrils or fibers of varying diameter. At some tissue sites, these collagens can be deposited in the same fiber, and it is possible that the relative proportion of the two collagens plays a role in determining fiber diameter (17).

In general, type I procollagen is rapidly processed to collagen. However, antibodies specific for the aminoterminal propeptide domain of type I also label fibers in newly deposited extracellular matrices. Interestingly, during the early phase of lung development, type I procollagen epitopes are preferentially expressed near the basement membrane zone surrounding the most distal fetal airways in the absence of a corresponding increase in cellular expression of transcripts for proα1(I) (18). Thus, it is possible that there are local alterations in the rate or efficiency of type I processing, or the clearance of liberated propeptides.

At most sites, including adult lung, type III procollagen is more slowly processed than type I and can retain one or more of its noncollagenous terminal domains following secretion (19–21). In vitro studies in other organ systems indicate that complete processing is not required for fiber formation. As for type I procollagen, the degree of processing could also play a role in regulating fiber diameter. The metabolic fate and possible biological properties of the liberated propeptides have not yet been elucidated. As in other tissues, oxidative deamination of specific lysyl residues is catalyzed by lysyl oxidase, leading to the formation of lysyl- and hydroxylysyl-derived cross links. However, there is evidence that type III collagen can also become rapidly cross linked by intertrimeric disulfide bonds via cysteine residues near the C-terminal end of the collagen domain (22).

### Type V Collagens

Type V collagens have been isolated from human lung and have been immunologically identified in the basement membrane (BM) zone (23) in both fetal and adult lung, but they are predominantly components of the interstitial or pericellular matrix. Type V collagens are assembled as homo- or heteropolymers of three chain types, and additional chains have been identified in some species. It is likely that there are tissue-specific differences in type V structure.

Based on cell culture experiments, there are several potential cellular sources of type V collagen. These include fibroblast-like interstitial cells, smooth muscle cells, and endothelial cells. Type V collagens are also synthesized by fetal lung epithelial cell lines (24), and freshly isolated type II cells. There are no data on the processing of lung type V, but in other tissues, type V collagen retains portions of its noncollagenous terminal domains. Types V and I collagen are extensively codistributed and in some tissues have been immunologically localized to the same fiber.

## Types II and XI Collagen

Not suprisingly, type II collagens have been isolated from large airway cartilage, and the synthesis of type II collagen has been demonstrated in organ cultures of tracheal hyaline cartilage (19). Based on Northern analysis, human fetal lung (15–19 weeks) may contain a predominance of the long form of the $pro\alpha1(II)$ chain (25). This splice variant contains exon 2, and it is the predominant transcript in several other predominantly noncartilagenous tissues (26).

Sandberg and co-workers also identified transcripts for $pro\alpha2(XI)$ in 15- to 19-week fetal human lung. In addition, the long-form mRNA encoding $pro\alpha1(XI)$ has been identified in developing mouse lung (27). Because the $\alpha3(XI)$ chain is identical to the $\alpha1(II)$ chain except for posttranslational modification and appears to be encoded by the same gene (7), type XI collagen could represent a major collagenous component of fetal airway cartilage. In this regard, it has been suggested that type XI collagen may form fine fibrils that can serve as a scaffolding for the deposition of type II collagen (10).

## Type VII Collagen

Type VII collagen is the major structural component of anchoring fibrils in the skin. Immunological studies of adult human lung using monoclonal antibodies have identified type VII collagen in a highly restricted distribution near the basement membrane zone of trachea, bronchi, and bronchioles (28). Based on studies of skin and certain blistering skin disorders (e.g., dystrophic epidermolysis bullosa), it is likely that type VII collagen helps to anchor the airway epithelium to the underlying matrix. It is possible that both basal epithelial cells and subepithelial fibroblast-like cells contribute to type VII deposition (29).

### *Sheet-Forming Collagens*

## Type IV Collagen

Type IV or basement membrane collagen is an integral component of all lung BMs. Lung type IV collagen comprises at least six genetically different chains (30), and at least five of the chains ($\alpha1-\alpha5$) have been biochemically or immunologically identified in adult human lung (31). Type IV is the major collagen synthesized by primary cultures of alveolar type II cells (32), and it is also synthesized by endothelial cells. In addition, strains of lung fibroblasts and embryonic mesenchymal cells and smooth muscle cells synthesize small amounts of type IV collagen in vitro (33,34). Interestingly, type IV collagen synthesized by dermal fibroblasts may contribute to the assembly of keratinocyte basement membranes (29). Type IV transcripts are also expressed by fetal lung mesenchymal cells in vivo (35).

Procollagen production appears to account for a high proportion of total lung collagen production in the neonatal and adult rat (36). The production of total lung type IV collagen and the concentration of type IV collagen mRNA are transiently decreased during the early postnatal period; possibly secondary to a combination of transcriptional and posttranscriptional mechanisms (36). Although the local accumulation of this collagen appears to be subject to complex regulation in prenatal lung development, there are no published studies examining the regional expression of type IV mRNAs in fetal lung.

Organ culture and isolated perfused organ studies of postnatal and adult rat lung indicate that type IV collagen does not undergo extracellular proteolytic processing (21,36,37). The secreted collagen is deposited as extended aggregates that are stabilized by noncovalent, antiparallel, interactions of the terminal domains as well as by intermolecular disulfide bonds and lysyl-derived cross links (20,36,38). These homologous interactions allow the formation of extended sheets. However, type IV deposited by mesenchyme also appears to be organized as fibrils (39). Type IV collagen binds to laminin, fibronectin (FN), heparan sulfate proteoglycan, and entactin in vitro (40), and such interactions are believed to contribute to basement membrane structure and function in vivo.

### *Microfibril-Forming Collagens*

#### Type VI Collagen

Type VI collagen has been localized to alveolar interstitial microfibrils of mature lung by immunofluoresence and electron microscopy (12,41). However, there are no data on the synthesis, processing, cross linking, or turnover of type VI collagens in adult or fetal lung matrix. Type VI is composed of at least three chain types, and at least two of the chains can be expressed in lung tissue. Type VI collagen is synthesized by smooth muscle cells and lung fibroblasts in culture.

Type VI collagen has large terminal globular domains that do not undergo significant proteolytic processing. The terminal domains mediate end-to-end interactions required for the assembly of microfibrils (42,43). Type VI collagen can promote cell attachment, is preferentially deposited in the cell layer in fibroblast cultures, and could represent a component of the interstitial pericellular matrix in vivo. It has also been suggested that type VI collagen can serve as a scaffolding that facilitates the deposition of types I and III collagen in fetal skin (44). It could also contribute to anchoring the basement membrane to the subjacent matrix.

#### Type VIII Collagen

Type VIII collagen is expressed in lung and is primarily deposited in the vascular subendothelium and in association with small pulmonary arteries and veins (45).

However, monoclonal antibodies to α1(VIII) have also demonstrated delicate fibrillar staining in association with with the pleura (46). These investigators suggested that type VIII collagen is deposited as microfibrils in association with some elastic fiber systems.

### Regulation of Collagen Production

The complexity of transcriptional and posttranslational control and extracellular processing and turnover of the collagens provides numerous levels of potential regulation. Furthermore, the precise regulatory mechanisms vary for different cell types, for different collagen types, and as a function of the local environment and proliferative state of the cell. The major controls for collagen production operate at the levels of collagen gene transcription, mRNA translation, and intracellular protein degradation (47–49). Posttranscriptional regulatory mechanisms also include age-dependent and tissue site–dependent differences in the expression or activity of hydroxylase and glycosyltransferase enzymes, collagen propeptidases, lysyl oxidase, and collagen-degrading enzymes and their inhibitors. For example, developmental changes in the profile of lysyl oxidase and total lung collagen cross links have been observed (50,51).

The developmentally regulated expression of specific growth factors such as transforming growth factor-β (TGF-β) isoforms and platelet-derived growth factor (PDGF) may play particularly important roles in regulating local collagen production and turnover. Other modulatory factors likely include local differences in the accumulation of other matrix proteins and the expression of various cellular receptors for collagen proteins.

### Extracellular Turnover of Collagens

Collagen degradation is determined by local regulation of levels of activated matrix metalloproteinases (MMPs) and specific enzyme inhibitors (52) (Table 3).The degradation of native and cross-linked collagens involves initial cleavage by specific collagenases, which are secreted in a proenzyme form requiring proteolytic activation. Activated collagenases are inhibited by specific tissue inhibitors of metalloproteinases (TIMPs). Collagenase enzymes and their tissue inhibitors are synthesized by a variety of pulmonary cell types, both mesenchymal and epithelial.

Collagen fibers consisting of type I and/or III collagen or type II collagen are substrates for interstitial collagenase (MMP-1). On the other hand, types IV and V collagen are not substrates for interstitial collagenase, but are efficiently degraded in vitro by the 72-kDa (MMP-2) and 92-kDa (MMP-9) collagenase/gelatinase, which do not cleave native types I and III collagen. Type IV collagen contains several interruptions in the central helical region that render it susceptible to degradation by a variety of less specific proteases, including stromelysin-1 (MMP-3).

**Table 3**  Matrix Metalloproteinases

| Enzyme | MMP[a] | Source(s) | Potential lung substrates[b] |
|---|---|---|---|
| Interstitial Collagenase (55 kDa) | 1 | Epithelial cells Connective tissue cells | Collagens I, II, III |
| Neutrophil Collagenase (75 kDa) | 8 | Neutrophils | Collagens I, II, III |
| Collagenase-3 (48 kDa) | 13 | ? Breast carcinomas | Collagens I, II, III |
| 72-kDa Collagenase | 2 | Interstitial cells Type II cells | Collagens IV, V, VI, XI; denatured collagens; E; EN; FN |
| 92-dKa Collagenase | 9 | Macrophages Eosinophils and neutrophils Epithelial cells | Same as MMP-2 |
| Stromelysin-1 (57 kDa) | 3 | Connective tissue cells Macrophages | Collagens IX, IV; denatured collagens LM, FN |
| Stromelysin-2 (57 kDa) | 10 | Epithelial cells | Same as MMP-3 |
| Matrilysin (PUMP; 28 kDa) | 7 | Activated epithelial cells Mononuclear phagocytes | Collagen IV; denatured collagens; FN, LM, PG, E, EN |
| Macrophage Metalloelastase | 12 | Macrophages | E, Collagen IV, denatured collagens |

[a]Standardized nomenclature for matrix metalloproteinases.
[b]Abbreviations: E, elastin; EN, entactin; FN, fibronectin; PG, proteoglycans; laminin, LM.

 

The gene expression and production of collagen-degrading enzymes can be modulated by a variety of hormones; growth factors such as fibroblast growth factor (FGF), TGF-$\beta$, and epidermal growth factor (EGF); and matrix components (53), and are likely subject to complex regulation within specific anatomical compartments during lung development. For example, Ganser et al. (54) demonstrated that EGF and TGF-$\alpha$ inhibited airway branching in lung rudiments. These effects were associated with an increase in the activity of 72-kDa collagenase, which can degrade types IV and V collagen, and are specifically inhibited with exogenous TIMP. TIMP activity is also subject to developmental regulation in the lung. For example, TIMP-1 expression was detectable in fetal baboon lung but showed a marked increase immediately after birth (55).

## IV.  Involvement of Collagens in Lung Development

There are striking changes in the expression of specific collagens within specific anatomical compartments during specific periods of lung development. Regulated deposition of specific collagen types contributes to airway branching and bronchial chondrogenesis, alveolar multiplication, and pulmonary angiogenesis as well as to subsequent growth and remodeling of the various anatomical compartments of the lung. Collagens may also play important informational roles in branching morphogenesis. Furthermore, cell culture studies suggest that collagen can modulate pneumocyte differentiation and function in vitro, suggesting that similar interactions may contribute to the regulation of epithelial differentiation.

### A.  Collagens and Branching Morphogenesis

Classic in vitro studies of airway branching, and ultrastructural studies of embryonic lung suggested a critical role for interstitial fibrous collagens in regulating airway branching. Branching of isolated lung rudiments was inhibited by certain inhibitors of collagen production such as *cis*-hydroxyproline, azetadine-2-carboxylic acid, and 2,2'-dipyridyl, or by collagen-degrading enzymes (56). Because quarter-staggered interstitial collagen fibers accumulate between branch points, it was inferred that type I collagen was the critical regulatory molecule. However, the independence of this aspect of morphogenesis from type I collagen has been definitively established in more recent experiments. Specifically, mice carrying an insertional null mutation of the type I collagen gene show normal airway branching in vivo (57).

Although the specificity of the prolyl analogues and collagenase enzymes used for these studies can be questioned, the effects of 2,2'-dipyridyl still strongly suggest that the synthesis of one or more collagenous proteins contributes to the regulation of airway branching. Basement membrane collagens, which are elaborated both by the epithelium and mesenchymal cells, are possible candidates. In this regard, electron microscopic studies of embryonic mouse lung show numerous discontinuities of the basement membrane near sites of branching which appear to permit direct interactions between epithelial cells and underlying mesenchymal cells and matrix (58,59). However, recent in situ hybridization studies failed to demonstrate any regional differences in proα1(IV) mRNA expression by mesenchymal or epithelial cells in branching rudiments, suggesting that regional differences in type IV synthesis are not required for branching (60). Although studies examining the expression of transcripts for the other type IV chains are required, it seems reasonable to speculate that the discontinuities form secondary to localized basement membrane degradation rather than regional differences in assembly. Finally, studies of branching morphogenesis of mouse submandibular gland have emphasized the possible importance of regional differences in type III collagen accumulation (61).

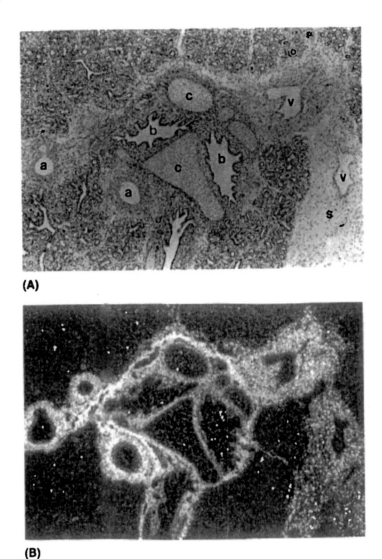

**(A)**

**(B)**

**Figure 1** Type I Procollagen in situ hybridization. (A, B) Canalicular period. Human lung shows strong labeling of arterial wall, bronchial adventitia, perichondrium, veins (v), and septum (s). (A) brightfield microscopy; (B) darkfield microscopy; a, artery; b, bronchus; c, cartilage (original magnification ×100). (C,D) Alveolar period. Muscular arteries of human lung show strong adventitial mRNA signal and weaker signal in the muscularis. (C) brightfield microscopy; (D) darkfield microscopy; a, artery; b, bronchiole (original magnification ×100). (E,F) Alveolar period. Strong PCI mRNA message is present in the lining mesothelium (arrowhead) and submesothelial cells (arrow) of human lung. (E) brightfield microscopy; (F) darkfield microscopy (original magnification ×200). (G,H) Alveolar period. Alveolar septae and crests (arrow) show strong signal in human lung (original magnification ×400). (From ref. 18.)

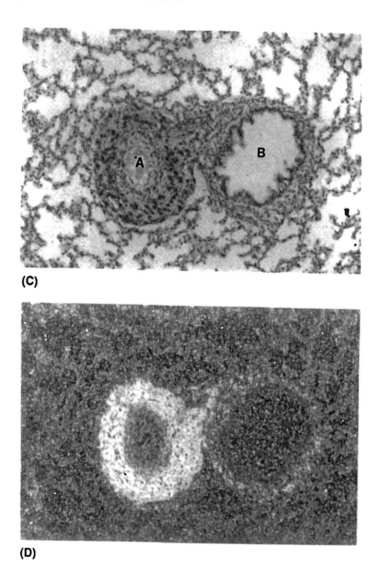

(C)

(D)

In any case, more recent organ culture studies indicate that noncollagenous matrix glycoproteins such as laminin and fibronectin also mediate critical interactions of mesenchyme with epithelial cell surface receptors (62). There is also indirect evidence that matrix expression at these sites is modulated by local expression of cytokines such as TGF-β (63). Thus, branching events likely involve the complex interactions between various collagenous and noncollagenous proteins associated with the periepithelial mesenchyme.

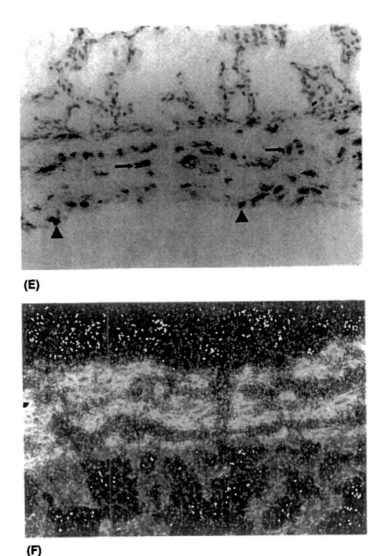

**(E)**

**(F)**

**Figure 1** Continued

## B. Collagens and the Development of Bronchial Cartilage

The pattern of collagen gene expression and matrix deposition appears to be modulated during airway development, with sequential changes occurring along the proximal-distal axis. During the early phase of cartilage development (±14 weeks), both perichondrial mesenchymal cells and chondrocytes show strong

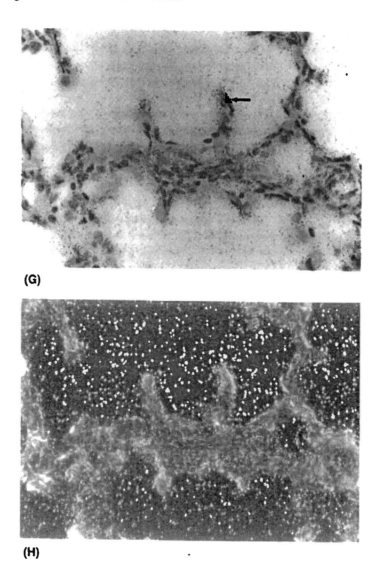

(G)

(H)

cellular expression of type I procollagen, as assessed by in situ hybridization, with an associated diffuse accumulation of procollagen epitopes in the surrounding matrices (18) (Fig. 1A,B). Subsequently, type I procollagen expression appears to be gradually extinguished within the cartilage beginning in the central regions of the largest plates. By 16 weeks, the central regions of the cartilage of the large lobar bronchi show no evidence of type I transcription with only weak staining of the central regions of the cartilagenous matrix. By contrast, the more distal cartilagenous airways continue to show diffuse cartilage staining for type I pro-collagen epitopes. During the late phase, matrix staining persists only at the periphery of the more distal plates. Presumably, decreases in type I expression are accompanied by an increase in the expression of type II procollagen, which is the predominant collagen synthesized in bronchial and tracheal cartilage during late fetal development (19). The perichondrium shows strong type I expression and procollagen accumulation throughout gestation and could still be detected in the postnatal lung.

### C.  Collagens and Pulmonary Vascular Development

Type I collagen, and presumably other interstitial and basement membrane col-lagens (types III, V, IV, VIII), are expressed throughout fetal vascular develop-ment. Beginning in the late early phase, individual compartments within the walls of the largest vessels can be readily identified. Throughout the remainder of gestation, the highest levels of type I gene expression and associated procollagen accumulation are found in the adventitia, with much weaker labeling of the media (18,64) (see Fig. 1A–D).

As observed for airway cartilage, the expression of type I procollagen in the pulmonary arteries appears to show complex regulation along the proximal-distal axis, as well as within specific compartments of the vascular wall. For example, the ratio of medial to adventitial labeling appears highest in the large elastic arteries and lowest in small muscular arteries, and expression appears to decrease first in the largest pulmonary arteries. Very little transcription is seen in the intima and any time of development. The expression of type I procollagen and pro-collagen accumulation also accompanies microvascular proliferation during the canalicular phase and is spatially concentrated near zones of crest formation (18) (see Fig. 1G–H).

### D.  Collagen and Pleural Development

Type I procollagen is expressed at high levels by submesothelial mesenchymal cells throughout fetal and early postnatal lung development (18) (see Fig. 1E,F). Particularly strong signals for procollagen mRNA and numerous immunoreactive connective tissue cells are seen as the submesothelial compartment expands during the late pseudoglandular period. Interestingly, there is also procollagen expression and production of immunoreactive protein by surface cuboidal meso-thelial cells, particularly during the pseudoglandular period and late gestation. The latter observation suggests that the lining epithelium may also contribute to the formation of the submesothelial fibrous matrix. During late gestation and the early postnatal period, pleural mesenchymal cells, together with connective tissue cells in the vascular adventitias and perichondrium, constitute the major cellular sites of type I procollagen gene expression.

### E.  Collagens and Alveolar Epithelial Differentiation

Matrix can in turn modify the morphology and biosynthetic phenotype of type II cells in culture (65–67). The differentiated phenotype of type II cells, which is rapidly lost by freshly isolated cells maintained on plastic in the presence of serum, is partially retained when cells are plated on certain defined matrices. Matrix components can markedly influence the morphology of alveolar epithelial cells; type II cells remain cuboidal on basement membrane components or contracting collagen gels, but they show marked spreading on fibronectin and certain other matrix components.

Although the nature of the cell and matrix interactions that contribute to lung development and cellular differentiation have not been defined, it seems likely that there are developmentally regulated interactions involving basement membrane as well as interstitial matrix components. Localized discontinuities in the basement membrane beneath cuboidal cells lining the primitive air spaces increase dramatically during late gestation—roughly correlating with the appearance of ultrastructurally identifiable type II cells and the onset of surfactant secretion (68,69). These discontinuities are sometimes associated with the formation of contacts between the surface epithelial cells and mesenchymal cells or other formed elements of the interstitial matrix. Thus, the discontinuities could modulate critical cell-cell or cell-matrix interactions. Local alterations in the subepithelial matrix could also modulate local concentrations of matrix associated growth factors such as basic FGF.

It is unclear whether the development of basement membrane discontinuities are primary or secondary events associated with epithelial differentiation. However, it is probable that they form as a consequence of localized basment membrane degradation mediated by the local elaboration of specific matrix-degrading metalloproteinases. For example, late fetal development in rats is associated with an increase in type IV collagen–degrading activity, which is associated with increased levels of 72-kDa collagenase (MMP-2) mRNA and increased enzyme activity by zymography (70). During this same period, there is no detectable increase in interstitial collagenase activity (70). The cellular source(s) of the MMP-2 have not been extablished. However, active 72- and 92-kDa gelatinases and TIMP are elaborated by adult rat type II cells in culture (71).

### F.  Mechanisms of Cellular Interactions with Collagens

Interactions of cells with the collagen matrix may play important roles in lung matrix metabolism by participating in the regulation of the synthesis and secretion of collagenous and noncollagenous proteins, by organizing the extracellular matrix, and by regulating the secretion and activity of various processing or degradative enzymes. Matrix receptors capable of interacting with collagens have been identified in association with lung epithelial cells in vivo and with isolated pneumocytes. These include integrins such as $\alpha 2\beta 1$ (72,73). Developmentally regulated alterations in the expression of such receptors could contribute to structural remodeling during development.

## V.  Elastic Fibers

The physiological importance of elastic fibers lies in the unique elastomeric properties of elastin, which is the protein that forms the functional component of the mature fiber. Elastin is of particular importance to the structural integrity and function of tissues in which reversible extensibility or deformability are crucial, such as the major arterial vessels, the lung, and the skin. The elastic fiber in lung, as well as in other tissues, is a complex structure that consists of two morphologically distinguishable components: 10- to 12-nm microfibrils that define fiber location and morphology and an abundant amorphous-appearing core formed by the protein elastin (74,75).

### A.  Elastin

Elastin is secreted from the cell as a soluble protein of approximately 70,000 molecular weight called tropoelastin. It has a low content of acidic amino acids and is correspondingly rich in hydrophobic amino acids, particularly valine. One third of the residues are glycine and one ninth are proline, and there is no methionine, tryptophan, histidine, or hydroxylysine, although small amounts of hydroxyproline are present. In the past few years, the complete amino acid sequence of tropoelastin from many different species has been determined (reviewed in refs. 76 and 77). These studies confirm that the tropoelastin molecule consists, for the most part, of alternating hydrophobic and cross-linking domains (Fig. 2).

#### Cross-Linking Domains

Of tropoelastin's 40 lysine residues, approximately 35 will serve as cross links. The domains in elastin that contain the cross-linking residues are of two types, with the most prevalent consisting of lysine pairs located in alanine-rich sequences. In the second type, proline or other hydrophobic residues are found between and around the lysines instead of the usual alanines. All but one of these proline-containing cross linking regions are found in the amino one third of the molecule (78).

Like cross links in collagen, cross links in elastin are formed through the oxidative deamination of lysine side chains in a reaction catalyzed by the enzyme lysyl oxidase (79). The reactive aldehyde that is formed by the deamination reaction condenses with a second aldehyde residue to form allysine aldol or with

## Tropoelastin

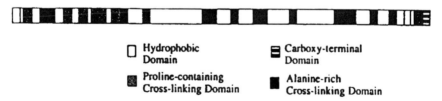

☐ Hydrophobic
   Domain

▦ Proline-containing
   Cross-linking Domain

◧ Carboxy-terminal
   Domain

■ Alanine-rich
   Cross-linking Domain

**Figure 2**  Domain structure of the bovine tropoelastin. The tropoelastin molecule consists of alternating cross-linking and hydrophobic domains. The cross-linking domains are either enriched in alanine or contain proline and hydrophobic residues. The carboxyterminus of the moledule is responsible for interactions with microfilbrils during elastic fiber assembly.

an ε-amino group on lysine to form dehydrolysinonorleucine. Allysine aldol and dehydrolysinonorleucine can then interact to form the pyridinium cross links desmosine and isodesmosine, both of which in vertebrates are unique to elastin and can be used as distinctive markers for the protein (reviewed in ref. 80). Gray (81) has proposed that the first step in desmosine formation is the creation of bifunctional "within chain" cross links which then condense "between chains" to form the tetrafunctional desmosines. This requirement for within chain cross-link intermediates is an intriguing explanation for why lysine residues in elastin occur in pairs. Several studies have documented that lysine residues in alanine-rich regions of the molecules are correctly positioned for side chain interaction (82,83). Lysine residues in the proline-rich domains, however, may serve to form cross links other than desmosine (84).

### Hydrophobic Domains

The hydrophobic domains of elastin are thought to contribute to the protein's ability to undergo elastic recoil (82,85). These domains are enriched in glycine and bulky hydrophobic amino acids (valine, leucine, and isoleucine) and most likely adopt β-turn structures (82,85). The unusually high hydrophobicity of these domains has led to models of elasticity that take into account the possibility that nonpolar side chains are exposed to water when elastin is stretched. Recoil then occurs when the nonpolar groups reaggregate and expel the water after the distending force is removed (86).

### Microfibril Interaction Domain

Another important domain is found at the carboxyterminus of the tropoelastin molecule. This domain contains the protein's only two cysteine residues which are disulfide bonded to form a loop structure and a highly basic pocket (87). In vitro studies have demonstrated that this domain mediates interactions between tropoelastin and microfibrillar components during assembly of the elastic fiber (88). Tropoelastin molecules that lack the carboxyterminus are not incorporated into fibers (89).

### Elastin Gene Structure and Regulation

Elastin is encoded by a single gene, situated in the human on the long arm of chromosome 7 (90). Expression of the elastin gene has been shown to be modulated by a variety of factors, including TGF-$\beta$, tumor necrosis factor-$\alpha$, insulin-like growth factor-1, various glucocorticosteroids, vitamin $D_3$ basic FGF, cyclic nucleotides, and retinoic acid (91–99). This regulation can occur at both the transcriptional and posttranscriptional levels. TGF-$\beta$, for example, has been shown to stabilize elastin mRNA resulting in increased steady-state levels (93). Furthermore, downregulation of elastin production by vitamin $D_3$ has been suggested to result from destabilization and increased turnover of elastin mRNA (99). Interleukin-1$\beta$ (IL-1$\beta$), in contrast, has been shown to increase elastin gene expression at the promoter level (100). A more complete discussion of transcriptional and posttranscription regulation of the elastin gene can be found in several recent reviews (77,101–103).

### Degradation and Turnover of Elastin

Elastin is one of the most stable proteins in the body, with a half-life approaching that of the animal (80,104–106). Thus, under normal conditions, very little remodeling of elastic fibers occurs in adult life. Increased elastin destruction does take place in certain pathological conditions either as a result of the release of powerful elastinolytic serine proteases (elastases) from inflammatory cells or bacteria or through the genetic deficiency of a naturally occurring elastase inhibitor such as in $\alpha_1$-antitrypsin deficiency. Although elastases from bacteria and inflammatory cells are unlikely to play a significant role in the normal regulation of the elastic matrix, it is clear that they contribute substantially to the pathogenesis of some human diseases, including pulmonary emphysema (reviewed in ref. 107), pollutional lung disease, atherosclerosis, and rheumatoid arthritis. Reactivation of elastin synthesis is observed in some disease states, although this often proceeds in a morphologically disordered manner with subsequent impairment of normal physiological functioning, as exemplified by the studies of Kuhn et al. (108) of elastase-induced emphysema in hamsters and in studies Fukuda et al. (109) of patients with emphysema.

There are many possible sources of elastolytic enzymes in the lung, including bacteria, inflammatory cells, and lung cells themselves. Neutrophil and macrohage elastases are of particular importance in this regard, and they have been the subject of much recent study. Full discussion of this subject is, however, outside the scope of this chapter, and reviews by Bieth (110), Shapiro et al. (111) and Snider et al. (112) should be consulted for further details.

## VI.  Microfibrils

Microfibrils are thought to align tropoelastin molecules in precise register so that cross linking regions are juxtaposed prior to oxidation by lysyl oxidase. This conclusion is based mostly on ultrastructural studies that show elastin molecules accumulate within bundles of microfibrils in developing tissues (74,75). Although the composition of microfibrils has proven difficult to determine, several constituent protein have recently been isolated and characterized. These proteins have interesting biological properties that suggest microfibrils have important functions in addition to their role in elastic fiber assembly.

Recently, three glycoproteins have been characterized that appear to be true constituents of microfibrils; ~350-kDa glycoproteins in the fibrillin family (113), a 31-kDa glycoprotein termed microfibril-associated glycoprotein (MAGP) (114), and a 58-kDa protein that is posttranslationally modified to a 32-kDa fragment called associated-microfibril protein (AMP) (115). Other proteins have been found to associated with microfibrils in some tissues, although their biological function has yet to be established. Microfibrils also associate with a number of other nonconstitutive proteins, including fibronectin (116), amyloid P component (117,118), and vitronectin (119).

### A.  Fibrillins

Fibrillin is found in nearly all tissues of the body as 10- to 12-nm microfibrils (113). Two fibrillin proteins have been identified that are encoded for by genes on human chromosomes 15 (fibrillin-1) and 5 (fibrillin-2). Interestingly, mutations in the fibrillin-1 gene have been linked to the connective tissue disease known as the Marfan syndrome (120,121), whereas mutations in fibrillin-2 have been linked to a Marfan-like syndrome, called congenital contractural arachnodactyly (122). The domain structure of the fibrillin family is shown in Figure 3. The molecules are made up of repeating domains that have homology to EGF and TGF-$\beta$1 binding protein. Several EGF-like repeats in fibrillin also have homology with the *Notch* gene in *Drosophila* and the *lin-12* gene in *C. elegans*. These repeats contain consensus sequences which have been associated with hydroxylation of asparagine or aspartic acid residues and participate in calcium binding (123). Furthermore, both fibrillin-1 and fibrillin-2 contain RGD sequences suggesting the potential for interaction with integrin receptors on the cell surface. In situ hybridization studies with developing mouse embryos have shown that fibrillin-2 expression occurs earlier in development than fibrillin-1 (discussed below). Accumulation of

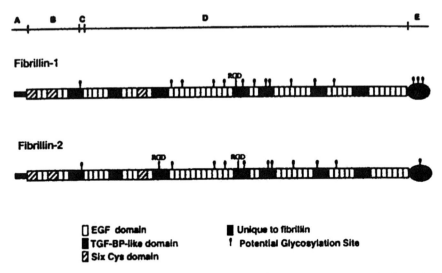

**Figure 3** Schematic diagram of fibrillin-1 and fibrillin-2. Letters at the top indicate the five structurally distinct regions of the molecule. The repeating structural elements are defined at the bottom of the figure as EGF-like calcium binding domains (EGF-CB), transforming growth factor-β binding protein–like domains (TGF-BP), and domains with structures unique to fibrillin. The location of RGD sequences and putative glycosylation sites are shown.

fibrillin-2 transcripts plateaus just before overt tissue differentiation and rapidly decreases or even disappears thereafter. In contrast, the amount of fibrillin-1 transcripts increases at an gradual rate throughout morphogenesis (124).

### B. Microfibril-Associated Glycoprotein

MAGP is a small (~20 kDa) glycoprotein that lacks the repeating domain structure characteristic of tropoelastin and fibrillin. There are, however, two structurally distinct regions in MAGP; an aminoterminal domain rich in glutamine, proline, and acidic amino acids and a carboxyterminal domain containing all 13 of the cysteine residues and most of the basic amino acids (114). Immunofluorescence and immunogold localization of MAGP with affinity purified antibodies has shown the distribution of the glycoprotein to correspond to that of both elastin- and nonelastin-associated microfibrils from a wide variety of tissues (125,126). Like fibrillin, the exact function and organization of MAGP within the microfibril structure is not known, although recent evidence suggests that it serves to bind elastin onto the microfibril during elastic fiber assembly (88). MAGP is also a substrate for transglutaminase, which may provide a mechanism for covalently linking microfibrillar components into a stable polymer (88).

In situ hybridization studies of MAGP expression in the developing mouse embryo found widespread expression in mesenchymal tissues as early as 8.5 days. At 13.5 days, MAGP expression was highest with strong hybridization occurring in loose connective tissues as well as the interstitium of the wall of the pulmonary artery and aorta, lung, and other tissues. Signal was not detected in the liver, heart, brain, and spinal cord (127). Interestingly, fibrillin-1 expression was not detected in the day 9 embryo, but after day 9 resembled expression of MAGP. These differences in gene expression are of interest becaue they suggest that the composition of microfibrils may vary during development and within different tissues.

## VII. Expression of Elastic Fiber Proteins in Developing Lung

### A. Tropoelastin Gene Expression

Elastogenesis in the lung has been extensively studied with the light and electron microscopes (1,4,128–130). Because most of the classic histological stains used to visualize elastin only interact with mature elastic fibers, newly deposited elastic fibers may not be detected using these reagents. To address this problem, in situ hybridization techniques have been employed to investigate more thoroughly elastin gene expression in the developing lung.

#### Elastin Expression and Vascular Development

Hybridization of fetal bovine lung from the pseudoglandular phase with a probe specific for tropoelastin showed that the strongest signal was associated with the muscular layer of large arteries (Fig. 4A,B). Similar findings were observed in developing rat lung where tropoelastin expression was first detected during the pseudoglandular stage (17 days) in the pulmonary vasculature and the bronchiolar wall (131).

During the ensuing canalicular period, the strongest signal was associated with the muscularis of arteries accompanying large cartilagenous airways, with weaker labeling of smaller vessels (see Fig. 4E,F). However, signal within the muscular wall was nonuniform, with larger numbers of strongly labeled cells concentrated in the outermost muscular layers. In addition, in the bovine lung, the largest arteries showed very strong labeling of the endothelium. The signal decreased along the proximal-distal axis with weak or no labeling present in the walls of arteries accompanying small bronchioles. Interestingly, the signal sometimes appeared to decrease abruptly near a branch point (see Fig. 4E,F). Signal was consistently identified in the walls of large veins, often in preferential association with the endothelium.

During the terminal sac/alveolar periods, a strong signal was still present in

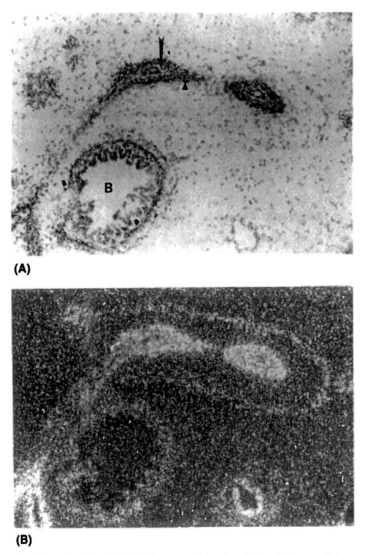

**(A)**

**(B)**

**Figure 4**  Tropoelastin in situ hybridization. (A,B) Pseudoglandular period. Strong signal is present in the vascular wall (arrow) and stromal cells at the periphery of the vessels (arrowhead) in bovine lung. Bronchus (B); (A) brightfield microscopy; (B) brightfield microscopy (original magnification ×100). (C,D) Pseudoglandular period. Bovine lung shows strong labeling in the bronchial wall (W) and perichondrium (arrow) of large bronchi. Bronchial lumen (L); (C) brightfield microscopy; (D) darkfield microscopy (original magnification ×100). (E,F) Canalicular period. Human lung shows strong mRNA signal in the arterial muscularis. The intensity signal decreases in smaller branches. (E) brightfield microscopy; (F) darkfield microscopy (original magnification ×100). (G,H) Alveolar period. Labeling is present in alveolar septa (arrow) and crests (arrowhead) of bovine lungs. (G) brightfield microscopy; (H) darkfield microscopy (original magnification ×400).

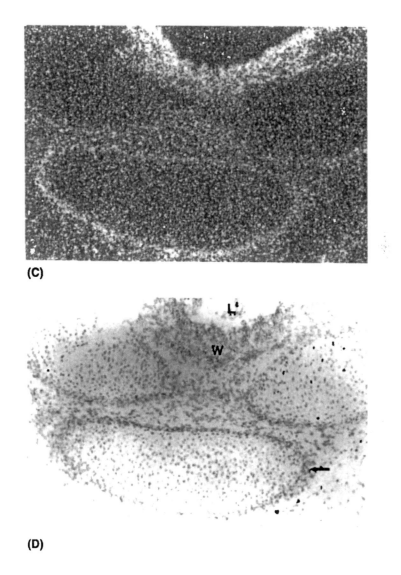

(C)

(D)

the muscularis and endothelium of elastic arteries. Weaker signal was also identi-fied in the muscular arteries, with focal labeling present in the adventitia of some vessels. In all species studied, peak elastin production occurs during the prenatal period. Tropoelastin production begins to decline in a pattern suggesting that cells in the outer layers of the vessel wall decrease their elastin production first followed by cells closer to the lumen (131,132).

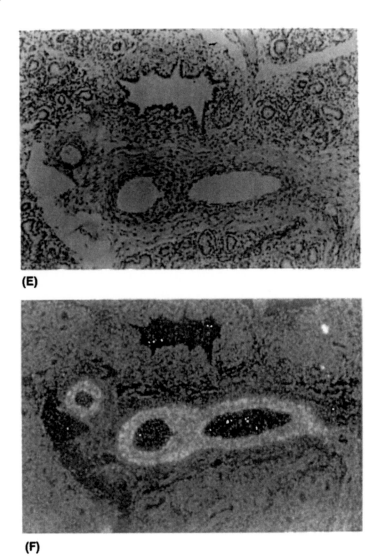

**(E)**

**(F)**

**Figure 3** Continued

### Elastin Expression and Alveolarization

Labeling also accompanied microvascular proliferation and alveolarization during the canalicular period. There was particularly strong labeling at sites of crest formation and at the septum where the airsac is formed (see Fig. 4G,H). In the rat, a variable degree of tropoelastin gene expression was observed at sites of septation (131). Spindle-shape cells subjacent to the epithelium at the tip of the septum

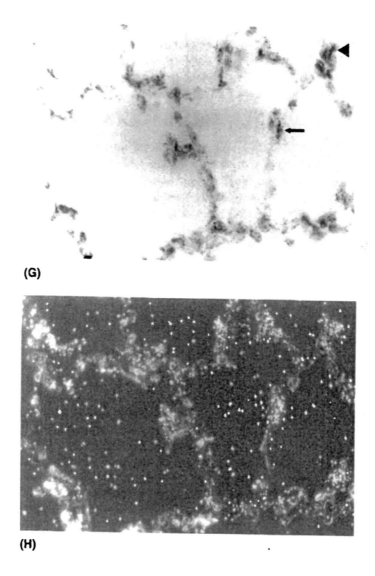

(G)

(H)

produced the most elastin. However, mesenchymal cells more remote from the septal tip showed a weak or negative hybridization signal, suggesting differentiation of a subset of elastogenic cells within the mesenchyme. Tropoelastin expression continued at the septal tips, reaching peak levels at postnatal days 7 and 11, which coincided with the peak of alveolarization.

### Elastin Expression in Large Airways and Pleura

Moderately strong labeling of was evident in the perichondrium of bronchial cartilage (see Fig. 4C,D) during the pseudoglandular phase. Only a weak signal was identified in the bronchial smooth muscle layer. Labeling of the perichondrium persisted in the canalicular period. In addition, there was weak to moderate labeling of cells associated with the muscularis of the large bronchi. In general, the intensity of labeling appeared to decrease along the proximal to distal axis. Although the pleural compartment is not well developed early in the pseudoglandular period, a weak signal was also identified in mesothelial cells of bovine lung. In the rat, pleural labeling was first observed in the canalicular period and persisted into the postnatal period (131).

### B.  Fibrillin Gene Expression

With the cloning and characterization of microfibrillar components, it is now possible to study their expression in developing lung using in situ hybridization. Zhang et al. (124) have recently studied fibrillin-1 and fibrillin-2 expression in developing mouse embryos. At 10.5 days gestation when lung buds are rapidly elongating, a strong fibrillin-2 signal was detected in the epithelial layer of the budding main bronchi along with a weaker and more diffuse signal in the primitive mesenchyme (Fig. 5A). A similarly weak fibrillin-1 signal was seen in the mesenchymal cells of the lung without additional expression in the bronchial epithelium (Fig. 5B). By day 13, branching of the segmental bronchi is the predominant feature of the forming lungs, and at this stage, the two fibrillin mRNAs accumulated to comparable levels in the mesenchyme. However, fibrillin-2 transcripts were seen in the epithelium of the developing segmental and main bronchi (Fig. 5E,G). At stage 16.5, the lungs are still compact and terminal bronchi lined with cuboidal cells begin to appear. Segmental bronchi at this stage displayed little fibrillin-2 mRNA accumulation, whereas the epithelial cells of the sprouting terminal bronchi were now the most active sites (Fig. 5I). Except for an increased but still low level of expression in the mesenchyme, fibrillin-1 transcripts could not be detected in the bronchial epithelium of this embryonic stage (Fig. 5J). The results of this study clearly suggest that (1) fibrillin-2 is selectively expressed in bronchial epithelium during the formation of bronchi, (2) both fibrillins are expressed by lung mesenchymal cells, and (3) the fibrillin-1/fibrillin-2 ratio progressively increases during the transition from the early to the late phases of lung morphogenesis.

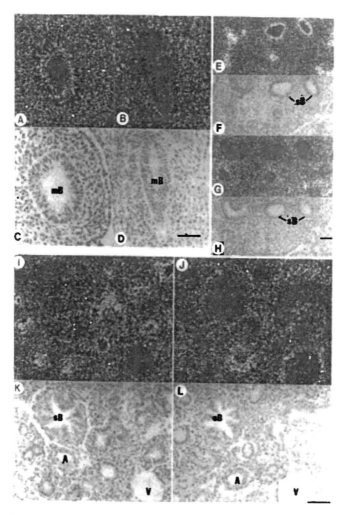

**Figure 5** In situ hybridization of developing lung in a 10.5-day (A–D), 13.5-day (E–H), and 16.5-day (I–L) mouse embryo with probe for fibrillin-2 (A,E,I) and fibrillin-1 (B,G,J). The epithelial cells of the main bronchi (mB), segmental bronchi (sB), and terminal bronchioles (arrow) specifically express fibrillin-2. By day 16.5, fibrillin-2 is no longer expressed in the segmental bronchi. Expression of fibrillin-1 at all stages is mostly in the lung parenchyma, arteriole (A), and venules (V). Bar, 50 μm. (From ref. 124.)

## VIII.   Questions and Future Strategies

Our knowledge of specific lung collagens and elastic fiber components, as well as the potential mechanisms responsible for regulating their production and turnover, have increased dramatically since the first edition of Development of the Lung. However, remarkably little is still known about the specific cellular and molecular events involved in regulating the assembly and turnover of collagenous and elastic matrices within various matrix compartments during the course of lung development. Specifically, how are the appropriate temporal and spatial expression of matrix proteins, matrix receptors, matrix-degrading enzymes and inhibitors, and growth factors regulated? Assuming that proximal-distal gradients (or regulatory blocks) of matrix protein gene expression contribute to airway and vascular development, how are these gradients generated? Are there specific homeotic gene products that participate in regulating positional differences in collagen and elastin gene expression?

Major advances in our understanding could come from fairly straightforward, although tedious and time-consuming, experiments that apply available molecular and immunological reagents to examine the expression of potentially interrelated gene products in appropriately processed human tissues of various known gestational ages. Genetic or functional knockouts of specific growth factors, growth factor receptors, and metalloproteinases should also provide important insights.

## References

1.  Loosli CG, Potter EL. Pre- and postnatal development of the respiratory portion of the human lung. Am Rev Respir Dis 1959; 80:5–23.
2.  Fukuda Y, Ferrans VJ, Crystal RG. Development of elastic fibers of nuchal ligament, aorta, and lung of fetal and postnatal sheep: An ultrastructural and electron microscopic immunohistochemical study. Am J Anat 1984; 170:597–629.
3.  Noguchi A, Reddy R, Kursar JD, Parks WC, Mecham RP. Smooth muscle isoactin and elastin in fetal bovine lung. Exp Lung Res 1989; 15:537–552.
4.  Fukuda Y, Ferrans VJ, Crystal RG. The development of alveolar septa in fetal sheep lung. An ultrastructural and immunohistochemical study. Am J Anat 1983; 167: 405–439.
5.  Emery JL. The postnatal development of the human lung and its implication for lung pathology. Respiration 1970; 27(suppl):41–50.
6.  Mercer RR, Crapo JD. Spatial distribution of collagen and elastin fibers in the lungs. J Appl Physiol 1990; 69:756–765.
7.  Burgeson RE, Nimni ME. Basic science and pathology. Collagen types: molecular structure and tissue distribution. Clin Orthoop 1992; 282:250–272.
8.  Hance AJ, Crystal RG. The connective tissue of lung. Am Rev Respir Dis 1975; 112:657–711.

9. Mayne R, Brewton RG. New members of the collagen superfamily. Curr Opin Cell Biol 1993; 5:883–890.

10. van der Rest M, Garrone R. Collagen family of proteins. FASEB J 1991; 5:2814–2823.

11. Oh SP, Kamagata Y, Muragaki Y, Timmons S, Ooshima A, Olsen BR. Isolation and sequencing of cDNAs for proteins with multiple domains of Gly-Xaa-Yaa repeats identify a distinct family of collagenous proteins. Proc Natl Acad Sci USA 1994; 91:4229–4233.

12. Amenta PS, Gil J, Martinez-Hernandez A. Connective tissue of rat lung. II: Ultra-structural localization of collagen types III, IV, and VI. J Histochem Cytochem 1988; 36:1167–1173.

13. Gil J, Martinez-Hernandez A. The connective tissue of the rat lung: electron immu-nohistochemical studies. J Histochem Cytochem 1984; 32:230–238.

14. Madri JA, Furthmayr H. Collagen polymorphism in the lung. An immunochemical study of pulmonary fibrosis. Hum Pathol 1980; 11:353–366.

15. Raghu G, Striker LJ, Hudson LD, Striker GE. Extracellular matrix in normal and fibrotic human lungs. Am Rev Respir Dis 1985; 131:281–289.

16. Bateman E, Turner-Warwick M, Adelmann-Grill BC. Immunohistochemical study of collagen types in human foetal lung and fibrotic lung disease. Thorax 1981; 36:645–653.

17. Burgeson RE. New collagens, new concepts. Annu Rev Cell Biol 1988; 4:551–577.

18. Davila RM, deMello D, Crouch EC. Ontogeny of type I procollagen expression during human fetal lung development. Am J Physiol 1995; 268(Lung Cell Mol Physiol 12):L309–L320.

19. Bradley K, McConnell-Breul S, Crystal RG. Lung collagen heterogeneity. Proc Natl Acad Sci USA 1974; 71:2828–2832.

20. Crouch EC, Chang D. Deposition and cross-linking of newly synthesized type IV procollagen in lung matrix. Am Rev Respir Dis 1987; 136:281–287.

21. Crouch EC, Moxley MA, Longmore WJ. Matrix deposition and extracellular proc-essing of newly synthesized collagens in the isolated perfused rat lung. Exp Lung Res 1988; 14:705–724.

22. Cheung DT, DiCesare P, Benya PD, Libaw E, Nimni ME. The presence of inter-molecular disulfide cross-links in type III collagen. J Biol Chem 1983; 258:7774–7778.

23. Clark JG, Kuhn C, McDonald JA, Mecham RP. Lung connective tissue. Int Rev Connect Tissue Res 1983; 10:249–330.

24. DiMari SJ, Howe AM, Haralson MA. Effects of transforming growth factor-beta on collagen synthesis by fetal rat lung epithelial cells. Am J Respir Cell Mol Biol 1991; 4:455–462.

25. Sandberg MM, Hirvonen HE, Elima KJ, Vuorio EI. Co-expression of collagens II and XI and alternative splicing of exon 2 of collagen II in several developing human tissues. Biochem J 1993; 294:595–602.

26. Horton WE, Wang L, Bradham D, Precht P, Balakir R. The control of expression of Type II collagen: relevance to cartilage disease. DNA Cell Biol 1992; 11:193–198.

27. Liu CY, Olsen BR, Kao WW. Developmental patterns of two alpha 1(IX) collagen mRNA isoforms in mouse. Dev Dyn 1993; 198:150–157.

28. Wetzels RHW, Schaafsma HE, Leigh IM, Lane EB, Troyanovsky SM, Wagenaar C, Vooijs GP, Ramaekers FCS. Laminin and type VII collagen distribution in different types of human lung carcinoma: correlation with expression of keratins 14, 16, 17, and 18. Histopathology 1992; 20:295–303.

29. Marinkovich MP, Keene DR, Rimberg CS, Burgeson RE. Cellular origin of the dermal-epidermal basement membrane. Dev Dyn 1993; 197:255–267.

30. Hudson BG, Reeders ST, Tryggvason K. Type IV collagen: structure, gene organization, and role in human disease. J Biol Chem 1993; 268:26033–26036.

31. Yoshioka K, Hino S, Takemura T, Maki S, Wieslander J, Takekoshi Y, Makino H, Kagawa M, Sado Y, Kashtan CE. Type IV collagen alpha 5 chain. Normal distribution and abnormalities in X-linked Alport syndrome revealed by monoclonal antibody. Am J Pathol 1994; 144:986–996.

32. Sage H, Farin FM, Striker GE, Fisher AB. Granular pneumocytes in primary culture secrete several major components of the extracellular matrix. Biochemistry 1983; 22:2148–2155.

33. Alitilo K. Product of bath interstitial and basement membrane procollagen by fibroblastic WI-38 cells from human embryonic lung. Biochem Biophys Res Commun 1980; 93:873–880.

34. Chen J-M, Little CD. Cells that emerge from embryonic explants product fibers of type IV collagen. J Cell Biol 1985; 101:1175–1181.

35. Thomas T, Dziadek M. Expression of collagen α1(IV), laminin and nidogen genes in the embryonic mouse lung: implications for branching morphogenesis. Mech Dev 1994; 45:193–201.

36. Blumberg B, Fessler LI, Kurkinen M, Fessler JH. Biosynthesis and supramolecular assembly of procollagen IV in neonatal lung. J Cell Biol 1986; 103:1711–1719.

37. Crouch EC, Quinones F, Chang D. Synthesis of type IV procollagen in lung explants. Am Rev Respir Dis 1986; 133:618–625.

38. Dixit SN, Stuart JM, Seyer JM, Risteli J, Timpl R, and Kang AH. Type IV collagens: isolation and characterization of 7S collagen from human kidney, liver and lung. Collagen Relat Res 1981; 1:549–556.

39. Chen J-M, Little CD. Cellular events associated with lung branching morphogenesis including the deposition of collagen type IV. Dev Biol 1987; 120:311–321.

40. Timpl R. Structure and biological activity of basement membrane proteins. Eur J Biochem 1989; 180:487–502.

41. Von der Mark H, Aumailley M, Wick G, Fleischmajer R, Timpl R. Immunochemistry, genuine size and tissue localization of collagen VI. J Biochem 1984; 142:493–502.

42. Engvall E, Hessle H, Gkier G. Molecular assembly secretion, and matrix deposition of type VI collagen. J Cell Biol 1986; 102:703–710.

43. Timpl R, Engel J. Type VI collagen. In: Mayne R, Burgeson RE, eds. Structure and Function of Collagen Types. Biology of extracellular matrix series. Orlando, FL: Academic Press, 1987:105–140.

44. Smith LT. Patterns of type VI collagen compared to types I, III and IV collagen in human embryonic and fetal skin and in fetal skin-derived cell cultures. Matrix Biol 1994; 14:159–170.

45. Kittelberger R, Davis PF, Flynn DW, Greenhill NS. Distribution of type VIII collagen in tissues: an immunohistochemical study. Connec Tissue Res 1990; 24: 303–318.

46. Sawada H, Konomi H. The alpha 1 chain of type VIII collagen is associated with many but not all microfibrils of elastic fiber system. Cell Struct Func 1991; 16: 455–456.

47. Brenner DA, Westwick J, Breindl M. Type I collagen gene regulation and the molecular pathogenesis of cirrhosis. Am J Physiol 1993; 264:G589–G595.

48. Sandell L, Boyd C. Extracellular Marix Genes. New York: Academic Press, 1989.

49. Slack JL, Liska DJ, Bornstein P. Regulation of expression of Type I collagen genes. Am J Med Genet 1993; 45:140–151.

50. Quaglino D, Fornieri C, Nanney LB, Davidson JM. Extracellular matrix modifications in rat tissues of different ages. Matrix 1993; 13:481–490.

51. Reiser KM, Last JA. A molecular marker for fibrotic collagen in lungs of infants with respiratory distress syndrome. Biochem Med Metab Biol 1987; 37:16–21.

52. Murphy G, Doucherty AJP. The matrix metalloproteinases and their inhibitors. Am J Respir Cell Mol Biol 1992; 7:120–125.

53. Matrisian LM, Hogan BL. Growth factor-regulated proteases and extracellular matrix remodeling during mammalian development. Curr Top Dev Biol 1990; 24: 219–259.

54. Ganser GL, Stricklin GP, Matrisian LM. EGF and TGFα influence *in vitro* lung development by the induction of matrix-degrading metalloproteinases. Int J Dev Biol 1991; 35:453–461.

55. Minoo P, Penn R, DeLemos DM, Coalson JJ, DeLemos RA. Tissue inhibitor of metalloproteinase-1 mRNA is specifically induced in lung tissue after birth. Pediatr Res 1993; 34:729–734.

56. Spooner BS, Thompson-Pletscher HA, Stokes B, Bassett KE. Extracellular matrix involvement in epithelial branching morphogenesis. In. Developmental Biology. Vol. 3. New York: Plenum, 1986:225–260.

57. Kratochwil K, Dziadek M, Löhler J, Harbers K, Jaenisch R. Normal epithelial branching morphogenesis in the absence of collagen 1. Dev Biol 1986; 117: 596–606.

58. Bluemink JG, van Maurik P, Lawson KA. Intimate cell contacts at the epithelial/ mesenchymal interface in embryonic mouse lung. J Ultrastruct Res 1976; 55: 257–270.

59. Jaskoll TF, Slavkin HC. Ultrastructural and immunofluorescence studies of basal-lamina alterations during mouse-lung morphogenesis. Differentiation 1984; 28: 36–48.

60. Thomas T, Dziadek M. Expression of collagen α1(IV), laminin and nidogen genes in the embryonic mouse lung: implications for branching morphogenesis. Mech Dev 1994; 45:193–201.

61. Nakanishi Y, Nogawa H, Hashimoto Y, Kishi JI, Hayakawa T. Accumulation of collagen III at the cleft points of developing mouse submandibular epithelium. Development 1988; 104:51–59.

62. Minoo P, King RJ. Epithelial-mesenchymal interactions in lung development. Annu Rev Physiol 1994; 56:13–45.
63. Heine UI, Munoz EF, Flanders KC, Roberts AB, Sporn MB. Colocalization of TGF-beta 1 and collagen I and III, fibronectin and glycosaminoglycans during lung branching morphogenesis. Development 1990; 109:29–36.
64. Mecham RP, Stenmark KR, Parks WC. Connective tissue production by vascular smooth muscle in development and disease. Chest 1991; 99:43S–47S.
65. Rannels DE, Rannels SR. Influence of the extracellular matrix on type 2 cell differentiation. Chest 1989; 96:165–173.
66. Shannon JM, Mason RJ, Jennings SD. Functional differentiation of alveolar type II epithelial cells *in vitro*: effects of cell shape, cell-matrix interactions and cello-cell interactions. Biochim Biophys Acta 1987; 932:143–156.
67. Shannon JM, Emrie PA, Fisher JH, Kuroki Y, Jennings SD, Mason RJ. Effect of a reconstituted basement membrane on expression of surfactant apoproteins in cultured adult rat alveolar type II cells. Am J Respir Cell Mol Biol 1990; 2:183–192.
68. Adamson IYR. Relationship of mesenchymal changes to alveolar epithelial cell differentiation in fetal rat lung. Anat Embryol 1992; 185:275–280.
69. Grant MM, Cutts NR, Brody JS. Influence of maternal diabetes on basement membranes, Type 2 cells, and capillaries in the developing rat lung. Dev Biol 1984; 104:469–476.
70. Arden MG, Spearman MA, Adamson IYR. Degradation of type IV collagen during the development of fetal rat lung. Am J Respir Cell Mol Biol 1993; 9:99–105.
71. Dunsmore SE, Parks WC, Senior RM, Welgus HG. Type II pulmonary epithelial cells produce matrix metalloproteinases in a differentiation-dependent manner. Am J Respir Cell Mol Biol 1995; 151:802A.
72. Papadopoulos T, Sirtl K, Dammrich J, Muller-Hermelink HK. Pattern of expression of integrins in alveolar epithelia of fetal and adult lungs and interstitial lung disease. Verh Dtsch Ges Pathol 1993; 77:292–295.
73. Zutter MM, Santoro SA. Widespread histologic distribution of the alpha 2 beta 1 integrin cell-surface collagen receptor. Am J Pathol 1990; 137:113–120.
74. Fahrenbach WH, Sandberg LB, Cleary EG. Ultrastructural studies on early elasto-genesis. Anat Rec 1966; 155:563–576.
75. Greenlee TKJ, Ross R, Hartman JL. The fine structure of elastic fibers. J Cell Biol 1966; 30:59–71.
76. Indik Z, Yeh H, Ornstein-Goldstein N, Rosenbloom J. Structure of the elastin gene and alternative splicing of elastin mRNA. In: Sandell L, Boyd C, eds. Genes for Extracellular Matrix Proteins. New York: Academic Press, 1990:221–250.
77. Parks WC, Pierce RA, Lee KA, Mecham RP. Elastin. In: Bittar EE, Kleinman HK, eds. Advances in Cell and Molecular Biology. No. 6. Greenwich, CT: JAI Press Inc. 1993:133–181.
78. Raju K, Anwar RA. Primary structures of bovine elastin a, b, and c deduced from the sequences of cDNA clones. J Biol Chem 1987; 262:5755–5762.
79. Kagan HM, Trackman PC. Properties and function of lysyl oxidase. Am J Respir Cell Mol Biol 1991; 5:206–210.

80. Rucker RB, Dubick MA. Elastin metabolism and chemistry: potential roles in lung development and structure. Environ Health Perspect 1984; 53:179–191.
81. Gray WR. Some kinetic aspects of crosslink biosynthesis. Adv Exp Med Biol 1977; 79:285–290.
82. Gray WR, Sandberg LB, Foster JA. Molecular model for elastin structure and function. Nature 1973; 246:461–466.
83. Mecham RP, Davis EC. Elastic Fiber Structure and Assembly. In: Yurchenko PD, Birk DE, Mecham RP, eds. Extracellular Matrix Assembly and Structure. San Diego: Academic Press, 1994:281–314.
84. Brown-Augsburger P, Broekelmann T, Mecham RP. Domain interactions in elastin crosslinking. 1995 (in press).
85. Urry DW. What is elastin; what is not. Ultrastruct Pathol 1983; 4:227–251.
86. Gosline JM. Hydrophobic interaction and a model for the elasticity of elastin. Biopolymers 1978; 17:677–695.
87. Brown PL, Mecham L, Tisdale C, Mecham R P. The cysteine residues in the carboxy-terminal domain of tropoelastin form an intrachain disulfide bond that stabilizes a loop structure and positively charged pocket. Biochem Biophys Res Commun 1992; 186:549–555.
88. Brown-Augsburger P, Broekelmann T, Mecham L, Mercer R, Gibson M A, Cleary EG, Abrams WR, Rosenbloom J, Mecham R P. Microfibril-associated glycoprotein (MAGP) binds to the carboxy-terminal domain of tropoelastin and is a substrate for transglutaminase. J Biol Chem 1994; 269:28443–28449.
89. Hinek A, Rabinovitch M. The ductus arteriosus migratory smooth muscle phenotype processes tropoelastin to a 52-kDa product associated with impaired assembly of elastic laminae. J Biol Chem 1993; 268:1405–1413.
90. Fazio MJ, Mattei MG, Passage E, Chu M-L, Black D, Solomon E, Davidson JM, Uitto J. Human elastin gene: new evidence for localization to the long arm of chromosome 7. Am J Hum Genet 1991; 48:696–703.
91. Brettell LM, McGowan SE. Basic fibroblast growth factor decreases elastin production by neonatal rat lung fibroblasts. Am J Respir Cell Mol Biol 1994; 10:306–315.
92. Kähäri VM, Chen YQ, Bashir M, Rosenbloom J, Uitto J. Tumor necrosis factor-α down regulates human elastin gene expression. J Biol Chem 1992; 267:26134–26141.
93. Kähäri VM, Olsen DR, Rhudy RW, Carrillo P, Chen YQ, Uitto J. Transforming growth factor-beta up-regulates elastin gene expression in human skin fibroblasts. Evidence for post-transcriptional modulation. Lab Invest 1992; 66:580–588.
94. Liu B, Harvey CS, McGowan SE. Retinoic acid increases elastin in neonatal rat lung fibroblast cultures. Am J Physiol. 1993; 265(5 Pt 1):L430–L437.
95. Liu J-M, Davidson JM. The elastogenic effect of recombinant transforming growth factor-beta on porcine aortic smooth muscle cells. Biophys Biochem Res Commun 1988; 154:895–901.
96. Mecham RP, Foster JA. Trypsin-like neutral protease associated with soluble elastin. Biochemistry 1977; 16:3825–3831.
97. Mecham RP, Levy BD, Morris SL, Madaras JG, Wrenn DS. Increased cyclic GMP

levels lead to a stimulation of elastin production in ligament fibroblasts that is reversed by cyclic AMP. J Biol Chem 1985; 260:3255–3258.

98. Mecham RP, Morris SL, Levy BD, Wrenn DS. Glucocorticoids stimulate elastin production in differentiated bovine ligament fibroblasts but do not induce elastin synthesis in undifferentiated cells. J Biol Chem 1984; 259:12414–12418.

99. Pierce RA, Kolodziej ME, Parks WC. 1,23-Dihydroxyvitamin D3 represses tropo-elastin expression by a posttranscriptional mechanism. J Biol Chem 1992; 267: 11593–11599.

100. Mauviel A, Chen YQ, Kahari VM, Ledo I, Wu M, Rudnicka L, Uitto J. Human recombinant interleukin-1 beta up-regulates elastin gene expression in dermal fibroblasts. Evidence for transcriptional regulation in vitro and in vivo. J Biol Chem 1993; 268:6520–6524.

101. Foster JA, Curtiss SW. The regulation of lung elastin synthesis. Am J Physiol 1990; 259:L13–L23.

102. McGowan SE. Extracellular matrix and the regulation of lung development and repair. FASEB J 1992; 6:2895–2904.

103. Rosenbloom J, Abrams WR, Mecham RP. The elastic fiber. FASEB J 1993; 7:1208–1218.

104. Davis EC. Stability of elastin in the developing mouse aorta: a quantitative radio-autographic study. Histochemistry 1993; 100:17–26.

105. Pierce JA, Ebert RV. Fibrosis network of the lung and its change with age. Thorax 1965; 20:469–476.

106. Shapiro SD, Endicott SK, Province MA, Pierce JA, Campbell EJ. Marked longevity of human lung parenchymal elastic fibers deduced from prevalence of D-aspartate and nuclear weapons-related radiocarbon. J Clin Invest 1991; 87:1818–1834.

107. Snider GL. Emphysema: The first two centuries - and beyond. A historical overview, with suggestions for future research: Parts 1 & 2. Am Rev Respir Dis 1992; 146: 1615–1622.

108. Kuhn CI, Yu SY, Chraplyvy M, Linder HE, Senior RM. The induction of emphysema with elastase. II. Changes in connective tissue. Lab Invest 1976; 34: 372–380.

109. Fukuda Y, Masuda Y, Ishizaki M, Masugi Y, Ferrans VJ. Morphogenesis of abnormal elastic fibers in panacinar and centriacinar emphysema. Hum Pathol 1989; 20: 652–659.

110. Bieth JG. Elastases: Catalytic and biological properties. In: Mecham RP, ed. Regulation of Matrix Accumulation. New York: Academic Press. 1986:217–320.

111. Shapiro SD, Campbell EJ, Welgus HG, Senior RM. Elastin degradation by mononuclear phagocytes. Ann NY Acad Sci 1991; 624:69–80.

112. Snider GL, Ciccolella DE, Morris SM, Stone PJ, Lucey EC. Putative role of neutrophil elastase in the pathogenesis of emphysema. Ann NY Acad Sci 1991; 624: 45–59.

113. Sakai LY, Keene DR, Engvall E. Fibrillin, a new 350-kD glycoprotein, is a component of extracellular microfibrils. J Cell Biol 1986; 103:2499–2509.

114. Gibson MA, Sandberg LB, Grosso LE, Cleary EG. Complementary DNA cloning

establishes microfibril-associated glycoprotein (MAGP) to be a discrete component of the elastin-associated microfibrils. J Biol Chem 1991; 266:7596–7601.

115. Horrigan SK, Rich CB, Streeten BW, Li ZY, Foster JA. Characterization of an associated microfibril protein through recombinant DNA techniques. J Biol Chem 1992; 267:10087–10095.

116. Goldfischer S, Coltoff SB, Goldfischer M. Microfibrils, elastic anchoring components of the extracellular matrix, are associated with fibronectin in the zonule of Zinn and aorta. Tissue Cell 1985; 17:441–450.

117. Breathnach SM, Pepys MF, Hintner H. Tissue amyloid P component in normal human dermis is non-covalently associated with elastic fiber microfibrils. J Invest Dermatol 1989; 92:53–58.

118. Inoue S, Leblond CP. The microfibrils of connective tissue. I. Ultrastructure. Am J Anat 1986; 176:121–138.

119. Dahlbäck K, Löfberg H, Alumets J, Dahlbäck B. Immunochemical demonstration of age-related deposition of vitronectin (S-protein of complement) and terminal complement complex on dermal elastic fibers. J Invest Dermatol 1989; 92:727–733.

120. Dietz HC, Cutting GR., Pyeritz RE, Maslen CL, Saai LY, Corson GM, Puffenberger EG, Hamosh A, Nanthakumar EJ, Curristin SM, Stetten G, Meyers DA, Francomano CA. Marfan syndrome caused by a recurrent de novo missense mutation in the fibrillin gene. Nature 1991; 352:37–339.

121. McKusick VA. The defect in Marfan syndrome. Nature 1991; 352:279–281.

122. Lee B, Goodfrey M, Vitale E, Hori H, Mattei M-G, Sarfarazi M, Tsipouras P, Ramirez F, Hollister DW. Linkage of Marfan syndrome and a phenotypically related disorder to two different fibrillin genes. Nature 1991; 352:330–334.

123. Corson GM, Chalberg SC, Dietz HC, Charbonneau NL, Sakai LY. Fibrillin binds calcium and is coded by cDNAs that reveal a multidomain structure and alternatively spliced exons at the 5' end. Genomics 1993; 17:476–484.

124. Zhang H, Hu W, Ramirez F. Developmental expression of fibrillin genes suggests heterogeneity of extracellular microfibrils J Cell Biol 1995; 129(4):1165–1176.

125. Gibson MA, Cleary EG. The immunohistochemical localization of microfibril-associated glycoprotein (MAGP) in elastic and non-elastic tissues. Immunol Cell Biol 1987; 65:345–356.

126. Kumaratilake JS, Gibson MA, Fanning JC, Cleary EG. The tissue distribution of microfibrils reacting with a monospecific antibody to MAGP, the major glycoprotein antigen of elastin-associated microfibrils. Eur J Cell Biol 1989; 50:117–127.

127. Chen Y, Faraco J, Yin W, Germiller J, Francke U, Bonadio J. Structure, chromosomal localization, and expression pattern of the murine *Magp* gene. J Biol Chem 1993; 268:27381–27389.

128. Amy RWM, Bowes D, Burri PH, Haines J, Thurlbeck WM. Postnatal growth of the mouse lung. J Anat 1977; 24:131–151.

129. Collett AJ, Des Biens G. Fine structure of myogenesis and elastogenesis in the developing rat lung. Anat Rec 1974; 179:343–360.

130. Jones AW, Barson AJ. Elastogenesis in the developing chick lung: a light and electron microscopical study. J Anat 1971; 110:1–15.

131.  Noguchi A, Firsching K, Kursar JD, Reddy R. Developmental changes in tropo-
      elastin gene expression in the rat lung studied by in situ hybridization. Am J Resp
      Cell Mol Biol 1991; 5:571–578.
132.  Stenmark KR, Dempsey EC, Badesch DB, Frid M, Mecham RP, Parks WC. Regula-
      tion of pulmonary vascular wall cell growth: Developmental and site-specific hetero-
      geneity. Eur Respir Rev 1993; 3:629–637.
133.  Rehn M, Pihlajaniemi T. Alpha 1(XVIII), a collagen chain with frequent interrup-
      tions in the collagenous sequence, a distinct tissue distribution, and homology with
      type XV collagen. Proc Natl Acad Sci 1994; 91:4234–4238.
134.  Juvonen M, Sandberg M, Pihlajaniemi T. Patterns of expression of the six alter-
      natively spliced exons affecting the structures of the COL1 and NC2 domains of the
      alpha 1(XIII) collagen chain in human tissues and cell lines. 1992; 267:24700–
      24707.

# 13

## Cell-Cell and Cell-Matrix Interactions in Development of the Lung Vasculature

**JESSE ROMAN**

Atlanta Veterans Affairs Medical Center
Decatur, Georgia
and Emory University School of Medicine
Atlanta, Georgia

## I. Introduction

The lung is composed of an extensive array of airways and vessels arranged to accomplish efficient transfer of gases from the air space to the bloodstream and vice versa. The factors involved in development of the lung from a single avascular bud into a complex structure containing a complex airway network, two complete circulatory systems, and millions of alveoli are the focus of intense investigation. With the aid of in vitro and in vivo models, much has been learned about the mechanisms involved in regulation of lung bud formation and airway branching morphogenesis. However, the mechanisms involved in vascular formation during lung development remain largely unknown. This is due in part to the fact that isolated congenital abnormalities (e.g., unilateral absence of a pulmonary artery) are very rare. Most abnormalities in pulmonary circulation are associated to major alterations in lung structure related to lung hypoplasia, dysplasia, and hyperplasia (1). This suggests that the factors controlling vessel formation in lung are linked to the formation of other structures (i.e., airways), and it indicates that perhaps a good understanding of vessel formation can be attained only after a better appreciation of the regulatory factors involved in the formation of these structures and the interdependence among the various processes responsible for their development.

Knowledge concerning the mechanisms involved in vessel formation has been greatly enhanced by the identification of novel polypeptides with angiogenic capabilities, the development of cell culture models of vasculogenesis (differentiation and organization of endothelial cells into vascular structures) and angiogenesis (extension of vessels by sprouting of endothelial cells) (Fig. 1), and advances in endothelial cell (EC) biology. Together with detailed studies examining the structure of developing lungs, advancement in these and other areas has allowed the development of the following conceptualization of lung vasculature formation. Vascular structures appear within the mesenchyme of embryonic lungs during the late stages of development. The formation of these structures appears to be preceded by the development of two separate vascular systems which become connected prior to birth. One vascular system is composed of the central pulmonary and bronchial arteries and veins which originate outside the lung, invade the lung parenchyma, and connect with the distal pulmonary circulation or microvasculature. The distal pulmonary circulation develops within the lung mesenchyme and is formed by ECs of nonpulmonary origin which have invaded the lung mesenchyme and ECs of pulmonary origin which result from the in situ differentiation of mesodermal cells. ECs of both origins cluster into discrete areas around the developing airways where they organize into elongated cords around a central lumen surrounded by cells that develop into smooth muscle. In this chapter, we discuss information available that has led to this conceptualization of lung vasculature development.

Development of the lung vasculature is dependent on control of EC differentiation and function (i.e., adhesion, migration, proliferation). Both cellular and extracellular signals appear important for vessel formation. The initial stages of vascular formation are likely dependent on genetic factors responsible for EC differentiation and their distribution to specific areas of the developing embryo. Events in later stages are believed to be modulated by extracellular signals provided by growth factors, extracellular matrices (ECMs), and other cells. This chapter focuses on extracellular signals considered important for lung vascular formation, since virtually nothing is known about the genetic factors involved in this process. It will provide a discussion of the factors that regulate vessel formation in vitro with emphasis on cell surface adhesive molecules involved in cell-cell and cell-matrix interactions. This discussion is intended to stimulate interest in this less well-studied area by providing a framework from which testable hypotheses may be generated.

## Vasculogenesis

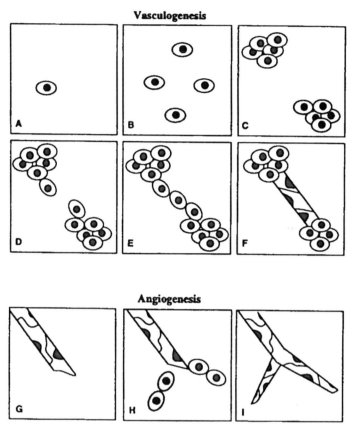

**Figure 1**  Scheme of vasculogenesis and angiogenesis. Vasculogenesis is the process by which vessels are formed from undifferentiated mesodermal cells. Once mesodermal cells differentiate into endothelial cells (ECs) (A), they proliferate (B), and organize into clusters or islands (C). These islands send out ECs that will connect them with adjacent islands (D). Cells present between islands develop tight cell-cell interactions (E) and organize around a central lumen forming a vessel (F). In angiogenesis, vascular structures are derived from existent vessels. These vessels send sprouts of ECs (G) that connect each other via cell-cell adhesion molecules (H) and organize around a lumen (I) extending the length of the vessel. Although both vasculogenesis and angiogenesis occur during embryogenesis, angiogenesis is considered to predominate in adult tissues, particularly during revascularization of injured tissues.

## II. Development of the Pulmonary Circulation

### A. Embryological Landmarks

Lung development can be divided into various stages based on the appearance of specific pulmonary structures such as the epithelial lung bud (embryonic stage), airways (pseudoglandular stage), vessels (canalicular stage), and alveoli (saccular and alveolar stages) (2,3). Although this classification is helpful for understanding lung development, significant overlap exists. Indeed, although intrapulmonary vascular structures are not present until the canalicular stage, the processes responsible for development of the pulmonary circulation are triggered much earlier and appear to be intimately related to airways formation (Table 1).

The human rudimentary lung bud is an epithelial evagination of the foregut during the embryonic stage of lung development (26 days to 6 weeks). During budding, the rudimentary epithelium brings with it loose connective tissue that contains primitive vascular structures present within the foregut (4). At the end of the embryonic stage, connections between the arterial supply and venous drainage of the lung (extrapulmonary structures at that point in time) are made with the right and left heart chambers, respectively. In addition, the central rudimentary extrapulmonary bronchial arteries, which develop earlier from the dorsal aorta,

**Table 1** Development of the Pulmonary Circulation

| Stage | Gestation | Events |
|---|---|---|
| Embryonic | 26 days to 6 weeks | Development of central bronchial arteries |
| Pseudoglandular | 6–16 weeks | Disappearance of central bronchial arteries and development of new bronchial arteries which arise from the aorta by 9–12 weeks |
| Canalicular | 16–28 weeks | Formation of acinus |
| | | Differentiation of acinar epithelium |
| | | Development of the distal circulation |
| | | Development of preacinar and resistant arteries |
| | | Connection of distal circulation with pulmonary arteries and veins |
| | | Thickness of blood-gas barrier is similar to adult |
| Saccular | 26–36 weeks | Subdivision of saccules by secondary crests containing capillaries |
| Alveolar | 36 weeks to term | Alveolar acquisition |
| Postnatal | Birth to 2 years | Formation of single capillary network |

disappear. On occasion, the primitive bronchial arteries persist, as seen when such an artery supplies a sequestered lung segment. During the pseudoglandular stage (6th to 16th weeks), the primitive bronchial tree is generated to the level of the terminal bronchioles by the process of lung branching morphogenesis (2,3). Coinciding with airway formation, new definitive bronchial arteries arise from the aorta and appear between the 9th and 12th week of gestation. By 16 weeks, airway branching is almost complete and the canalicular stage (also termed vascular stage) of lung development begins (16–28 weeks). Formation of the acinus, differentiation of the acinar epithelium, and development of the distal pulmonary circulation take place during this stage. Preacinar and resistant arteries are present by the 28th week, but their muscularization continues to term. Capillary networks derived from EC precursors (also termed angioblasts) extend from and around distal air spaces and connect with the developing pulmonary arteries and veins. At the end of the canalicular stage, the mesenchyme becomes thinner and the vascular system closely opposes the airspaces. By the 28th week, the thickness of the alveolar-capillary membrane is similar to that of the adult (5,6).

Between 26 and 36 weeks of gestation, the terminal airway structures termed saccules are subdivided by crests emerging from the parenchyma and bringing with them extensions of capillaries. This represents the beginning of the saccular stage of lung development. Further subdivisions of the saccules precede the formation of alveoli during the alveolar stage (36 weeks to term). Thinning of the interstitium continues during the alveolar stage of lung development, bringing capillary networks from adjacent alveoli into close apposition and thereby leading to a double capillary network around the primitive alveolar structures. Near birth, capillaries from opposing networks fuse to form a single network, and capillary volume increases with continuing growth and expansion (7,8). Fusion of the capillaries is almost complete by 18 months of postnatal age.

The fully matured lung has a complete circulatory system characterized by double arterial supplies and venous drainage systems (1). The arterial supply is derived from the pulmonary and bronchial arteries. The pulmonary artery branches with the airways, supplies the acinar structures, and provides a capillary bed to the respiratory bronchioles and the pleura. The bronchial artery extends from the aorta and supplies the capillary bed within the bronchial wall and perihilar structures. Two types of arterial branches have been described: *conventional* and *supernumerary* (9). The conventional arteries run with the airways extending toward the terminal bronchioles where they form an extensive capillary network. The *supernumerary arteries* are located between conventional arteries, are greater in number, and run a short course supplying a capillary bed to the alveoli adjacent to the airway. All intrapulmonary structures drain into the pulmonary vein, whereas hilar structures drain into bronchial veins and then the azygous system.

## III.  Basic Mechanisms of Vessel Formation

In general, organogenesis is dependent on the regulation of organ growth (cell proliferation), maturation (cell differentiation), and pattern formation (organization of cells into a multicellular structure). These functions are also necessary for vascularization of the lung and are considered important components of two distinct processes responsible for vessel formation: vasculogenesis and angiogenesis (10,11). In this chapter, *vasculogenesis* is defined as the process by which randomly distributed mesodermal cells differentiate into ECs, proliferate, and organize into multicellular structures singularly arranged around a central lumen (see Fig. 1). *Angiogenesis* is defined as the process by which differentiated ECs proliferate and sprout from previously formed vessels to form new vascular structures. Although these processes are considered responsible for different aspects of organ vascularization, a clear distinction between them is not always evident in the literature. Furthermore, factors that enhance the migration, proliferation, and differentiation of cultured ECs are often considered angiogenic factors despite ample evidence showing that these capabilities do not predict induction of vessel formation in vitro or in vivo. Therefore, when possible, we shall discuss these processes separately.

Much of our knowledge related to vessel formation is derived from studies using EC lines in migration and proliferation assays as well as in vitro assays of vasculogenesis and angiogenesis. In the vasculogenesis assay, ECs are cultured on two- or three-dimensional substrates containing one or more extracellular matrix (ECM) components in the presence of serum or well-defined growth factors (Fig. 2). Studies using this system have shown that in vitro capillary tube or "cord" formation is characterized by a series of morphological changes that include EC migration, invasion of the ECM, and development of cell-cell connections. Once the cords are formed, cellular retraction and elevation above the surface of the rigid substrate are followed by involution of cells around a lumen (12). Other assays examine angiogenesis by culturing previously formed vascular structures such as aortic vessel wall (13) or rat corneal explants on three-dimensional ECM substrates (14).

As expected, experiments performed in such assays reveal that EC adhesion to the substrate, migration, and proliferation are necessary for the initiation and progression of both vasculogenesis and angiogenesis. These processes are regulated by soluble and insoluble extracellular signals (15,16). Soluble molecules believed to modulate organ vascularization include platelet-derived growth factor, transforming growth factor-β, and heparin-binding growth factors (17,18). Insoluble factors affecting organ vascularization include components of the ECM (e.g., collagen types I, III, IV and V, laminin, and fibronectin) (12). Although both signals are critical, studies directed at examining in vitro EC cord formation suggest the influence of ECMs predominates (15). More recently, attention has

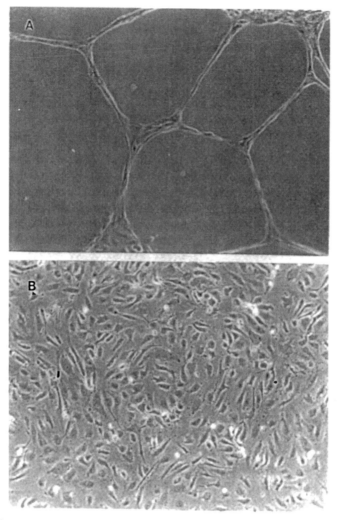

**Figure 2** Human umbilical endothelial cells (HUVECs) form cords when cultured on Matrigel but not on plastic. HUVECs were cultured on Matrigel (A) or on plastic (B) for 12 hr in the presence of 10% bovine calf serum. Note that on Matrigel, HUVECs organized into capillary-like structures or cords. Reorientation of cells into polygones was noticed as early as 3 hr after culture suggesting that, although proliferation is important, the matrix can drive the organization of cells into cords in the absence of significant proliferation. In contrast to cells cultured on Matrigel, HUVECs cultured on plastic (B) did not organize into cords and remained as a monolayer.

been given to the potential role of cell-cell interactions in vessel formation (19). The following sections deal with information available concerning the role of cell-matrix and cell-cell interactions and growth factors in vessel formation.

## IV. Role of Cell-Matrix Interactions in Vessel Formation

### A. Effects of Extracellular Matrices on Endothelial Cell Function

Embryogenesis is characterized by complex structural and compositional changes in the ECM of developing organs (20–22). In the lung, laminin and collagen are present very early during development and their amount increases steadily during embryogenesis (23). In rabbit, chick, and murine lungs, fibronectin concentration increases during the mid pseudoglandular stage of lung development coinciding with branching morphogenesis; and it decreases thereafter coinciding with vessel formation during the canalicular stage (23–25) (Fig. 3). In contrast, some thrombospondin variants increase during the late stages of lung development (26). Like thrombospondin, very little elastin content is found in lungs during the pseudoglandular stage, but it increases markedly during the saccular and alveolar stages (22, 27). The types and amounts of glycosaminoglycans also change dramatically during lung development. In chick lung, hyaluronic acid is the predominant species in mesenchyme and the content of sulfated glycosaminoglycans increases as development progresses (28). Although the consequences of these and other alterations in composition of the ECM in embryonic lungs are unknown, it seems likely that they influence airway and vessel formation.

In vitro, ECMs stimulate directional and nondirectional migration of cultured human umbilical ECs and bovine aortic ECs, to name just a few (29–33). ECMs also influence the growth of cultured ECs (34,35). In addition, insoluble ECMs provide an adhesive scaffold for building of elongated vascular structures in vitro (36,37). For example, fibronectin, a major component of the ECM of developing microvessels (38,39), promotes vessel elongation during angiogenesis (40). Collagen matrices promote EC organization into capillary-like networks (41). Matrigel, a reconstituted basement membrane product of Engelbreth-Holm-Swarm tumor which is composed mainly of laminin, collagen type IV, and nidogen, is a potent inducer of cord formation in vitro (12). Thrombospondin, a matrix component with antiadhesive properties, does not affect EC proliferation but promotes angiogenesis of explants of rat aorta, particularly when incorporated into fibrin and collagen gels (42). In rabbit cornea, the induction of angiogenesis by fibroblasts growth factors is enhanced by thrombospondin (43). Conversely, others have demonstrated that thrombospondin-1 inhibits neovascularization and EC migration (44). In fibroblasts, control of thrombospondin-1 secretion is controlled by the tumor suppressor gene p53 (45). The relevance of these observations

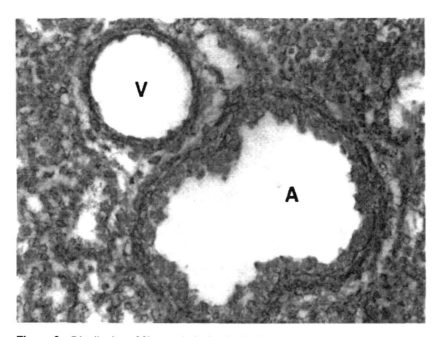

**Figure 3** Distribution of fibronectin in developing lung. Lungs were obtained at 16 days of gestation, frozen, and processed for immunostaining with polyclonal antibodies to fibronectin. Afterward, a photograph of the tissue was submitted to electronic digital continuous tone imaging using Macintosh Photoshop 2.5 (Adobe Systems Inc., Mountain View, CA). During the canalicular stage of gestation, fibronectin is detected with mesenchymal cells, in particular, cells localized around the developing airways (A) and vessels (V). These cells are known to express markers of smooth muscle differentiation (25 and 164).

to lung development is unclear. SPARC, another matrix-associated glycoprotein transiently expressed during development and implicated in morphogenesis, stimulates angiogenesis of bovine aortic ECs (46). The angiogenic activity of SPARC is contained in a small peptide sequence (Lys-Gly-His-Lys) that can be released during tissue remodeling by various enzymes, including plasmin and elastase. Another two peptides, containing the adhesive sequence YIGSR (Tyr-Ile-Gly-Ser-Arg) present in B1 chain of laminin, and PA 21 present in the A chain, prevent in vitro cord formation on Matrigel (36).

The ability to stimulate in vitro cord formation is not limited to the aforementioned matrix components. In fact, many matrix proteins tested to date are capable of inducing or sustaining this process if enough time is allowed (from hours to weeks). How this finding relates to the in vivo situation is unknown, particularly in view that lipopolysaccharide, a contaminant frequently found in experimental reagents, has recently been shown to promote angiogenesis (43). Nevertheless, the effect of ECMs on EC phenotype in vitro appears to be real and is dependent on time of exposure, cell type, configuration and composition of the matrix, as well as EC density, and the presence or absence of growth factors (12). Altogether, these studies suggest that switching of ECs between differentiation, growth, and spatial organization during vascular formation in developing lungs may be influenced by alterations in the adhesive or mechanical integrity of their ECM (12).

## B.  Cell-Matrix Adhesion Molecules In Vessel Formation

### Integrins

The effects of ECMs on EC function are mediated via cell surface receptors expressed by ECs both in culture and in vivo (Table 2), (Fig. 4) (reviewed in ref. 47). Of these, integrins are considered the main surface proteins responsible for cell-substrate adhesion. Integrins are glycoproteins composed of $\alpha$ and $\beta$ subunits that assemble noncovalently into a transmembrane complex (48–51). These $\alpha\beta$ heterodimers bind their extracellular ligands in a divalent cation-dependent manner (52) and interact with cytoskeletal structures intracellularly (53–55). Ligand binding specificity is conferred by the $\alpha$ subunit, although the identity of the $\beta$ subunit, which is shared by other integrins, seems important. Integrins are classified into subfamilies depending on their $\beta$ subunit ($\beta$1, 2, 3, and so forth). At least 30 $\alpha$ subunits and 7 $\beta$ subunits have been described. Certain $\alpha$ subunits may associate with more than one $\beta$ subunit (56–58).

The best-characterized matrix binding integrins are members of the $\beta$1 subfamily (also termed VLAs for very late activation antigens) and include receptors for laminin ($\alpha1\beta1$, $\alpha3\beta1$, and $\alpha6\beta1$), collagen ($\alpha1\beta1$, $\alpha2\beta1$, and $\alpha3\beta1$), and fibronectin ($\alpha5\beta1$, $\alpha3\beta1$, and $\alpha4\beta1$) (58–63). ECs express all the above receptors except for $\alpha4\beta1$ (64). Some of these receptors bind more than one type of ECM protein. Although not studied extensively in ECs, some $\beta$1 integrins can demonstrate different ligand specificities when expressed on different cell types (65).

Integrins in the $\beta$2 (CD18) subfamily (leucams) are mainly involved in cell-cell interactions. However, some $\beta$2 integrins have been found to bind fibrin (i.e., CD11b/CD18 and CD11c/CD18 (66,67). Although $\beta$2 integrins are expressed mainly by white blood cells, their ligands are present in ECs as well (see below).

Integrins in the $\beta$3 subfamily or cytoadhesins are expressed by ECs and platelets and include receptors for vitronectin, fibrinogen, fibronectin, von Willebrand's factor, and thrombospondin (68). Integrins containing the $\alpha$v subunit are quite heterogeneous with respect to their ligand specificities. Although the $\alpha$v$\beta$3

**Table 2**  Cell-Matrix Adhesion Molecules

| Family/molecule | Ligand(s) |
|---|---|
| Integrins | |
| β1 *Subfamily* | |
| α1β1 (VLA-1) | Laminin, collagen |
| α2β1 (VLA-2) | Collagen, laminin |
| α3β1 (VLA-3) | Collagen, laminin, fibronectin |
| α4β1 (VLA-4)[a] | Fibronectin, VCAM-1[b] |
| α5β1 (VLA-5) | Fibronectin |
| α6β1 (VLA-6) | Laminin |
| αvβ1 | Fibronectin |
| β3 *Subfamily* | |
| αvβ3 | Vitronectin, fibrinogen, fibronectin von Willebrand factor, thrombospondin, laminin |
| αIIb/β3[a] | Fibronectin, vitronectin, fibrinogen von Willebrand factor, thrombospondin |
| *Other* | |
| α6β4 | Laminin |
| αvβ5 | Vitronectin |
| αvβ6 | Fibronectin |
| α4β7 | Fibronectin, VCAM-1 |
| Nonintegrins | |
| CD44[a] | Hyaluronic acid, addressins |
| Syndecan[a] | Collagen, fibronectin |
| 67- to 69-kDa protein | Laminin, elastin, collagen |

[a]Not expressed by ECs.
[b]Vascular cell adhesion molecule-1.

and αvβ5 complexes bind vitronectin preferentially in certain cell types, αvβ1 binds fibronectin (69,70).

Integrin function-may be modulated by differential expression of splicing variants (56) and lipid composition of the membrane (71). The mechanisms by which an extracellular signal is transferred from ECMs into the cell via integrin receptors are unclear. Several reports have demonstrated regulation of gene expression by ligand binding to integrins (72). Intracellular signaling processes implicated in integrin-mediated signal transduction include activation of tyrosine kinases (73,74), receptor phosphorylation (75), protein kinase C (76), calcium fluxes (77), and cytoskeletal arrangements (12,78,79). Although most of these processes have been investigated in cells other than ECs, some signal transduction events triggered by ligand binding to integrins have been clarified in ECs. For example, EC proliferation on fibronectin substrates is associated with cell spread-

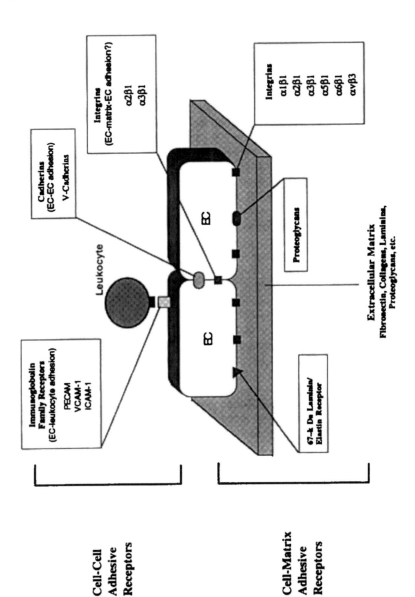

**Figure 4**

ing and activation of Na/H antiporters which leads to an increase in intracellular pH (80).

Although the role of integrin-mediated intracellular signals in vessel formation is unclear, many of the aforementioned signaling pathways have been implicated in vessel formation. For example, inhibition of expression of messenger RNA and protein production prevents a human endothelium-derived permanent cell line (EAhy926) from undergoing cord formation (81). Similar observations were made when G-protein function was blocked with pertussis toxin (81). Protein kinase C inhibitors blocked and phorbol esters stimulated cord formation of human umbilical endothelial cells (82). Vanadate, an inhibitor of phosphotyrosine-specific phosphatases, stimulated capillary endothelial cells to invade collagen matrices and form cords suggesting a role for tyrosine phosphorylation in vessel formation (83). It should be noted that, in general, the effects on in vitro cord formation by reagents that affect the signals described above are independent of their effects on EC adhesion to their substrate (81).

### Nonintegrins

Proteoglycans are also considered important in substrate adhesion and transmission of signals from the ECM. Hyaluronidase-sensitive proteoglycans predominate in migrating ECs of sprouting capillaries, whereas heparinase-sensitive proteoglycans predominate in quiescent ECs (84). This difference in expression of various groups of proteoglycans in proliferating and migrating ECs versus ECs present in quiescent capillaries suggests a role in vessel formation. A well-studied proteoglycan with matrix binding activity is Syndecan, which binds to collagen and fibronectin (85). However, Syndecan is mainly expressed in epithelial cells and not endothelium. Another well-characterized matrix-binding nonintegrin receptor is the 67- to 69-kDa receptor that binds to laminin, elastin, and collagen (86). This protein binds with high affinity to the amino acid sequence Tyr-Ile-Gly-Ser-Arg (YIGSR) contained in the B1 chain of laminin (87).

### C. Potential Role of Matrix-Binding Receptors in Lung Vessel Formation

Compelling evidence that favors a role for integrins in vessel formation during lung development is derived from descriptive studies examining the temporal and

---

**Figure 4** Adhesion molecules involved in cell-cell and cell-matrix interactions in endothelial cells (ECs). The basal surface of ECs is in contact with matrix components present in the basement membrane. Attachment of ECs to the underlying matrix is mediated via integrin and non-integrin receptors (see Table 2). On their luminal and lateral surfaces, ECs express receptors involved in cell-cell interactions. Some of these receptors mediate EC-EC interactions (e.g., cadherins), whereas others mediate EC-leukocyte interactions (e.g., immunoglobulin family receptors, carbohydrates) (see Table 3).

spatial distribution of integrins and functional studies using specific reagents that inhibit integrin function. β1 and β3 integrins are detected in developing lungs at very early stages of gestation. The α5 subunit present in the fibronectin binding α5β1 complex is detected in mesenchymal cells of murine lungs as early as 11 days of gestation and is expressed in vascular structures as soon as they appear (25). The α4 subunit of the α4β1 receptor is also detected in vascular structures, mainly in muscle cells (unpublished observations). This receptor and one of its ligands, vascular cell adhesion molecule-1, or VCAM-1 (α4β1 also binds fibronectin), are considered important in muscle differentiation (88). The α3 subunit is expressed in epithelial cells of developing airways and αvβ3 receptors are present in epithelial and mesenchymal cells, including vessels (89). More recently, it has been reported in preliminary form that integrin subunits α1, α2, and α6 (90) and α9 (91) are present in developing lungs as well.

Many integrins, particularly some members of the β1 and β3 subfamilies, bind an RGD (Arg-Gly-Asp) amino acid sequence present in their ligands (92–95). The RGD sequence is found in various matrix proteins, including fibronectin, thrombospondin, fibrinogen, vitronectin, laminin, and type I collagen (94). This observation has been extremely important, as synthetic peptides containing this sequence inhibit ligand binding to integrin receptors and have been used to study the role of integrins in multiple biological systems (89,96–98). Through inhibition of EC integrin adhesion to matrices, RGD-containing peptides prevent the formation of microvessels from aortic explants placed on collagen gels (99) as well as cord formation of ECs placed on a reconstituted basement membrane (36). Polymeric peptides based on the RGD sequence inhibit neovascularization of tumors in mouse lungs (100).

Antibodies to various integrin subunits have also been used successfully to prevent vascular formation in vitro. Anti-αvβ3 antibodies have recently been shown to block growth factor–induced angiogenesis in the chick chorioallantoic membrane model (14). In contrast, antibodies to α2β1 and αvβ3 integrin receptors enhance capillary tube formation in vitro (101). This seemingly paradoxical observation suggests that, although EC adhesion to the matrix is important for vessel formation, antiadhesive events are also necessary, since they allow detachment of the EC from their substrate and presumably facilitate mitosis and migration. This is reminiscent of other observations showing that changes in adhesivity induced by alterations in the density of ECM molecules can affect capillary tube formation (12).

### D. ECMs and Proteinases in Vascular Formation

Although in situ differentiation of mesodermal cells into ECs appears to be a major mechanism for vascularization of developing organs, invasion of avascular tissues by well-differentiated ECs which may then become incorporated into developing vessels is considered important as well. Tissue invasion by ECs requires the production of proteolytic enzymes necessary for traversing basement membranes and reorganizing ECM components (102). The expression of interstitial collagenases and u-PA in cultured capillary ECs is enhanced by growth factors such as basic fibroblast growth factor (bFGF) (103). Type IV collagenase is another enzyme expressed by ECs with ECM-degrading activity (104). Some of these enzymes reside in the ECM and are released during tissue remodeling (106–109). In addition, ECMs may themselves stimulate the production of proteinases by lung fibroblasts. Fibronectin, for example, stimulates WI-38 and IMR-90 fetal lung fibroblastic cells to express both stromelysin and collagenase by binding to the integrin $\alpha 5\beta 1$ (72). Thus, ECMs may affect regional expression of proteolytic enzymes by stimulating their production in mesenchymal cells other than ECs.

## V. Role of Cell-Cell Interactions in Vessel Formation

Cell-cell junctions between ECs have been classified in communicating (gap) junctions, adherens junctions, and occluding (tight) junctions, and are crucial for maintenance of tissue integrity and formation of tight permeability barriers (105). ECs interact physically with endothelial and other cell types via specific surface receptors (47). Similar to the cell-matrix receptors, cell-cell adhesion molecules interact with cytoplasmic proteins, including the cytoskeleton. Unlike the cell-matrix receptors, some receptors that mediate cell-cell interactions are involved in homophilic interactions (i.e., cadherins); in other words, they bind to similar molecules on other cells. In general, cell-cell-adhesion molecules expressed by ECs are members of the cadherin, integrin, and immunoglobulin families (Table 3) (see Fig. 4).

Cadherins are surface receptors composed of a single transmembrane polypeptide chain (111). Similar to the integrins, cadherin-cadherin interactions are dependent on extracellular calcium concentration (112). Cadherins have been classified in four subgroups: the epithelial or E-cadherins (found mainly in epithelial cells), neural or N-cadherins (found in adult neural tissues and muscle), the placental or P-cadherins (found in placenta and epithelial cells), and the vascular or V-cadherins (expressed mainly in ECs). A role for these molecules in cell-cell adhesion is suggested by in vitro studies showing that neutralizing anti–E-cadherin antibodies and peptides that mimic the N-terminal portion of V-cadherins increased epithelial (110) and endothelial (113) monolayer permeability.

Some members of the integrin family may also be important in cell-cell adhesion events between ECs. $\beta 2$ integrins are expressed mainly in leukocytes, whereas $\beta 1$ and $\beta 3$ integrins can be found on ECs. The $\beta 1$ integrins, $\alpha 2\beta 1$ and $\alpha 3\beta 1$, have been found to be localized at cell-cell contact sites in cultured keratinocytes (114), and $\alpha 2\beta 1$ and $\alpha 5\beta 1$ have been localized to the same sites in

**Table 3** Cell-Cell Adhesion Molecules

| Family/molecule | Ligand(s) |
| --- | --- |
| Cadherins | |
| E-cadherin (uvomorulin) | E-cadherin |
| P-cadherin | P-cadherin |
| V-cadherin | ? |
| Integrins | |
| β1 *Subfamily* | |
| α2β1 | Matrix protein ? |
| α3β1 | Epiligrin |
| α5β1 | |
| β2 *Subfamily* | |
| α1β2 (CD11a/CD18, LFA-1)[a] | ICAM-1, ICAM-2 |
| αmβ2 (CD11b/CD18, Mac-1)[a] | ICAM-1, fibrinogen, C3bi |
| αxβ2 (CD11c/CD18)[a] | Fibrinogen, C3bi |
| Immunoglobulin Family | |
| PECAM-1 | PECAM-1, glycosaminoglycans |
| ICAM-1[b] | α1β2, αmβ2 |
| ICAM-2 | α1β2 |
| VCAM-1[b] | α4β1 |
| Selectins | |
| E-selectin[b] | Sialyl Lewis x, sialyl Lewis a, L-selectin |
| P-selectin[b] | Sialyl Lewis x, L-selectin |
| L-selectin[a] | E- and P-selectin, MECA 79 antigen |
| Carbohydrates | |
| Sialyl Lewis x (CD15) | E- and P-selectin |

[a]Not expressed by ECs.
[b]Inducible.

ECs (115). This characteristic distribution suggested a role in cell-cell adhesion which was further supported by studies showing that antibodies specific for these integrin subunits disrupt cell-cell adhesion. The exact nature of the cell-cell interactions mediated via integrins in ECs is unknown. They are unlikely to be involved in homophilic interactions. Instead, they may bind to ECM proteins present between cells. This seems to be the case for the α3β1 receptor which binds to the extracellular molecule epiligrin (116). Thus, matrix-binding integrins may strengthen the adhesion of cells by binding to ECM proteins which serve as bridges between integrins expressed on the surface of different cells.

Platelet-EC adhesion molecule-1, or PECAM-1, is also considered important for cell-cell adhesion in ECs (117). This transmembrane glycoprotein is a member of the immunoglobulin superfamily and is expressed in ECs, leukocytes, and platelets (47). As expected, immunofluorescent staining of PECAM in ECs is localized to cell-cell contact sites (19). In contrast, this staining pattern is lost in migrating ECs. Identical findings were made in NIH3T3 cells transfected with PECAM. This together with the observed decrease in the migration of PECAM-transfected NIH3T3 cells compared with nontransfected cells suggest that cell-cell contacts between ECs may modulate the migration of ECs. One might speculate that tight cell-cell adhesions between ECs may prevent their migration and therefore inhibit their invasion into tissues and reorganization into vascular structures during development.

## VI. Role of Growth Factors in Vessel Formation

The angiogenic activity of multifunctional peptide growth factors has been studied extensively (17). Particular attention has been given to heparin-binding growth factors such as acidic fibroblast growth factor (aFGF) and basic fibroblast growth factor (bFGF) (118). Heparin-binding angiogenic growth factors have been isolated from embryonic tissues, including kidney (119), limb bud (120), brain (118), and chorioallantoic membrane (121). The angiogenic activity of FGFs is further enhanced by ECM components such as heparan sulfate proteoglycans (122). It must be noted that although FGFs are potent angiogenic factors, expression of FGF receptors in embryonic lung ECs has not been firmly established using in situ hybridization techniques, and therefore the function of these factors in organ vascularization is unclear (123,124).

A recently discovered heparin binding growth factor with mitogenic and angiogenic activity is vascular endothelial growth factor (VEGF) (125–128). Unlike other angiogenic factors, this 46-kDa polypeptide is specific for ECs. Expression of VEGF and VEGF binding sites is regulated during lung development, increasing during late stages of gestation in blood vessels (129). In addition to its ability to increase vascular permeability (for which it is also known as vascular permeability factor, or VPF) (130), VEGF has been shown to promote angiogenesis in rat cornea and chicken chorioallantoic membrane assays (125, 131,132). The effects of VEGF are mediated via at least two tyrosine kinase receptors: flt-1 (133) and flk-1/kdr (134). The limited expression of these receptors to ECs has led to their consideration as good markers of EC precursors (135).

Platelet-derived growth factor A and B chain (PDGF A and PDGF B) mRNAs are present in microvascular ECs (136,137). Although PDGF AA has no mitogenic activity on microvascular ECs, PDGF AB has a small but significant effect, and PDGF BB has the strongest effect. The expression of PDGF receptors in these cells is downregulated during induction of cord formation in three-dimensional collagen gels, whereas they are upregulated in two-dimentional cultures. This may explain why EC differentiation and organization into cords, which correlates with downregulation of PDGF receptors, is associated with reduced proliferation (138).

Other growth factors implicated in vasculogenesis include platelet-derived EC growth factor (PD-ECGF) which is present in human placenta (139), stimulates EC proliferation and chemotaxis in vitro, and enhances angiogenesis in vivo (140). Transforming growth factor-β (TGF-β) inhibits the proliferation of ECs but induces a potent angiogenic response (141) depending on the cell substrate composition and organization (142). Both transforming growth factor-α (TGF-α) and epidermal growth factor stimulate microvascular EC proliferation (143). TGF-α has been shown to have angiogenic activity in rat airways (144). Other growth factors with angiogenic activity are the granulocyte-monocyte/Colony-stimulating/Factor (145) and angiogenin (146).

Many of these growth factors reside in the ECM of developing and adult organs (108) and their binding to ECM components may synergize their growth-promoting effects (147). It should be noted that we have observed organization of HUVECs into cords as early as 3 hr after plating on Matrigel. In the absence of serum-derived growth factors, this process begins but is not sustained after 10–12 hr (unpublished observations). This suggests that ECMs may drive EC organization into cords in the absence of serum-derived growth factors, but that growth factors are needed for sustaining this process, perhaps by stimulating EC proliferation. Our conclusion must be tempered by the possibility that Matrigel contains growth factors embedded in the insoluble matrix that may help initiate EC organization.

## VII. Development of the Vasculature in Developing Lungs

The relative contribution of vasculogenesis and angiogenesis to the development of the pulmonary vasculature has been studied in transplantation experiments performed in developing chick, quail, and more recently mouse tissues. These studies suggest that, although some organs such as the brain and kidney are vascularized by sprouting of ECs from vessels that invade the rudiments (angiogenesis), vasculogenesis is the predominant method of vascularization in lung (reviewed in ref. 148). As described before, lung vasculogenesis is dependent on the differentiation of mesodermal cells into ECs and their organization into multicellular structures. These vascular structures are not apparent until the canalicular stage of lung development, and therefore one might predict that cells expressing EC markers would appear much earlier, perhaps during the pseudo-glandular stage. ECs or EC precursors may derive from the invasion of extra-pulmonary ECs into the lung and/or the in situ differentiation of lung mesenchymal cells. In an attempt to begin to define the mechanisms of vessel formation in lung, we have made the following observations.

Immunohistochemical staining of murine lung rudiments with antibodies to the EC-specific antigen von Willebrand's factor (vWF) and the lectin BSLB4, which binds to a-galactose residues on ECs (166), revealed staining in few lung mesenchymal cells in 12- and 13-day-old lung rudiments (early pseudoglandular stage; offsprings are born at 21 days of gestation). The number of vWF-positive cells increased with maturation, became coalescent with other vWF-positive cells, and were later found staining the endothelium of vascular structures at about 16 days of gestation (149) (Fig. 5). This is consistent with other studies where distribution of the EC-specific antigen flk, a receptor for VEGF, was observed in mesenchymal cells surrounding the developing airways at about the same time (150). Although these studies do not clarify the origin of pulmonary ECs, they do demonstrate that ECs appear during the early pseudoglandular stage of lung development prior to the detection of vascular structures.

Examination of isolated cells obtained by trypsinization of 11-day-old murine lung rudiments revealed 1–2% of BSLB4-positive cells. After 72 hr in culture, the percentage of BSLB4-positive cells doubled. However, this percentage was not significantly affected when cells were cultured on various matrix components suggesting that EC differentiation and/or proliferation was not affected by ECM composition (unpublished observations). Of note, mesenchymal cells obtained from 11-day-old murine lung rudiments clumped and underwent cord formation in vitro when cultured on Matrigel for 6 days (Fig. 6) suggesting that ECMs may drive vasculogenesis of lung mesodermal cells as has been shown for ECs of other origins. However, in contrast to HUVECs (see Fig. 2), very few cords were observed which were short and rarely connected two or more EC islands. Cord formation was not apparent, however, when cells were cultured on fibronectin, fibrin clots, or gels made of type I collagen. These findings are intriguing, particularly in view that, although EC differentiation may be complete during the pseudoglandular stage, conditions necessary for vessel formation in vivo are not established until the canalicular stage. Conditions favorable for vasculogenesis may depend on appropriate ECM composition and growth factor expression. On the other hand, it may depend mainly on the proliferation of ECs.

Thus, development of the pulmonary circulation appears to be dependent on invasion of lung parenchyma by extrapulmonary vessels during angiogenesis, and linkage of these vessels with distal capillary networks formed via vasculogenesis of EC precursors present within the lung mesenchyme (1). The idea that the pulmonary circulation develops as two separate systems is supported by reports of neonates showing isolated absence of pulmonary artery capillaries or no connection between capillaries and the central pulmonary arteries (151–153).

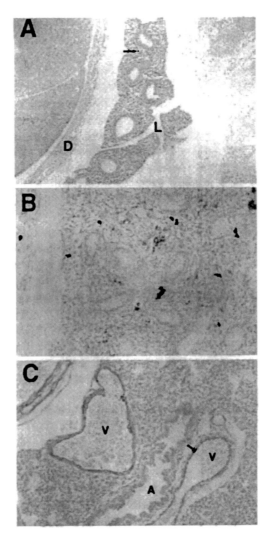

**Figure 5**   Distribution of endothelial cells in developing murine lung. Lungs were obtained at 13 (A), 15 (B), and 16 (C) days of gestation, fixed, immunostained with an
antibody to von Willebrands factor (vWF) and processed as described for Figure 3. (A) At
13 days of gestation (mid pseudoglandular stage), vascular structures were absent. During
this stage, few cells expressing vWF were detected within the mesenchyme (arrow).
Staining was detected in some cells in the liver but not in the diaphragm (D). (B) At 15 days
of gestation, endothelial cells were detected in clusters or islands within the mesenchyme
localized adjacent to developing airways. (C) At day 16 (the beginning of the canalicular
stage), when vascular structures are evident, staining was detected within endothelial cells
in vessels (arrows).

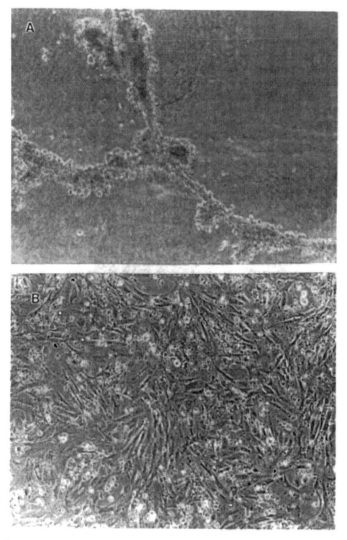

**Figure 6** Lung mesenchymal cells undergo in vitro cord formation when cultured on Matrigel. Lung mesenchymal cells were obtained by trypsinization of 11-day-old murine lungs and cultured for 6 days on Matrigel (A) or plastic (B). In contrast to HUVECs, lung mesenchymal cells did not undergo cord formation early and, although they organized into clusters which developed extensions, few capillary-like structures were observed. When present, the cords were short and surrounded by multiple mesenchymal cells of unknown origin (A). In contrast to cells cultured on Matrigel, cord formation was not observed in lung mesenchymal cells cultured on plastic (B).

## VIII.  Summary and Research Needs

The studies described above are part of the growing literature that is shaping our understanding of lung development. Information about the development of the vasculature in the lung has led to the following conceptualization. The central pulmonary vessels are formed outside the lung during the early stages of lung development. These extrapulmonary structures invade the lung via angiogenesis and connect with distal capillary networks. The distal circulation, on the other hand, is developed by vasculogenesis which requires the differentiation in situ of mesodermal cells into ECs and their organization into capillaries within the acinus. In vitro studies suggest that both lung angiogenesis and vasculogenesis are influenced by extracellular signals provided by growth factors and ECMs. Although the influence of ECMs seems to predominate, both signals may affect EC differentiation, migration, proliferation, and organization into vascular structures. Once EC differentiation takes place, ECMs appear to drive EC migration and reorganization into multicellular vascular structures, whereas growth factors may be necessary to sustain the process by stimulating EC proliferation and perhaps to induce their expression of ECMs (154) as well as cell surface receptors which are necessary for EC responsiveness to extracellular signals (155). Cell-cell interactions between ECs may slow down migration thereby inhibiting vessel formation. However, once individual ECs make contact with each other, their organization into multicellular structures requires intact cell-cell interactions.

Several pieces of information are missing. For example, what effect does airway formation have on vascular formation? Most congenital malformations leading to aberrant pulmonary circulation are associated with major alterations in overall lung structure. This may be explained by the intricate relationship between lung vascularization and airway formation summarized in the third law of lung development as originally described by Lynne M. Reid and colleagues (reviewed in ref. 165). This together with the observation that vessels follow the overall distribution of airways suggest that lung vascularization during the canalicular stage is dependent on events coinciding with branching morphogenesis during the pseudoglandular stage. Thus, it is reasonable to postulate that many of the events responsible for lung branching may somehow affect vasculogenesis and angiogenesis. Since airway formation occurs earlier during development, and EC differentiation appears to follow the distribution of the airways, ECMs and growth factors derived from airway epithelial and mesenchymal cells may drive EC differentiation and vessel formation. Future work directed at studying vessel formation in the lung should consider the processes involved in lung branching.

The factors responsible for EC differentiation during lung development are also unknown. What phenotypic changes accompany EC differentiation and what is their role in vascular formation? Once the factors involved in EC differentiation in the lung are identified, it will be important to determine if they play similar roles in other organs. In doing so, it would suggest that vascularization of organs during embryogenesis follows a general scheme with common mechanisms of action.

Our studies showing that ECs present in avascular lungs are capable of undergoing vasculogenesis in vitro but not in vivo suggest that conditions are not ideal for in vivo vasculogenesis until the canalicular stage of lung development. This may be due to the absence of angiogenic/vasculogenic factors or the presence of inhibitors of these processes. For example, angiogenic inhibitors are produced by certain tumor cells, but it is unknown whether similar factors are produced in developing tissues. More recently, attention has focused on bioactive peptides derived from neuroendocrine cells. One such peptide, endothelin 1, has been found to be highly expressed in developing lungs, particularly at late stages of gestation; however, its role in vessel formation is unknown (156). On the other hand, lung vascularization may depend on multiple factors coming spatially and temporally together. Identifying these factors and how they interact to permit vascular formation during lung development will be a major task for developmental biologists.

Another important aspect that is poorly understood is that of vascular smooth muscle differentiation and EC-smooth muscle interactions. Both ECMs (157) and growth factors (158) can affect muscle differentiation, but it is unknown if vascular smooth muscle differentiation is tied to EC differentiation and vascular formation. It is also unknown whether vascular and airway smooth muscle cells follow similar pathways of differentiation and organization around endothelial and epithelial structures, respectively. What surface molecules mediate EC-smooth muscle cell interactions in developing lungs will need to be investigated as well.

Once the air spaces and vessels are formed, apposition of these structures needs to occur. This process takes place during the late stages of lung development and is crucial for developing functional gas-exchanging units. A major part of this process is the clearing of mesenchymal cells and connective tissue present between the developing airways and vessels. We have observed that the number of mesenchymal cells undergoing programmed cell death (apoptosis) increases in the mouse lung during the saccular stage of development, whereas no apoptotic cells are detected during the pseudoglandular stage (Sundell and Roman, unpublished observations) (Fig. 7). Similar observations were made when we examined the distribution of Gelatinase A and B, metalloproteases capable of degrading ECM proteins (C. Sundell and J. Roman, unpublished observations). Thus, activation of mechanisms leading to apoptosis and expression of matrix-degrading enzymes during the late stages of development may be crucial for the formation of functional alveoli-capillaries barriers.

Another intriguing question is related to EC invasion of the lung, migration, and connection with vascular structures. ECs appear to migrate long distances to be able to connect with forming vessels. One might speculate that EC migration is

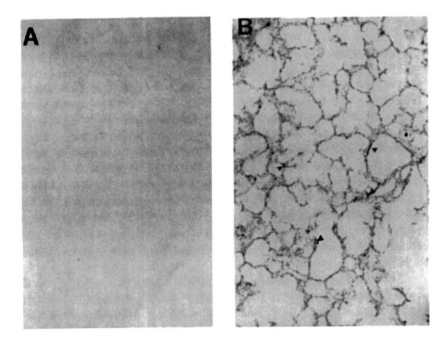

**Figure 7** Apoptosis in lung development. Murine lungs were obtained at 14 (pseudoglandular stage) (A) and 18 days of gestation (saccular) (B), stained with an antibody that detects cells undergoing apoptosis or programmed cell death, and processed as described for Figure 3. Apoptotic cells were not present in pseudoglandular stage lungs (A) but were markedly increased in mesenchymal cells of 18-day-old lungs (B). The function of apoptosis in lung development is unknown. However, it is conceivable that programmed cell death is activated during late stages of development to rid the lung of excess mesenchymal cells and allow apposition of vessels and airspaces to form a thin alveolar-capillary barrier.

driven by soluble (chemotaxis) and insoluble (haptotaxis) gradients present within the lung. The factors that drive these processes and the embryonic clock that triggers their expression need to be identified.

Finally, it is important to determine what controls overall lung development. For example, what triggers the formation of the lung bud? What genes (e.g., homeobox genes; see ref. 159) control lung pattern formation? Why do vessels and airways demonstrate scale invariance symmetry (invariant structure under changes in scale of the picture) which is characteristic of fractals? Fractal patterns like the one observed in the lung vasculature are common in other organs, including salivary glands, pancreatic duct system, liver biliary tree, urinary collecting duct, and the His-Purkinje nerve fiber network in the heart (160,161). The universality of fractal patterns in nature (snowflakes, lightning-like paths of electricity, tree branches) and the ability of relatively simple computer models to simulate fractals suggest that nonequilibrium growth processes of living and inanimate objects share similar mechanisms (162). Advances in quantum mechanics, thermodynamics, and chaos theory (and their application to biological problems) are likely to have an impact in the study of lung development in the future.

Appropriate answers to these questions can not be obtained in the absence of appropriate models of organ formation and vascularization. We anticipate these models will become available within the next decade. Technological advances in this and other areas will accelerate our understanding of vasculature development in the lung. This new information will likely affect the way we approach congenital lung malformations and other processes such as regulation of angiogenesis by tumors. In addition, they may contribute to our understanding of revascularization after lung injury which appears to trigger the expression of angiogenic factors that may be common to developing lungs (163).

## Acknowledgments

The authors thank Drs. Cinthia Sundell, Rafael Perez, Samuel Aguayo, and Roland Ingram for careful review of the manuscript; Dr. Cinthia Sundell for insightful comments, data collection, and photographic work; and Doug Durham for image analysis of photographs. This work was supported by a Merit Review Grant from the Department of Veterans Affairs.

## REFERENCES

1.  deMello DE, Reid LM. Pre- and postnatal development of the pulmonary circulation. In: Chernick V, Mellins RB, eds. Basic Mechanisms of Pediatric Respiratory Disease: Cellular and Integrative. Philadelphia: Decker, 1991:36–54.
2.  Ten-Have-Opbroek AAW. The development of the lung in mammals: an analysis of concepts and findings. Am J Anat, 1981; 162:201–219.
3.  Thurlbeck WM. Pre- and postnatal organ development. In: Chernick V, Mellins RB, eds. Basic Mechanisms of Pediatric Respiratory Disease: Cellular and Integrative. Philadelphia: Decker, 1991:23–35.
4.  Weibel ER. Design of airways and blood vessels considered as branching trees. In: Crystal R, West J, Cherniack R, Weibel ER, eds. The Lung: Scientific Foundations. New York: Raven Press, 1991:711–720.
5.  Hislop A, Reid L. Growth and development of the respiratory system-anatomical development. In: Davis JA, Dobbing J, eds. Scientific Foundations of Pediatrics. London: Heinemann, 1974:214–254.
6.  Hislop A, Reid L. Lung development in relationship to gas exchange capacity. Bull Physio-Pathol Respir 1973; 9:1317–1343.

7.  Zeltner TB, Caduff JH, Gehr T, Pfenninger J, Burri PH. The postnatal development and growth of the human lung. 1. Morphol Respir Physiol 1987; 67:247–267.
8.  Zeltner TB, Burri PH. The postnatal development and growth of the human lung. 2. Morphol Respir Physiol 1987; 67:269–283.
9.  Elliott FM, Reid L. Some new facts about the pulmonary artery and its branching pattern. Clin Radiol 1965; 16:193–198.
10. Poole TJ, Coffin JD. Vasculogenesis and angiogenesis: two distinct morphogenetic mechanisms establish embryonic vascular pattern. J Exp Zool 1989; 251:224–231.
11. Coffin JD, Harrison J, Schwartz S, Heimark R. Angioblast differentiation and morphogenesis of the vascular endothelium in the mouse embryo. Dev Biol 1991; 148:51–62.
12. Ingber DE, Folkman J. Mechanochemical switching between growth and differentiation during fibroblast growth factor-stimulated angiogenesis in vitro: role of extracellular matrix. J Cell Biol 1989; 109:317–330.
13. Nicosia RF, Ottinetti A. Growth of microvessels in serum-free matrix culture of rat aorta. Lab Invest 1990; 63:115–122.
14. Brooks PC, Clark RAF, Cheresh DA. Requirement of vascular integrin $\alpha v \beta 3$ for angiogenesis. Science 1994; 264:569–571.
15. Ingber DE, Folkman J. How does extracellular matrix control capillary morphogenesis? Cell 1989; 58:803–805.
16. Furcht L. Critical factors controlling angiogenesis: Cell products, cell matrix and growth factors. Lab Invest 1986; 55:505–509.
17. Risau W. Embryonic angiogenesis factors. Pharm Ther, 1991; 51:371–376.
18. D'Amore PA. Mechanisms of endothelial cell growth. Am J Respir Cell Mol Biol 1992; 6:1–8.
19. Schimmenti LA, Yan H-C, Madri JA, Albelda SM. Platelet endothelial cell adhesion molecule, PECAM-1, modulates cell migration. J Cell Physiol 1992; 153:417–428.
20. Hay ED. Collagen and Embryonic Development. New York: Plenum, 1981: 379–405.
21. McGowan SE. Extracellular matrix and the regulation of lung development and repair. FASEB J 1992; 6:2895–2904.
22. Guzowski DE, Blau H, Bienkowski RS. Extracellular matrix in developing lung. Philadelphia: Lea & Febiger, 1990:83–105.
23. Chen WT, Chen JM, Mueller SC. Coupled expression and colocalization of 140K cell adhesion molecules, fibronectin, and laminin during morphogenesis and cytodifferentiation of chick lung cells. J Cell Biol 1986; 103:1073–1090.
24. Snyder J, O'Brien J, Rodgers H. Localization and accumulation of fibronectin in rabbit fetal lung tissue. Differentiation 1987; 34:32–39.
25. Roman J, McDonald JA. Expression of fibronectin, the integrin VLA-5 and $\alpha$-smooth muscle actin in lung and heart development. Am J Respir Cell Mol Biol 1992; 6:472–480.
26. Iruela-Arispe ML, Liska DJ, Sage EH, Bornstein P. Differential expression of thrombospondin 1, 2, and 3 during murine development. Dev Dyn 1993; 197:40–56.
27. Myers B, Dubick M, Last JA, Rucker RB. Elastin synthesis during perinatal lung development in the rat. Biochim Biophys Acta 1983; 761:17–22.

28. Becchetti E, Evangelisti R, Stabellini G, Pagliarini A, Borrello ED, Castrini C, Carinci P. Developmental heterogeneity of mesenchymal glycosaminoglycans (GAG) distribution in chick embryo lung anlagen. Am J Anat 1988; 181:33–42.

29. Madri JA, Pratt BM, Yannariello-Brown J. Matrix-driven cell size change modulates aortic endothelial cell proliferation and sheet migration. Am J Pathol 1988; 132:18–27.

30. Madri JA, Pratt BM, Yannariello-Brown J. Endothelial cell-extracellular matrix interactions: matrix as a modulator of cell function. In: Simionescu N, Simionescu M, eds. Endothelial Cell Biology. New York: Plenum, 1988:167–190.

31. Dejana O, Colella S, Conforti G, Abbadini M, Gaboli M, Marchisio PC. Fibronectin and vitronectin regulate the organization of their respective Arg-Gly-Asp receptors in cultured human endothelial cells. J Cell Biol 1988; 107:1215–1223.

32. Gospodarowicz D, Vlodavsky I, Savion N. The extracellular matrix and the control of proliferation of vascular endothelial and smooth muscle cells. J Supramol Struct 1980; 13:339–372.

33. Bowersox JC, Sorgente N. Chemotaxis of aortic endothelial cells in response to fibronectin. Cancer Res 1982; 42:2547–2551.

34. Ingber DE, Madri JA, Folkman J. Endothelial growth factors and extracellular matrix regulate DNA synthesis through modulation of cell and nuclear expansion. In Vitro Cell Dev Biol 1987; 23:387–394.

35. Form DM, Pratt BM, Madri JA. Endothelial cell proliferation during angiogenesis. In vitro modulation of basement membrane components. Lab Invest 1986; 55:521–530.

36. Grant DS, Tashiro K, Sequi-Real B, Yamada Y, Martin GR, Kleinman HK. Two different laminin domains mediate the differentiation of human endothelial cells into capillary-like structures in vitro. Cell 1989; 58:933–943.

37. Kubota Y, Kleinman HK, Martin GR, Lawley TJ. Role of laminin and basement membrane in the morphological differentiation of human endothelial cells into capillary-like structures. J Cell Biol 1988; 107:1589–1598.

38. Tonnesen MG, Jenkins D, Seibel SL, Lee LA, Huff JC, Clark RAF. Expression of fibronectin, laminin, and factor VIII–related antigen during development of the human cutaneous microvasculature. J Invest Dermatol 1985; 85:564–568.

39. Risau W, Lemmon V. Changes in the vascular extracellular matrix during embryonic vasculogenesis and angiogenesis. Dev Biol 1988; 125:441–450.

40. Nicosia RF, Bonanno E, Smith M. Fibronectin promotes the elongation of microvessels during angiogenesis in vitro. J Cell Physiol 1993; 154:654–661.

41. Montesano R, Orci L, Vasalli P. In vitro rapid organization of endothelial cells into capillary-like networks is promoted by collagen matrices. J Cell Biol 1983; 97:1648–1652.

42. Nicosia RF, Tuszynski GP. Matrix-bound thrombospondin promotes angiogenesis in vitro. J Cell Biol 1994; 124:183–193.

43. BenEzra D, Griffin BW, Maftzir G, Aharonov O. Thrombospondin and in vivo angiogenesis induced by basic fibroblast growth factor or lipopolysaccharide. Invest Ophthalmol Vis Sci 1993; 34:3601–3608.

44. Good DJ, Polverini PJ, Rastinejad F, Beau MML, Lemons RS, Frazier WA, Bouck

NP. A tumor suppressor-dependent inhibitor of angiogenesis is immunologically and functionally indistinguishable from a fragment of thrombospondin. Proc Natl Acad Sci USA 1990; 87:6624–6628.

45. Dameron KM, Volpert OV, Tainsky MA, Bouck N. Control of angiogenesis in fibroblasts by p53 regulation of thrombospondin-1. Science 1994; 265:1582–1584.

46. Lane TF, Iruela-Arispe L, Johnson RS, Sage EH. SPARC is a source of copper-binding proteins that stimulate angiogenesis. J Cell Biol 1994; 125:929–943.

47. Albelda SM. Endothelial and epithelial cell adhesion molecules. Am J Respir Cell Mol Biol 1991; 4:195–203.

48. Albelda SM, Buck CA. Integrins and other cell adhesion molecules. FASEB J 1990; 4:2868–2880.

49. McDonald JA. Receptors for extracellular matrix components. Am J Physiol 1989; 257:331–337.

50. Ruoslahti E. Integrins. J Clin Invest 1991; 87:1–5.

51. Akiyama SK, Nagata K, Yamada KM. Cell surface receptors for extracellular matrix components. Biochim Biophys Acta 1990; 1031:91–110.

52. Gailit J, Ruoslahti E. Regulation of the fibronectin receptor affinity by divalent cations. J Biol Chem 1988; 26:12927–12932.

53. Burridge K, Molony L, Kelly T. Adhesion plaques: Sites of transmembrane interaction between the extracellular matrix and the actin cytoskeleton. J Cell Sci 1987; 8:211–229.

54. Buck CA, Horwitz AF. Cell surface receptors for extracellular matrix molecules. Ann Rev Cell Biol 1987; 3:179–205.

55. Roman J, LaChance RM, Broekelmann TJ, Kennedy CJR, Wayner EA, Carter WJ, McDonald JA. The fibronectin receptor is organized by extracellular matrix fibronectin: implications for oncogenic transformation and for cell recognition of fibronectin matrices. J Cell Biol 1989; 108:2529–2543.

56. Cheresh DA. Structural and biologic properties of integrin-mediated cell adhesion. Clin Lab Med 1992; 12:217–236.

57. Cheresh D, Smith J, Cooper H, Quaranta V. A novel vitronectin receptor integrin ($\alpha v \beta 1$) is responsible for distinct adhesive properties of carcinoma cells. Cell 1989; 57:59–69.

58. Wayner EA, Orlando RA, Cheresh DA. Integrins $\alpha v \beta 3$ and $\alpha v \beta 5$ contribute to cell attachment to vitronectin but differentially distribute on the cell surface. J Cell Biol 1991; 113:919–929.

59. Hemler ME. VLA proteins in the integrin family: Structures, functions, and their role on leukocytes. Ann Rev Immunol 1990; 8:365–400.

60. Hemler ME, Huang C, Schwarz L. The VLA protein family: Characterization of five distinct cell surface heterodimers each with a common 130,000 molecular weight $\beta$ subunit. J Biol Chem 1987; 262:3300–3309.

61. Wayner EA, Garcia-Pardo A, Humphries M, McDonald JA, Carter WG. Identification and characterization of the T lymphocyte adhesion receptor for an alternative cell attachment domain (CS-1) in plasma fibronectin. J Cell Biol 109:1321–1330.

62. Wayner EA, Carter WG. Identification of multiple cell adhesion receptors for

collagen and fibronectin in human fibrosarcoma cells possessing unique alpha and common beta subunits. J Cell Biol 1987; 105:1873–1884.

63. Wayner EA, Carter WG, Piotrowicz RS, Kunicki TJ. The function of multiple extracellular matrix receptors (ECMRs) in mediating cell adhesion to extracellular matrix: preparation of monoclonal antibodies to the fibronectin receptor that specifically inhibit cell adhesion to fibronectin and react with platelet glycoproteins Ic-IIa. J Cell Biol 1988; 107:1881–1891.

64. Defilippi P, Hinsbergh VV, Bertolotto A, Rossino P, Silengo L, Tarone G. Differential distribution and modulation of expression of alpha 1/beta 1 integrin on human endothelial cells. J. Cell Biol 1991; 114:855–863.

65. Elices MJ, Hemler ME. The human integrin VLA-2 is a collagen receptor on some cells and a collagen-laminin receptor on others. Proc Natl Acad Sci USA 1989; 86:9906–9910.

66. Arnaout MA. Structure and function of the leukocyte adhesion molecules CD11/CD18. Blood 1990; 75:1037–1050.

67. Springer TA. Adhesion receptors of the immune system. Nature 1990; 346:425–434.

68. Ginsburg M, Loftus J, Plow ED. Cytoadhesins, integrins, and platelets. Thromb Haemost 1988; 59:1–6.

69. Smith JW, Vestal DJ, Irwin SV, Burke TA, Cherish DA. Purification and functional characterization of integrin $\alpha v\beta 5$. J Biol Chem 1990; 265:11008–11013.

70. Horton M. Current status review: vitronectin receptor: tissue specific expression or adaptation to culture. Int J Exp Pathol 1990; 71:741–759.

71. Conforti G, Zanetti A, Pasquali-Ronchetti I, Quaglino D, Neyroz P, Dejana E. Modulation of vitronectin receptor binding by membrane lipid composition. J Biol Chem 1990; 265:4011–4019.

72. Werb Z, Tremble PM, Behrendtsen O, Crowley E, Damsky CH. Signal transduction through the fibronectin receptor induces collagenase and stromelysin gene expression. J Cell Biol 1989; 109:877–889.

73. Shattil SJ, Brugge JS. Protein tyrosine phosphorylation and the adhesive functions of platelets. Curr Opin Cell Biol 1991; 3:869–879.

74. Hynes RO. Integrins: versatility, modulation, and signaling in cell adhesion. Cell 1992; 69:11–25.

75. Valmu L, Autero M, Siljander P, Patarroyo M, Gahmberg CG. Phosphorylation of the $\beta$-subunit of CD11/CD18 integrins by protein kinase C correlates with leukocyte adhesion. Eur J Immunol 1991; 21:2857–2862.

76. Chang ZL, Beezhold DH, Personius CD, Shen ZL. Fibronectin cell-binding domain triggered transmembrane signal transduction in human monocytes. J Leukoc Biol 1993; 53:79–85.

77. Ng-Sikorski J, Andersson R, Patarroyo M, Andersson T. Calcium signaling capacity of the CD11b/CD18 integrin on human neutrophils. Exp Cell Res 1991; 195: 504–508.

78. Ingber DE. Integrins as mechanochemical transducers. Curr Opin Cell Biol 1991; 3:841–848.

79. Otey CA, Pavalko FM, Burridge K. An interaction between a-actinin and the $\beta 1$ subunit in vitro. J Cell Biol 1990; 111:721–729.

80. Schwartz MA, Lechene C, Ingber DE. Insoluble fibronectin activates the Na/H antiporter by clustering and immobilizing integrin α5β1, independent of cell shape. Proc Natl Acad Sci USA 1991; 88:7849–7853.

81. Bauer J, Margolis M, Schreiner C, Edgell C, Azizkhan J, Lazarowski E, Juliano RL. In vitro model of angiogenesis using a human endothelium-derived permanent cell line: Contributions of induced gene expression, G-proteins, and integrins. J Cell Physiol 1992; 153:437–449.

82. Davis CM, Danehower A, Laurenza A, Molony JL. Indentification of a role of the vitronectin receptor and protein kinase C in induction of endothelial cell vascular formation. J Cell Biochem 1993; 5:206–218.

83. Montesano R, Pepper MS, Belin D, Vassall J, Orci L. Induction of angiogenesis in vitro by vanadate, an inhibitor of phosphotyrosine phosphatases. J Cell Physiol 1988; 134:460–466.

84. Ausprunk DH, Boudreau CL, Nelson DA. Proteoglycans in the microvasculature. II. Histochemical localization of in proliferating capillaries of the rabbit cornea. Am J Pathol 1981; 103:367–375.

85. Saunders S, Jalkanen M, O'Farrell S, Bernfeld M. Molecular cloning of syndecan, an integral membrane proteoglycan. J Cell Biol 1989; 108:1547–1556.

86. Mecham RP, Hinek A, Griffin GL, Senior RM, Liotta LA. The elastin receptor shows structural and functional similarities to the 67-kDa tumor cell laminin receptor. J Biol Chem 1989; 264:16652–16657.

87. Liotta LA, Wewer UM, Rao CN, Bryant G. Laminin receptor. In: Edelman GM, Thiery J-P, eds. The Cell in Contact: Adhesions and Junctions as Morphogenetic Determinants. New York: Wiley, 1985:333–334.

88. Rosen GR, Sanes JR, LaChance R, Cunningham JM, Roman J, Dean DC. Roles for the integrin VLA-4 and its counter receptor VCAM-1 in myogenesis. Cell 1992; 69:1107–1119.

89. Roman J, Little CW, McDonald JA. Potential role of RGD-binding integrins in mammalian lung branching morphogenesis. Development 1991; 112:551–558.

90. Edelman JM, Buck CE, Ballard PL, Buck CA. Integrin expression in human lung development (abstr). Am J Respir Crit Care Med 1994; 149:A714.

91. Wang A, Patrone L, McDonald JA, Sheppard D. Expression of α9 subunit in the murine embryo (abstr). Am J Respir Crit Care Med, 1994; 149:A1003.

92. Piersbacher MD, Hayman EG, Ruoslahti E. Location of the cell-attachment site in fibronectin with monoclonal antibodies and proteolytic fragments of the molecule. Cell 1981; 26:259–267.

93. Ruoslahti E, Pierschbacher MD. Arg-Gly-Asp: A versatile cell recognition signal. Cell 1986; 44:517–518.

94. Ruoslahti E, Pierschbacher MD. New perspectives in cell adhesion: RGD and integrins. Science 1987; 238:491–497.

95. Ruoslahti E. Fibronectin and its receptors. Ann Rev Biochem 1988; 57:375–413.

96. Boucaut JC, Darribere T, Poole TJ, Aoyama H, Yamada KM. Biologically active synthetic peptides as probes of embryonic development: a competitive peptide inhibitor of fibronectin function inhibits gastrulation in amphibian embryos and neural crest cell migration in avian embryos. J Cell Biol 1984; 99:1822–1830.

97. Naidet C, Semeriva M, Yamada KM, Thiery JP. Peptides containing the cell-attachment recognition signal Arg-Gly-Asp prevent gastrulation in *Drosophila* embryos. Nature 1987; 325:348–350.

98. Darribere T, Boucher D, Lacrois JC, Boucaut JC. Fibronectin synthesis during oogenesis and early development of the amphibian *Pleurodeles waltlii*. Cell Diff 1984; 14:171–177.

99. Nicosia RF, Bonanno E. Inhibition of angiogenesis in vitro by Arg-Gly-Asp-containing synthetic peptide. Am J Pathol 1991; 138:829–833.

100. Saiki I, Murata J, Makabe T, Nishi N, Tokura S, Azuma I. Inhibition of tumor angiogenesis by a synthetic cell-adhesive polypeptide containing the Arg-Gly-Asp (RGD) sequence of fibronectin, poly (RGD). Jpn J Cancer Res 1990; 81: 668–675.

101. Gamble JR, Matthias LJ, Meyer G, Kaur P, Russ G, Russ G, Faull R, Berndt MC, Vadas MA. Regulation of in vitro capillary tube formation by anti-integrin antibodies. J Cell Biol 1993; 121:931–943.

102. Matrisian LM, Hogan BLM. Growth factor-regulated proteases and extracellular matrix remodeling during mammalian development. In: Nilsen-Hamilton M, eds. Growth Factors and Development. San Diego: Academic Press, 1990:219–259.

103. Gross JL, Moscatelli D, Rifkin DB. Increased capillary endothelial cell protease activity in response to angiogenic stimuli in vitro. Proc Natl Acad Sci USA 1983; 80:2623–2627.

104. Kalebic T, Garbisa S, Glaser B, Liotta LA. Basement membrane collagen: degradation by migrating endothelial cells. Science 1983; 221:281–283.

105. Dejana, E. Endothelial cell adhesive receptors. J Cardiovasc Pharmacol 1993; 21:S18–S21.

106. Folkman J, Haudenschild C. Angiogenesis *in vitro*. Nature 1980; 288:551–556.

107. Folkman J. How is blood vessel growth regulated in normal and neoplastic tissue? Cancer Res 1986; 46:467–473.

108. Vlodavsky I, Korner G, Ishai-Michaeli R, Bashkin P, Bar-Shavit R. Extracellular matrix–resident growth factors and enzymes: possible involvement in tumor metastasis and angiogenesis. Cancer Metast Rev 1990; 9:203–206.

109. Moscatelli D, Rifkin DB. Membrane and matrix localization of proteinases: A common theme in tumor cell invasion and angiogenesis. Biochim Biophys Acta 1988; 948:1648–1652.

110. Behrens J, Birchmeir W, Goodman SL, Imhof BA. Dissociation of Madin-Darby canine kidney epithelial cells by the monoclonal antibody anti-Arc-1: mechanistic aspects and identification of the antigen as a component related to uvomorulin. J Cell Biol 1985; 101:1307–1315.

111. Takeichi M. Cadherins: a molecular family important in selective cell-cell adhesion. Annu Rev Biochem 1990; 59:237–252.

112. Chen W, Obrink B. Cell-cell contacts mediated by E-cadherin (uvomorulin) restrict invasive behavior of L-cells. J Cell Biol 1991; 114:319–327.

113. Liaw CW, Tomaselli KJ, Cannon C. Distribution of MDCK and bovine endothelial cell tight junctions with cadherins synthetic peptides (abstr). J Cell Biol 1990; 111:408.

114. Carter WG, Wayner EA, Bouchard TS, Kaur P. The role of integrins α2β1 and α3β1 in cell-cell and cell-substrate adhesion of human epidermal cells. J Cell Biol 1990; 110:1387–1408.

115. Lampugnani MG, Resnati M, Dejana E, Marchisio PC. The role of integrins in the maintenance of endothelial monolayer integrity. J Cell Biol 1991; 112:479–490.

116. Carter WG, Ryan MC, Gahr PJ, Epiligrin, a new cell adhesion ligand for integrin α3β1 in epithelial basement membranes. Cell 1991; 65:599–610.

117. Albelda SM, Oliver PD, Romer LH, Buck CA. EndoCAM: a novel endothelial cell-cell adhesion molecule. J Cell Biol 1990; 110:1227–1237.

118. Risau W. Developing brain produces an angiogenesis factor. Proc Natl Acad Sci USA 1986; 83:3855–3959.

119. Risau W, Ekblom P. Production of a heparin-binding angiogenesis factor by the embryonic kidney. J Cell Biol 1986; 103:1101–1107.

120. Munaim SE, Klagsbrun M, Toole BP. Developmental changes in fibroblast growth factor in the chicken embryo limb bud. Proc Natl Acad Sci USA 1988; 85:8091–8093.

121. Flamme I, Schulze-Osthoff K, Jacob HJ. Mitogenic activity of chicken chorioallantoic fluid is temporally correlated to vascular growth in the chorioallantoic membrane and related to fibroblast growth-factors. Development 1991; 111:683–690.

122. Gospodarowicz D, Massoglia S, Cheng J, Fujii DK. Effect of fibroblast growth factor and lipoproteins on the proliferation of endothelial cells derived from bovine adrenal cortex, brain cortex, and corpus luteum capillaries. J Cell Physiol 1986; 127:121–136.

123. Wanaka A, Milbrandt J, Johnson EM. Expression of FGF receptor gene in rat development. Development 1991; 111:455–468.

124. Reid HH, Wilks AG, Bernard O. Two forms of the basic fibroblast growth-factor receptor-like messenger-RNA are expressed in the developing mouse brain. Proc Natl Acad Sci USA 1990; 87:1596–1600.

125. Senger D, Connolly D, Water LVD, Feder J, Dvorak H. Purification of NH2-terminal amino acid sequence of guinea pig tumor-secreted vascular permeability factor. Cancer Res 1990; 50:1774–1778.

126. Connolly D, Heuvelman D, Nelson R, Olander J, Eppley B, Delfino J, Siegel N, Leimgruber R. Tumor vascular permeability factor stimulates endothelial cell growth and angiogenesis. J Clin Invest 1989; 84:1470–1478.

127. Ferrara N, Henzel W. Pituitary follicular cells secrete a novel heparin-binding growth factor specific for vascular endothelial cells. Biochem Biophys Res Commun 1989; 161:851–858.

128. Gospodarowicz D, Abraham J, Schilling J. Isolation and characterization of a vascular endothelial cell mitogen produced by pituitary-derived folliculo stellite cells. Proc Natl Acad Sci USA 1989; 86:7311–7315.

129. Jakeman LB, Armanini M, Phillips HS, Ferrara N. Developmental expression of binding sites and messenger ribonucleic acid for vascular endothelial growth factor suggests a role for this protein in vasculogenesis and angiogenesis. Endocrinology 1993; 133:848–858.

130. Keck PJ, Hauser SD, Krivi G, Sanzo K, Warren T, Feder J, Connolly DT. Vascular

permeability factor, an endothelial cell mitogen related to PDGF. Science 1989; 246:1309–1312.

131. Leung D, Cachianes G, Kuang WJ, Goeddel D, Ferrara N. Vascular endothelial growth factor is a secreted angiogenic mitogen. Science 1989; 246:1306–1309.

132. Plouet J, Schilling J, Gospodarowicz D. Isolation and characterization of a newly identified endothelial cell mitogen produced by AtT-20 cells. EMBO J 1989; 8:3801–3806.

133. Shibuya M, Yamaguchi S, Yamane A, Ikada T, Matsushine HT, Sato M. Nucleotide sequence and expression of a novel human receptor-type tyrosine kinase (flt) closely related to the fms family. Oncogene 1990; 8:519–527.

134. Matthews W, Jordan CT, Gavin M, Jenkins NA, Copeland NG, Lemischka IR. A receptor tyrosine-kinase cDNA isolated from a population of enriched primitive hematopoietic cells and exhibiting close genetic linkage to c-kit. Proc Natl Acad Sci USA 1991; 88:9026–9030.

135. Yamaguchi TP, Dumont DJ, Conion RA, Breitman ML, Rossant J. flk-1, an flt-related receptor tyrosine kinase is an early marker for endothelial cell precursors. Development 1993; 118:489–498.

136. DiCorleto PE, Bowen-Pope DF. Cultured endothelial cells produce a platelet-derived growth factor-like protein. Proc Natl Acad Sci USA 1983; 80:1919–1923.

137. Collins T, Ginsburg D, Boss JM, Orkins SH, Pober JS. Cultured human endothelial cells express platelet-derived growth factor B-chain: cDNA cloning and structural analysis. Nature 1985; 261:748–750.

138. Marx M, Perlmutter RA, Madri JA. Modulation of platelet-derived growth factor receptor expression in microvascular endothelial cells during in vitro angiogenesis. J Clin Invest 1994; 93:131–139.

139. Usuki K, Norberg L, Larsson E, Miyazono K, Hellman U, Wernstedt C, Rubin K, Heldin CH. Localization of platelet-derived endothelial-cell growth-factor in human placenta and purification of an alternatively processed form. Cell Reg 1990; 1: 577–584.

140. Ishikawa F, Miyazono K, Hellman U, Drexler H, Wernstedt C, Hagiwara K, Usuki K, Takaku F, Risau W, Heldin CH. Identification of angiogenic activity and the cloning and expression of platelet-derived endothelial-cell growth-factor. Nature 1989; 338:557–562.

141. Roberts AB, Sporn MB, Assoian RK, Smith JM, Roche NS, Wakefild D, Heine UI, Liotta LA, Falanga V, Kehrl JH, Fauci A. Transforming growth factor type B: rapid induction of tufts and angiogenesis in vivo and stimulation of collagen formation in vitro. Proc Natl Acad Sci USA 1986; 83:4167–4172.

142. Madri JA, Pratt BM, Tucker AM. Phenotypic modulation of endothelial cells by transforming growth factor-β depends upon composition and organization of the extracellular matrix. J Cell Biol 1988; 106:1375–1384.

143. Schreiber AB, Winkler ME, Derynck R. Transforming growth factor-a: a more potent angiogenic mediator than epidermal growth factor. Science 1986; 232:1250–1253.

144. Schraufnagel DE, Arzouman DA, Sekosan M, Ho. The effect of transforming

growth factor-alpha on airway angiogenesis. J Thorac Cardiovasc Surg 1992; 104(6):1582–1588.

145. Bussolino F, Wang JM, Defilippi P, Turrini F, Sanavio F, Edgell CJS, Aglietta M, Arese P, Mantovani A. Granulocyte- and granulocyte-macrophage–colony stimulating induce human endothelial cells to migrate and proliferate. Nature 1989; 337:471–473.

146. Folkman J, Klagsbrun M. Angiogenic factors. Science 1987; 235:442–447.

147. End P, Engel J. Multidomain proteins of the extracellular matrix and cellular growth. In: McDonald JA, Mecham RP, eds. Receptors for extracellular matrices. San Diego: Academic Press, 1991:79–129.

148. Noden DM. Embryonic origins and assembly of blood vessels. Am Rev Respir Dis 1989; 140:1097–1103.

149. Sundell CL, Roman J. Control of lung vasculogenesis by extracellular matrix composition (abstr). Mol Biol Cell 1994; 5:179a.

150. Millauer B, Wizigmann-Voos S, Schnurch H, Martinez R, Moller NPH, Risau W, Ullrich A. High affinity VEGF binding and development expression suggest Flk-1 as a major regulator of vasculogenesis and angiogenesis. Cell 1993; 72:835–846.

151. Janney CG, Askin FB, Kuhn C. Congenital alveolar capillary dysplasia—an unusual cause of respiratory distress syndrome in the newborn. Am J Clin Pathol 1981; 76:722–727.

152. Cater G, Thibeault DW, E. C. Beatty EA. Misalignment of lung vessels and alveolar capillary dysplasia: a cause of persistent pulmonary hypertension. J Pediatr 1989; 114:293–300.

153. Wagenvoort CA. Misalignment of lung vessels: a syndrome causing persistent neonatal pulmonary hypertension. Hum Pathol 1986; 17:727–730.

154. Ignotz RA, Massague J. Transforming growth factor-β stimulates the expression of fibronectin and collagen and their incorporation into the extracellular matrix. J Biol Chem 1986; 261:4337–4345.

155. Roberts CJ, Birkenmeier TM, McQuillan JJ, Akiyama SK, Yamada SS, Chen WT, Yamada KM, McDonald JA. Transforming growth factor β stimulates the expression of fibronectin and of both subunits of the human fibronectin receptor by cultured human lung fibroblasts. J Biol Chem 1988; 263:4586–4592.

156. Giaid A, Polak JM, Gaitonde V, Hamid QA, Moscoso G, Legon S, Uwanogho D, Roncalli M, Shinmi O, T. Sawamura SK, Yanagisawa M, Masaki T, Springall DR. Distribution of endothelin-like immunoreactivity and mRNA in developing and adult human lung. Am J Respir Cell Mol Biol 1991; 4:50–58.

157. Menko AS, Boettiger D. Occupation of the extracellular matrix receptor, integrin, is a control point for myogenic differentiation. Cell 1987; 51:51–57.

158. Seed J, Hauschka SD. Clonal analysis of vertebral myogenesis. VII. Fibroblast growth factor (FGF)–dependent and FGF-independent muscle colony types during chick wing development. Dev Biol 1988; 128:40–49.

159. Sassoon D. Hox genes: a role for tissue development. Am J Respir Cell Mol Biol 1992; 7:1–2.

160. Sander LM. Fractal growth processes. Nature 1986; 322:789–793.

161. Gleick J. Chaos: Making a New Science. New York: Penguin Books, 1987.

162. Mandelbrot B. The Fractal Geometry of Nature. San Francisco: Freeman, 1982.
163. Henke C, Fiegel V, Peterson M, Wick M, Knighton D, McCarthy J, Bitterman P. Identification and partial characterization of angiogenesis bioactivity in the lower respiratory tract after acute lung injury. J Clin Invest 1991; 88:1386–1395.
164. Mitchell JJ, Reynolds SE, Leslie KO, Low RB, Woodcock-Mitchell J. Smooth muscle cell markers in developing rat lung. Am J Respir Cell Mol Biol 1990; 3: 515–523.
165. Zwerdling R. Abnormalities of lung growth and development. In: Shirley M, Katz R, eds. Clinics in Chest Medicine. Philadelphia: Saunders, 1987:711–720.
166. Coffin JD, Harrison J, Schwartz, S, Heimark, R. Angioblast differentiation and morphogenesis of the vascular endothelium in the mouse embryo. Dev Biol 148: 51–62.

# 14

## Neuropeptides and Lung Development

MARY E. SUNDAY

Harvard Medical School
and Brigham and Women's Hospital
and Children's Hospital
Boston, Massachusetts

## I. Introduction

It has been recognized for over 50 years that lung tumors can elaborate hormonal substances, including catecholamines and multiple bioactive peptides (1). Often referred to as "ectopic hormones," these substances may infrequently give rise to secondary paraneoplastic syndromes such as Cushing's syndrome due to production of bombesin-like peptide (BLP) or adrenocorticotropic hormone (ACTH) by small cell carcinomas of the lung (SCLCs) or pulmonary carcinoid tumors (2,3). However, many of the same substances have been identified in normal or nonneoplastic lung, with highest levels often being observed during fetal gestation.

The concept of the lung as an endocrine organ was especially appealing to me for several reasons. First, having previously studied the role of helper and suppressor factors in immunoregulation (4), I had begun to view all organ systems as part of a global endocrine/paracrine network. It seemed very reasonable that circulating or diffusible bioactive substances derived from different cell types might have effects on neighboring cells and/or distant organs. This has become increasingly recognized over the past decade as numerous peptides have been demonstrated to have differing biological effects on distinct cell types (5). In further recognition of this tenet, "lymphokines" were renamed "cytokines," because they were found to have effects on cells outside the classic immune system. Second, the lung was ideally suited to such a function, because it receives 100% of the blood supply and contains multiple different cell types, including epithelial, mesenchymal, and hematopoietic cells, capable of elaborating bioactive substances. Third, there was relatively little known about cell proliferation and differentiation during lung development compared with the hematopoietic or immune systems. With regard to human lung development, this was in part due to the difficulty in obtaining normal human fetal and neonatal lung tissues for study (6). Also, there was a paucity of animal models for developmental lung disorders, which could be related to lethal phenotypes resulting from mutations in genes critical for lung embryogenesis and maturation. Fourth, the study of fetal lung development has obvious clinical implications for promoting the survival of infants at risk for respiratory distress syndrome (7). Finally, it was apparent that relatively little was known about the cell biology, physiology, and pathology of normal pulmonary neuroendocrine cells (PNECs) (8,9), and what was known had been learned mostly from studies of SCLC cell lines, which have highly abnormal karyotypes (10,11). Although PNECs have been recognized since 1939 (see below), the first National Institutes of Health (NIH) Workshop on PNECs in Health and Disease was not held until 1991 (12). This is a relatively unexplored area of cell and developmental biology.

Most of the cumulative knowledge concerning fetal lung development has been derived from studies in rodents; predominantly rats and mice (13–21). Most of these studies have focused on the biology and biochemistry of type II pneumocytes, which produce surfactant phospholipids and proteins. Recently, there has been a surge in interest about the role of specific growth factors in regulating the maturation of type II pneumocytes and other epithelial cells. In recognition of this widespread interest, this chapter begins with a brief overview of the prevailing theories pertaining to nonneuropeptide growth factors in fetal lung. After defining the nomenclature and pulmonary sources of neuropeptides, some general principles of neuropeptide physiology in extrapulmonary systems and in postnatal lung are then reviewed. Most of this chapter is an in-depth state of the art discussion of the potential role of bioactive neuropeptides in fetal lung development.

### A. Nonneuropeptide Growth and Differentiation Factors Involved in Lung Development

Lung development, including morphogenesis, growth, and differentiation or maturation (22,23), is a complex process involving multiple interactions between different cell types and hormones, where epithelial-mesenchymal interactions have been best characterized (19) (see Chapter 4). Peptide growth factors (24) such as epidermal growth factor (EGF) (25) as well as extracellular matrix components (26), in particular collagen, fibronectin, and laminin (27), are all critical components regulating branching morphogenesis. Cellular interactions with extracellular matrix and proteoglycan molecules via integrins (28) are also important in cell proliferation and differentiation. Glucocorticoids (exogenous or from fetal adrenal cortex) trigger increased production of fibroblast-pneumono-cyte factor (FPF) from pulmonary fibroblasts, leading to increased surfactant production by type II pneumonocytes, but with growth arrest (which is reversible after ~2 weeks in the rabbit model) (19,29); this process can be enhanced by thyroid hormone (30) or inhibited by androgens (31–33). Although FPF has never been isolated, recent data suggest that it could be a lipid rather than a protein (34). EGF, transforming growth factor-α (TGF-α) and amphiregulin (35), which are all ligands for the EGF receptor (36,37), are produced by nonneuroendocrine (non-NE) epithelium and/or mesenchymal cells in fetal lung (37–39), stimulating branching morphogenesis, cell growth, and type II cell maturation (40). EGF may also act via FPF (41). Basic fibroblast growth factor (bFGF) (42,43) and platelet-derived growth factor (PDGF) (44) are also produced by non-NE epithelium and have also been demonstrated to augment branching morphogenesis, cell differen-tiation, and cell proliferation via specific receptors in developing lung (43,45). Transforming growth factor-β (TGF-β) isoforms, synthesized by both nonneuro-endocrine epithelium and mesenchymal cells, function to inhibit FPF-induced (46) and/or EGF-induced type II cell maturation growth and maturation (40). Insulin-like growth factors (IGFs) (47) are produced by mesenchymal cells and have also been implicated in lung growth during development. However, until recently, there was no developmental role in lung development identified for any of the neuropeptides normally secreted in the lung.

### B. Pulmonary Sources of Neuropeptides

The two major pulmonary sources of neuropeptides are the PNECs (8,48,49) and intrapulmonary nerve fibers (50,51). The nomenclature used to describe these components are summarized in Table 1. Each of these will be discussed in the following sections. There are several outstanding recent reviews on both PNECs and neuropeptides in lung physiology and pathology: the encyclopedic overview by Sorokin and Hoyt in 1989, which was a previous volume in this series (8); more current overviews of PNECs as specifically related to lung development and pediatric lung diseases by Dana Johnson (48) and Ernest Cutz (9); and general physiological roles of the diverse bioactive peptides produced in the lung, with particular focus on peptides derived from nerve fibers and potential roles for these in the pathophysiology of asthma, by Peter Barnes et al. (50,52,53) and David Springall et al. (54). In addition, recent experimental work has revealed several nonclassic sources of neuropeptides in the lung, primarily non-NE epithelial cells

**Table 1**  Pulmonary Sources of
Neuropeptides: Nomenclature

---

Pulmonary neuroendocrine cells
  isolated or solitary neuroendocrine (NE) cells
    small granule cells
    argyrophil cells
    APUD cells
    Kultschitzky-like cells
    enterochromaffin-like cells
  neuroepithelial body (NEB)
    innervated PNEC cluster
    intraepithelial organoid
Nerve Fibers
  extrinsic
    parasympathetic
    sympathetic
    nonadrenergic, noncholinergic
    sensory
  intrinsic
    parasympathetic

---

(see Section III.B below). Several methods which have been used to detect, quantitate, and/or localize specific neuropeptide gene expression within an organ such as the lung are given in Table 2. "Gene expression" per se usually refers to the process of transcription, which may be constitutive (basal or constant level) or may be regulated developmentally or by specific agents such as glucocorticoids or retinoids (55,56). Relative levels of specific mRNAs in a given tissue may be quantitated using any of several different RNA analyses, given in order of ascending sensitivity: Northern blot analyses; RNAse protection or S1 nuclease protection assays; and semiquantitative reverse-transcribed polymerase chain reaction (RT-PCR). Localization of cells producing a given mRNA species is usually carried out using the technique of in situ hybridization (ISH) (57), in which the greatest sensitivity is achieved using cRNA probes. Details of these experimental methods are given elsewhere (57–61). A schematic diagram illustrating the major features of ISH are given in Figure 1. Recently, in situ RT-PCR has been developed as a highly sensitive alternative method for detecting low-level gene expression in tissue sections, but it has the drawbacks of being relatively untested (used by very few investigators) and being very costly (62).

Similarly, peptide levels in a given tissue may be quantitated absolutely (for instance, in fentomoles per gram wet weight of tissue) using radioimmunoassays (RIAs) or enzyme-linked immunosorbent assays (63–66). Many such assay sys-

**Table 2** Methods for Detection and/or Quantitation of Gene Expression in the Lung

| | |
|---|---|
| mRNA | |
| quantitation: | Northern blots, S1 nuclease, RNAse protection, RT-PRC |
| localization: | in situ hybridization, in situ PCR |
| Peptide | |
| quantitation: | RIA, ELISA, immunoPCR |
| localization: | immunohistochemistry, enzyme histochemistry |

tems are now commercially available for bioactive peptides. ImmunoPCR has been described as an alternative highly sensitive technique for detecting as little as one molecule of a substance per well of an assay plate (67). Localization of specific peptides or proteins stored in specific cells in a tissue section has been accomplished using immunohistochemistry, with either immunoperoxidase or immunofluorescence as the most common tools for this purpose. The immuno-peroxidase assay used in our laboratory is based on the avidin-biotin complex approach (57) and is schematically depicted in Figure 2.

Additional methods for the detection of neural or neuroendocrine (NE) cells are summarized in Table 3. Electron microscopy (EM) is still widely used for demonstrating dense-core vesicles of various sizes as a complex phenotypic marker of NE cells in the lung and other organs (8,68–70). Scanning EM may be

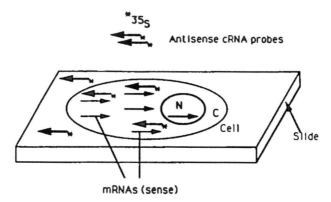

**Figure 1** In situ hybridization. Schematic representation of in situ hybridization using antisense cRNAs (labeled with *35S) complementary to mRNAs (shown in sense orientation) a cell in a tissue section (N, nucleus; C, cytoplasm). Nonhybridized probes, such as those present on the glass slide adjacent to the tissue section, would be removed by RNAse treatment and washes posthybridization.

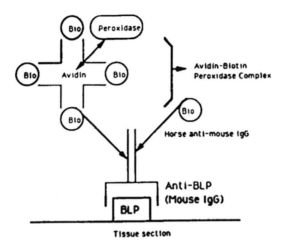

Tissue section

**Figure 2** Immunoperoxidase analyses using the avidin-biotin-complex (ABC) technique. Schematic representation of immunoperoxidase analyses of a tissue section containing a BLP antigen. The primary anti-BLP antibody exemplified is the mouse monoclonal IgG$_1$ 2A11 (250). The secondary antibody is biotinylated horse antimouse IgG, which is followed by the ABC immunoperoxidase reagent (Vector Laboratories, Burlingame, CA). Amplification of the signal occurs with the likelihood of multiple secondary antimouse IgG$_1$ antibodies and multiple ABCs at the site of each BLP antigen (space permitting). The peroxidase is developed using a substrate such as diaminobenzidine.

**Table 3** Methods for Demonstrating Neural and/or Neuroendocrine Cells in Tissue Sections

Electron microscopy (EM)
Immuno–electron microscopy (ImmunoEM)
Silver Staining: Grimelius (argyrophil reaction), Fontana-Masson (argentaffin reaction)
Formaldehyde-induced fluorescence
Lead hematoxylin
PAS–lead hematoxylin
Nonspecific esterase histochemistry
Immunohistochemistry[a]

[a]For PNEC-specific markers, see Table 4.

used to identify three-dimensional structural changes in morphology (71). ImmunoEM can be used to localize specific peptides or other antigens at the subcellular level, which may provide information of functional relevance. For instance, housekeeping enzymes such as neuron-specific enolase (NSE) and creatine phosphokinase BB isoform are early cytoplasmic markers of NE cells, whereas many of the neurosecretory granule markers are bioactive peptides which are secreted via fusion of dense core vesicles membranes with the basal cell membrane followed by exocytosis (48). Many of these bioactive peptides may play multiple roles as paracrine growth and differentiation factors for neighboring cells (24). Colocalization of two or more peptides to the same neurosecretory granules suggests a possible functional interdependence and/or regulatory effects (72,73). The main drawback of EM is that PNECs are so sparsely distributed in the pulmonary epithelium that multiple sections may be required to demonstrate only a few cells or neuroepithelial bodies (NEBs).

However, except for EM, most of the techniques listed in Table 3 are now mainly of historical interest and are described in detail elsewhere (8). Silver staining methods react with amine-containing cells, including both NE cells and neurons. PNECs (high in 5-hydroxytryptamine [5-HT]) and pulmonary nerve fibers are usually strongly positive for argyrophilic silver staining by the Grimelius method in which cell components spontaneously reduce silver nitrate; only rare PNECs stain using the argentaffin reaction of Fontana-Masson in which cell components require the presence of silver salts and an exogenous reducing agent. Formaldehyde-induced or formaldehyde vapor–induced fluorescence also depends on the presence of amines, either catecholamines or 5-HT, and has been the principal methodology historically used to establish the presence of the amine precursor uptake and decarboxylation (or APUD) characteristic in NE cells (see below); however, immunostaining and RIA for 5-HT is even more sensitive than formaldehyde condensation reactions and has therefore replaced them in histochemical investigations. Lead hematoxylin is also selective for cells containing neurosecretory granules, where lead acts as a mordant that binds to the granules and forms a lake with hematoxylin; however, nonselective staining of nucleoli, nuclear chromatin, keratohyalin granules, centrioles, and other structures is a limiting feature. PAS-lead hematoxylin adds a further dimension of selectivity (8), because the granules of many PNECs are only weakly stained by lead hematoxylin and yet may contain diastase-resistant carbohydrates or glycoproteins stainable by the periodic acid–Schiff (PAS) procedure for peripheral glycols or glycol amino groups. In developing lungs, PNEC precursors are identified by lack of PAS staining such that the PNECs stand out as negative images among undifferentiated epithelial cells that contain glycogen (8). Later, as dense core vesicles accumulate, PNECs become stained by PAS and/or lead hematoxylin. Enzyme histochemistry has focused primarily on the activity of nonspecific esterases and acetylcholinesterases, but the greater sensitivity and selectivity of immunostaining for neuron-specific enolase (74) and other enzymes such as dihydroxyphenylalanine (DOPA) decarboxylase (75) has replaced classical histochemical staining methods.

During the past decade, much attention has been focused on the role of bioactive peptides derived from pulmonary nerve fibers with regard to the pathophysiology of neurogenic inflammation and reactive airways disease or asthma (50,76). Relatively little is known about the possible physiological and/or pathophysiological roles of peptides derived from PNECs, especially with regard to normal fetal lung development, which will be discussed below.

### C. General Principles of Neuroendocrine/Neural Systems and Neuropeptide Physiology in the Gastrointestinal Tract and Brain

Historically, epithelial endocrine cells were first recognized as cells in the gastrointestinal tract with granular or clear cytoplasm by Heidenhain in 1870 (77), in spite of which these cells are referred to as Kultschitzky cells following Kultschitzky's paper in 1897. The gut endocrine cells were also called enterochromaffin cells, because they closely resembled the chromaffin cells of the adrenal medulla (78). They have been extensively studied in the gastrointestinal tract and pancreas for almost a century. In 1914, Masson noted the affinity of these cells for silver salts (argentaffinity) and suggested that they might subserve an endocrine function. This system was initially considered to involve only a single cell type producing a single hormonal substance, 5-HT (79). However, subsequent studies revealed that these endocrine cells demonstrated wide histochemical variability with regard to argentaffinity, argyrophilia, autofluorescence after formaldehyde fixation, and masked metachromasia. This staining heterogeneity was eventually correlated with intracellular stores of peptide and polypeptide hormones as well as amines. The diffuse neuroendocrine system in multiple organs was described formally in the middle 1960s by Pearse (80–82), who noted a number of histochemical and ultrastructural similarities between insulin- and glucagon-producing cells of the pancreatic islets, calcitonin-producing C cells of the thyroid and ultimobranchial body, and ACTH and melanocyte-stimulating hormone (MSH)–producing cells of the anterior pituitary. Subsequent histochemical, immunohistochemical, and ultrastructural analyses led to recognition of at least 19 distinct cell types in the gut and pancreas (83).

In the gut, these epithelial NE cells have been demonstrated clearly to arise from the endoderm in chick-quail chimera experiments by Le Douarin and coworkers (84). This approach involves the transplantation of neural tube and associated neural crest cells from quail embryos to replace the corresponding region removed from a host chick embryo; the subsequent migration of the neural crest can be traced in the host embryo, because the nucleus of quail cells contains a large perinucleolar mass of heterochromatin, which is absent from the nucleus of chicks (84). Whereas C cells within the ultimobranchial body and thyroid gland all contain the quail marker and thus migrate from neural crest (85), similar to the myenteric plexus of intrinsic neurons throughout the gut, quail cells were never found in the endodermal epithelium of the gut or pancreas (86,87). This conclusion was supported by more definitive investigations in the chick in which endoderm and adhering mesoderm from presumptive gut was grafted onto the chorioallantoic membrane of host embryos: in those experiments, endocrine cells appeared in the epithelium whether grafts were made before or after the probable time that neural crest cells reach the gut (88). This thesis is supported by the finding that cultured normal gastric mucous cells (83) or clonal colonic adenocarcinoma cell lines (89) can demonstrate divergent differentiation into both NE and non-NE phenotypes, suggesting that multiple major cell types arise from a common precursor cell.

Regardless of the histogenesis of NE cells in a given organ and their precise peptide/amine profile, their differentiated NE phenotype is strikingly similar (Table 4, discussed in detail below). Thus, most NE cells contain vasoactive amines, either epinephrine/norepinephrine or 5-HT, cytoplasmic enzyme markers

**Table 4**  Markers of Normal and/or Hyperplastic
Pulmonary Neuroendocrine Cells

---

Cell surface
  CD10/neutral endopeptidase 24.11 (CD10/NEP)
  neural cell adhesion molecule (N-CAM)
  leukocyte -7/human natural killer cell antigen (Leu 7)
Cytoplasmic
  neuron-specific enolase (NSE)
  protein gene product 9.5 (PGP 9.5)
  creatine phosphokinase BB isoform
  DOPA decarboxylase
Neurosecretory granules
  chromogranin A (CGA)
  synaptophysin
  serotonin (5-HT)
  gastrin-releasing peptide/bombesin-like peptide (GRP/BLP)
  calcitonin gene–related peptide (CGRP)
  calcitonin
  cholecystokinin (CCK)
  substance P
  enkephalin
  ACTH
  hCG

---

such as NSE, and markers of neurosecretory granules such as chromogranins and a wide variety of neuropeptides. Although none of the peptides are entirely organ specific, they may be sometimes species dependent. For instance, islet cells in rat pancreas express the gastrin gene transiently during development (90), and gastrin may act as a growth factor for pancreas. Similar expression of gastrin has not been reported in human pancreas, although it is likely that this has not been systematically investigated.

In neurons, there may also be stage-specific peptide gene expression. We have observed high levels of gastrin-releasing peptide (GRP) gene expression in intrinsic neurons of human fetal colon (91), although this peptide is undetectable in adult colon (83). Thus, transient expression of genes encoding peptides or their receptors by NE cells and/or peripheral neurons may indicate involvement in developmental processes. This tenet may be a general rule, but it may require comprehensive analyses of gene expression during ontogeny for confirmation.

A corollary of this generalization is that peak relative numbers of peptide-positive neuroendocrine cells or intrinsic neurons may occur in any species during fetal or neonatal development of peripheral organs such as the gut (92), pancreas (90), or thyroid (66). In contrast, expression of neuropeptides in the brain may reach peak levels at or about the time of birth, subsequently plateauing at that level rather than declining (92,93). The corresponding neuropeptide receptor gene expression may be regulated in parallel with the peptide mRNA levels (93).

These observations are consistent with the thesis that in the central or peripheral nervous systems or the diffuse neuroendocrine system, neuropeptides may subserve fundamentally distinct roles at different times during ontogeny (5). In early development, neuroendocrine/neuronal peptide mRNAs may peak during organogenesis, suggesting a role as factors stimulating morphogenesis, cell proliferation, and/or differention. For instance, gastrin (90) and/or GRP (94) may function as growth factors for the gastrointestinal tract during ontogeny, whereas the same peptides function as neuroregulatory factors in adult enteropancreatic systems (91). Similarly, numerous brain-gut peptides have been identified in the gut and/or pancreas as neurotransmitters involved in paracrine regulation of hormone secretion and the regulation of smooth muscle contraction responsible for gut motility (83).

### D. Classic Functions of Neuropeptides and Amines in Normal Postnatal Lung

Most of the current knowledge about the effects of neuropeptides and amines on postnatal lung is focused on molecules derived from intrapulmonary nerve fibers (50,52). Sensory nerve fibers in the lung are believed to play a physiological role as irritant receptors linked to the cough reflex regulating respiratory skeletal muscle and bronchial smooth muscle contractility (53). These sensory nerves contain a variety of neuropeptides, especially tachykinins, which have been most extensively studied with regard to their contribution to the pathogenesis of neurogenic inflammation and/or asthma (see Section IV.D below). Thus, the classic functions of neuropeptides and amines in postnatal lung have mainly been determined for those agents derived from the intrapulmonary nerve fibers, as summarized in Table 5.

Intrinsic parasympathetic and extrinsic sympathetic nerve fibers originating from the extrapulmonary ganglia are believed to regulate bronchoconstriction and vascular resistance through feedback mechanisms in a similar fashion (51,53,54). Increased mucous glandular secretion, ciliary beat frequency, contraction of bronchial musculature, and vasodilation are stimulated by vagal (parasympathetic, cholinergic) fibers; the opposite effects are triggered by sympathetic (adrenergic) fibers as well as by humoral catecholamines (endogenous or exogenous epinephrine or other $\beta_2$-adrenergic agonists). Vasoactive intestinal peptide (VIP) has been shown to have the same effects as acetylcholine except for its action as a bronchial smooth muscle relaxant (53). The classic teachings of the neural control of breathing are detailed elsewhere (53,54).

Neuroendocrine cells might also be implicated in cough reflexes, bronchial and vascular smooth muscle tone, or glandular secretion. In 1990, Lundgren et al. (95) demonstrated that the bombesin-like peptides (BLPs), including GRP and

**Table 5** Classic Functions of Neuropeptides and Amines in Postnatal Lung

---

Sensory (Tachykinins, CGRP)
  cough (irritant reflex afferents)
  vasodilator
  bronchoconstriction
  increased glandular secretion and ciliary motility
Cholinergic (vasoactive intestinal peptide, VIP)
  vasodilator (bronchial and pulmonary blood vessels)
  bronchial smooth muscle relaxant
Cholinergic (acetylcholine)
  vasodilator
  bronchoconstriction
  increased glandular secretion and ciliary motility
Adrenergic (epinephrine/isoproterenol/other $\beta^2$ stimulators)[a]
  vasoconstriction
  bronchial smooth muscle relaxant
  inhibit glandular secretion

---

[a]Opposite effects of epinephrine and norepinephrine are mediated via α-adrenergic receptors.

bombesin, can stimulate glandular secretion of respiratory glycoconjugate in the feline trachea, similar to BLP-induced stimulation of glandular secretion in the gastrointestinal tract (91) (see below). In a follow-up study, Baraniuk et al. (96) administered BLPs topically to human nasal mucosa in vivo and observed dose-dependent stimulation of both serous (lactoferrin) and mucous (glycoconjugate) secretion, similar to prior experiments with nasal mucosal explants in vitro. These data suggest that GRP released from trigeminal sensory nerves may bind to BLP receptors on respiratory epithelial cells and submucosal glands to promote neurogenic inflammation.

The role of PNECs as oxygen chemosensors in postnatal life will be discussed in Section III below.

## II. Pulmonary Neuroendocrine Cells

### A. History and Markers

The concept of endocrine cells as normal components of the lung was introduced by Feyrter in 1938 (97), who observed epithelial clear cells (*helle zellen*) which he noted to occur predominantly at airway branch points. Considering their similarities to the Kultschitzky cells in the gut, he speculated that these cells in the lung might subserve an endocrine function (98). In 1969, Lauweryns first described innervated clusters of silver-stained NE cells in human infant airway epithelium, which he called neuroepithelial bodies (NEBs) (99). In 1973, Lauweryns observed that these cells produce the vasoactive amine 5-HT (100). PNECs were thus confimed to be part of the diffuse neuroendocrine system of APUD cells described by Pearse in the late 1960s (80,81), constituting the pulmonary equivalent of Kultschitzky cells or enterochromaffin cells in the gut.

In 1978, BLP was identified in human fetal lung by Wharton, Polak, and coworkers (101) as the first neuropeptide immunoreactivity localized to PNECs. Since then, a wide spectrum of peptides, amines, and other markers have been identified in PNECs from species ranging from amphibians and reptiles to diverse mammalian species, including primates (8,102,103); the species distribution of these markers have been summarized in the Proceedings of the First NIH Workshop on PNECs in Health and Disease (12). NE cells have also been described in fish gills (12), suggesting a common function related to respiratory control.

A listing of current markers of normal (nonneoplastic) PNECs is given in Table 4. The major neuropeptides present in developing normal PNECs are BLP GRP (91) and calcitonin gene–related peptide (CGRP) (8) at 10–14 weeks' gestation; calcitonin is not detected until the second trimester (104). There are single reports also demonstrating cholecystokinin (CCK) (105) and endothelin (106) in normal human fetal lung. Leu-enkephalin (104), human chorionic gonadotropin (hCG) (107,108), and ACTH (109,110) have been demonstrated in injured postnatal lung but are not known to occur with any frequency in normal fetal lung.

### B.  PNEC Terminology

The terminology for PNECs includes several different names derived from their appearance, histochemical reactivity, or putative functions (see Table 1) (8, 111,112). The use of a single term for all pulmonary epithelial cells with NE properties suggests that these cells are morphologically and functionally equivalent, which may be incorrect. Feyrter described isolated, noninnervated PNECs which are now sometimes referred to as Kultschitzky cells or K cells, because of their similarity to NE cells in the gastrointestinal tract (20,1777). Alternatively, isolated PNECs may be referred to as solitary small-granule cells, because ultrastructural analyses reveal that they contain small (100–300 nm) membrane-bound cytoplasmic dense-core neurosecretory-type granules where secretory peptides and the amine 5-HT are stored (8). Lauweryns made the important observation in human (113) and rabbit (100) newborn lung that PNECs also occur as complex clusters, most of which become innervated, giving rise to the name NEB for the resulting intraepithelial organoid. Hoyt and co-workers defined *nodal* NEBs as those occurring at branchpoints and *internodal* NEBs as those in the airway between branchpoints (114). Both clustered and isolated PNECs react with a specific silver stain (Grimelius's "argyrophilia" method) that detect amines; PNECs are therefore sometimes referred to as argyrophil cells (8).

### C.  Morphology and Ontogeny

*Embryological Origins of PNECs*

All mature PNECs, both solitary and clustered, share numerous structural and chemical similarities which suggest that they are derived from the same precursor cell (Table 6). Both isolated PNECs and NEBs are localized above the epithelial basement membrane. Definitive cell lineage analyses of pulmonary NE cells have never been published in spite of the likelihood that such information is available in embryonic preparations (8). In brief, it is most likely that PNECs are derived from the endoderm, because the lung epithelium originates from the endodermal lining of the foregut (6) and enteropancreatic NE cells have been demonstrated to derive from endoderm (88). Furthermore, detailed thymidine labeling studies of fetal hamster lung by Hoyt and colleagues demonstrated labeling of both isolated PNECs and NEBs at 23% of the labeling index of non-NE epithelial cells; in contrast, there was absolutely no labeling of intrinsic bronchial ganglia, supporting a relationship between PNECs and non-NE pulmonary epithelial cells, both of which were distinct from neural crest derivatives (114). The intrinsic myenteric

**Table 6** Key Features of PNECs

Epithelial localization
Isolated vs NEBs
Endodermal origin
Dense-core granules by EM (basal, diverse)
Amine: 5-HT
Peptides: e.g., GRP, CGRP, calcitonin (see Table 4)
Other markers: NSE, CGA (see Table 4)
Low mitotic rate
Paracrine effects on neighboring epithelial cells

plexuses of the gut and intrinsic bronchial ganglia are known to be derived from the neural crest (8) (detailed above). Studies of teratomas support the hypothesis that PNECs differentiate and presumably descend directly from respiratory epithelium, because there was no association between PNECs and brain tissue (115).

### Ontogeny of Pulmonary Epithelial Cell Differentiation

During human embryonic development, simple lung buds lined by undifferentiated pulmonary epithelium initially are formed by invagination of the endodermal lining of the foregut at gestational week 3 and all bronchopulmonary segments are started by week 7 (116). The first epithelial cells to differentiate in both human (6) and rodent (8,13) fetal airways are the PNECs (Fig. 3). Isolated PNECs are demonstrated by ultrastructural (117), immunohistochemical, and in situ hybridization analyses (104) at human gestational week 8–9 (Fig. 4A,B). It is not until 11 weeks' gestation that presecretory and preciliated cells are detectable by immunostaining and morphology (6). This suggests that well-differentiated NE cells may be functionally important for facilitating differentiation of other non-NE bronchial epithelial cell types which appear later on. This concept is supported by the light microscopic observation of basally oriented PNECs with dendritic processes extending along the basement membrane between adjacent epithelial cells (48,118) (Fig. 4C), which is consistent with paracrine secretion of neurosecretory granules along the basolateral aspects of the cell. These dendritic cells are more frequently identified in developing fetal airways, suggesting that they could also represent immature cells that have yet to contact the future airway lumen (8,48).

By light microscopy, PNECs first appear in the most proximal airways of human fetal lung at 8 weeks' gestation as isolated pyramidal- or spindle-shaped cells with their basal surface resting on the basement membrane and a thin cytoplasmic process extending to the future airway lumen (see Fig. 4A) (48). This cytoplasmic process is believed to be involved in sensing oxygen levels in the airway, which is an important function in postnatal life (see below). At 8–9 weeks,

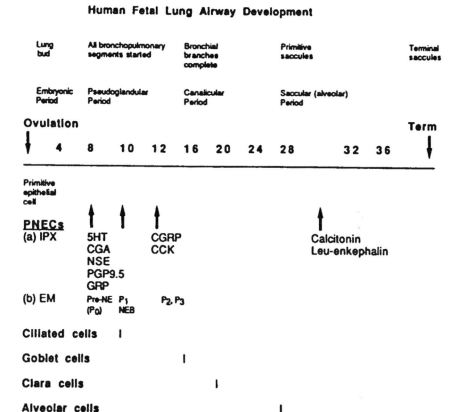

**Figure 3** Summary of the milestones in human fetal lung development. Airway development is shown above the time course from ovulation (time = 0 weeks) to term (40 weeks). The appearance of differentiated epithelial cells is given according to immunoperoxidase (IPX) and ultrastructural (EM) analyses (bars). (Modified from ref. 6.)

the earliest stage of detection, many of these cells immunostain for BLP, 5-HT, chromogranin A (CGA), NSE, and protein gene product 9.5 (PGP 9.5). At 8–9 weeks, GRP mRNAs also are demonstrated in a similar distribution using in situ hybridization (see Fig. 4B) (119). Peak immunostaining for NSE and PGP 9.5 occurs at 12–14 weeks' gestation, which is consistent with cytoplasmic markers being present in early NE cells which are just beginning to express granule markers (120). In contrast, CGA peaks later, at 18–22 weeks, similar to CGRP,

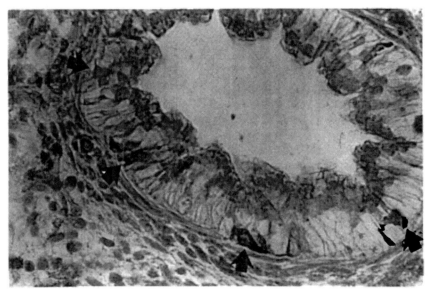

**(A)**

**Figure 4**   Immunohistochemical analyses of PNECs in developing human fetal lung. (A) BLP-positive isolated PNECs (arrows) in a large airway from a 9-week-gestation human fetal lung (×400). (B) Cells containing GRP mRNAs are demonstrated in large (proximal, P) airways that have begun to branch using GRP in situ hybridization with antisense cRNA probes (arrows). Note that smaller unbranching distal airways (D) are devoid of an mRNA signal (×200). (C) BLP-positive PNECs in large bronchiole from a 20-week-gestation human fetal lung (L, airway lumen), demonstrating NEBs (arrows) and dendritic processes (arrowheads) (×100).

5-HT, BLPs, and other early neurosecretory granule markers (see Table 4). Calcitonin, leu-enkephalin and ACTH have only been observed in the lungs of infants on chronic respirator therapy with secondary lung disease (104,109).

Light Microscopic Analyses of NEB Formation and Distribution

The formation of NEBs begins with an increase in numbers of NE cells per cluster (8,102). In human fetal lung, NEBs begin to form at 9–10 weeks' of gestation, and by 20 weeks' gestation, NE cell clusters account for the majority of NE cells (see Fig. 4C) (8,121). In contrast, isolated NE cells are almost exclusively found within the trachea (122,123). After NE clusters begin to form within the developing fetal lung, the clusters become innervated by both sympathetic and sensory (nonadrenergic, noncholinergic) nerve fibers (50,52,54,117,124,125).

The dynamics of NEB formation have been most extensively investigated

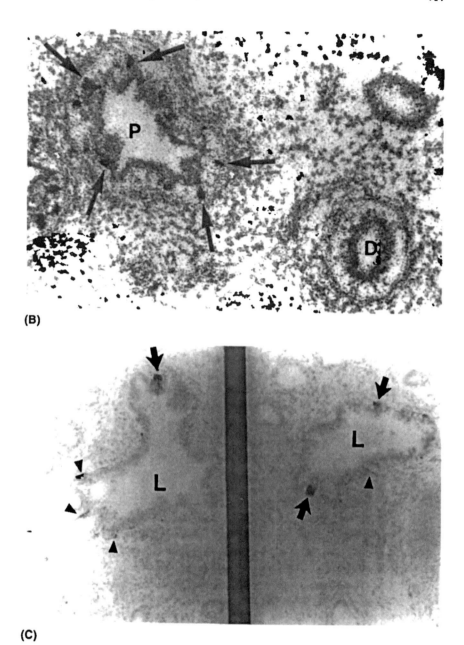

(B)

(C)

by Hoyt et al. in developing hamster lung (114,126). Those studies suggest that NE clusters could arise because of cell differentiation from adjacent precursor cells (126), together with a very slow rate of cell proliferation (114) and prolonged cell survival, similar to neurons. Following exposure to [³H]thymidine for the final 4.5 days of a normal 16-day gestation, total label of NEBs was only 23% of that in non-NE cells, and all non-NE cells were labeled, whereas many NE cells were not (114). The mean label in non-NE cells and internodal NEBs (in airway epithelium between branch points) rose 10-fold between the hilum and the periphery; however, nodal NEBs (at branch points, see Section II.B above) were more lightly labeled than internodal NEBs, which is consistent with their earlier differentiation (114). They concluded that NEBs are derived from cells from the endoderm (see Section II.C above) which are programmed to stop dividing before other non-NE epithelial cells; thus, the formation of NEBs is linked closely to the early proliferation of the bronchial tree.

Cutz et al. (127) carried out an extensive three-dimensional reconstruction of the distribution of NEBs immunostained for 5-HT in fetal rabbit lung. They found that the overall number and size of NEBs increased during the immediate perinatal period, peaking at 6 days and 11 days, respectively; by 56 days of age, NEBs became significantly smaller. They demonstrated that about half of all NEBs were localized within the small peripheral airways at all ages examined, and up to 64% of NEBs occur at branch points (127). These findings suggest that NEBs may be functionally most active in the perinatal period, which may be important during adaptation to extrauterine life. Functional responses of PNECs and/or NEBs to altered oxygen levels and the role of PNEC-derived substances in lung development will be discussed at greater length below.

### Electron Microscopy of PNECs and NEBs in Normal and Abnormal Developing Lungs

Ultrastructurally, both solitary and clustered PNECs contain dense-core neurosecretory granules characteristic of cells within the APUD series. Precursor NE cells (pre-NE cells, termed $P_0$ (6,70,104,117), containing primordial dense-core granules (64–245 nm) are evident as early as gestational week 8 in larger potential airways of human fetal lung (6,70,104,117) (see Table 6). By 10 weeks, pre-NE cells are still predominant but more well differentiated NE cells (nonvesicular $P_{1A}$ and vesicular $P_{1V}$) both isolated and in clusters (developing NEBs, see below) are also beginning to appear in future conducting airways. PNEC subtypes $P_2$ and $P_3$ containing larger granules are usually evident by 14 weeks' gestation. The differentiated PNECs are more electron dense than the surrounding glycogen-rich columnar epithelium and are located basally in the epithelium. Some sections demonstrate dendritic cytoplasmic processes running along the basement membrane beneath adjoining cells or in the intercellular spaces (117,128), consistent with the observation of similar processes by immunostaining (Fig. 4D). Five subtypes of NE cells are identifiable ultrastructurally based on the size and morphology of dense core vesicles, as summarized in Table 7 (72,117). Using immunoEM, BLP, calcitonin, and CGRP have been localized to large-granule $P_3$-type PNECs in which all three peptides are localized to the same neurosecretory granules; these are seen predominantly in lungs from infants who died with either hyaline membrane disease (HMD) or chronic lung disease, usually broncho-pulmonary dysplasia (BPD, see below) (72,73). NE cells containing a predominance of large granules may contain BLP, calcitonin, CGRP, or combinations of these peptides; few of those with small granules contain either of these two peptides; at least two other morphological populations of NE cells were not labeled for either peptide, suggesting that as yet unidentified peptides and/or amines are contained in their granules. The presence of up to three peptides in a single granule implies that their release may be simultaneous rather than sequential, and that their action might be concerted. Possible implications of this hypothesis are to be discussed in the following sections on lung development and asthma.

### D. Role of PNECs as Chemosensors in Postnatal Adaptation: Effects of Oxygen, Nicotine, and Nitrosamines In Vivo and In Culture Systems

*Acute Hypoxia*

In 1973, Lauweryns and Cokelaere provided the first definitive evidence that innervated PNECs (NEBs) function as airway sensors (129), which supported previous hypotheses. Using a cross-circulation model in newborn rabbits, they demonstrated that NEB respond to acute airway hypoxia, but not to hypoxemia without airway hypoxia, by increased secretion of the contents of dense-core vesicles and decreased amine fluorescence consistent with amine release by PNECs (129). These observations indicated that PNECs are likely to function as intrapulmonary chemoreceptors in postnatal life. In subsequent studies, Lauweryns et al. also demonstrated that hypercapnia, but not hyperoxia, produced increased exocytosis and the uptake of biogenic amines; they went on to point out that the occurrence of NEBs at airway branch points (113,127) would be optimal for modulation of airway and vascular smooth muscle tone in response to airway hypoxia in order to alter local ventilation-perfusion ratios (130). Pulmonary NE cells are strongly conserved throughout phylogeny (8), including amphibians and birds, further suggesting that these cells might serve a critical role in respiratory physiology. Fish gills are also known to contain cells similar to PNECs (12,131), raising the possibility that NE cells may be important as oxygen chemosensors even in non–air breathing vertebrates.

A major breakthrough in our understanding of PNEC responses to acute hypoxia was recently reported by Cutz and coworkers (132). That investigation utilizing patch-clamp technology was made possible by the discovery that rabbit PNECs are selectively stained by the vital dye neutral red and hence can be visualized in mixed pulmonary cell cultures which have been enriched for NE cells (132). Cultured NEBs isolated from rabbit fetal lungs were exposed to acute hypoxia in culture: Significant (43%) reduction in outward $K^+$ current was observed when the cell was first exposed (less than 1 sec) to hypoxic medium (Po$_2$: 25–30 vs 150 mm Hg in normoxic media); following recovery in normoxia, a second exposure to hypoxia produced a similar reduction in $K^+$ current. There is definitive evidence that the $O_2$-sensor protein is a membrane-bound NADPH oxidase similar to that present in neutrophils: NEBs immunostain for the NADPH oxidase p91 polypeptide; and a specific inhibitor of NADPH oxidase (DPI) caused a reduction in the $K^+$ current in NEB cells similar in magnitude to that seen with hypoxia; further, NEB cells no longer responded to hypoxic stimulus, after treatment with DPI. These results support a chemoreceptive function for NEB which operates through $K^+$ channels to activate the secretion of bioactive amines and peptides. Because NEBs are known to release amines on hypoxic stimulation, Cutz et al. suggest that the closing of $K^+$ channels by hypoxia may initiate depolarization of the NEB cell membrane which could open voltage-sensitive $Ca^{2+}$ channels and lead to increased $Ca^{2+}$ influx and neurotransmitter release.

### Chronic Hypoxia

Further evidence supporting a role of PNECs as airway chemosensors is provided by several animal models of chronic hypoxia. It has been recognized for some time that some species of animals living at constant hypoxia at high altitude may demonstrate increased numbers of PNECs immunostaining for 5-HT or CGRP (133). This has been referred to as PNEC "hyperplasia," based on the assumption that increased numbers of immunopositive PNECs represents a proliferative response. However, the findings are somewhat controversial, with possible influencing factors including the age of the animals, the length of in hypoxic exposure time, and the species. For instance, Hernandez-Vasquez et al. (134) observed a decrease in the number of argyrophilic PNECs and NEBs in fetal rabbit lung exposed to short-term (10–15 days) chronic hypoxemia. It has been suggested that some of this variability may depend on whether the animal is genetically adapted or simply acclimatized to living in a hypoxic environment (133). Pack et al. (135) have shown that adult Sprague-Dawley but not Wistar rats exposed to 10% hypoxia had a significant increase in the size and number of NEBs. An increased number of PNECs has also been reported in rats or neonatal rabbits kept in experimental hypoxia (136,137) or in rabbits and guinea pigs maintained at high altitude (133,138,139).

The biological implication of PNEC responses to chronic hypoxia in vivo has been investigated in an elegant and systematic manner by Springall and co-workers (136,140,141). Those studies used rats with short-term (3–21 days) chronic exposure to 10% hypoxia to demonstrate that immunostaining of PNECs for CGRP increases, although PGP 9.5 immunostaining does not change, suggesting that latent PNECs are turning on CGRP gene expression rather than proliferating (136). Subsequently, Montuenga et al. (140) used 5′-bromodeoxyuridine labeling to confirm that CGRP-containing PNECs or their precursors are capable of low-level proliferation, but that the proliferation is not increased significantly in hypoxia. A detailed time course carried out by Polak's laboratory (141) demonstrated significant increases in CGRP immunoreactivity after only 4 hr of hypoxia, which preceded changes associated with vascular remodeling as assessed by the number of vessels with evidence of vascular proliferation and muscularization at 1–20 days. Thus, it is possible that PNEC-derived neuropeptides such as CGRP may be implicated in the etiology of pulmonary hypertensive arteriopathy in experimental hypoxia (142).

### Chemical Stimuli for PNEC Hyperplasia in Vivo and in Vitro

It is likely that other PNEC hyperplasia responses to chemical stimuli both in vivo and in tissue culture may also represent primarily NE differentiation rather than proliferation. PNEC hyperplasia has been described in response to ozone, although there was no significant difference in nuclear labeling for bromodeoxyuridine (BrdU) (143). Amine- or peptide-positive PNECs have been shown to increase in hamster lung following treatment with nitrosamine carcinogens, nicotine, or cigarette smoke either alone or together with chronic hyperoxia in vivo (144–147). One level of control in these systems may be at cholinergic-nicotinic receptors on PNECs, as demonstrated by monitoring calcitonin production by PNECs in vivo or in culture (147). Recent work in our laboratory has confirmed that this presumptive hyperplasia is likely to represent predominantly a NE cell differentiation response rather than PNEC proliferation (148), because only rare PNECs labeled by immunostaining for proliferating cell nuclear antigen (PCNA), whereas about 25% or more of the non-NE pulmonary epithelial cells were PCNA positive (148). These data are consistent with the observation of almost exclusively non-NE lung tumors in nitrosamine-treated rodents (149). It is possible that such PNEC differentiation may be sustained for weeks or even years after the initial stimulus is withdrawn, as occurs following acute inhalation burn injury (150).

The PNEC differentiation response that occurs normally during fetal lung development may be similarly studied in culture systems (151) which may be utilized to clarify molecular mechanisms of normal regulation of NE cell growth and peptide secretion. For instance, Nylen et al. (147) have demonstrated that transplacental nicotine pretreatments resulted in a significant increase in calcitonin levels in newborn hamster lungs which could be sustained in culture for weeks by the addition of nicotine to the culture medium; this was blocked by nicotinic but not by muscarinic cholinergic antagonists. Similarly, Ebina et al. (152) demonstrated that calcium and ionophore A23187 lead to lower numbers of CGRP-positive PNECs in fetal rat lung cultures, suggesting that these cells secrete peptide hormones in response to calcium influx across the plasma membrane.

Speirs and Cutz (126,153,154) and Linnoila et al. (144,155) have developed isolation methods and long-term selective culture conditions for PNECs which should help to clarify the responses of PNECs to a variety of chemical stimuli. For instance, the addition of GRP to rabbit fetal PNEC cultures at 24 days of gestation but not 20 or 28 days of gestation, led to an increase in 5-HT–positive PNECs in spite of no change in [$^3$H]thymidine labeling of PNECs (126), which is consistent with observations of Polak et al. (140,141); this effect coincided with the detection of mRNA for GRP receptors in fetal rabbit lung at 24 days but not 20 or 28 days. It should be noted that all primary PNEC cultures contain other non-NE epithelial cells and fibroblasts, which appear to be important in maintaining the viability of PNECs (126,154).

### E. What Has Been Learned About PNECs from Studies of Small Cell Carcinoma of the Lung

In addition to primary PNEC cultures and fetal lung organ cultures, much has been learned about normal PNEC markers and biology using cell lines derived from small cell carcinomas of the lung, most of which express NE-specific markers. The major limitations that must be kept in mind, however, are that these cell lines have highly unstable chromosomes, with numerous karyotypic abnormalities and consequently a constantly shifting phenotype even if clonal lines are developed (10,156,157). Most of these studies have been specifically directed at lung tumor cell biology, and yet this body of work does shed light on some of the similarities and differences between malignant and normal PNECs. For instance, several genes thought to play a role in normal cell proliferation are over-expressed in human lung cancer. These include the c-*myc* proto-oncogene (10,158) and numerous growth factors which may function in an autocrine or paracrine fashion (159). Other genes important for development and also expressed at high levels in lung cancer include DNA-binding homeobox proteins that are involved in the regulation of gene expression during embryonic development (160) and may function themselves to promote cell proliferation (161). Conversely, lung cancer cells may be resistant to the induction of normal differentiation and growth cessation, such as terminal squamous differentiation induced by TGF-β (162) and mucosecretory differentiation induced by retinoic acid (163,164). In dysplasias and neoplasms, there is frequently a loss or mutation of genes involved in orderly regulation of growth and differentiation programs (165–168), including *Rb*, p53, and as yet unidentified tumor suppressor genes on chromosome 3p which may be deleted or mutated in a variety of tumor cells (169,170).

A number of classic molecular markers of normal PNEC maturation (see Table 4) have also been described in small cell lung carcinoma (SCLC), including:

1.  Neuropeptides, amines, and other neurosecretory granule components (reviewed in refs. 8 and 48): CGA (171,172), 5-HT, GRP/BLP, calcitonin, and leu-enkephalin (72,104,172), CGRP (173), ACTH (109, 174), hCG (107,108), endothelin (106), neurotensin (175), synaptophysin (176), and enzymes involved in processing peptides such as peptide amidation enzymes (PAM) (177,178) which amidate many neuropeptides to their bioactive forms, and prohormone convertase (179). Some of these peptides have been demonstrated to act as significant growth factors for SCLC and/or normal bronchial epithelial cells, including GRP/BLP (91) (see below), neurotensin (175,180), endothelin (180), and CGRP (181).
2.  NE cytoplasmic markers: neuron-specific enolase (NSE) (74,174), L-DOPA decarboxylase (DDC) (75,156), creatine kinase BB isoform (69), and PGP 9.5 (182), the neural/NE isoform of ubiquitin C-terminal hydroxylase, are present in resting adult PNECs (136) and may be markers of early PNECs.
3.  NE cell surface markers: neural cell adhesion molecule (N-CAM), which is a marker of well-differentiated NE cells and SCLCs (183–185) and may be implicated in developmental processes (186,187); and Leu 7 (188).

Several novel NE antigens have been identified recently. The Second Small Cell Lung Cancer Workshop held in 1990 reported 87 well-characterized monoclonal antibodies (MoAbs), many of which could be clustered into groups based on similar patterns of immunoreactivity (189). The cluster 1 antigen has been identified as N-CAM, which is restricted to neural and NE cell types (190). Other clusters recognize general epithelial cell or stromal cell antigens (191). Most of the MoAbs reported in the Second Workshop have already been localized in human fetal lung (191), and with the exception of N-CAM, few are NE specific. The 7B2 protein also appears to be a marker of NE differentiation (192). Some cluster 4 (MoAb SWA21) and cluster 5 (MoAbs SWA23 and SEN12) antigens are also expressed on neural and epithelial components (191,193,194). The temporal expression of these SCLC antigens in fetal lung has not been explored.

There are additional antigens associated with either SCLCs and/or NE cells which are not NE specific but may play a role in cell proliferation and/or differentiation during tumorigenesis or lung development. Several such cell surface molecules are listed below:

1. Low levels of CD10/NEP are present on SCLCs and normal NE cells (195) in which it may be involved in regulating the bioavailability of specific regulatory peptides such as tachykinins and BLPs (76,195, 196).
2. Receptors specific for GRP/BLP (197,198), the BLP-related peptide neuromedin B (NMB) (199), unknown BLPs (200,201), calcitonin (202), CGRP (203), and 5-HT (204) are likely to be involved in modulation of growth processes: calcitonin might induce different biological responses in target cells depending on their positions in the cell cycle (205); and in NE cell lines, calcitonin mRNA is lowest and CGRP is highest during rapid growth (206); 5-HT has been demonstrated to act as a growth factor in both neuronal and nonneuronal systems (207).
3. Laminin receptors may contribute to the aggressive tumorigenicity and metastatic capability of SCLCs (208,209) as well as play a role in normal developmental processes such as morphogenesis (210,211).

There is a need for clarifying lineages of bronchial epithelial cells, which give rise to the vast majority of human lung cancers. In the WHO classification, only SCLC and carcinoids are considered to be NE (212–214). However, many non-SCLCs are now known to express NE markers, suggesting a common lineage for most of the major forms of lung cancer (11,215,216). This is believed to reflect the inherent plasticity of airway epithelium (217), where epithelial metaplasia occurs frequently in injured lung. We found proGRP to be a tumor marker of large cell undifferentiated lung carcinoma (LCLC) as well as SCLC (172), which is consistent with the belief that LCLCs are predominantly NE if poorly differentiated squamous cell and adenocarcinomas are excluded (216). N-CAM (184) or a panel of NE markers may predict which non-SCLCs will behave more like SCLCs with regard to prognosis (184), response to chemotherapy (188,218), or tumor stage (219). Thus, SCLC and non-SCLC tumors may have direct histogenic links along a common differentiation pathway operative in the bronchial epithelium (Fig. 5) (218,220). SCLC thus appears to be derived from an undifferentiated cell either identical to or close to the stem cell which bears a partial NE phenotype, which is consistent with immunostaining of undifferentiated fetal airway epithelial cells with a few NE cell markers (PGP 9.5, NSE, and CGRP) (120,221). It is not surprising that tumor progression of SCLC, such as occurs following chemotherapy (222) or upon *myc* gene transfection (223), may involve movement toward a more complex phenotype with non-SCLC features (69,157). SCLC progression and direct conversion of SCLC to a non-SCLC phenotype may also occur following transfection of the v-Ha-*ras* oncogene which is normally not expressed in SCLCs (224–226). Clinical progression of lung cancer may recapitulate normal differentiation or dedifferentiation pathways.

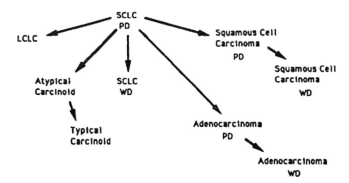

**Figure 5** Hypothetical bronchial epithelial differentiation pathway. The phenotype and behavior of lung cancers may reflect the developmental stage at which tumor cells are arrested due to a block in normal differentiative capacity (PD, poorly differentiated; WD, well differentiated).

### F. Bombesin-Like Peptides as Growth Factors for Small Cell Carcinoma of the Lung, Non-SCLC, and Normal Adult Pulmonary Cells

Bombesin is a 14–amino acid peptide originally identified by Erspamer in 1971 in the skin of the frog *Bombina bombina* (91,227). Using antibodies to amphibian bombesin, a 27–amino acid mammalian homologue of bombesin was identified by McDonald as GRP (228). GRP and bombesin share a highly conserved seven–amino acid C-terminus (Fig. 6) which is required for immunogenicity and for high-affinity binding to physiological receptors. GRP, the major known pulmonary BLP, is synthesized as a larger precursor hormone, proGRP, two cDNAs of which were originally cloned from a human pulmonary carcinoid tumor by Spindel et al. (229,230); later, Battey and co-workers identified the third human GRP cDNA from a SCLC cell line (Fig. 7) (231). All three transcripts are derived from one gene via alternative splicing at the junction of exons two and three; all three transcripts occur together in the same proportions in all positive tissues and cell lines examined, including SCLC cell lines and human fetal lung (119,232). GRP has multiple physiological effects which are essentially identical to the effects of its amphibian peptide homologue bombesin (Fig. 8) (91). These have been studied most extensively in the brain, gut, pancreas, and thyroid (233–242) and include both neuroregulatory and growth-modulating effects (91). At this point, only a few major points of relevance to understanding the effects of BLPs in developing lung will be mentioned. The growth-promoting effects in the gut and pancreas may be mediated in part via release of CCK and/or gastrin (90,236,243–

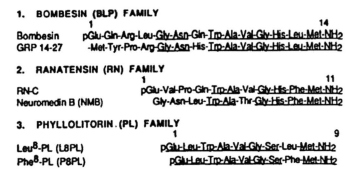

**1. BOMBESIN (BLP) FAMILY**

Bombesin    pGlu-Gln-Arg-Leu-Gly-Asn-Gln-Trp-Ala-Val-Gly-His-Leu-Met-NH₂
GRP 14-27   -Met-Tyr-Pro-Arg-Gly-Asn-His-Trp-Ala-Val-Gly-His-Leu-Met-NH₂

**2. RANATENSIN (RN) FAMILY**

RN-C                pGlu-Val-Pro-Gln-Trp-Ala-Val-Gly-His-Phe-Met-NH₂
Neuromedin B (NMB)  Gly-Asn-Leu-Trp-Ala-Thr-Gly-His-Phe-Met-NH₂

**3. PHYLLOLITORIN (PL) FAMILY**

Leu⁸-PL (L8PL)    pGlu-Leu-Trp-Ala-Val-Gly-Ser-Leu-Met-NH₂
Phe⁸-PL (P8PL)    pGlu-Leu-Trp-Ala-Val-Gly-Ser-Phe-Met-NH₂

**Figure 6**  The three major groups of BLPs and related peptides. Key C-terminal amino acid similarities within each group are underlined. Note that the C-terminal met is amidated in all three groups.

245). Neuroregulatory effects of GRP derived from thyroidal C cells (66) may include stimulation of calcitonin secretion (246) and thyroid hormone secretion (240), in contrast to calcitonin and CGRP which inhibit thyroid hormone secretion (240). The BLP-related peptide neuromedin B (NMB) has indirect effects on thyroid function via direct actions on the release of thyroid-stimulating hormone (TSH) that vary depending on the thyroid status of the animal (247).

A few years after BLP was localized to NE cells in human fetal lung in 1978 by Wharton et al., two lines of investigation were followed to determine the function of BLP in normal and neoplastic cell growth. After Rozengurt and Sinnett-Smith showed that bombesin was a potent mitogen, stimulating proliferation and DNA synthesis in Swiss 3T3 murine fibroblast cells, Willey used a soft agar clonogenic assay to demonstrate that GRP and its bioactive carboxylterminal peptide induced the growth of normal adult human bronchial epithelial cells (248). At about the same time, two different laboratories independently showed that BLPs are potent mitogens for SCLC: Weber et al. (249) used [³H]thymidine incorporation and cell counts to show a mitogenic effect of GRP on two SCLC cell lines but neither of two non-SCLC cell lines; and Cuttitta et al. (250) demonstrated stimulation of growth of several SCLC cell lines by bombesin in a soft agar clonogenic assay and in nude mice in vivo. Cuttitta also made the important observation that the unstimulated growth of two different lines could be blocked either in culture or in nude mice by MoAbs to bombesin (250). Because many of these SCLC lines both secrete BLPs and bear BLP receptors (250), an autocrine-positive feedback effect on SCLC growth was implicated. Since then, multiple BLP receptor-specific antagonists have been demonstrated to inhibit the growth of several SCLC cell lines (251). In an ongoing clinical trial using the 2A11-blocking

ProGRP

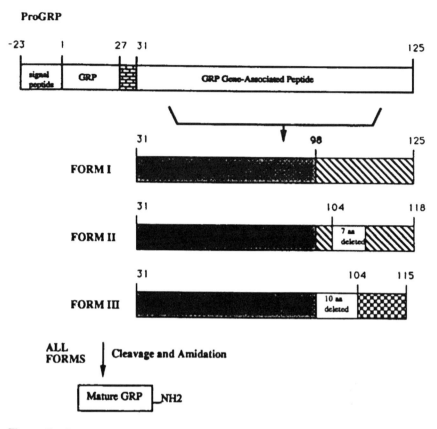

**Figure 7** Structure and processing of the prohormone form(s) of GRP. In humans, there is one GRP gene which is alternatively spliced to yield three forms of proGRP in humans (all of which encode GRP but differ in the GRP gene-associated peptide) (231); all three forms of proGRP are present in the same ratios in all GRP-positive tissues examined, including both normal and neoplastic cell types (232). In rats, there is only one proGRP which is homologous to the human proGRP form 3 (as shown) (445). In order to generate mature bioactive GRP, the prohormone must be cleaved and amidated (178).

antibombesin monoclonal antibody, 1 of 14 patients has gone into complete remission with no evidence of further disease (159). These observations indicate that a subset of SCLCs may be inhibited by anti-BLP antibodies. Some SCLCs similarly produce NMB (252). However, tumor responsiveness to 2A11 did not correlate with BLP receptor mRNA expression (253).

Extending the earlier analyses, Shipp et al. (195) demonstrated that SCLCs express low levels of the cell surface metalloendopeptidase CD10/neutral endo-

## BLP Effects: Postnatal Tissues

**Neuroregulatory**
**CNS:** Secretion of
 ACTH, PRL, GH;
 Satiety;
 Scratching;
 Sympathetic Drive;
 Hypothermia.
**GI:** Increased Gut Motility,
 Secretion of Gastrin,
 Glucagon, PP;
 Decreased Secretion
 of Insulin
**Thyroid:** Secretion of
 Calcitonin,
 Thyroid Hormone

**Mitogenic**
**In Vitro:**
 Bronchial Epithelium,
 SCLC Cell Lines
 Pulmonary Fibroblasts
 Thyroid follicular cells
**In Vivo:**
 Gut and Pancreatic Epithelium
 SCLC Cell Lines

**Figure 8** Key effects of BLPs as neuroregulatory peptides and as mitogens in postnatal tissues. Central nervous system (CNS) effects include stimulation of secretion of pituitary peptides, increased sympathetic output leading to hypothermia due to heat loss, and behavioral effects, including anorexia. Gastrointestinal (GI) effects are due predominantly to GRP released by intrinsic neurons and include increased gut motility and modulation of secretion of enteropancreatic hormones, with elevated gastrin, glucagon, and pancreatic polypeptide (PP) secretion and suppression of insulin release, leading to increased blood glucose. Thyroidal effects are believed to be linked to GRP production by NE cells, the C cells (66).

peptidase 24.11 (CD10/NEP, common acute lymphoblastic leukemia antigen, CALLA) and that this enzyme hydrolyzes BLPs at two sites within the bioactive C-terminal seven–amino acid sequence, which is consistent with earlier analyses of the BLP-related peptide NMB (254). The growth of BLP-responsive SCLC cell lines was investigated using a soft agar clonogenic assay and [$^3$H]thymidine incorporation into DNA. SCLC growth was inhibited by CD10/NEP and potentiated by CD10/NEP inhibition. A specific BLP receptor antagonist, [13-psi-14-CH$_2$NH]bombesin (255), inhibited SCLC colony formation resulting from the addition of either phosphoramidon or bombesin. Thus, CD10/NEP inhibition led to effectively increased levels of endogenous BLP which then acted in an autocrine fashion to promote clonal SCLC growth.

In addition to SCLCs, the proliferation of normal human bronchial epithelium (256) and many non–small cell carcinomas (NSCLCs) (257,258) may be regulated by BLPs or CD10/NEP inhibition (258). BLP/GRP receptors have been isolated (259) and cloned (260) from H345, a human SCLC cell line which responds to multiple growth factors (159), and from Swiss 3T3 fibroblasts (197,198,261). In addition, high-affinity receptors for BLPs have been characterized by binding studies in normal guinea pig lung membranes (262) and novel

BLP binding proteins have been identified in normal mouse lung (263). Proliferative responses of SCLC and NSCLC cell lines and normal bronchial epithelial cells to bombesin or GRP are often maximal at ~50 nM (256), suggesting that the receptor involved in these functional effects may be different from the BLP/GRP receptor cloned from 3T3 fibroblasts, which has a $K_d$ ~1nM or less (198). DeMichele et al. (264) and Ganju et al. (258) have demonstrated that, similar to SCLCs, the majority of NSCLCs and cultured normal bronchial epithelial cells express the gene-encoding receptors for NMB (199), a BLP-related peptide which is the mammalian homologue of amphibian ranatensin (see Fig. 6). BLP and NMB are closely enough related that they each bind reasonably well to both BLP receptors and NMB receptors, albeit with somewhat different affinities (261). Although most SCLCs, NSCLCs, and cultured human bronchial epithelial cells produce mRNA for the BLP/GRP–preferring receptor, this gene was not expressed in any of five primary bronchial biopsies in spite of the use of highly sensitive RT-PCR analyses (which did detect NMB receptor transcripts in the same samples) (264). These data suggest that the GRP receptor gene is not expressed in normal adult bronchial epithelium but may be induced in tissue culture. mRNA for the third bombesin-like receptor subtype (BRS-3) is detected in only a minority of lung tumors or bronchial epithelial cell cultures and neither of two normal bronchial biopsies (264). The stimulatory effects of BLPs were observed on human adult bronchial epithelial cells from 8 of 13 donors in a colony-forming assay, including three with chronic obstructive lung disease (COPD); the inhibitory effects of BLPs were observed with the remaining 5 donors (256). These widely varying effects of BLPs on normal adult bronchial epithelial cultures do not correlate with the smoking status of the donor but might be heightened in disease states involving a proliferation of PNECs.

NSCLCs may be also capable of producing GRP, suggesting that there may be a common stem cell for both SCLC and NSCLC (258). These observations are consistent with the thesis that undifferentiated fetal lung epithelial cells may express the GRP gene even in the absence of other differentiated NE features such as dense-core granules (120,221).

### G. Bombesin-Like Peptides in Fetal Lung Development

*Cell Proliferation and Differentiation*

In 1978, mammalian BLP was identified as the first neuropeptide hormone localized to PNECs, with highest levels being detected by RIA in human fetal lung (101). BLP appears in human PNECs as soon as the cells are detectable at 8–9 weeks' gestation (119). Peak relative numbers of BLP-positive PNECs occur at about mid gestation in human fetal lung (91,119), which is also the time of maximal GRP gene expression (detailed below). One study has described GRP-immunoreactive nerve fibers in the respiratory tract, the tracheobronchial wall, and the nasal mucosa, but the antiserum used was not fully characterized and could be cross reactive with NMB, which is the BLP-like peptide shown by several others to be present in intrapulmonary nerve fibers (50,265).

The BLPs GRP and bombesin (Fig. 8), described in Section II.F above, have essentially identical dose-response curves for physiological effects (91), acting both as neuroregulatory peptides and as growth factors. BLPs stimulate serous and mucous secretion in the upper respiratory tract and clonal proliferation of normal adult bronchial epithelial cells (248,256), human pulmonary fibroblasts (266), and several SCLC cell lines (see above).

Considering the abundance of BLP in PNECs, the high numbers of PNECs in human fetal lung, and the potentially important role of BLPs as growth factors in lung development, I began to study GRP gene expression in human fetal lung in the laboratories of Joel Habener and William Chin. A cDNA spanning most of the proGRP cDNA (hence, detecting all three splice variants) (see Fig. 7) had been cloned from a human pulmonary carcinoid tumor by Spindel (229). A cRNA probe derived from this cDNA was used for Northern blot analyses and in situ hybridization (ISH) analyses (119). GRP mRNAs were first detectable in fetal lung at 9–10 weeks' gestation, plateaued at levels 25-fold higher than in adult lungs from 16 to ~30 weeks, coinciding with the pseudoglandular and canalicular periods of lung development, and then declined to near adult levels by 34 weeks' gestation. Using ISH, we demonstrated transient expression of GRP mRNAs in PNECs (from 9 weeks' gestation [see Fig. 4B] to ~22 weeks) in a proximal to distal fashion in parallel with the growth of fetal airways (119). In contrast, BLP immunostaining was detectable at 9.5 weeks' gestation and remained elevated until several months after birth. A direct comparison of ISH and immuno-histochemical studies on serial sections showed that (1) GRP mRNA and BLP peptide consistently colocalized in early gestation lung; (2) at only 9.5 weeks' gestation, there were about 20% more cells detected by ISH than by BLP immuno-staining, suggesting that a lag period might occur between the time of initial GRP gene transcription and the processing of proGRP via cleavage and amidation into mature GRP; and (3) in neonatal lung, many cells containing BLP immunostain-ing no longer contained detectable GRP mRNA. It is likely that this dissociation between GRP mRNA and BLP peptide is due to the storage of GRP peptide in dense-core granules of resting PNECs. However, we cannot exclude the possi-bility that GRP is not the only pulmonary BLP and that another mammalian BLP-like peptide gene may be expressed in the perinatal period, such as a mammalian phyllolitorin analog (see Fig. 6).

My major interest was then to pursue the functional relevance of BLPs in fetal lung development. Up to that time, the role of neuropeptides in developing lung was essentially unknown. I used three distinct experimental approaches:

1. Administration of exogenous BLPs (267)

2. Treatment with a well-characterized blocking MoAb (2A11) to BLPs (267,268)
3. Potentiation of tissue levels of endogenous BLP by blocking peptide degradation (269,270)

For these investigations, we felt it would be most helpful to have a readily available, cost-effective, well-characterized, and rapid assay system for screening large numbers of peptides or combinations of peptides for the effects on mammalian lung development. We screened fetal murine lung for BLP immunoreactivity by RIA and determined that peak BLP levels occur between embryonic day 16 (e16) and neonatal day 3 (Fig. 9), similar to peak BLP levels in human fetal lung which peak between mid gestation and the early neonatal period (91,119, 127). GRP mRNA was detected as early as e16 in fetal murine lung using Northern blot analyses of poly(A)$^+$ RNA, with peak expression occurring just before birth (Fig. 10) (267); levels drop off substantially after birth (Fig. 10). Thus, the mouse demonstrates transient expression of the GRP gene analogous to what was observed in human fetal lung. Although at first glance this appears to be a different time course of expression in mouse versus humans, it is quite similar according to the chronology of major developmental events (Fig. 11). Thus, GRP gene expression most closely coincides with the onset of surfactant synthesis and type II pneumocyte maturation, which occurs over the last 2 days before birth in the mouse but in the last half of human fetal gestation. Classic experiments by Buckingham and Avery analyzed type II pneumocyte differentiation and surfac-

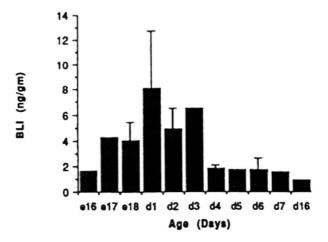

**Figure 9** Levels of BLPs in developing murine lung by radioimmunoassay. Results represent pooled tissues from at least four litters per time point. (Reprinted with permission from Anat Rec, ref. 268.)

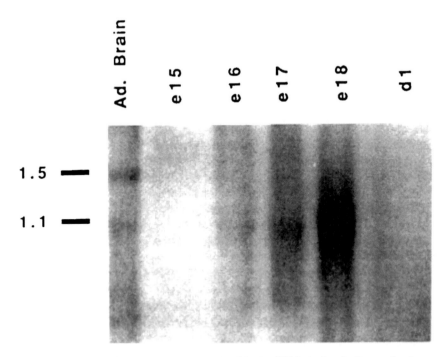

**Figure 10**   Poly(A)$^+$ Northern Blot analysis of GRP mRNAs in developing murine lung. Adult murine brain is the positive control showing a 1.5-kb brain-specific mRNA and the 1.1-kb band present in peripheral tissues. Fetal lungs were taken from e15 to e18 (day of birth); postnatal day 1 is also given (267). (Reprinted with permission from Am J Respir Cell Mol Biol, ref. 267.)

tant production first in mice and found surface-active material at highest levels during the 2 days prior to birth (271); these first experiments were an important prelude to more lengthy and costly experiments in rabbits and lambs. We chose the mouse as the first experimental animal system for our analyses because it constitutes an important and valid model for a first analysis of mammalian lung development: The short gestational period of the mouse allows questions to be answered with a fast turnaround time; and mice are well-characterized in terms of basic embryology, lung cell biology, and genetics.

The three experimental systems we are using to analyze mammalian lung development are:

1.   Fetal murine lung in organ culture to provide a rapid screening tool for assessing the effects of peptides on cell proliferation and differentiation;
2.   Fetal murine lung in utero, to address specifically questions related to

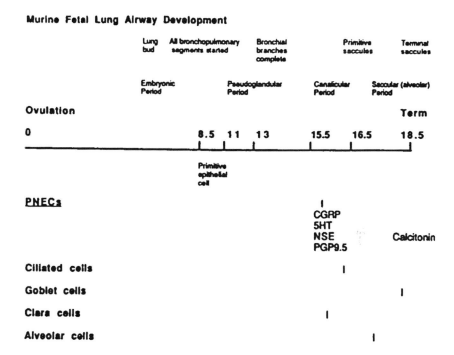

**Figure 11** Summary of the milestones in murine fetal lung development. Airway development is shown above the time course from ovulation (between midnight and 2 AM on day of mating, defined as day 0) to term (18.5 days). The appearance of differentiated epithelial cells is given according to immunoperoxidase (IPX) and ultrastructural (EM) analyses (bars). (Modified from refs. 8 and 13.)

placental peptide transfer and type II pneumocyte maturational effects in vivo and hence potential clinical applicability

3. Human fetal lung in organ culture, which provides the gold standard for understanding human fetal lung development with the ultimate goal of clinical usefulness in the prevention of respiratory distress syndrome in premature infants

In the first series of experiments reported in 1990, exogenous bombesin was administered to cultured human fetal lung and fetal murine lung both in utero and in organ cultures (267). We determined that bombesin does cross the placenta by immunoprecipitation of fetal and maternal soft tissues (minus placentas) 1 hr after administering $^{125}$I-bombesin to the mother by a single intraperitoneal injection;

identical specific activity was precipitated from both maternal and fetal tissues. Following in utero bombesin administration, increased parameters of both growth and lung organ maturation were observed according to both biochemical and ultrastructural analyses (267).

Growth, or pulmonary cell proliferation, was evaluated using [³H]thymidine incorporation into acid-precipitable nuclear DNA normalized for DNA content; total DNA and protein content per lung; and nuclear autoradiography following [³H]thymidine administration in vivo. There were significant dose-dependent increases in [³H]thymidine incorporation following in utero bombesin administration on both e17 and e18, which occurred together with elevated total protein and total DNA per lung (Fig. 12). Tissue autoradiography demonstrated increased labeling of mesenchymal cells as well as epithelial cells in airways and primitive alveoli, indicating a broad-ranging proliferative effect (Fig. 13). These data are consistent with bombesin being a direct growth factor for bronchial epithelial cells and pulmonary fibroblasts.

Maturation, or type II cell differentiation, was assessed by [³H]choline incorporation into saturated phosphatidylcholine (SPC), the rate-limiting step in surfactant phospholipid synthesis (272), normalized for protein content; total SPC content per lung; and electron microscopy for glycogen, which disappears with

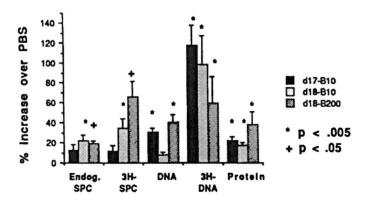

**Figure 12**  Histogram of biochemical effects of bombesin on fetal murine lung development in utero. Mice were treated with either 10 or 200 μg/kg of bombesin (B10 and B200 in figure) from e14 to e17 or e18, and lungs were harvested on e17 or e18. Values shown represent increases over the baseline values ± standard error (SE). Parameters of maturation are total saturated phosphatidylcholine (SPC) content per lung and [³H]choline uptake into SPC (normalized for protein content), both of which were only significant on e18. Parameters of growth are total DNA and total protein content per lung and [³H]thymidine uptake (normalized for DNA content), all of which are elevated on both e17 and e18 (267). (From ref. 267.)

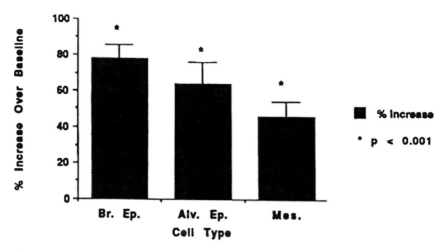

**Figure 13** Proliferation of pulmonary cells in response to bombesin administered in utero. Bombesin (10 μ/kg) was given from e14 to e18; 24 hr prior to harvest, 1 mCi of [³H]thymidine was given as a single intraperitoneal bolus to each pregnant mouse. After harvest, tissue sections were dipped in photographic emulsion. Nuclei labeled on the resulting autoradiograms were quantitated in the three major compartments: bronchial and bronchiolar epithelium (Br. Ep.), alveolar epithelium (Alv. Ep.), and mesenchymal cells (Mes.). The data (267) are expressed as percentage increase over mice given saline vehicle instead of bombesin.

epithelial cell differentiation, and for content of lamellar bodies (LBs), one of the major morphological manifestations of pulmonary surfactant. Bombesin treatment in utero induced significant dose-dependent elevations in [³H]choline uptake and total SPC content per lung which was evident only on e18 (see Fig. 12). Ultrastructurally, there was a dose-dependent increase in the number of cells containing lamellar bodies (differentiated type II cells) on e18, but there was no difference in the number of LBs per type II cell. These data suggest that total surfactant production per cell is comparable, but that there is an effect of bombesin on type II cell differentiation and/or proliferation. However, it is unknown whether the effect on type II cells was direct or requires an intermediary cell such as a fibroblast to be observed; for instance, via a fibroblast-pneumonocyte factor (18,29,273). Studies by Fraslon and Bourbon (274) (see below) suggest that the effect on type II cell differentiation and proliferation are likely to be direct. Of particular interest, the effects on [³H]thymidine and [³H]choline uptake which we observed appeared to be dissociable, with the choline effect being observed only on e18 in utero, suggesting that the cell proliferation and differentiation responses may occur by independent mechanisms. It is unlikely that the bombesin effects in

utero were mediated by endogenous glucocorticoids, because there was no difference in fetal mouse serum corticosterone levels. Finally, the same effects on
thymidine and choline incorporation were observed in both human and murine
fetal lung organ cultures, and the effects of bombesin were blocked by a specific
antibombesin MoAb (2A11), indicating that at least part of the in utero effect was
mediated by bombesin acting directly on fetal lung. The effect of bombesin on
human fetal lung was comparable in magnitude to that observed with peak
concentrations of dexamethasone (10 nM) in the same cultured lung.

In the second series of experiments, anti-BLP MoAb 2A11 was used to test
for the blocking function of endogenous BLPs. First, 2A11 ($IgG_1$) alone blocked
fetal murine lung automaturation in serum-free lung organ cultures by ~60% as
compared with control cultures incubated with only an irrelevant $IgG_1$ (MOPC) as
assessed by choline incorporation ($p < .001$) (267); there was no effect of 2A11
on thymidine incorporation in the same cultures. We then tested the effect of 2A11
on fetal lung maturation in utero and observed a dose-dependent inhibition of lung
maturation on e18 (up to ~35% inhibition) as assessed by choline uptake consistent with the prior observation of a maturational effect on e18 in utero (268).
Again, there was no effect of 2A11 on thymidine incorporation on e18, suggesting
that other lung growth factors may compensate if endogenous BLP levels drop
substantially. Paradoxically, on e17 antibody 2A11 given either in utero or in
serum-containing lung organ cultures led to increased thymidine and choline
incorporation; this effect could be blocked by antibodies to the EGF receptor and
reconstituted by exogenous EGF, suggesting that dropping endogenous BLP
levels on e17 leads to compensatory feedback with EGF receptor upregulation and
consequent increased parameters of growth and maturation. These observations
support a paracrine role for BLPs together with hormonal products of other
epithelial cells in endogenous fetal lung development and underscore the complexity of the whole process.

In the third series of experiments, our aim was to raise the tissue levels of
endogenous BLPs by inhibiting their degradation and then to test for specific
effects which could, in turn, be blocked by specific BLP receptor antagonists (Fig.
14). We chose to potentiate endogenous tissue levels of BLPs by inhibiting BLP
degradation by the cell membrane–associated enzyme CD10/neutral endopeptidase 24.11 (CD10/NEP). CD10/NEP is present on target cells bearing peptide
receptors in multiple organ systems in which it hydrolyzes a number of naturally
occurring peptides. Thus, the enzyme functions to downregulate induced responses to peptide hormones (76,275,276), including leu-enkephalin, substance P,
neurotensin, bradykinin, angiotensin, and endothelin. CD10/NEP is expressed at
high levels in the lung, where it modulates responses to tachykinins such as
substance P that mediate neurogenic inflammation (277). Inhibition of CD10/NEP
dramatically increases both the binding of substance P to bronchial membranes
and the resulting proinflammatory physiological effects. This experimental ap-

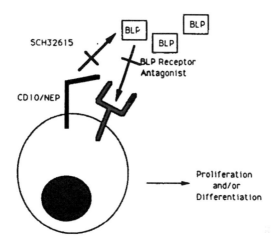

**Figure 14**  Hypothetical model of target cell bearing BLP receptors and CD10/NEP. Inhibition of CD10/NEP (which degrades BLPs and other bioactive peptides) by agents such as SCH32615 would lead to longer tissue half-life of BLPs. The resulting higher tissue levels of BLPs are postulated to result in increased cell proliferation and/or differentiation. The specificity of these enhanced responses may be demonstrate by blocking the enhanced effects using specific BLP receptor antagonists.

proach has been instrumental in clarifying the role of these pulmonary peptides in the pathogenesis of certain disease states, including asthma (50,278). CD10/NEP had been demonstrated to hydrolyze BLPs (195,254) and to modulate growth of BLP-dependent SCLCs (see above) (195). Thus, CD10/NEP inhibition would be a valid approach for investigating the possible role of endogenous BLPs in fetal lung development (Fig. 14).

Before embarking on functional studies of human fetal lung, we used immunoperoxidase and ISH analyses to localize CD10/NEP and its mRNAs to human fetal airway epithelial cells, including PNECs (195,269). Especially high levels of CD10/NEP were present on undifferentiated airway epithelial cells and airway-associated mesenchyme, including smooth muscle in the older fetuses (269), which are likely targets for BLPs. We reasoned that inhibition of CD10/NEP was likely to be a useful approach to study the role of PNEC-derived neuropeptides such as BLPs in lung development. Observations from our laboratory have confirmed the validity of this approach (269,270). CD10/NEP gene expression occurs during the same developmental window as GRP in both human fetal (269) and murine fetal lung (270). In human fetal lung organ cultures, CD10/NEP inhibition by either of two chemically dissimilar agents (SCH32615 and phosphoramidon) resulted in more than a doubling of [$^3$H]thymidine incorpora-

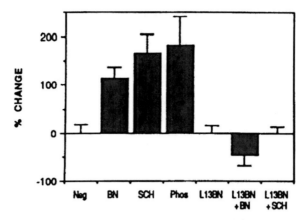

**Figure 15** Increased [³H]thymidine uptake into nuclear DNA induced by CD10/NEP inhibition is due to endogenous BLPs. Human fetal lungs at gestational weeks 14–15 were maintained in organ culture for 48 hr with media alone (Neg); with bombesin alone (BN 100 nM), which resulted in a doubling of [³H]thymidine uptake, with two different CD10/NEP inhibitors (SCH 32615 and phosphoramidon, 5 µM each), which led to more than a doubling of [³H]thymidine uptake; with a BLP receptor antagonist (L13BN 100 nM), which alone had no effect but did completely block proliferation induced by either bombesin or CD10/NEP inhibition (269). Values represent pooled results from three different fetal lungs and are expressed as percentage increase over baseline (media alone). (Reprinted with permission from J Clin Invest, ref. 269.)

tion, which was completely prevented by treatment with a highly specific BLP receptor antagonist [Leu ¹³-psi(CH₂NH) Leu ¹⁴]bombesin (L13BN) (269) (Fig. 15). These experiments support a role for endogenous BLPs in mediating cell proliferation in human fetal lung early in the second trimester.

In order specifically to address questions of the effects on lung organ maturation, we extended our experiments on CD10/NEP inhibition to the mouse in utero. These experiments were made feasible by availability of a long-acting CD10/NEP inhibitor that could be administered to laboratory animals in vivo (279). First, using semiquantitative RT-PCR, we demonstrated CD10/NEP mRNA in fetal murine lung from e15 to e18 (270). CD10/NEP inhibition by SCH32615 given in utero from e12 to e14 resulted in significantly increased thymidine uptake only from e15 to e18, which is consistent with an effect corresponding to the time course of CD10/NEP mRNA expression. Similar to treatment with exogenous BLPs, CD10/NEP inhibition from e15 to e17 in utero was found to elevate parameters of fetal lung growth and maturation on e18, including the following:

1. Increasing [³H]thymidine into nuclear DNA and [³H]choline incorporation into saturated phosphatidylcholine in 48-hr organ cultures (Fig. 16).

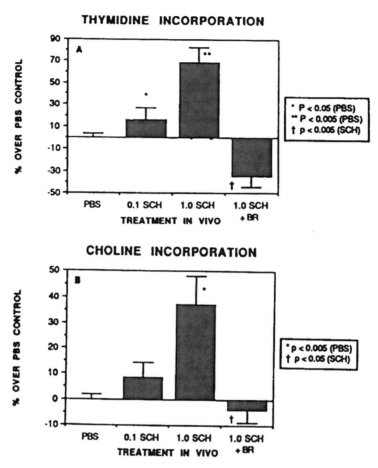

**Figure 16** Increased pulmonary DNA synthesis and surfactant phospholipid synthesis in fetal murine lung after CD10/NEP inhibition in utero. Pregnant mice were treated with saline, SCH32615 alone (0.1 or 1.0 mg/kg), or SCH32615 (1 mg/kg) plus BLP receptor antagonist ([D-Phe12,Leu14]-bombesin, BR) from e15 to e17, and lungs were harvested as previously described (270). Values for [$^3$H]thymidine incorporation (normalized for DNA content) and [$^3$H]choline incorporation (normalized for protein content) are given as percentage increase over baseline (negative control given phosphate-buffered saline (PBS) alone) with *p* values as indicated. (Reprinted with permission from J Clin Invest, ref. 270.)

Tissue autoradiography for nuclear labeling by [$^3$H]thymidine demonstrated significantly increased labeling of type II pneumocytes (K. King and M. Sunday, unpublished data).

2. Ultrastructural evidence of a trend toward increased relative numbers of type II cells (defined as lamellar body–containing cells) in primitive alveoli and a dose-dependent significant decrease in the number of lamellar bodies per type II cell consistent with surfactant secretion (Fig. 17).

3. Fivefold increased levels of surfactant protein A (SP-A) transcripts ($p < .05$) (270). The effects on proliferation and type II cell differentiation were completely blocked by a BLP receptor–specific antagonist, [D-Phe$^{12}$,Leu$^{14}$]bombesin (see Fig. 16), suggesting that CD10/NEP modulates fetal lung development mediated by endogenous BLPs. The lack of an effect with BLP receptor antagonists given alone either in human fetal lung organ cultures (269) or in mice in utero (270) is likely to be related to partial agonist function of the antagonists which would counteract inhibitory effects. This could also be interpreted as indicating the presence of novel and as yet undiscovered BLP receptors (280).

Other laboratories have demonstrated similar enhancement of lung growth and maturational events by BLPs (126,274,281,282). In 1992, Fraslon and Bourbon (274) demonstrated that 1 nM or less of GRP stimulated the proliferation of isolated fetal rat type II cells on e19.5 as determined by measuring total DNA content and thymidine incorporation. GRP at 10 nM or more was inhibitory for growth of both type II cells and fibroblasts, which is consistent with GRP receptor downregulation. Furthermore, 10 nM GRP stimulated [$^3$H]choline incorporation into both surfactant phospholipids (phosphatidylcholine) and nonsurfactant (residual) phospholipids in isolated e19.5 rat type II cells by ~40%. These results are entirely consistent with our own observations, and suggest that the effects we observed in utero and in lung organ cultures could be due to direct stimulation of type II cell surfactant synthesis (267). However, trace contamination of these cultures by fibroblasts cannot be ruled out.

In a similar fashion, Asokananthan and Cake (281) demonstrated that BLPs stimulate surfactant phospholipid secretion from cultured e19 fetal rat type II cells. These data are consistent with our EM results showing decreased LBs in type II cells of fetal mice treated with the CD10/NEP inhibitor SCH32615 to potentiate endogenous BLPs (270), which we had interpreted to suggest increased surfactant secretion. BLPs studied by Cake and Asokananthan included GRP, bombesin, and the BLP-like peptide NMB: Peak effects were observed at 3 nM GRP or bombesin versus 30 nM NMB, supporting the concept that GRP/bombesin–preferring receptors might be physiologically most important in these processes. Interestingly, the magnitude of the stimulatory effect on surfactant

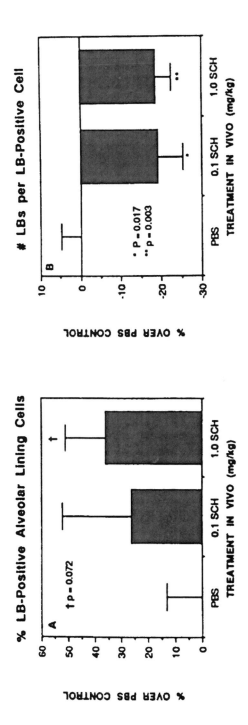

**Figure 17** Ultrastructural analyses for lamellar bodies (LBs) in murine fetal lung following CD10/NEP inhibition. Pregnant mice were treated with saline or SCH32615 (0.1 or 1.0 mg/kg) from e15 to e17 and morphometric analyses carried out as previously described to determine (A) the percentage of alveolar lining cells containing LBs and (B) the number of LBs per LB-positive cell. Results are expressed as percentage change over baseline with *p* values as indicated. (Reprinted with permission from J Clin Invest, ref. 270.)

secretion observed with GRP was about a fourfold increase over baseline as compared with a twofold increase with bombesin. This suggests that there might be conformational differences between these two BLPs such that pulmonary BLP receptors favor the native pulmonary GRP. Furthermore, GRP-enhanced surfactant secretion was blocked 86% by a specific protein kinase C inhibitor (calphostin) and 18% by inhibitors of the calcium/calmodulin–dependent protein kinase but not at all by inhibitors of protein kinase A. These observations indicate that the signal transduction mechanism in type II cells involves intracellular calcium and protein kinase C, similar to what has been observed in 3T3 fibroblasts (283).

BLPs may also function as autocrine differentiation factors for PNECs. Cutz and co-workers (126) have used fetal rabbit PNEC-enriched cultures to study the growth and differentiation of PNECs using [³H]thymidine incorporation and 5-HT immunostaining. GRP stimulated an increase in numbers of 5-HT–positive cells without any effect on thymidine labeling of PNECs. These results are consistent with recruitment of either undifferentiated stem cells or immature PNECs not yet expressing the full PNEC phenotype. GRP did stimulate proliferation of non-PNECs; predominantly mesenchymal cells (126).

Li et al. have carried out functional investigations of BLP induced proliferation in fetal rhesus monkey lung (282). Fetal rhesus monkeys express the GRP gene in lung at mid gestation as determined by Northern blot analyses, similar to human fetal lung (119), indicating that this might be a good animal model for direct comparison with human fetal lung development. GRP receptors are expressed with a similar time course, as shown by RNAse protection analyses, with GRP receptor mRNAs localized primarily to airway epithelium. These results differ somewhat from in situ hybridization studies in other laboratories analyzing fetal human (284), rat (285), and mouse (286) lung (see below) which have localized GRP receptor mRNAs at the highest levels to airway-associated mesenchyme. However, Cutz et al. (284) do identify low levels of GRP receptor mRNAs in the epithelium as well as in the non–airway-associated mesenchyme, suggesting that all of the published in situ studies are correct.

Li et al. (282) also localized GRP mRNAs to airway epithelium of the smallest budding airways as well as to PNECs, although there is no sense control on a serial section for comparison; BLP or proGRP immunostaining was not detectable. If this is real, it is intriguing and would agree with studies in the laboratories of Warburton (221) and Sunday (120) demonstrating CGRP and PGP 9.5 together with the Clara cell marker CC10 in undifferentiated airway epithelium. These observations support a partial NE and Clara cell phenotype of the undifferentiated airway epithelium, which could represent totipotential airway epithelial precursor cells. Li et al. also carried out functional studies with 1-mm cubes of fetal monkey lung in organ culture for 5 days. The addition of bombesin (either 1 or 10 nM) significantly increased DNA synthesis in airway epithelial cells, as determined by BrdU labeling, and apparently significantly increased the airway size and number. Although it is conceptually difficult to understand how an increased number of airways would occur in a 1-mm cube of tissue taken at 60–80 days' gestation, which is after completion of airway branching, the data on increased airway epithelial cell growth and increased airway size are well presented and appear statistically sound.

The major disadvantages of using nonhuman primates are the high cost and limited availability. Rhesus monkeys (*Macaca mulatta*) do develop respiratory distress syndrome (RDS) with HMD when delivered prematurely at ~80% of gestation (287), similar to rabbits (288,289), lambs (290), macaques (*Macaca nemestrina*) (291–293), and baboons (294). However, only baboons have been shown to develop the chronic sequelae to HMD, bronchopulmonary dysplasia (BPD), which is similar to humans physiologically, radiographically, and morphologically (295–298). Macaques do not appear to develop chronic lung disease (299). The reasons for this discrepancy are not known, but it suggests that baboons would be preferable to rhesus monkeys as a nonhuman primate model of fetal lung development.

### Branching Morphogenesis

PNECs are localized predominantly at airway branch points. In our prior work, we showed that GRP and GRP mRNAs occurred in well-differentiated PNECs exclusively in branching human fetal airways. To analyze GRP receptor mRNAs in embryonic and fetal murine lung where the amounts of tissue available are small, we carried out RT-PCR analyses. Katherine King in my laboratory found that GRP and GRP receptor genes are expressed in fetal murine lung as early as embryonic day 12 (e12); when lung buds are beginning to branch. By ISH, GRP receptor transcripts were at the highest levels in mesenchymal cells at cleft regions of branching airways and blood vessels (Fig. 18). To explore the possibility that bombesin-like peptides might play a role in branching morphogenesis, e12 lung buds were cultured for 48 hr in serum-free medium. In the presence of 0.10–10 $\mu$M bombesin, branching was significantly augmented as compared with control cultures, with a peak of 94% above control values at 1 $\mu$M ($p < .005$) (Fig. 19). The bombesin receptor antagonist [Leu$^{13}$-psi(CH$_2$NH)Leu$^{14}$]bombesin (L13BN) alone (100 nM) had no effect on baseline branching but completely abolished bombesin-induced branching (Fig. 19). A bombesin-related peptide [Leu$^8$]-phyllolitorin (L8PL), also increased branching (65% above controls at 10 nM, $p < .005$) (Fig. 20). L8PL (10–100 nM) also significantly augmented thymidine incorporation in cultured lung buds. Fibronectin, which is known to be abundant at branchpoints, induces GRP gene expression in H82, an undifferentiated SCLC cell line. These observations suggest that bombesin-like peptides could contribute to lung branching morphogenesis. Furthermore, components of branch points such as fibronectin might induce pulmonary NE cell differentiation as part of a positive feedback loop, which could account in part for the high prevalence of these cells at branch points.

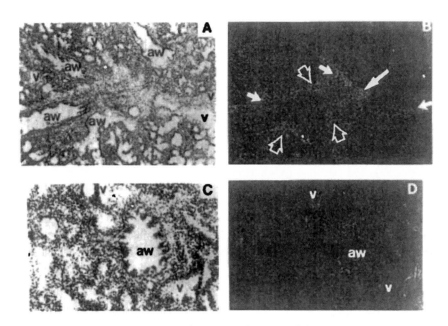

**Figure 18**   In situ hybridization of fetal murine lung for GRP receptor transcripts. Each pair of photographs represents the same field viewed by bright field microscopy to demonstrate histology (left: A,C) and darkfield microscopy to demonstrate autoradiographic grains (right: B,D). (A,B) Probed with GRP receptor antisense cRNA (×40). Note hybridization is most intense in mesenchyme of the cleft regions of airways (aw, outlined arrows), blood vessels (v, small solid arrows), and a region with branching airways and blood vessels (long solid arrow). (C,D) Probed with control GRP receptor sense cRNA (×100). Note lack of a specific hybridization signal. (Reprinted with permission from Proc Natl Acad Sci USA, ref. 446.)

Similarly, Agauyo et al. (300) independently identified bombesin/GRP–preferring receptors in e13 murine lung and observed a trend toward increased murine branching morphogenesis with 1–100 nm of bombesin in serum-containing media. They also observed modest augmentation of branching in the presence of phosphoramidon, a CD10/NEP inhibitor, either alone or together with exogenous bombesin, which was decreased by bombesin receptor antagonists. In our system using serum-free media, we have been unable to demonstrate any significant effects of phosphoramidon on branching morphogenesis in either of two experiments, which is consistent with the lack of detectable CD10/NEP mRNAs at e12–e14 (270).

Mechanisms for BLP-induced branching are likely to be similar for epithelial and vascular systems and include altered cell adhesion and/or cell motility (27,28,301) and/or differential cell proliferation (25,302–305). The importance of

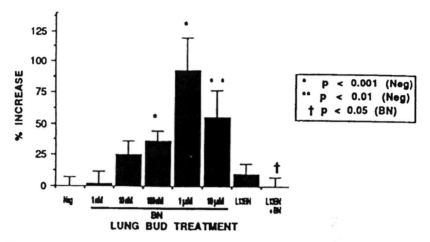

**Figure 19** Quantitation of lung branching morphogenesis in serum-free medium with varying doses of bombesin (BN) or the specific bombesin receptor antagonist, L13BN. e12 Lung buds were photographed and cultured in serum free medium alone (Neg) or in medium containing 1–10 μM bombesin, 100 nM L13BN, or 100 nM bombesin plus 100 nM L13BN. On e14, lung buds were photographed and the percentage increase in peripheral branch points was determined. Values are normalized with respect to baseline (medium alone) which was defined as zero. Data shown represent pooled results from 15 experiments, ± SE. *P* values are given with *$p$ < .001 and **$p$ < .01 as compared with the negative control with medium alone; and †$p$ < .05 compared with 100 nM bombesin alone. (Reprinted with permission from Proc Natl Acad Sci USA, ref. 446.)

mesenchyme for morphogenesis is well recognized (301,306–309). Fibronectin and other extracellular matrix components are localized predominantly at airway branch points (310,311); specific blocking peptides or MoAbs to fibronectin or laminin inhibit branching (210,312). Multiple extracellular matrix components (27,28), including proteoglycans such as syndecan (301,313), may affect branching by altering cell adhesion, cell motility, and/or growth factor availability. EGF and TGF-α augment branching by a mechanism involving increased cell proliferation (25,304,305); preliminary data suggest that the same is true of platelet-derived growth factor (314).

In addition, BLPs might alter epithelial cell migration directly. Bombesin has been reported to stimulate chemotaxis of macrophages and SCLC (epithelial) cell lines (315). BLPs could trigger the release of a soluble branching factor such as hepatocyte growth factor (307), bFGF (302), or epimorphin (308) from pulmonary fibroblasts or primitive mesenchymal cells, which might act in a secondary manner to promote branching by altering cell migration. However, bFGF appears to regulate branching morphogenesis of developing blood vessels in vitro

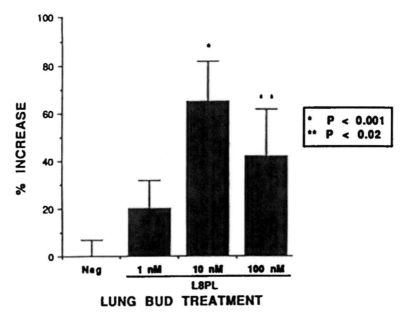

**Figure 20**  Quantitation of lung branching morphogenesis in serum-free medium with varying doses of Leu8-phyllolitorin (L8PL). e12 Lung buds were cultured in medium alone or in medium containing 1–100 nM L8PL. Values within each experiment are expressed as percentage increased branching above baseline. *P* values are given with *$p$ < .001 and **$p$ < .01 as compared with medium alone. (Reprinted with permission from Proc Natl Acad Sci USA, ref. 446.)

by a complex mechanism including both chemotaxis and proliferation (302,303). Peptides such as BLPs, hepatocyte growth factor, epimorphin, or bFGF could function as well by stimulating homeobox gene transcription, analogous to activin triggering of mesoderm induction in *Xenopus* oocytes (316).

### H.  Possible Roles for Other Neuropeptides and Amines from Neuroendocrine Cells in Fetal and Neonatal Lung Physiology

*CGRP and Calcitonin*

In the lung, CGRP occurs in intrapulmonary sensory nerves (50,52,54,317), undifferentiated airway epithelium (see below) (221), and serous glands of the trachea (318) as well as in PNECs (317,319); calcitonin is found only in PNECs (104). CGRP is derived from the same gene as calcitonin by alternative splicing (320) (Fig. 21) but is preferentially expressed by PNECs early in fetal lung

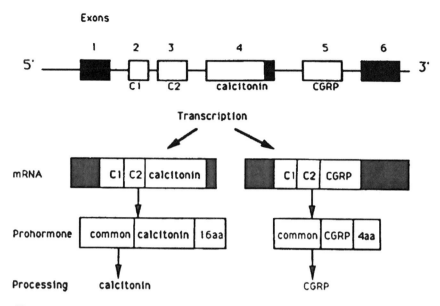

**Figure 21** Alternative splicing of the calcitonin/calcitonin–gene related peptide gene. (Modified from ref. 54.)

development in both rodents (319) and humans (173). Most of the functional analyses have focused on CGRP as a potential growth factor in the lung. CGRP is likely to be responsible in part for the growth-promoting effects of NEBs on non-NE airway epithelial cells (321) which was mapped by Sorokin and co-workers (322). White et al. (181) also have carried out proliferative analyses of normal adult guinea pig tracheal epithelium in the presence or absence of exogenous CGRP. Peak BrdU incorporation in guinea pig tracheal epithelium was observed at 24 hr after 0.01 nM CGRP for only 4 hr in culture, with the magnitude of this response being threefold greater than that in control cultures lacking CGRP; similar effects on absolute cell numbers in 3-day cultures were also observed. All of these growth effects were blocked by a CGRP receptor antagonist, hCGRP-(8-37), in a dose-dependent fashion.

CGRP (203) and calcitonin (202) receptors also could be involved in the modulation of growth processes. CGRP receptor autoradiography in human and guinea pig lung demonstrated dense binding over bronchial and pulmonary blood vessels of all sizes and alveolar walls and more sparse labeling of smooth muscle and airway epithelium (203). Calcitonin might induce different biological responses in target cells depending on their position in the cell cycle: The calcitonin receptor is linked to the cAMP transduction pathway via the cholera toxin-

sensitive Gs protein and to the protein kinase C pathway via the pertussis toxin–
sensitive Gi protein, and selective activation of one or the other pathway is cell
cycle dependent (205). In NE cell lines, calcitonin mRNA is lowest and CGRP is
highest during rapid growth (206); apparently by reversible alterations in alternative RNA-processing patterns dependent on growth conditions in vitro. Similarly,
high CGRP levels in developing PNECs early in ontogeny could be linked to the
rapid growth phase of lung development, with calcitonin becoming more prevalent only when PNECs are fully differentiated (104). The precise roles for CGRP
and calcitonin in developing fetal lung remain to be established.

Furthermore, additive, synergistic, or antagonistic effects may occur between CGRP, calcitonin, and BLP, especially because all three of these peptides
are contained in the same neurosecretory granules (73). Stahlman and Gray (73)
have suggested that these three peptides could act in concert, or perhaps one
peptide may act in a paracrine role (e.g., on bronchial or bronchiolar smooth
muscle) and the second peptide acting in an autocrine fashion on the parent cell
(e.g., in the regulation of granule production or release). In analyses of smooth
muscle contraction induced by 5-HT or carbamylcholine in rat isolated airway
smooth muscle (323) or BLP and substance P in guinea pigs in vivo (324), CGRP
and/or calcitonin were able effectively to inhibit increases in airway tone. In the
first study (323), the inhibitory action of CGRP was not mediated by the release of
endogenous prostaglandins, since indomethacin had no effect; and the action of
CGRP was not related to the discharge of neuronal action potentials or β-adreno-
receptor activation, because tetrodotoxin or propranolol had no effect. It has been
suggested that CGRP and/or calcitonin prevent airway smooth muscle contraction
by interfering with BLP- or substance P-induced changes in intracellular calcium
concentration (324).

### Enkephalins, ACTH, and Corticotropin-Releasing Hormone

Leu-enkephalin is expressed by occasional PNECs in the postnatal lung of infants
with chronic respirator lung disease (104). Leu-enkephalin is an opioid peptide
which is synthesized as part of a larger molecule, proenkephalin (325), and may
function to regulate growth processes induced by BLP or other peptides in the
developing lung. In the gastrointestinal tract, met-enkephalin and β-endorphin
effectively antagonized the gut-contracting effect of BLPs (326), shifting the
dose-response curves to the right and depressing the maximum response to BLP.
Opioid peptides also mediate growth inhibitory effects on human lung cancer cell
lines, both SCLC and NSCLC, and this inhibitory effect can be reversed by
nicotine (327). These growth-inhibitory effects appear to be mediated via nonconventional opioid binding sites distinct from those found in the brain (328).

The opioid peptide β-endorphin is synthesized as part of a larger molecule,
proopiomelanocortin (POMC), which also gives rise to ACTH by proteolytic
cleavage. ACTH, a 39–amino acid peptide, and POMC-derived peptides, includ-

ing β-endorphin, are absent from normal fetal or adult human lung but have been localized to rare PNECs in postnatal lung from infants with chronic respirator lung disease (104,109). The POMC gene is expressed in rat and human lung (329–331). ACTH and BLP immunoreactivities have been localized to distinct PNEC subpopulations (109). ACTH and POMC-derived peptides have also been identified in SCLC (110,330). The identification of corticotropin-releasing hormone (CRH) and ACTH (2,109,332–335), as well as CRH receptors (336) on lung tumor cell lines suggest a potential role in the regulation of cell proliferation and/or differentiation. CRH has been demonstrated to stimulate cAMP and the clonal growth of lung cancer cells (337).

It is possible that ACTH and CRH from lung, brain, and/or pituitary may have direct effects on lung neuromuscular development, cell differentiation, and/or indirect effects on fetal lung development (109,110) via increased endogenous glucocorticoid production from the fetal adrenal (338). This hypothesis is supported by new observations in CRH knockout mice (see below). CRH, a 41–amino acid neuropeptide produced in the paraventricular nucleus of the hypothalamus and many regions of cerebral cortex, is a key regulator of the mammalian stress response mediated via the hypothalamic-pituitary-adrenal axis (338). It is transported from the hypothalamus to the pituitary, where it stimulates the release of ACTH. ACTH, in turn, stimulates the adrenal cortex to produce glucocorticoids, which mediate adaptive responses to stress. Like ACTH, CRH is produced in the fetal lung (339). Although the cell of origin has not been precisely mapped, CRH mRNAs are transiently expressed from e12.5 to e17.5 in epithelial cells in the region of the branching bronchioles, corresponding to the late pseudoglandular and early canalicular phases of lung development (339). CRH might be localized to PNECs in the fetal lung.

To define the importance of CRH in the response of the hypothalamic-pituitary-axis to stress, Muglia et al. (340) constructed a mammalian model of CRH deficiency by targeted mutation in embryonic stem cells. All CRH-deficient mice demonstrate a fetal glucocorticoid requirement for lung maturation. Homozygous CRH-deficient mice born to heterozygous mothers have no detectable abnormalities in spite of evidence of impaired adrenal response to stress postnatally, with plasma corticosterone levels up to 28% of wild type in females and up to 4% of wild type in males (340). Despite this impaired response to stress, male and female CRH-deficient mice exhibit normal viability and fertility without glucocorticoid replacement. Matings between CRH-deficient mice result in apparently normal pregnancies, but after a full gestation, the progeny all die within the first 12 hr of life despite a normal external appearance. Histological examination of newborn lungs revealed thickened alveolar septae and a paucity of air spaces in knockout animals compared with wild type, and surfactant apoprotein B (SP-B) mRNA levels were only 44% of the wild-type value on e18.5 (340). Administration of corticosterone to pregnant homozygous females from e12 to postpartum day 14 completely reversed the abnormal lung architecture and SP-B deficiency in homozygous deficient mice from homozygous matings. This resulted in the production of viable litters which survived without subsequent postnatal glucocorticoid treatment. These observations indicate an absolute requirement for glucocorticoids in the lung during fetal rather than postnatal life. These results are consistent with in vivo and in vitro studies showing the ability of glucocorticoids to promote lung maturation (23,29,341–343).

### Cholecystokinin

Cholecystokinin (CCK) has been recently identified in solitary PNECs and in NEBs in the developing lung in humans and seven other mammalian species (344). In the human and monkey lung, CCK-positive cells are less abundant than BLP-positive PNECs, but BLP frequently colocalizes in the same PNECs as CCK. Using immunoEM analyses, CCK-like immunoreactivity is in dense-core vesicles, in some of which 5-HT is also present. CCK could act as either a classic hormone, released into the circulation, or as a neurotransmitter in central and peripheral neurons (344,345). In the gut and pancreas, CCK-like peptides promote gastric emptying, gallbladder motility, satiety, and exocrine pancreatic secretion (346). CCK is the most potent inducer of pancreatic growth; the effects of BLP on pancreatic growth and secretion may be mediated via synthesis and release of CCK (238,243,245). Conversely, CCK can downregulate the binding of BLP to BLP receptors in pancreatic acini (347). Both CCK and BLP stimulate c-*fos*, c-*jun*, and c-*myc* gene expression in rat pancreatic acini, suggesting that these peptides activate early-response genes similarly prior to stimulating DNA synthesis and cell division (244). Finally, in the brainstem, CCK modulates the firing rate of dopaminergic neurons (348) and alters the affinity and number of dopamine $D_2$ receptors (349). In the carotid body, CCK reduces dopamine-induced inhibition of the carotid body response to hypoxia (350).

Considering the parallels between the effects of CCK and BLP in the gastrointestinal tract, it is plausible that CCK has effects similar to BLP as both a growth and differentiation factor in developing fetal lung. CCK is as effective as GRP in promoting clonal growth of SCLC cell lines (180). In one study of a panel of SCLC and NSCLC cell lines, neither specific BLP nor specific CCK antagonists given alone were able effectively to inhibit tumor cell growth, whereas the more broad-spectrum substance P agonists did inhibit tumor growth (351). These data suggest that CCK and BLP may act in a reciprocal fashion to compensate for a decline in the levels of one or the other. Such mechanisms could include receptor transregulation as well as altered peptide synthesis and/or secretion.

### 5-HT

5-HT has been demonstrated to act as a direct growth factor in both neuronal and nonneuronal systems (207), including rodent fibroblasts, apparently via a

G-protein–coupled pathway. Specific 5-HT receptors have been identified in the brain (204). Ectopic expression of brain-specific 5-HT receptors (subtype 1c) in murine 3T3 fibroblasts surprisingly results in a high frequency of malignant transformation (204), suggesting that 5-HT receptors could act as proto-oncogenes. Other 5-HT receptor subtypes trigger mitogenesis in aortic smooth muscle cells and human B cells (reviewed in ref. 204). Extrapolating to fetal lung, one can speculate that 5-HT might act as a mesenchymal growth factor and possibly also as an epithelial cell growth and differentiation factor analogous to BLP.

### Endothelin

Endothelin immunoreactivity and mRNA have been localized to PNECs of the developing fetal and postnatal human lung (106) and newborn cat, rat, hamster, and mouse (352). Immunoreactivity is also detectable in the bronchial epithelium of about 50% of human adults as well as in the endothelium; its expression in normal adults may be associated with asthma (54). In addition to being the most potent vasoconstrictor peptide known, endothelin stimulates contraction of smooth muscle in airways and the gut (353,354), has neurotransmitter function in the central nervous system, and stimulates proliferation of fibroblasts and airway smooth muscle (355,356). Its potential roles in lung development have not yet been analyzed.

## III. Non-PNEC Neuropeptides in Fetal Lung

### A. Intrapulmonary Nerve Fibers

The major neuropeptide and enzyme markers of intrapulmonary nerve fibers are summarized in Table 7. The history, morphology, and ontogeny of lung innervation, recently reviewed by Springall et al. (54) and Barnes et al. (50,52), are discussed in depth in Chapter 9 and will not be covered here. The possible roles of selected neuropeptides in lung development will be considered in the following section. It is unlikely that nerve fiber–derived peptides play a role in branching morphogenesis, because the lung innervation is not established until later in development (8). CGRP, synthesized and secreted by both PNECs and sensory nerves, is covered in the discussion in Section II.H above.

### Tachykinins

Substance P, neurokinin A, and neuropeptide K are all derived from a single preprotachykinin gene by alternative splicing of seven exons (Fig. 22) (54). Together with CGRP (see above), the tachykinins are the major peptides expressed in sensory nerves. In addition, substance P has been demonstrated in human PNECs, both isolated PNECs and NEBs, especially in fetal lung (357). The presence of substance P–positive cytoplasmic processes which interdigitate with

**Table 7**  Markers of Intrapulmonary Nerve Fibers

---

Sympathetic, adrenergic: cervical and thoracic ganglia
  neuropeptide Y
  tyrosine hydroxylase
  dopamine-B-hydroxylase
  PNMT
Parasympathetic, cholinergic: vagus preganglionic, nodose ganglion, intrinsic ganglia
  vasoactive intestinal peptide (VIP)
  peptide histidine-isoleucine (PHI)
  galanin
  cholinesterase
  neuropeptide Y
Sensory, nonadrenergic noncholinergic: dorsal root and vagal, nodose ganglia
  CGRP
  Tachykinins: neurokinin A, neurokinin B, eledoisin, neuropeptide K, substance P
All nerve fibers
  PGP 9.5

---

the other epithelial cells suggests possible paracrine effects on neighboring cells. The inhibition of the growth of SCLC and NSCLC cell lines by substance P analogues (351) suggests that substance P may modulate lung epithelial cell proliferation. Substance P may play a role in the neural control of hair growth (358), which may serve as an animal model. Both substance P and neurokinin A stimulate DNA synthesis in cultured arterial smooth muscle cells and human skin fibroblasts (359); substance P and neurokinin A were less effective in stimulating DNA synthesis if the cells were simultaneously stimulated with suboptimal concentrations of PDGF, suggesting similar mechanisms of action of these neuropeptides and growth factors. Because PDGF is known to act as a mediator of branching morphogenesis, growth, and type II cell differentiation in developing lung, the tachykinins could have similar effects (338,360,361).

### Galanin

Galanin has been mapped to the parasympathetic (intrinsic) nerve fibers in the mammalian lung (54,362), where it is relatively sparse and coexists with VIP and peptide histidine-isoleucine (PHI). Originally identified in porcine gastrointestinal tract, galanin consists of 29 amino acids, and its name is derived from the first and last amino acids of the peptide (glycine and alanine) (54,363). Galanin functions both as a growth factor and as a neuroregulatory hormone (363). Its effects on growth may be mediated via the release of other substances such as epinephrine and growth hormone (364). In neuroregulatory reponses, galanin functions in an

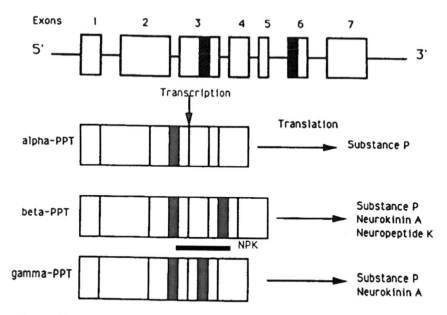

**Figure 22** Preprotachykinin (PPT) gene expression. Alternative splicing yields three different transcripts which are translated to substance P, neurokinin A, and/or neuropeptide K as indicated. (Modified from ref. 54.)

opposite fashion to BLPs, modulating insulin and gastrin secretion (346,363,365). It is feasible that galanin may act to regulate the growth and differentiation effects of BLP and other peptides. Whereas VIP inhibits the leukotriene-induced contraction of airway smooth muscle, galanin has no effect in the same system, indicating that its function is not necessarily linked to that of other cholinergic neuropeptides (53). Galanin is known also to be capable of acting as a direct clonal growth factor for SCLC cell lines (180), in which it acts via stimulating calcium mobilization and inositol phosphate accumulation (366). It may act as a lung growth factor. The galanin receptor distribution and functions of galanin in developing lung have yet to be elucidated.

### VIP

Similar to galanin, VIP has been localized to the parasympathetic nerves of the lung (54). VIP has been demonstrated to act as a potent growth factor for multiple tissues in postimplantation mouse embryo cultures via multiple VIP receptors that exhibit tissue-specific responses (367). After a 4-hr incubation, VIP stimulates growth, increasing somite number, embryonic volume, DNA and protein content, and the number of cells in S phase (367); a VIP antagonist significantly modulates the effects on growth, completely suppressing VIP-stimulated mitosis in the brain but decreasing growth by only about 40% in nonneuronal tissues. This same antagonist is highly effective at inhibiting the growth of NSCLC (368), in which VIP could act as an autocrine growth factor (258,368). VIP also elevates intracellular cAMP and increases the secretion rate of BLP from SCLC cell lines (369). It would not be surprising to find that VIP could function as a growth and/or differentiation factor similar to BLP in fetal lung.

### B. Immunostaining of Undifferentiated Epithelium for NE Markers

A second pattern of cytoplasmic immunostaining of the most distal undifferentiated airway epithelium has been observed during the pseudoglandular period of lung development for PGP 9.5, but not CGA, in human fetal lung (120) (Fig. 23), and both CGRP and the Clara cell–specific marker CC10 in murine fetal lung (221) (see Fig. 4D). The similar detection of GRP mRNAs in the undifferentiated airway epithelium of fetal rhesus monkey lung has been demonstrated using ISH (282), but there is no immunostaining for mature BLP corresponding to this. Similarly, we were not able to detect BLP immunostaining in the undifferentiated epithelium of human fetal lung (K. Haley and M. Sunday, unpublished data). These data suggest that the GRP gene is expressed but very little of the prohormone is cleaved and amidated to yield mature GRP. The meaning of this novel pattern of cytoplasmic immunostaining of undifferentiated epithelium for partial NE and Clara cell markers is not understood, but it may simply reflect the phenotype of a totipotential precursor cell. The undifferentiated epithelium is known to be devoid of dense-core granules (128).

### C. Exogenous Thyrotropin

Endogenous thyrotropin (TRH) has not been identified in mammalian lung (338), but its localization in NE cells of the pancreas and stomach (370) suggests that it might occur in PNECs as well. Exogenous TRH has been utilized in rabbits (371), rats (372), lambs (373,374), and humans (375,376) to promote lung maturation in prematurely delivered animals. TRH has been used to promote lung maturation, because it readily passes from the maternal to the fetal circulation and presumptively causes thyroid axis stimulation (376), resulting in increased pulmonary surfactant production, functional and morphological fetal lung maturation, and increased duration of neonatal survival after premature delivery (372). The mechanism of the TRH effect has been thought to be via induction of thyroid hormone (338) and/or prolactin (374,376) secretion. However, Devaskar et al. (372) found the same effects as TRH using a TRH analogue which did not induce the production of prolactin or thyroid-stimulating hormone from the anterior pituitary,

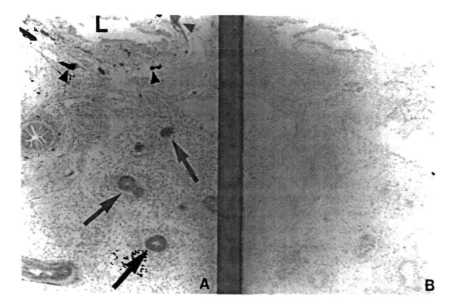

**Figure 23** PGP 9.5 immunostaining in undifferentiated epithelium of 10-week-gestation human fetal lung. (A) Immunostaining for PGP 9.5 is shown with large arrows indicating PGP 9.5–positive epithelium lining small undifferentiated airways. Arrowheads indicate nerve fiber bundles surrounding a large proximal airway (L) (×40). (B) Serial section run in parallel using PGP 9.5 antiserum preabsorbed with PGP 9.5 antigen. (Reprinted with permission from Miscrosc Res Techn, ref. 120.)

supporting a role for TRH in fetal lung development that is either direct or mediated via neurotransmitter stimulation of parasympathetic nervous system activity (372,377,378). TRH has the advantage of stimulating maturation of the antioxidant enzyme response to hyperoxic injury in contrast to thyroid hormone, which delays antioxidant enzyme system development (371). Its direct effect on lung development in fetal lung organ cultures has not been tested.

## IV. PNECs in Developmental Lung Disorders: Clinical Associations and Animal Models

### A. Pulmonary Hypoplasia and Dysmaturity

The common perinatal condition, pulmonary hypoplasia, may be caused by any of several different factors, including oligohydramnios, polyhydramnios, congenital diaphragmatic hernia, renal agenesis, and anencephaly (379,380). We used immunostaining for BLP and CGA and ISH for GRP to study lung tissue from three infants with pulmonary hypoplasia (91): one with multiple congenital anomalies, including renal agenesis; one with polyhydramnios; and one with anencephaly. The first two of the infants had decreased or absent PNECs; this relative lack of GRP and CGA supports the thesis that PNECs, and in particular GRP, may be required for normal growth and maturation of the lungs. In contrast, the infant with anencephaly and pulmonary hypoplasia had markedly elevated numbers of GRP-positive PNECs. One additional infant with anencephaly without pulmonary hypoplasia had normal numbers of PNECs. Other investigators have observed similar variability in the number of GRP-positive PNECs associated with pulmonary hypoplasia (9). These data suggest that PNECs and GRP may be necessary but not sufficient for normal growth and maturation of the lungs.

Pulmonary dysmaturity, or Wilson-Mikity syndrome (WMS), is a chronic neonatal lung disorder of unknown etiology predominantly affecting premature infants (9,381). In contrast to the respiratory distress observed immediately after birth in infants with HMD, patients with WMS do not develop respiratory distress until several days after birth. Histopathologically, there are multiple areas of respiratory bronchioles and alveolae with impaired maturation and alveolar collapse. The airways appear normal except for a distinct PNEC hyperplasia, with a normal number of PNEC-positive airways but a striking increase in the number of PNECs per positive airway. There is no obvious relationship between the foci of PNEC hyperplasia and areas of alveolar collapse. However, NEBs within the respiratory bronchioles and alveolar ducts are a distinguishing feature of WMS rarely seen in control infants, which may indicate that PNEC hyperplasia is related to hypoxia.

### B.  Hyaline Membrane Disease and Bronchopulmonary Dysplasia

Studies of cellular and molecular mechanisms of fetal lung development have obvious implications for improving treatment and clinical outcome of premature infants by preventing or minimizing the severity of RDS with HMD and BPD (382,383) (see Chapter 16).

Pulmonary BLP levels are altered in a variety of perinatal disease states, especially in infants with HMD and BPD (91,384). Lungs of infants with HMD have low levels of BLPs and low numbers of BLP-positive PNECs (104,385,386). In the acute lung injury associated with HMD, airway hypoxia is believed to lead to degranulation of PNECs releasing 5-HT, BLPs, and other vasoactive substances with resulting alterations in vasomotor and/or bronchomotor tone (104). Teleologically, this may represent a key mechanism for shifting ventilation-perfusion mismatches. Similar changes have been demonstrated in response to airway hypoxia in sheep (387). It is also possible that necrosis and sloughing of airway epithelium contribute to lower BLP levels in HMD (388). In contrast, if infants with RDS survive the acute lung injury and develop BPD, markedly increased numbers of BLP-positive PNECs occur as compared with control infants of a similar age (385). The PNEC hyperplasia associated with BPD has a significantly decreased percentage of immunopositive airways in contrast to WMS, where the percentage of immunopositive airways was similar to age-matched controls (see above).

Using immunoperoxidase and ISH analyses, we observed lower numbers of PNECs containing BLP and GRP mRNAs in three of four infants with HMD as compared with control infants (91), which is similar to observations in other laboratories (104,385,386). In addition, in our series, one infant with only a few BLP-positive PNECs by immunostaining exhibited abundant GRP mRNA-containing cells by ISH (91), suggesting that GRP gene expression might be turned on as an early component of the response to acute lung injury. In our study, both of two infants with BPD had normal to high levels of both GRP immunoreactivity and also GRP mRNAs (91). Carefully controlled animal studies will be required to clarify the time course of GRP gene activation in relation to airway regeneration.

The association of PNEC hyperplasia with airway epithelial regeneration during the transition to BPD suggests that BLPs derived from PNECs may be critical growth and differentiation factors involved in airway epithelial regeneration (389).

Alternatively, it has been suggested that excessive secretion of BLPs could actually be a cause of the peribronchiolar fibrosis, obliterative bronchiolitis, and hypertrophy of peribronchial smooth muscle which are characteristic of BPD (384,390). Similar histopathological changes are present in adult patients with primary hyperplasia of PNECs (391). Increased reactive airways disease in infants surviving BPD may also be linked pathophysiologically to PNEC hyperplasia which has been shown to develop in animals sensitized for an asthmatic response (392), because BLPs, including bombesin and the immunologically crossreactive amphibian phyllolitorin peptides, have been demonstrated to induce smooth muscle contraction (393,394). Both BPD and WMS share the features of PNEC hyperplasia and increased incidence of sudden and unexpected death (9), similar to some infants who die of sudden infant death syndrome (SIDS, see below).

## C. Chronic Perinatal Lung Diseases

Increased PNECs in both children and adults is also associated with hypoxia (136), hyperoxia (91,148), advanced primary pulmonary hypertension (395), and a variety of chronic lung diseases (91), including cystic fibrosis and following prolonged assisted ventilation (396). These observations support the concept that PNEC hyperplasia may occur as part of a regenerative response following prolonged lung injury and/or in response to chronic hypoxia, such as occurs with BPD or in the advanced stages of pulmonary hypertensive arteriopathy (390). This concept is supported by our observations of the induction of intense PNEC hyperplasia in a hamster model of chronic lung injury induced by nitrosamines plus hyperoxia (145,148). Such PNEC hyperplasia appears to represent predominantly cellular differentiation, because only rare PNECs immunostain for PCNA, whereas numerous non-NE epithelial cells immunostained for both PCNA and c-*myc* oncoprotein (148). These data suggest that PNECs might subserve a role as a paracrine effector cell, secreting growth and differentiation peptides such as BLPs that may act to promote regeneration of a variety of neighboring cell types. Primary or idiopathic PNEC hyperplasia could also occur in association with obstructive airways disease and peribronchiolar fibrosis, which are postulated to be due to excessive secretion of neuropeptides by PNECs (397).

### D. Asthma

There is increasing evidence that abnormal PNEC development may be implicated in the pathophysiology of asthma in children. However, it must be kept in mind that there is no ideal animal model of asthma, and one cannot talk about asthmatic animals but only of animals with bronchospasm (398). Also, patients with bronchial asthma have an increased airway responsiveness to various bronchoconstrictor stimuli, including chemical agents such as histamine, neurokinin A and methacholine, and "nonspecific" physical agents such as cold air and exercise (399). The bronchoconstrictor response may be mediated via direct interaction with receptors on smooth muscle cells, via stimulation of mediator release from inflammatory cells, or by stimulation of sensory nerve receptors leading to local axon reflexes or vagally mediated reflexes. Many of the studies cited below have utilized tracheal smooth muscle, which may be the most accessible airway smooth muscle for studies of constrictor responses, but it may be functionally distinct from the smooth muscle associated with the large and/or small airways in the lung. This point is especially relevant to the effects of PNEC-derived peptides (398), because most of the PNEC increase following systemic immunization of experimental animals occurs in the bronchioles (see below) (400,401).

Maternal smoking could have effects on fetal PNECs during lung development, which in turn might potentiate asthmatic responses. In an ultrastructural study of human newborn lungs obtained at autopsy by Chen et al., enlarged polypoid NE cell clusters were observed with decreased dense-core granules (suggesting degranulation) in infants with prenatal smoke exposure (402). In a subsequent investigation, Chen et al. (403) found an apparent lack of influence of maternal smoking during pregnancy on the expression of GRP gene products in human fetal PNECs. However, there are several problems with the design of that follow-up study: There were only 20 cases in total; there was no consideration of the number of cigarettes smoked by the mother; and no mention is made of past medical history or family history of asthma or allergies, which could skew the data.

The possibility of abnormal NE cells in the lungs of fetuses whose mothers smoke is especially interesting in view of the strong, consistent epidemiological association between maternal smoking and asthma. Children of mothers who smoke cigarettes are 1.5 to 2.6 times more likely to be diagnosed with asthma compared with children of nonsmoking mothers. Correlations between asthma and maternal smoking are particularly strong for children less than 5 years of age (404), and maternal smoking has a greater impact than paternal smoking (405). A recent study addressed the issue of possible prenatal tobacco effects: Hanrahan et al. showed decreases in tidal volume, expiratory flow rates, and residual capacity in infants of smoking mothers as early as 4 weeks after birth (406).

Animal models support the concept of altered NE cells in fetal lung following maternal smoke exposure. In a mouse model, Wang et al. (71) demonstrated NE cell hyperplasia following maternal nicotine exposure. Chen and co-workers (407) used a similar rabbit model of nicotine injections during gestational and lactating periods to study ultrastructural changes in fetal lungs, which had larger and more numerous NEBs. NE cell hyperplasia occurs in rodents following hypoxia (408) and tobacco metabolite exposure (148). Animal studies have shown fetal hypoxia after maternal nicotine exposure (409), which is probably due to catecholamine-induced decreases in uterine blood flow. Thus, NE cell hyperplasia could be either secondary to chronic hypoxia or induced by tobacco constituents such as nicotine or nitrosamine carcinogens.

The most convincing direct evidence linking NE cell hyperplasia to the pathophysiology of asthma was first demonstrated by Marchevsky et al. (400) and later confirmed by Bousbaa and co-workers (401,410) using a guinea pig model. Marchevsky et al. (400) immunized guinea pigs in the footpads with ovalbumin and 21 days later challenged animals with an intracardiac injection of ovalbumin (experimental group) or saline (negative control for challenge). PNECs were identified by silver staining using the Grimelius method. Saline-challenged animals exhibited a 10-fold increase in numbers of isolated PNECs in the bronchioles compared with nonimmunized age-matched animals versus a 2-fold increase in the trachea or no change in the bronchi or ileum. Animals that survived the challenge and were harvested 10 min after intracardiac injection had a significant decrease in argyrophilic cells (to ~3% of control values) whether the results were expressed as number of APUD cells per millimeters of organ perimeter or as the ratio of APUD cells per 100 epithelial cells, which is consistent with degranulation; all of this APUD cell degranulation occurred in the bronchioles, which would be an appropriate anatomical site for significantly altering airflow resistance, because a small decrease in bronchiolar airway diameter could lead to a large increase in total airflow resistance. The major limitations of this study are that

NEBs were not quantitated and the intracardiac route of challenge is not typical for induction of an asthmatic response.

In two follow-up studies, Bousbaa and co-workers (401,410) immunized guinea pigs systemically with two intraperitoneal injections of ovalbumin over a 3-week period of sensitization. After this period of time, there was a 1.7-fold increase in numbers of argyrophilic PNECs (401). When animals were given an aerosol challenge of ovalbumin antigen, the NE cells degranulated, with a significant decrease to ~50% of control values (measured as number of argyrophilic cells per millimeter of bronchial wall) at 24 hr after challenge. Subsequent quantitation of CGA-positive cells in the same system by Bousbaa and co-workers showed about a 2.3-fold increase in CGA-positive PNECs (410) following sensitization and significantly decreased CGA-positive cells 24 hr after challenge; there was no difference in numbers of cells immunostaining for NSE. These results suggest that the numbers of PNECs containing neurosecretory granule components such as amines and chromogranins is increased by immunization, whereas the number of "latent" PNECs containing the cytoplasmic enzyme marker NSE is unchanged. This suggests that immunization may trigger an increase in PNEC differentiation.

Bousbaa and Fleury-Feith also observed a significant influx of eosinophils in cartilaginous bronchial walls in animals following sensitization that was further augmented by challenge (401). However, the early study (401) did not take into account the anatomical site of the PNECs within the airways and also did not assess NEBs in spite of discussing the background literature that "only the innervated groups of PNECs, ... the NEBs, have been demonstrated to have a neurochemoreceptor function in reponse to hypoxia in the lung." In the more recent report (410), they state that most of the CGA-positive cells were in the large bronchi, rarely in the bronchioles, and that single PNECs were quantitated, because NEBs were difficult to identify in guinea pigs. They suggest a causal connection between the PNEC degranulation and eosinophil influx in spite of the fact that they evaluate eosinophils only in the large airways, in which there was no evidence of PNEC degranulation in Marchevsky's study (400). It is likely that PNEC-derived peptides may induce chemotaxis of eosinophils: CGRP is a direct eosinophil chemotactic factor which becomes more potent after cleavage by pulmonary endopeptidases (411); and Aguayo et al. have observed a 10-fold increase in BLP-positive PNECs in airway epithelium in patients with eosinophilic granuloma compared with both asymptomatic smokers and patients with idiopathic pulmonary fibrosis (266).

The quantitative differences between the studies of Marchevsky et al. (400) and Bousbaa and co-workers (401,410) could be related to the pooling of bronchial and bronchiolar PNEC data in the latter study, the different routes of antigen administration and different genetic backgrounds of the outbred guinea pigs used. Because of the aerosol challenge used, the studies of Bousbaa et al. (401,410) are probably more relevant as an animal model for asthma. However, although these observations are intriguing, the functional significance of a twofold increase in PNECs is unclear; in particular because the immunostaining detects total peptide stores and not simply what is available for secretion (412). PNECs have many similarities to mast cells (413); about one third of the mast cell granules are released on degranulation. Similarly, PNEC degranulation could be incomplete and could be regulated by exogenous factors (401). The mechanisms of this regulation and the functional significance of PNECs in hyperreactive airways disease remain to be investigated in depth, but BLPs and CGRP are two candidate neuropeptides involved in these responses.

In 1973, only 2 years after the discovery of bombesin and 5 years before BLP was identified in the lung, Impicciatore and Bertaccini demonstrated that bombesin is a potent bronchoconstrictor in guinea pig lung (414). Evidence from several other laboratories has shown that NE cell–associated peptides have bronchoconstrictor activity. BLPs given via the jugular vein exert a potent constrictor response on bronchiolar muscle of anesthetized Guinea pigs which is not blocked by antagonists of acetylcholine, histamine or 5-HT (414); these data are consistent with high levels of GRP receptor mRNAs in bronchial and bronchiolar smooth muscle (284–286). BLPs, including bombesin, GRP, and the immunologically cross-reactive amphibian phyllolitorin peptides, have been demonstrated to induce smooth muscle contraction in guinea pig gastric smooth muscle cells (393) and have been isolated and in situ smooth muscle from rat and guinea pig gut and bladder (394). Increased reactive airways disease in infants surviving BPD could also be linked pathophysiologically to BLP-positive PNEC hyperplasia (390). Amino acid sequence analyses have demonstrated that phyllolitorin-like peptides can account for most of the elevated BLP immunoreactivity in bronchoalveolar lavage fluid of asymptomatic adult smokers (415), and phyllolitorins have been shown to mediate branching morphogenesis in murine lung buds (286). Cumulatively, these observations suggest that there could be mammalian phyllolitorins derived from NE cells which might be important in lung pathophysiology.

CGRP is present in both sensory nerve fibers and in PNECs. The data for CGRP effects on airway smooth muscle constriction are more complex than those of BLPs. CGRP induces contraction of human bronchial smooth muscle rings (416) and tracheal smooth muscle strips (417). CGRP also appears to mediate the epithelium-dependent contractile response of guinea pig tracheal strips to capsaicin (418). Springall and co-workers have demonstrated that capsaicin induces PNEC degranulation as well as sensory nerve discharge (419). CGRP is also detected in capsaicin-treated isolated perfused lung concurrent with bronchoconstriction, suggesting local release (420). The data with CGRP are variable, however, with bronchoconstriction being reported on isolated smooth muscle (416–418) but no effects in whole lung organ assays giving peptides or capsaicin via a bolus into the guinea pig pulmonary artery (420) or on parenchymal strips including both airway and vascular smooth muscle (323). It is likely that the controversial data for CGRP may be due, at least in part, to the relaxing effect of CGRP on vascular smooth muscle in the whole organ preparations, which would oppose the bronchoconstrictor effects, yielding no net effect (324,421). In contrast, bombesin is a potent vasoconstrictor as well as bronchoconstrictor (421). Furthermore, additivity or antagonism between multiple agents may occur. CGRP is able to inhibit 5-HT–induced contraction in rat isolated airways (323). In another study, either calcitonin or CGRP blocked bombesin-induced and substance P–induced increases in airway tone in guinea pig lung in vivo (324). It is likely that in vivo animal models that recapitulate the complex in vivo events occurring in human asthma will be most valuable in clarifying the role of PNEC-derived neuropeptides in asthma.

The role of neuropeptides derived from the intrapulmonary nerve fibers in the etiopathogenesis of asthma has been presented recently in reviews by Barnes et al. (50,52) and Springall et al. (54). That work will not be discussed here except to mention that >99% of the research on neuropeptides in reactive airways disease has not taken PNEC-derived peptides such as BLP into account.

### E. Transplacental Lung Tumorigenesis

Although lung cancer is extremely rare in children, there is an epidemiological association between maternal smoking and lung cancer in the offspring in later life (422). Pulmonary NE cell hyperplasia also may be induced in fetal lung in utero by maternal smoking (see discussion in Section IV.D above). This may be due to several components of tobacco smoke, including nicotine and tobacco-specific nitrosamine carcinogens (147,423).

In addition to its possible epidemiological significance, transplacental carcinogenesis has been used as a proven experimental model for determining the effects of carcinogens on different cell populations in developing lung (423–426). For instance, nitrosamine carcinogens administered to the mother several days before birth leads to PNEC hyperplasia (423) and non-NE tumors of the respiratory tract in hamsters and mice (426,427). The tobacco-specific nitrosamine 4-(methylnitrosamino)-1-(3-pyridyl)-1-butanone (NNK) has been shown to cross the placenta into fetal tissues, including the lung (428). NNK is activated in fetal tissues to genotoxic intermediates, leading to DNA methylation and chromosome aberrations (428). These data suggest that early carcinogenic influences could be clinically relevant, perhaps via stem cell somatic mutations in essential tumor suppressor genes such as *p53* or the retinoblastoma gene *Rb* (425,429).

These experimental models might recapitulate events that occur in human lung during early carcinogenesis. It has been suggested that the subset of smokers that is genetically predisposed to developing NE cell hyperplasia and/or hypersecreting BLPs into bronchoalveolar lavage could be the same group of individuals that develops small airway fibrosis, reactive airways disease, and/or lung cancer (430,431). This hypothesis remains purely speculative but deserves serious appraisal because of the long-ranging clinical implications. It has been shown in several clinical studies that adult smokers with abnormally low FEV1.0 values are the highest risk group of smokers for ultimately developing lung cancer, suggesting that there may be a common mechanism underlying the pathophysiology of obstructive airways disease and carcinogenesis. PNEC hyperplasia may represent part of that mechanism (430). However, the link between PNEC hyperplasia and lung carcinogenesis remains to be established.

### F. Sudden Infant Death Syndrome

SIDS, which is defined as death occurring in infants less than 1 year of age for no apparent reason, may be due to abnormal PNEC development and function (9,432,433). Recently, Cutz and co-workers (9,433) have presented compelling histochemical evidence that abnormalities of PNECs may be present in infants dying of SIDS as compared with age-matched controls. Perrin et al. (434) studied BLP-positive PNECs, both single cells and NEBs, and demonstrated a significant increase in total cytoplasmic BLP immunostaining expressed as a ratio to the total epithelial cytoplasm of the same airway. They also found significantly larger NEBs. RIA for BLP confirmed the quantitative morphometry data.

Gillan and co-workers (231) carried out morphometry in a different fashion but arrived at the same conclusions. They quantitated airways containing argyrophilic PNECs in a minimum of two random sections of lung and expressed the results as percentage positive airways; the resulting percentage was above the range of normals in 21 of the 25 SIDS cases. They also counted the number of PNECs per positive airway, which was also higher in the SIDS patients, although there was overlap with the controls. Furthermore, SIDS lungs contained frequent PNECs and a few NEBs within respiratory brinchioles and alveolar ducts, which were not present in any of the controls, and suggests enhanced PNEC differentiation induced by hypoxia.

In one investigation by Cutz and co-workers (435), Northern blot analyses were used to identify increased levels of GRP mRNA in the lungs of 12 SIDS patients as compared with 8 controls. In contrast, CCK gene expression was similar to that of controls. This upregulation of BLP gene expression suggests increased synthesis of peptide by PNECs rather than simply failure of BLP release.

Although these changes may be only secondary, it is feasible that they may be a mechanism for sudden death if widespread bronchoconstriction occurs secondary to PNEC degranulation. However, SIDS is not associated with the typical histopathological changes found in lungs from patients dying with status asthmaticus or from chronic asthmatics with clinically inactive disease, such as basement membrane thickening and smooth muscle constriction leading to exaggerated epithelial folding (436). The lack of a convincing animal model for SIDS and the potential for clinical heterogeneity has hampered progress in understanding its pathophysiology. The magnitude of PNEC change in SIDS exceeds that described in brainstem-damaged infants (437). Neonates with severe hypoxic ischemic encephalopathy due to birth asphyxia, whose brainstem respiratory centers had ceased to function, showed a marked increase in BLP immunostaining and argyrophilic PNECs over controls (437). This observation has been interpreted as meaning that disruption of neurogenic modulation leads to impaired PNEC degranulation, thus explaining the significant increase in detectable PNECs containing stored peptides. However, neurogenic insults do not explain the prominence of PNEC distal to the terminal bronchioles (9), which is more likely to represent hypoxia-induced PNEC hyperplasia.

In fact, both brainstem dysfunction and hypoxia-induced PNEC hyperplasia could be operating: Impaired neural control of respiration could cause hypoxia secondary to intrapulmonary hypoventilation, which in turn might lead to PNEC hyperplasia. Increased BLP levels could provide a marker for SIDS and also might explain the increased peribronchiolar connective tissue present in SIDS patients (438). As suggested by Southall et al. (439), increased intrapulmonary vascular shunting, mediated via NEBs, could feasibly precipitate death in SIDS. Whether there is a primary abnormality of PNECs remains to be explored.

## V.  Summary and Conclusions

I would like to propose a working model of the role of PNEC-derived neuropeptides in fetal lung development. A summary diagram is given in Figure 24, which corresponds to events on e17–e18 in fetal murine lung (Fig. 25) or ~20 weeks' gestation in human fetal lung. This model is focused on NEBs in the smaller airways and/or alveolar ducts, although the same principles could apply to isolated PNECs in larger airways. Bioactive peptides such as BLPs secreted by PNECs (* in Fig. 24) act as a mitogenic signal to neighboring non-NE airway epithelial cells (pathway 1 in Fig. 24). It is possible, but not yet demonstrated, that differentiation of non-NE airway epithelial cells could also be promoted. In a similar fashion, proliferation and/or differentiation of airway-associated smooth muscle cells (pathway 2 in Fig. 24) might be augmented, which could account in part for the smooth muscle cell hyperplasia which appears to be present in airways of infants with BPD as well as many asthmatics (440). GRP receptors have been localized to airway-associated mesenchymal cells, including smooth muscle in three mammalian species (284–286). The influence of BLPs on proliferation and

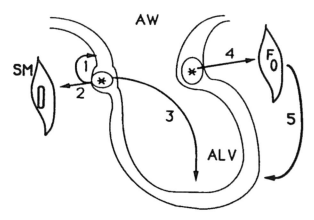

**Figure 24** Schematic diagram summarizing possible effects of BLPs on cells in fetal lung. A developing airway (AW) is shown leading into a primitive alveolus (ALV) lined by epithelium containing NEBs (*). BLPs derived from PNECs in NEBs may act directly on adjacent epithelial cells (pathway 1), on airway-associated smooth muscle cells (SM, pathway 2), or directly on type II pneumocytes via the future airway lumen (pathway 3). Alternatively, BLPs may first trigger a pulmonary mesenchymal cell such as a fibroblast (F, pathway 4) which, in turn, may produce a soluble mediator such as FPF to induce maturation of type II cells.

differentiation of type II pneumocytes has been demonstrated in vivo by ultrastructural and biochemical analyses by our laboratory (267) and directly in primary type II cell cultures (pathway 3 in Fig. 24) by the laboratories of Cake (281) and Fraslon (274), as detailed above. It is likely that at least some of the contents of dense-core vesicles gain access to the future airway lumen, in which they would

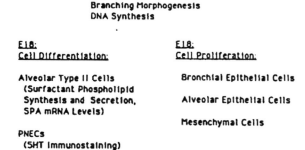

**Figure 25** Summary of major effects of BLPs (endogenous and/or exogenous) on embryonic (e11–e14) or fetal (e18) murine lung.

be capable of spreading over long distances very rapidly owing to the presence of even small amounts of surfactant (441). This differs from the classic teachings that PNECs degranulate only along the basolateral surfaces of the cell but not along the apical membrane which is in contact with the future airway lumen (112). It is possible that a fraction of the peptides secreted basolaterally leaks out to the future airway lumen because of incomplete tight junctions. Support for the postulate that BLPs are present in airways is the finding by Aguayo et al. that adult BAL fluid contains very high levels of BLP immunoreactivity (415). The second hypothesis is that PNECs may influence type II pneumocyte growth and/or differentiation via a mesenchymal cell intermediary (pathways 4 and 5 in Fig. 24). It has been shown that glucocorticoids and EGF can trigger type II cell maturation via a soluble fibroblast-derived factor (18,29,41). BLPs have been reported to stimulate proliferation of adult human pulmonary fibroblasts (266) and BLP receptors have been localized to airway-associated mesenchyme (284–286), supporting pathway 4 (see Fig. 24). A factor such as FPF could subsequently trigger type II cell responses (pathway 5 (see Fig. 24). In the kidney, hepatocyte growth factor has been demonstrated to function as a soluble mesenchyme-derived factor capable of stimulating epithelial cell branching morphogenesis. It is also possible that both pathways in Figure 24 (3 versus 4 plus 5) are operational.

Although light is beginning to dawn on the role of neuropeptides such as BLPs in fetal lung development (280), all that has been learned thus far represents only the tip of the iceberg. Much remains to be learned about the interactions between multiple cell types and between multiple bioactive peptides. In both lung development and in lung injury, there are numerous growth factors and cytokines to consider which may modulate cell proliferation, differentiation, secretion, and/ or receptor function. For instance, increased concentrations of BLPs appear to downregulate EGF receptors (442), and, conversely, functional blocking of BLP receptors by anti-BLP monoclonal antibodies leads to upregulation of EGF receptor function (268). The role of peptidases such as CD10/NEP (269,270) and extracellular matrix molecules such as fibronectin (286) will also have to be factored in. Innervation of NEBs may also be required to facilitate peptide secretion by PNECs (437). The use of normal PNEC culture systems, such as the enriched PNEC cultures described by Cutz (153,154) and Linnoila (155) and fetal lung organ cultures described by Hoyt and others (151) should prove to be invaluable tools for exploring the responses of PNECs to specific chemical and physical stimuli. Changes in parameters of growth and maturation due to specific neuropeptides may be determined in utero using animal models and in organ cultures using human or animal fetal lung.

The definitive experiment to answer many of these questions would involve selective ablation of PNECs at different times during development to determine what would be the consequences on lung development. At the present, this experiment is not feasible, because there is no marker expressed exclusively by PNECs: Most PNEC markers are expressed throughout the diffuse NE system as well as in the central nervous system. It is likely that hormones derived from the hypothalamus, pituitary, adrenal, and thyroid glands may have effects on fetal lung development. We propose that ablation of fully differentiated PNECs during the canalicular phase (e16–e18 in the mouse) would greatly diminish proliferation and differentiation of non-NE cells, both epithelial and mesenchymal. There is likely to be a redundancy of growth factors, with similar effects on cell proliferation induced by BLPs or non-PNEC–derived factors, including EGF, PDGF, or bFGF. In that case, as in our experiments blocking the effects of endogenous BLPs using anti-BLP monoclonal antibodies (268), there may be diminished cell differentiation without inhibition of cell proliferation. The major role of PNECs may be to determine epithelial cell fate by local concentrations of BLPs or other PNEC-derived peptides. For instance, type II cell differentiation might peak at <1 nM BLP (a more distant paracrine effect), whereas PNEC differentiation may occur optimally at 10–50 nM BLP (an autocrine or intracrine effect). It is likely that such differences in cellular responses could be correlated with different BLP receptors as well as distinct subtypes of BLPs.

New questions are now being raised about the significance of NE gene expression (CGRP, PGP 9.5, and NSE immunostaining and GRP mRNAs) in undifferentiated pulmonary epithelium. There has been some concern that this might require redefinition of what constitutes a PNEC. We believe that these data do not invalidate any of the previous theories pertaining to NE cells, nor does this mean that undifferentiated airways are populated by committed NE cells. In addition to selected NE cell markers, undifferentiated epithelium immunostains for the Clara cell marker CC10 (443) and an SP-C transgene (444) which are later expressed only by differentiated Clara cells or type II pneumocytes, respectively. These data suggest that the early pulmonary epithelium may be composed of multipotential precursor cells which have not yet become committed to either NE or non-NE cell lineages. It would then follow that peptides which promote branching morphogenesis, such as BLPs, may be expressed in embryonic lung by all primitive epithelial cells. Although peptides derived from the GRP gene or other BLP-related peptides such as a mammalian phyllolitorin have not yet been detected in early lung buds by immunostaining, it is nonetheless possible that sufficient levels of the relevant bioactive peptide(s) are secreted to trigger a response at physiological receptors; testing of this hypothesis will depend on the demonstration of peptides using a more sensitive method, such as immunoPCR (67). Thus, the formation of a branchpoint might occur where the density of mesenchymal BLP receptors is highest.

Perhaps the most challenging enigmas are those related to the role of PNECs in developmental lung disorders, especially BPD, SIDS, and pediatric asthma, which are three major unsolved problems in pediatric medicine. If excess PNECs are implicated in the pathophysiology of these disorders, it is possible that gene therapy directed at repressing PNEC differentiation might arrest the sequence of events before irreversible structural changes occur. Conversely, if insufficient PNECs are a cause of pulmonary hypoplasia, therapy could be directed at restoring normal numbers of PNECs by inducing their differentiation with specific cytokines or peptides such as BLPs. A key area for future research is understanding the signal transduction of PNEC differentiation and survival during normal development and in lung injury. These investigations should also shed light on mechanisms of neurogenesis and neuronal survival, as well as abnormal differentiation and growth during lung carcinogenesis.

## REFERENCES

1. Netter FH. The CIBA Collection of Medical Illustrations. 7th ed. Summit, NJ: CIBA, 1988.
2. Malchoff CD, Orth DN, Abboud C, Carney JA, Pairolero PC, Carey RM. Ectopic ACTH syndrome caused by a bronchial carcinoid tumor responsive to dexamethasone, metyrapone, and corticotropin-releasing factor. Am J Med 1988; 84:760–764.
3. Howlett TA, Hale AC, Price J, et al. Pituitary ACTH-dependent Cushing's syndrome due to ectopic production of a bombesin-like peptide by a medullary carcinoma of the thyroid. Clin Endocrinol 1985; 22:91–96.
4. Sunday ME, Benacerraf B, Dorf ME. Hapten-specific T cell responses to 4-hydroxy-3-nitrophenyl acetyl. VIII. Suppressor cell pathways in cutaneous sensitivity responses. J Exp Med 1981; 153:811–822.
5. Sporn MB, Roberts AB. Peptide growth factors are multifunctional. Nature 1988; 332:217–219.
6. Cutz E. Cytomorphology and differentiation of airway epithelium in developing human lung. In: McDowell EM, ed. Lung Carcinomas: Current Problems in Tumor Pathology. Edinburgh: Churchill Livingstone, 1987:1–41.
7. Hallman M, Merritt TA, Akino T, Bry K. Surfactant protein A, phosphatidylcholine, and surfactant inhibitors in epithelial lining fluid: Correlation with surface activity, severity of respiratory distress syndrome, and outcome in small premature infants. Am Rev Respir Dis 1991; 144:1376–1384.
8. Sorokin SP, Hoyt RF. Neuroepithelial bodies and solitary small-granule cells. In: Massaro D, ed. Lung Cell Biology. Lung Biology in Health and Disease. Vol. 41. New York: Dekker, 1989:191–344.
9. Cutz E, Gillan JE, Perrin DG. Pulmonary neuroendocrine cell system: an overview of cell biology and pathology with emphasis on pediatric lung disease. Perspect Pediatr Pathol 1995; 18:32–70.
10. Birrer MJ, Minna JD. Molecular genetics of lung cancer. Semin Oncol 1990; 15: 226–235.
11. Warren WH, Memoli VA, Kittle CF, Jensik RJ, Faber LP, Gould VE. The biological implications of bronchial tumors. J Thorac Cardiovasc Surg 1984; 87:274–282.

12. Polak JM, Becker KL, Cutz E, et al. Lung endocrine cell markers, peptides, and amines. Anat Rec 1993; 236:169–171.

13. Ten Have-Opbroek AAW. Lung development in the mouse embryo. Exp Lung Res 1991; 17:111–130.

14. Gross I, Wilson CM, Fetal rat lung maturation: initiation and modulation. J Appl Physiol Respir Environ Exerc Physiol 1983; 55:1725–1732.

15. Adamson IYR, King GM. Epithelial-interstitial cell interactions in fetal rat lung development accelerated by steroids. Lab Invest 1986; 55:145–154.

16. Tanswell AK, Joneja MG, Vreeken E, Lindsay J. Differentiation-arrested rat fetal lung in primary monolayer cell culture II. Dexamethasone, triiodothyronine, and insulin effects on different gestational age cultures. Exp Lung Res 1983; 5:49–60.

17. Gross I, Wilson CM, Floros J, Dynia DW. Initiation of fetal rat lung phospholipid and surfactant-associated protein A mRNA synthesis. Pediatr Res 1989; 25:239–244.

18. Post M, Floros J, Smith BT. Inhibition of lung maturation by monoclonal antibodies against fibroblast-pneumonocyte factor. Nature 1984; 308:284–286.

19. Smith BT. Lung maturation in the fetal rat: acceleration by injection of fibroblast-pneumonocyte factor. Science 1979; 204:1094–1095.

20. Phelps DS, Floros J. Localization of pulmonary surfactant proteins using immuno-histochemistry and tissue *in situ* hybridization. Exp Lung Res 1991; 17:985–995.

21. Caniggia I, Tseu I, Han RNN. Smith BT, Tanswell K, Post M. Spatial and temporal differences in fibroblast behavior in fetal rat lung. Am Physiol 1991; 261:L424–L433.

22. Gross I. Regulation of fetal lung maturation. Am J Physiol 1990; 259:L337–L344.

23. Ballard PL. Hormonal regulation of pulmonary surfactant. Endocr Rev 1989; 10:165–181.

24. King RJ, Jones MB, Minoo P. Regulation of lung cell proliferation by polypeptide growth factors. Am J Physiol 1989; 257:L23–L38.

25. Warburton D, Seth R, Shum L, et al. Epigenetic role of epidermal growth factor expression and signalling in embryonic mouse lung morphogenesis. Dev Biol 1992; 149:123–133.

26. Lin CQ, Bissell MJ. Multi-faceted regulation of cell differentiation by extracellular matrix. FASEB J 1993; 7:737–743.

27. McGowan SE. Extracellular matrix and the regulation of lung development and repair. FASEB J 1992; 6:2895–2904.

28. Hynes RO. Integrins: Versatility, modulation, and signaling in cell adhesion. Cell 1992; 69:11–25.

29. Post M, Barsoumian A, Smith BT. The cellular mechanism of glucocorticoid accel-eration of fetal lung maturation: fibroblast-pneumonocyte factor stimulates choline-phosphate cytidylyltransferase activity. J Biol Chem 1986; 261:2179–2184.

30. Gross I, Wilson CM, Ingleson LD, Brehier A, Rooney SA. Fetal lung in organ culture. III. Comparison of dexamethasone, thyroxine and methylxanthines. J Appl Physiol 1980; 48:872–878.

31. Floros J, Nielsen HC, Torday JS. Dihydrotestosterone blocks fetal lung fibroblast-pneumonocyte factor at a pretranslational level. J Biol Chem 1987; 262:13592–13598.

32. Nielsen HC. Androgen receptors influence the production of pulmonary surfactant in the testicular feminization mouse fetus. J Clin Invest 1985; 76:177–181.

33. Adamson IYR, King GM. Sex differences in development of fetal rat lung. I. Autoradiographic and biochemical studies. Lab Invest 1984; 50:456–460.

34. Torday J, Hua J, Slavin R. Metabolism and fate of neutral lipids of fetal lung fibroblast origin. Biochim Biophys Acta 1995; 1254:198–206.

35. Shoyab M, Plowman GD, McDonald VL, Bradley JG, Todaro GJ. Structure and function of human amphiregulin: a member of the epidermal growth factor family. Science 1989; 243:1074–1076.

36. Carpenter G, Zendegui JG. Epidermal growth factor, its receptor, and related proteins. Exp Cell Res 1986; 164:1–10.

37. Johnson MD, Gray ME, Carpenter G, Pepinsky RB, Stahlman MT. Ontogeny of epidermal growth factor receptor and lipocortin-1 in fetal and neonatal human lungs. Hum Pathol 1990; 21:182–191.

38. Stahlman MT, Orth DN, Gray ME. Immunocytochemical localization of epidermal growth factor in the developing human respiratory system and in acute and chronic lung disease in the neonate. Lab Invest 1989; 60:539–547.

39. Gross I, Rooney SA, Smart DA, et al. Influence of epidermal growth factor on fetal rat lung development *in vitro*. Pediatr Res 1986; 20(5):473–477.

40. Whitsett JA, Weaver TE, Lieberman MA, Clark JC, Daugherty C. Differential effects of epidermal growth factor and transforming growth factor-beta on synthesis of Mr=35,000 surfactant associated protein in fetal lung. J Biol Chem 1987; 262: 7908–7913.

41. Sen N, Cake MH. Enhancement of disaturated phosphatidylcholine synthesis by epidermal growth factor in cultured fetal lung cells involves a fibroblast-epithelial cell interaction. Am J Respir Cell Mol Biol 1991; 5:337–343.

42. Peters K, Werner S, Liao X, Wert S, Whitsett J, Williams L. Targeted expression of a dominant negative FGF receptor blocks branching morphogenesis and epithelial differentiation of the mouse lung. EMBO J 1994; 13:3296–3301.

43. Han RNN, Liu J, Tanswell AK, Post M. Expression of basic fibroblast growth factor and receptor: immunolocalization studies in developing rat fetal lung. Pediatr Res 1992; 31:435–440.

44. Han RNN, Mawdsley C, Souza P, Tanswell AK, Post M. Platelet-derived growth factors and growth-related genes in rat lung. III. Immunolocalization during fetal development. Pediatr Res 1992; 31:323–329.

45. Caniggia I, Liu J, Han R, et al. Fetal lung epithelial cells express receptors for platelet-derived growth factor. Am J Respir Cell Mol Biol 1993; 9:54–63.

46. Torday JS, Kourembanas S. Fetal rat lung fibroblasts produce a TGF-β homolog that blocks alveolar type II cell maturation. Dev Biol 1990; 139:35–41.

47. Stiles AD, D'Ercole AJ. The insulin-like growth factors and the lung. Am J Respir Cell Mol Biol 1990; 3:93–100.

48. Johnson DE. Pulmonary neuroendocrine cells. In: Farmer SG, Hay DWP, eds. The Airway Epithelium. 55th ed. New York: Dekker, 1991:335–381.

49. Scheuermann DW. Neuroendocrine cells. In: Crystal RG, West JB, Barnes PJ, Cherniack NS, Weibel ER, eds. The Lung: Scientific Foundations. New York: Raven Press, 1991:289–300.

50. Barnes PJ, Baraniuk, JN, Belvisi MG. State of the art: neuropeptides in the respiratory tract. Part I. Am Rev Respir Dis 1991; 144:1187–1198.
51. Laitinen LA, Laitinen A. Neural system. In: Crystal RG, West JB, Barnes PJ, Cherniack NS, Weibel ER, eds. The Lung: Scientific Foundations. New York: Raven Press, 1991:759–766.
52. Barnes PJ, Baraniuk JN, Belvisi MG. State of the art: neuropeptides in the respiratory tract. Part II. Am Rev Respir Dis 1991; 144:1391–1399.
53. Barnes PJ. Neural control of airway smooth muscle. In: Crystal RG, West JB, Barnes PJ, Cherniack NS, Weibel ER, eds. The Lung: Scientific Foundations. New York: Raven Press, 1991:903–916.
54. Springall DR, Bloom SR, Polak JM. Neural, endocrine, and endothelial regulatory peptides. In: Crystal RG, West JB, Barnes PJ, Cherniak NS, Weibel ER, eds. The Lung: Scientific Foundations. New York: Raven Press, 1991:69–90.
55. Venkatesh VC, Ballard PL. Glucocorticoids and gene expression. Am J Respir Cell Mol Biol 1991; 4:301–303.
56. De Luca LM. Reinoids and their receptors in differentiation, embryogenesis, and neoplasia. FASEB J 1991; 5:2924–2933.
57. Sunday ME. Cell-specific localization of neuropeptide gene expression: gastrin-releasing peptide (GRP; mammalian bombesin). Methods Neurosci 1991; 5:123–136.
58. Ausubel FM, Brent R, Kingston RE, et al. Current Protocols in Molecular Biology. New York: Greene and Wiley-Interscience, 1987.
59. Davis LG, Dibner MD, Battey JF. Basic Methods in Molecular Biology. New York: Elsevier, 1986:1–388.
60. Lloyd RV. *In situ* hybridization. In: Endocrine Pathology. New York: Springer-Verlag, 1990:241–253.
61. Hofler H, DeLellis RA, Wolfe HJ. In situ hybridization and immunohistochemistry. In: DeLellis RA, ed. Advances in Immunohistochemistry. New York: Raven Press, 1988:47–66.
62. Martínez A, Miller MJ, Quinn K, Unsworth EJ, Ebina M, Cuttitta F. Non-radioactive localization of nucleic acids by direct *in situ* PCR and *in situ* RT-PCR in paraffin-embedded sections. J Histochem Cytochem 1995; 43:739–747.
63. Yam LT, Janckila AJ, Li C-Y. The immunoalkaline phosphatase methods. In: DeLellis RA, ed. Advances in Immunohistochemistry. New York: Raven Press, 1988:1–29.
64. Tijssen P, Adam A. Enzyme-linked immunosorbent assays and developments in techniques using latex beads. Curr Opin Immunol 1991; 3:233–237.
65. Yalow RS. The Nobel lectures in immunology. The Nobel prize for physiology or medicine. Scand J Immunol 1992; 35:1–23.
66. Sunday ME, Wolfe HJ, Roos BA, Chin WW, Spindel ER. Gastrin-releasing peptide gene expression in developing, hyperplastic, and neoplastic human thyroidal C-cells. Endocrinology 1988; 122:1551–1558.
67. Sano T, Smith CL, Cantor CR. Immuno-PCR: Very sensitive antigen detection by means of specific antibody-DNA conjugates. Science 1992; 258:120–122.
68. Bensch KG, Gordon GB, Miller LR. Electron microscopic and biochemical studies on the bronchial carcinoid tumor. Cancer 1965; 18:592–602.
69. Carney DN, Gazdar AF, Bepler G, et al. Establishment and identification of small

cell lung cancer cell lines having classic and variant features. Cancer Res 1985; 45:2913–2923.

70.  Hage E. Histochemistry and fine structure of endocrine cells in foetal lungs of the rabbit, mouse and Guinea-pig. Cell Tissue Res 1974; 149:513–524.

71.  Wang NS, Chen MF, Schraufnagel DE. The cumulative scanning electron microscopic changes in baby mouse lungs following prenatal and postnatal exposures to nicotine. J Pathol 1984; 144:89–100.

72.  Stahlman MT, Jones M, Gray ME, Kasselberg AG, Vaughn WK. Ontogeny of neuroendocrine cells in human fetal lung: III. An electron microscopic immunohistochemical study. Lab Invest 1987; 56:629–641.

73.  Stahlman MT, Gray ME. Colocalization of peptide hormones in neuroendocrine cells of human fetal and newborn lungs: an electron microscopic study. Anat Rec 1993; 236:206–212.

74.  Wharton J, Polak JM, Cole GA, Marangos PJ, Pearse AGE. Neuron-specific enolase as an immunocytochemical marker for the diffuse neuroendocrine system in human fetal lung. J Histochem Cytochem 1981; 29:1359–1364.

75.  Lauweryns JM, Van Ranst L. Immunocytochemical localization of aromatic L-amino acid decarboxylase in human, rat, and mouse bronchopulmonary and gastrointestinal endocrine cells. J Histochem Cytochem 1988; 36:1181–1186.

76.  Shipp MA, Stefano GB, Scharrer B, Reinherz EL. CD10 (CALLA, common acute lymphoblastic leukemia antigen)/neutral endopeptidase 24.11 (NEP, "enkephalinase"): molecular structure and role in regulating met-enkephalin mediated inflammatory responses. Adv Neuroimmunol 1991; 1:139–149.

77.  Heidenhain R. Untersuchungen uber den Bau des Darmkanals. Arch Mikrosk Anat 1870; 6:368–372.

78.  Ciaccio C. Sopra speciali cellule granulose della mucosa intestinale. Arch Ital Anat Embriol 1907; 6:482–484.

79.  Erspamer V. Cellule enterochromaffinie cellule argentophile nel pancreas dell'uomo e die mammiferi. Z Anat Entwicklungs-gesch 1937; 107:574–576.

80.  Pearse AGE. Common cytochemical and ultrastructural characteristics of cells producing polypeptide hormones (the APUD series) and their relevance to thyroid and ultimobranchial C cells and calcitonin. Proc R Soc B 1968; 170:71–80.

81.  Pearse AGE. The cytochemistry and ultrastructure of polypeptide hormone producing cells of the APUD series and the embryologic physiologic and pathologic implications of the concept. Histochem Cytochem 1969; 17:303.

82.  Pearse AG. The diffuse neuroendocrine system and the APUD concept: related "endocrine" peptides in brain, intestine, pituitary, placenta, and anuran cutaneous glands. Med Biol 1977; 55:115–125.

83.  Dayal Y. Neuroendocrine cells of the gastrointestinal tract: introduction and historical perspectives. In: Dayal Y, ed. Endocrine Pathology of the Gut and Pancreas. Boca Raton, FL: CRC Press, 1991:1–32.

84.  Le Douarin N. Particularites du noyau interphasique chez la caille japonaise (Coturnix coturnix japonica). Utilisation de ces particularities comme 'marque biologique' dans les recherches sur les interactions tissulaires et les migrations cellulaires au cours de l'ontogenese. Bull Biol Fr Belg 1969; 103:435–452.

85. Le Douarin N, Le Lievre C. Demonstration de l'origine neurale des cellules a calcitonine du corps ultimobranchial chez l'embryon de poulet. CR Acad Sci Paris 1970; 270:2857–2860.
86. Le Douarin N, Teillet M-A. The migration of neural crest cells to the wall of the digestive tract in avian embryo. J Embryol Exp Morphol 1973; 30:31–48.
87. Pictet RL, Rall LB, Phelps P, Rutter WJ. The neural crest and the origin of the insulin-producing and other gastrointestinal hormone-producing cells. Science 1976; 191:191–192.
88. Andrew A. Further evidence that enterochromaffin cells are not derived from the neural crest. J Embryol Exp Morphol 1974; 31:589–598.
89. Cutz E. Neuro-endocrine cells of the lung: an overview of morphologic characteristics and development. Exp Lung Res 1982; 3:185–208.
90. Brand SJ, Fuller PJ. Differential gastrin gene expression in rat gastrointestinal tract and pancreas during neonatal development. J Biol Chem 1988; 263:5341–5347.
91. Sunday ME, Kaplan LM, Motoyama E, Chin WW, Spindel ER. Biology of disease: gastrin-releasing peptide (mammalian bombesin) gene expression in health and disease. Lab Invest 1988; 59:5–24.
92. Gabriel SM, Kaplan LM, Martin JB, Koenig JI. Tissue-specific sex differences in galanin-like immunoreactivity and galanin mRNA during development in the rat. Peptides 1989; 10:369–374.
93. Gillati MT, Moody TW. The development of rat brain bombesin-like peptides and their receptors. Dev Brain Res 1984; 15:286–289.
94. Lehy T, Puccio F, Chariot J, Gres L, Lewin MJM. Influence of rGRF and bombesin on the growth of lung and digestive tract in suckling rats. In: Lewin MJM, Bonfils S, eds. Regulatory Peptides in Digestive, Nervous and Endocrine Systems. Amsterdam: Elsevier Science, 1985:413–416.
95. Lundgren JD, Baraniuk JN, Ostrowski NL, Kaliner MA, Shelhamer JH. Gastrin-releasing peptide stimulates glycoconjugate release from feline trachea. Am J Physiol 1990; 258:L68–L74.
96. Baraniuk JN, Silver PB, Lundgren JD, Cole P, Kaliner MA, Barnes PJ. Bombesin stimulates human nasal mucous and serous cell secretion *in vivo.* Am J Physiol 1992; 262:L48–52.
97. Feyrter F. Ueber diffuse endokrine epitheliale Organe. Leipzig: Barth, 1938.
98. Feyrter F. Zur pathologie des argyrophilen helle-zellen-organes im bronchialbaum des menschen. Virchows Archiv 1954; 325:723–732.
99. Lauweryns JM, Peuskens JC. Neuro-epithelial bodies (neuroreceptor or secretory organs?) in human infant bronchial and bronchiolar epithelium. Anat Rec 1971; 172:471–482.
100. Lauweryns JM, Cokelaere M, Theunynck P. Serotonin producing neuroepithelial bodies in rabbit respiratory mucosa. Science 1973; 180:410–414.
101. Wharton J, Polak JM, Bloom SR, et al. Bombesin-like immunoreactivity in the lung. Nature 1978; 273:769–770.
102. Sorokin SP, Hoyt RF, Pearsall AD. Comparative biology of small granule cells and neuroepithelial bodies in the respiratory system. Am Rev Respir Dis 1983; 128:S26–S31.

103. Cutz E, Gillan JE, Track NS. Pulmonary endocrine cells in the developing human lung and during neonatal adaption. In: Becker KL, Gazdar AF, eds. The Endocrine Lung in Health and Disease. Philadelphia: Saunders, 1984:210–231.

104. Stahlman MT, Kasselberg AG, Orth DN, Gray ME. Ontogeny of neuroendocrine cells in human fetal lung: II. An immunohistochemical study. Lab Invest 1985; 52: 52–60.

105. Wang YY, Cutz E. Localization of cholecystokinin-like peptide in neuroendocrine cells of mammalian lungs: A light and electron microscopic immunohistochemical study. Anat Rec 1993; 236:198–205.

106. Giaid A, Polak JM, Gaitonde V, et al. Distribution of endothelin-like immunoreactivity and mRNA in the developing and adult human lung. Am J Respir Cell Mol Biol 1991; 4:50–58.

107. Fukayama M, Hayashi Y, Shiozawa Y, Furukawa E, Funata N, Koike M. Human chorionic gonadotropin alpha-subunit in endocrine cells of fibrotic and neoplastic lung: Its mode of localization and the size profile of granules. Lab Invest 1990; 62: 444–451.

108. Fukayama M, Hayashi Y, Koike M, Hajikano H, Endo S, Okumura H. Human chorionic gonadotropin in lung and lung tumors: immunohistochemical study on unbalanced distribution of subunits. Lab Invest 1986; 55:433–443.

109. Tsutsumi Y, Osamura Y, Watanabe K, Yanaihara N. Immunohistochemical studies on gastrin-releasing peptide- and adrenocorticotropic hormone-containing cells in the human lung. Lab Invest 1983; 48:623–632.

110. Osamura RY, Tsutsumi Y, Watanabe K. Light and electron microscopic localization of ACTH and proopiomelanocortin-derived peptides in human development and neoplastic cells. J Histochem Cytochem 1984; 32:885–893.

111. Becker KL. The endocrine lung. In: Becker KL, Gazdar AF, eds. The Endocrine Lung in Health and Disease. Philadelphia: Saunders, 1984:3–46.

112. Adriaensen D, Scheuermann DW. Neuroendocrine cells and nerves of the lung. Anat Rec 1993; 236:70–85.

113. Lauweryns JM, Peuskens JC. Argyrophil (kinin and amine producing?) cells in human infant airway epithelium. Life Sci 1969; 8:577–585.

114. Hoyt RF, McNelly NA, Sorokin SP. Dynamics of neuroepithelial body (NEB) formation in developing hamster lung: light microscopic autoradiography after $^3$H-thymidine labeling *in vivo*. Anat Rec 1990; 227:340–350.

115. Bosman FT, Louwerens JWK. APUD cells in teratomas. Am J Pathol 1981; 104: 174–180.

116. O'Rahilly R. The early prenatal development of the human respiratory system. In: Nelson GH, ed. Pulmonary Development: Transition from Intrauterine to Extrauterine Life. New York: Dekker, 1985:3–18.

117. Stahlman MT, Gray ME. Ontogeny of neuroendocrine cells in human fetal lung. An electron microscopic study. Lab Invest 1984; 51:449–463.

118. Hage E. Morphology and histochemistry of the normal and abnormal pulmonary endocrine cell. In: Becker KL, Gazdar AF, eds. The Endocrine Lung in Health and Disease. Philadelphia: Saunders, 1984:193–209.

119. Spindel ER, Sunday ME, Hofler H, Wolfe HJ, Habener JF, Chin WW. Transient

elevation of mRNAs encoding gastrin-releasing peptide (GRP), a putative pulmonary growth factor, in human fetal lung. J Clin Invest 1987; 80:1172–1179.

120. Haley KJ, Drazen JF, Osathanondt R, Sunday ME. Comparison of the ontogeny of protein gene product 9.5, chromogranin A, and proliferating cell nuclear antigen in developing human lung. Microsc Res Techn 1996 (in press).

121. Watanabe H. Pathological studies of neuroendocrine cells in human embryonic and fetal lung. Acta Pathol Jpn 1988; 38:59–74.

122. McDowell EM, Sorokin SP, Hoyt RF. Ontogeny of endocrine cells in the respiratory system of Syrian golden hamsters. I. Larynx and trachea. Cell Tissue Res 1994; 275: 143–156.

123. McDowell EM, Hoyt RF, Sorokin SP. Ontogeny of endocrine cells in the respiratory system of Syrian golden hamsters. II. Intrapulmonary airways and alveoli. Cell Tissue Res 1994; 275:157–167.

124. Van Lommel ATL, Lauweryns JM. Ultrastructure and innervation of neuroepithelial bodies in the lungs of newborn cats. Anat Rec 1993; 236:181–190.

125. Lauweryns JM, Van Lommel A. The intrapulmonary neuroepithelial bodies after vagotomy: demonstration of their sensory neuroreceptor-like innervation. Experientia 1983; 39:1123–1124.

126. Speirs V, Bienkowski E, Wong V, Cutz E. Paracrine effects of bombesin/gastrin-releasing peptide and other growth factors on pulmonary neuroendocrine cells *in vitro*. Anat Rec 1993; 236:53–61.

127. Cho T, Chan W, Cutz E. Distribution and frequency of neuroepithelial bodies in postnatal rabbit lung: quantitative study with monoclonal antibody against serotonin. Cell Tissue Res 1989; 255:353–362.

128. Cutz E, Conen PE. Endocrine-like cells in human fetal lungs: an electron microscopic study. Anat Rec 1972; 173:115.

129. Lauweryns JM, Cokelaere M. Hypoxia-sensitive neuro-epithelial bodies. Intrapulmonary secretory neuroreceptors, modulated by the CNS. Cell Tissue Res 1973; 145:521–540.

130. Lauweryns JM, Cokelaere M, Deleersynder M, Liebens M. Intrapulmonary neuroepithelial bodies in newborn rabbits. Influence of hypoxia, hyperoxia, hypercapnia, nicotine, reserpine, L-DOPA and 5-HTP. Cell Tissue Res 1977; 182:425–440.

131. Fritsch HAR, Van Noorden S, Pearse AGE. Substance P-, neurotensin- and bombesin-like immunoreactivities in the gill epithelium of Ciona intestinalis L. Cell Tissue Res 1980; 208:467–473.

132. Youngson C, Nurse C, Yeger H, Cutz E. Oxygen sensing in airway chemoreceptors: demonstration of hypoxia-sensitive $K^+$ current and $O_2$-sensor protein. Nature 1993; 365:153–155.

133. Gosney JR. Pulmonary neuroendocrine cells in species at high altitude. Anat Rec 1993; 236:105–107.

134. Hernandez-Vasquez A, Will JA, Guay WB. Quantitative characteristics of the Feyrter cells and neuroepithelial bodies of the fetal rabbit lung in normoxia and short term chronic hypoxia. Cell Tissue Res 1978; 189:179–186.

135. Pack RJ, Barker S, Howe A. The effect of hypoxia on the number of amine-containing cells in the lung of the adult rat. Eur Respir J 1986; 68:121–130.

136. Springall DR, Collina G, Barer G, Suggett AJ, Bee D, Polak JM. Increased intracellular levels of calcitonin gene-related peptide-like immunoreactivity in pulmonary endocrine cells of hypoxic rats. J Pathol 1988; 155:259–267.

137. Keith IM, Will JA. Hypoxia and the neonatal rabbit lung: neuroendocrine cell numbers, 5-HT fluorescence intensity, and the relationship to arterial thickness. Thorax 1981; 36:767–773.

138. Taylor W. Pulmonary argyrophil cells at high altitude. J Pathol 1977; 122:137–144.

139. Gosney JR. Pulmonary endocrine cells in native Peruvian Guinea pigs at low and high altitude. J Comp Pathol 1990; 102:7–12.

140. Montuenga LM, Springall DR, Gaer J, et al. CGRP-immunoreactive endocrine cell proliferation in normal and hypoxic rat lung studied by immunocytochemical detection of incorporation of 5'-bromodeoxyuridine. Cell Tissue Res 1992; 268:9–15.

141. Roncalli M, Springall DR, Maggioni M, et al. Early changes in the calcitonin gene-related peptide (CGRP) content of pulmonary endocrine cells concomitant with vascular remodeling in the hypoxic rat. Am J Respir Cell Mol Biol 1993; 9:467–474.

142. Springall DR, Polak JM. Calcitonin gene-related peptide and pulmonary hypertension in experimental hypoxia. Anat Rec 1993; 236:96–104.

143. Ito T, Ikemi Y, Ohmori K, Kitamura H, Kanisawa M. Airway epithelial cell changes in rats exposed to 0.25 ppm ozone for 20 months. Exp Toxic Pathol 1994; 46:1–6.

144. Linnoila RI, Nettesheim P, DiAugustine RP. Lung endocrine-like cells in hamsters treated with diethylnitrosamine: Alterations *in vivo* and in cell culture. Proc Natl Acad Sci USA 1981; 78:5170–5174.

145. Sunday ME, Willett CG. Induction and spontaneous regression of intense pulmonary neuroendocrine cell differentiation in a model of preneoplastic lung injury. Cancer Res 1992; 52(suppl):2677s–2686s.

146. Nylen ES, Becker KL. Chronic hyperoxia and hamster pulmonary neuroendocrine cell bombesin and calcitonin. Anat Rec 1993; 236:248–252.

147. Nylen ES, Becker KL, Snider RH, Tabassian AR, Cassidy MM, Linnoila RI. Cholinergic-nicotinic control of growth and secretion of cultured pulmonary neuroendocrine cells. Anat Rec 1993; 236:129–135.

148. Sunday ME, Willett CG, Patidar K, Graham SA, Kelly D. Modulation of oncogene and tumor suppressor gene expression in a hamster model of chronic lung injury with varying degrees of pulmonary neuroendocrine cell hyperplasia. Lab Invest 1994; 70:875–888.

149. Oreffo VIC, Lin HW, Gumerlock PH, Kraegel SA, Witschi HP. Mutational analysis of a dominant oncogene (c-Ki-*ras*-2) and a tumor suppressor gene (p53) in hamster lung tumorigenesis. Mol Carcinog 1992; 6:199–202.

150. Becker KL, O'Neill WJ, Snider RH, et al. Hypercalcitoninemia in inhalation burn injury: a response of the pulmonary neuroendocrine cell? Anat Rec 1993; 236:136–138.

151. Sorokin SP, Ebina M, Hoyt RF. Development of PGP 9.5- and calcitonin gene-related peptide-like immunoreactivity in organ cultured fetal rat lungs. Anat Rec 1993; 236:213–225.

152. Ebina M, Hoyt RF, Sorokin SP, McNelly NA. Calcium and ionophore A23187 lower calcitonin gene-related peptide-like immunoreactivity in endocrine cells of organ cultured fetal rat lungs. Anat Rec 1993; 236:226–230.

153. Speirs V, Cutz E. An overview of culture and isolation methods suitable for *in vitro* studies on pulmonary neuroendocrine cells. Anat Rec 1993; 236:35–40.

154. Cutz E, Speirs V, Yeger H, Newman C, Wang D, Perrin DG. Cell biology of pulmonary neuroepithelial bodies—validation of an *in vitro* model. I. Effects of hypoxia and $Ca^{2+}$ ionophore on serotonin content and exocytosis of dense core vesicles. Anat Rec 1993; 236:41–52.

155. Linnoila RI, Gazdar AF, Funa K, Becker KL. Long-term selective culture of hamster pulmonary endocrine cells. Anat Rec 1993; 236:231–240.

156. Gazdar AF, Carney DN, Russell EK, et al. Establishment of continuous, clonable cultures of small cell carcinoma of the lung which have amine precursor uptake and decarboxylation cell properties. Cancer Res 1980; 40:3502–3507.

157. Gazdar AF, Carney DN, Nau MM, Minna JD. Characterization of variant subclasses of cell lines derived from small cell lung cancer having distinctive biochemical, morphological, and growth properties. Cancer Res 1985; 45:2924–2930.

158. Little CD, Nau MM, Carney DN, Gazdar AF, Minna JD. Amplification and expression of the c-myc oncogene in human lung cancer cell lines. Nature 1983; 306:194–196.

159. Minna JD, Cuttitta F, Battey JF, et al. Gastrin-releasing peptide and other autocrine growth factors in lung cancer: pathogenetic and treatment implications. In: DeVita VT, Hellman S, Rosenberg SA, eds. Important Advances in Oncology. First ed. Philadelphia: Lippincott, 1988:55–64.

160. Wewer UM, Mercurio AM, Chung SY, Albrechtsen R. Deoxyribonucleic-binding homeobox proteins are augmented in human cancer. Lab Invest 1990; 63:447–454.

161. Castrillo J-L, Theill LE, Karin M. Function of the homeodomain protein GHF1 in pituitary cell proliferation. Science 1991; 253:197–199.

162. Jetten AM, Shirley JE, Stoner G. Regulation of proliferation and differentiation of respiratory tract epithelial cells by TGF-β. Exp Cell Res 1986; 167:539–549.

163. Nervi C, Vollberg TM, George MD, Zelent A, Chambon P, Jetten AM. Expression of nuclear retinoic acid receptors in normal tracheobronchial cells and in lung carcinoma cells. Exp Cell Res 1991; 195:163–170.

164. Gebert JF, Moghal N, Frangioni JV, Sugarbaker DJ, Neel BG. High frequency of retinoic acid receptor beta abnormalities in human lung cancer. Oncogene 1991; 6: 1859–1868.

165. Marceau N. Biology of disease: Cell lineages and differentiation programs in epidermal, urothelial and hepatic tissues and their neoplasms. Lab Invest 1990; 63:4–20.

166. Dulbecco R. Experimental studies in mammary development and cancer. Adv Oncol 1989; 5:3–6.

167. Gould VE, Linnoila RI, Memoli VA, Warren WH. Biology of disease: Neuroendocrine components of the bronchopulmonary tract: hyperplasias, dysplasias, and neoplasms. Lab Invest 1983; 49:519–537.

168. Teitelman G, Alpert S, Hanahan D. Proliferation, senescence, and neoplastic progression of beta cells in hyperplastic pancreatic islets. Cell 1988; 52:97–105.

169. Solomon E, Borrow J, Goddard AD. Chromosome aberrations and cancer. Science 1991; 254:1153–1160.

170. Weinberg RA. Tumor suppressor genes. Science 1991; 254:1138–1146.

171. Lloyd RV, Wilson BS. Specific endocrine tissue marker defined by a monoclonal antibody. Science 1983; 222:628–630.

172. Sunday ME, Choi N, Spindel ER, Chin WW, Mark E. Gastrin-releasing peptide gene expression in small cell and large cell undifferentiated lung carcinomas. Hum Pathol 1991; 22:1030–1039.

173. Johnson MD, Gray ME, Stahlman MT. Calcitonin gene–related peptide in human fetal lung and in neonatal lung disease. J Histochem Cytochem 1988; 36:199–204.

174. Blobel GA, Gould VE, Moll R, et al. Coexpression of neuroendocrine markers and epithelial cytoskeletal proteins in bronchopulmonary neuroendocrine neoplasms. Lab Invest 1985; 52:39–51.

175. Davis TP, Crowell S, McInturff B, Louis R, Gillespie T. Neurotensin may function as a regulatory peptide in small cell lung cancer. Peptides 1991; 12:17–23.

176. Lee I, Gould VE, Moll R, Wiedenmann B, Franke WW. Synaptophysin expressed in the bronchopulmonary tract: neuroendocrine cells, neuroepithelial bodies, and neuroendocrine neoplasms. Differentiation 1987; 34:115–125.

177. Treston AM, Mulshine JL, Cuttitta F. Control of tumor cell biology via regulation of peptide hormone processing. Monographs—National Cancer Institute 1992; 169–175.

178. Cuttitta F. Peptide amidation: signature of bioactivity. Anat Rec 1993; 236:87–93.

179. Smeekens SP, Chan SJ, Steiner DF. The biosynthesis and processing of neuroendocrine peptides: identification of proprotein convertases involved in intravesicular processing. Prog Brain Res 1992; 92:235–246.

180. Sethi T, Rozengurt E. Multiple neuropeptides stimulate clonal growth of small cell lung cancer: effects of bradykinin, vasopressin, cholecystokinin, galanin, and neurotensin. Cancer Res 1991; 51:3621–3623.

181. White SR, Hershenson MB, Sigrist KS, Zimmermann A, Solway J. Proliferation of guinea pig tracheal epithelial cells induced by calcitonin gene–related peptide. Am J Respir Cell Mol Biol 1993; 8:592–596.

182. Thompson RJ, Doran JF, Jackson P, Dhillon AP, Rode J. PGP 9.5—a new marker for vertebrate neurons and neuroendocrine cells. Brain Res 1983; 278:224–228.

183. Speirs V, Eich-Bender S, Youngson R, Cutz E. Localization of MOC-1 cell surface antigen in small-cell lung carcinoma cell lines: an immunohistochemical and immunoelectron microscopic study. J Histochem Cytochem 1993; 41:1303–1310.

184. Kibbelaar RE, Moolenaar KEC, Michalides RJAM, et al. Neural cell adhesion molecule expression, neuroendocrine differentiation and prognosis in lung carcinoma. Eur J Cancer 1991; 27:431–435.

185. Jin L, Hemperly JJ, Lloyd RV. Expression of neural cell adhesion molecule in normal and neoplastic human neuroendocrine tissues. Am J Pathol 1991; 138:961–969.

186. Edelman GM. Expression of cell adhesion molecules during embryogenesis and regeneration. Exp Cell Res 1985; 161:1–16.

187. Hoffman S, Crossin KL, Prediger EA, Cunningham BA, Edelman GM. Expression and function of cell adhesion molecules during the early development of the heart. Ann NY Acad Sci 1990; 588:73–86.

188. Graziano SL, Mazid R, Newman N, et al. The use of neuroendocrine immunoperoxidase markers to predict chemotherapy response in patients with non-small-cell lung cancer. J Clin Oncol 1989; 7:1398–1406.

189. Beverley PCL, Olabiran Y, Ledermann JA, Bobrow LG, Souhami RL. Results of the central data analysis. Br J Cancer 1991; 63(suppl 14):10–19.
190. Patel K, Frost G, Kiely F, Phimister E, Coakham HB, Kemshead JT. Expression of the cluster 1 antigen (neural cell adhesion molecule) in neuroectodermal tumours. Br J Cancer 1991; 63(suppl 14):20–23.
191. Bobrow LG, Happerfield L, Patel K. The expression of small cell lung cancer related antigens in foetal lung and kidney. Br J Cancer 1991; 63(suppl 14):56–58.
192. Van Duijnhoven HLP, Vissers PMAM, Timmer EDJ, Groeneveld A, Van de Ven WJM. The 7B2 protein as marker for neuroendocrine differentiation in human lung cancer. Br J Cancer 1991; 63(suppl 14):82.
193. Manderino GL, Leicht JC, Mulshine JL, Gooch GT. Cross validation of cluster analysis using immunostained multi-tissue tumour block slides. Br J Cancer 1991; 63(suppl 14):60–63.
194. Waibel R, O'Hara CJ, Stahel RA. Monoclonal antibodies defining the cluster-5A small cell lung carcinoma antigen. Br J Cancer 1991; 63(suppl. 14):29–32.
195. Shipp MA, Tarr GE, Chen C-Y, et al. CD10/NEP hydrolyzes bombesin-like peptides and regulates the growth of small cell carcinomas of the lung. Proc Natl Acad Sci USA 1991; 88:10662–10666.
196. Shipp MA, Stefano GB, D'Adamio L, et al. Downregulation of enkephalin-mediated inflammatory responses by CD10/neutral endopeptidase 24.11. Nature 1990; 347: 394–396.
197. Spindel ER, Giladi E, Brehm P, Goodman RH, Segerson TP. Cloning and functional characterization of a complementary DNA encoding the murine fibroblast bombesin/ gastrin-releasing peptide receptor. Mol Endocrinol 1990; 4:1956–1963.
198. Battey JF, Way JM, Corjay MH, et al. Molecular cloning of the bombesin/gastrin-releasing peptide receptor from Swiss 3T3 cells. Proc Natl Acad Sci USA 1991; 88: 395–399.
199. Wada E, Way J, Shapira H, et al. cDNA cloning, characterization, and brain region–specific expression of a neuromedin-B-preferring bombesin receptor. Neuron 1991; 6:421–430.
200. Gorbulev V, Akhundova A, Buchner H, Farenholz F. Molecular cloning of a new bombesin receptor subtype expressed in uterus during pregnancy. Eur J Biochem 1992; 208:405–410.
201. Fathi Z, Corjay MH, Shapira H, et al. BRS-3: A novel bombesin receptor subtype selectively expressed in testis and lung carcinoma cells. J Biol Chem 1993; 268: 5979–5984.
202. Lin HY, Harris TL, Flannery MS, et al. Expression cloning of an adenylate-cyclase–coupled calcitonin receptor. Science 1991; 254:1022–1024.
203. Mak JC, Barnes PJ. Autoradiographic localization of calcitonin gene–related peptide (CGRP) binding sites in human and guinea pig lung. Peptides 1988; 9:957–963.
204. Julius D, Livelli TJ, Jessell TM, Axel R. Ectopic expression of the serotonin 1c receptor and the triggering of malignant transformation. Science 1989; 244:1057–1062.
205. Chakraborty M, Chatterjee D, Kellokumpu S, Rasmussen H, Baron R. Cell cycle-dependent coupling of the calcitonin receptor to different G proteins. Science 1991; 251:1078–1082.

206. Nelkin BD, Chen KY, de Bustros A, Roos BA, Baylin SB. Changes in calcitonin gene RNA processing during growth of a human medullary thyroid carcinoma cell line. Cancer Res 1989; 49:6949–6952.

207. Seuwen K, Pouyssegur J. Serotonin as a growth factor. Biochem Pharmacol 1990; 39:985–990.

208. Tagliabue E, Martignone S, Mastroianni A, Ménard S, Pellegrini R, Colnaghi MI. Laminin receptors on SCLC cells. Br J Cancer 1991; 63(suppl 14):83–85.

209. Fridman R, Giaccone G, Kanemoto T, Martin GR, Gazdar AF, Mulshine JL. Reconstituted basement membrane (Matrigel) and laminin can enhance the tumorigenicity and the drug resistance of small cell lung cancer cell lines. Proc Natl Acad Sci USA 1990; 87:6698–6702.

210. Schuger L, O'Shea S, Rheinheimer J, Varani J. Laminin in lung development: Effects of anti-laminin antibody in murine lung morphogenesis. Dev Biol 1990; 137: 26–32.

211. Fraser MB. An antibody to a receptor for fibronectin and laminin perturbs cranial neural crest development *in vivo*. Dev Biol 1986; 117:528–536.

212. de Bruine AP, Bosman FT. Neuroendocrine tumors in the respiratory tract. Acta Histochem 1990; 38(suppl):S99–S105.

213. Paladugu RR, Benfield JR, Pak HY, Ross RK, Teplitz RL. Bronchopulmonary Kulchitzky cell carcinomas: a new classification scheme for typical and atypical carcinoids. Cancer 1985; 55:1303–1311.

214. Yousem SA. Pulmonary carcinoid tumors and well-differentiated neuroendocrine carcinomas: Is there room for an atypical carcinoid? Am J Clin Pathol 1991; 95: 763–764.

215. Berendsen HH, de Leij L, Poppema S, et al. Clinical characterization of non–small-cell lung cancer tumors showing neuroendocrine differentiation features. J Clin Oncol 1989; 7:1614–1620.

216. Hammond ME, Sause WT. Large cell neuroendocrine tumors of the lung: clinical significance and histopathologic definition. Cancer 1985; 56:1624–1629.

217. Basbaum C, Jany B. Plasticity in the airway epithelium. Am J Physiol 1990; 259: L38–L46.

218. Baylin SB. Neuroendocrine differentiation: a prognostic feature of non–small-cell lung cancer? J Clin Oncol 1989; 7:1375–1376.

219. Sundaresan V, Reeve JG, Stenning S, Stewart S, Bleehen NM. Neuroendocrine differentiation and clinical behaviour in non-small cell lung tumors. Br J Cancer 1991; 64:333–338.

220. Goodwin G, Shaper JH, Abeloff MD, Mendelsohn G, Baylin SB. Analysis of cell surface proteins delineates a differentiation pathway linking endocrine and nonendocrine human lung cancers. Proc Natl Acad Sci USA 1983; 80:3807–3811.

221. Wuenschell CW, Sunday ME, Singh G, Minoo P, Slavkin HC, Warburton D. Embryonic mouse lung epithelial progenitor cells co-express immunohistochemical markers of diverse mature cell lineages. J Histochem Cytochem 1995; 44:113–123.

222. Brambilla E, Moro D, Gazzeri S, et al. Cytotoxic chemotherapy induces cell differentiation in small-cell lung carcinoma. J Clin Oncol 1991; 9:50–61.

223. Johnson BE, Battey J, Linnoila I, et al. Changes in the phenotype of human small cell lung cancer cell lines after transfection and expression of the c-myc proto-oncogene. J Clin Invest 1986; 78:525–532.

224. Doyle LA, Mabry M, Stahel RA, Waibel R, Goldstein LH. Modulation of neuroendocrine surface antigens in oncogene-activated small cell lung cancer lines. Br J Cancer 1991; 63(suppl 14):39–42.

225. Mabry M, Nakagawa T, Baylin S, Pettengill O, Sorenson G, Nelkin B. Insertion of the v-Ha-ras oncogene induces differentiation of calcitonin-producing human small cell lung cancer. J Clin Invest 1989; 84:194–199.

226. Mabry M, Nakagawa T, Nelkin BD, et al. v-Ha-ras oncogene insertion: a model for tumor progression of human small cell lung cancer. Proc Natl Acad Sci USA 1988; 85:6523–6527.

227. Erspamer V. Amphibian skin peptides in mammals—looking ahead. Trends Neurosci 1983; 6:200–201.

228. McDonald TJ, Jornvall H, Nilsson G, et al. Characterization of a gastrin-releasing peptide from porcine non-antral gastric tissue. Biochem Biophys Res Commun 1979; 90:227–233.

229. Spindel ER, Chin WW, Price J, Rees LH, Besser GM, Habener JF. Cloning and characterization of cDNAs encoding human gastrin-releasing peptide. Proc Natl Acad Sci USA 1984; 81:5699–5703.

230. Gillan JE, Cutz E. Abnormal pulmonary bombesin immunoreactive cells in Wilson-Mikity syndrome and bronchopulmonary dysplasia. Pediatr Pathol 1993; 13: 165–180.

231. Gillan JE, Curran C, O'Reilly E. Abnormal patterns of pulmonary neuroendocrine cells in victims of sudden infant death syndrome. Pediatrics 1989; 84:828–834.

232. Cuttitta F, Fedorko J, Gu J, Lebacq-Verheyden A, Linnoila I, Battey JF. Gastrin-releasing peptide gene-associated peptides are expressed in normal human fetal lung and small cell lung cancer: A novel peptide family found in man. J Clin Endocrinol Metab 1988; 67:576–583.

233. Masui A, Kato N, Itoshima T, Tsunashima K, Nakajima T, Yanaihara N. Scratching behavior induced by bombesin-related peptides. Comparison of bombesin, gastrin-releasing peptide and phyllolitorins. Eur J Pharmacol 1993; 238:297–301.

234. Malendowicz LK, Lesniewska B, Baranowska B, Nowak M, Majchrzak M. Effect of bombesin on the structure and function of the rat adrenal cortex. Res Exp Med 1991; 191:121–128.

235. Tornquist K. 1,25-Dihydroxycholecalciferol enhances both the bombesin-induced transient in intracellular free $Ca2+$ and the bombesin-induced secretion of prolactin in $GH_4C_1$ pituitary cells. Endocrinology 1991; 128:2175–2182.

236. Nealon WH, Beauchamp RD, Townsend CM, Thompson JC. Role of cholecystokinin in canine pancreatic exocrine response to bombesin stimulation. Am J Surg 1987; 153:96–101.

237. Flowe KM, Welling TH, Mulholland MW. Gastrin-releasing peptide stimulation of amylase release from rat pancreatic lobules involves intrapancreatic neurons. Pancreas 1994; 9:513–517.

238. Jansen JB, deJong AJ, Singer MV, Niebel W, Rovati LC, Lamers CB. Role of cholecystokinin in bombesin- and meal-stimulated pancreatic polypeptide secretion in dogs. Dig Dis Sci 1990; 35:1073–1077.

239. Represa JJ, Miner C, Barbosa E, Giraldez F. Bombesin and other growth factors activate cell proliferation in chick embryo otic visicles in culture. Development 1988; 102:87–96.

240. Ahren B. Regulatory peptides in the thyroid gland-a review on their localization and function. Acta Endocrinol 1991; 124:225–232.

241. Pang XP, Hershman JM. Differential effects of growth factors on thymidine incorporation and iodine uptake in FRTL-5 rat thyroid cells. Proc Soc Exp Biol Med 1990; 194:240–244.

242. Lewinski A, Sewerynek E, Wajs E, Baranowska B, Zerek-Melen G. Inhibitory effect of bombesin and SMS 201-995 on DNA synthesis in the rat thyroid lobes incubated *in vitro*. Biochem Biophys Res Commun 1991; 178:520–525.

243. Kanayama S, Liddle RA. Regulation of intestinal cholecystokinin and somatostatin mRNA by bombesin in rats. Am J Physiol 1991; 261:G71–77.

244. Lu L, Logsdon CD. CCK, bombesin, and carbachol stimulate c-fos, c-jun, and c-myc oncogene expression in rat pancreatic acini. Am J Physiol 1992; 263: G327–332.

245. Liehr RM, Rosewicz S, Reidelberger RD, Solomon TE. Direct vs. indirect effects of bombesin on pancreatic growth. Digestion 1990; 46:202–207.

246. Abe Y, Kanamori A, Yajima Y, Kameya T. Increase in cytoplasmic $Ca^{2+}$ and stimulation of calcitonin secretion from human medullary thyroid carcinoma cells by the gastrin-releasing peptide. Biochem Biophys Res Commun 1992; 185:833–838.

247. Rettori V, Pazos-Moura CC, Moura EG, Polak J, McCann SM. Role of neuromedin B in control of the release of thyrotropin in hypothyroid and hyperthyroid rats. Proc Natl Acad Sci USA 1992; 89:3035–3039.

248. Willey JC, Lechener JF, Harris CC. Bombesin and the C-terminal tetradecapeptide of gastrin-releasing peptide are growth factors for normal human bronchial epithelial cells. Exp Cell Res 1984; 153:245–248.

249. Weber S, Zuckerman JE, Bostwick DG, Bensch KG, Sikic BI, Raffin TA. Gastrin releasing peptide is a selective mitogen for small cell lung carcinoma *in vitro*. J Clin Invest 1985; 75:306–309.

250. Cuttitta F, Carney DN, Mulshine J, et al. Bombesin-like peptides can function as autocrine growth factors in human small cell cancer. Nature 1985; 316:823–826.

251. Mahmoud S, Staley J, Taylor J, et al. [Psi[13,14]] bombesin analogues inhibit growth of small cell lung cancer *in vitro* and *in vivo*. Cancer Res 1991; 51:1798–1802.

252. Cardona C, Rabbitts PH, Spindel ER, et al. Production of neuromedin B and neuromedin B gene expression in human lung tumor cell lines. Cancer Res 1991; 51: 5205–5211.

253. Yang HK, Kelley MJ, Battey JF, et al. Correlation of gastrin-releasing peptide (GRP), gastrin-releasing peptide receptor (GRP-R) and neuromedin B receptor (NMB-R) mRNA expression in small cell lung cancer (SCLC) cell lines with *in vitro* response to antibombesin monoclonal antibody (2A11) (meeting abstr). Proc Annu Meet Am Assoc Cancer Res 1993; 34:A2042.

254. Bunnett NW, Kobayashi R, Orloff MS, Reeve JR, Turner AJ, Walsh JH. Catabolism of gastrin releasing peptide and substance P by gastric membrane–bound peptidases. Peptides 1985; 6:277–283.
255. Coy DH, Taylor JE, Jiang N-Y, et al. Short-chain pseudopeptide bombesin receptor antagonists with enhanced binding affinities for pancreatic acinar and Swiss 3T3 cells display strong antimitotic activity. J Biol Chem 1989; 264:14691–14697.
256. Siegfried JM, Guentert PJ, Gaither AL. Effects of bombesin and gastrin-releasing peptide on human bronchial epithelial cells from a series of donors: individual variation and modulation by bombesin analogs. Anat Rec 1993; 236:241–247.
257. Siegfried JM, Han YH, DeMichele MA, Hunt JD, Gaither AL, Cuttitta F. Production of gastrin-releasing peptide by a non-small cell lung carcinoma cell line adapted to serum-free and growth factor-free conditions. J Biol Chem 1994; 269:8596–8603.
258. Ganju RK, Sunday ME, Tsarwhas DG, Card A, Shipp MA. The expression of CD10/NEP in non-small cell lung carcinomas: relationship to cellular proliferation. J Clin Invest 1994; 94:1784–1791.
259. Kane MA, Aguayo SM, Portanova LB, et al. Isolation of the bombesin/gastrin–releasing peptide receptor from human small cell lung carcinoma NCI-H345 cells. J Biol Chem 1991; 266:9486–9493.
260. Corjay MH, Dobrzanski DJ, Way JM, et al. Two distinct bombesin receptor subtypes are expressed and functional in human lung carcinoma cells. J Biol Chem 1991; 266:18771–18779.
261. Battey J, Wada E. Two distinct receptor subtypes for mammalian bombesin-like peptides. Trends Neurosci 1991; 14:524–528.
262. Lach E, Trifilieff A, Landry Y, Gies JP. High-affinity receptors for bombesin-like peptides in normal guinea pig lung membranes. Life Sci 1991; 48:2571–2578.
263. Geraci MW, Miller YE, Escobedo-Morse A, Kane MA. Novel bombesin-like peptide binding proteins from lung. Am J Respir Cell Mol Biol 1994; 10:331–338.
264. DeMichele MA, Gaither Davis AL, Hunt JD, Landreneau RJ, Siegfried JM. Expression of mRNA for three bombesin receptor subtypes in human bronchial epithelial cells. Am J Respir Cell Mol Biol 1994; 11:66–74.
265. Uddman R, Moghimzadeh E, Sundler F. Occurrence and distribution of GRP-immunoreactive nerve fibres in the respiratory tract. Arch Otorhinolaryngol 1984; 239:145–151.
266. Aguayo SM, King TE, Waldron JA, Sherritt KM, Kane MA, Miller YE. Increased pulmonary neuroendocrine cells with bombesin-like immunoreactivity in adult patients with eosinophilic granuloma. J Clin Invest 1990; 86:838–844.
267. Sunday ME, Hua J, Dai HB, Nusrat A, Torday JS. Bombesin increases fetal lung growth and maturation *in utero* and in organ culture. Am J Respir Cell Mol Biol 1990; 3:199–205.
268. Sunday ME, Hua J, Reyes B, Masui H, Torday JS. Anti-bombesin antibodies modulate fetal murine lung growth and maturation *in utero* and in organ cultures. Anat Rec 1993; 236:25–32.
269. Sunday ME, Hua J, Torday J, Reyes B, Shipp MA. CD10/Neutral endopeptidase 24.11 in developing human fetal lung: patterns of expression and modulation of peptide-mediated proliferation. J Clin Invest 1992; 90:2517–2525.

270. King KA, Hua J, Torday JS, et al. CD10/Neutral endopeptidase regulates fetal lung growth and maturation *in utero*. J Clin Invest 1993; 91:1969–1973.

271. Buckingham S, Avery ME. Time of appearance of lung surfactant in the fetal mouse. Nature 1962; 193:688–689.

272. Rooney SA. The surfactant system and lung phospholipid biochemistry. Am Rev Respir Dis 1985; 131:439–460.

273. Post M, Torday JS, Smith BT. Alveolar type II cells isolated from fetal rat lung organotypic cultures synthesize and secrete surfactant-associated phospholipids and respond to fibroblast-pneumonocyte factor. Exp Lung Res 1984; 7:53–65.

274. Fraslon C, Bourbon JR. Comparison of effects of epidermal and insulin-like growth factors, gastrin releasing peptide and retinoic acid on fetal lung cell growth and maturation *in vitro*. Biochim Biophys Acta 1992; 1123:65–75.

275. Erdos EG, Skidgel RA. Neutral endopeptidase 24.11 (enkephalinase) and related regulators of peptide hormones. FASEB J 1989; 3:145–151.

276. LeBien TW, McCormack RT. The common acute lymphoblastic leukemia antigen (CD10)—emancipation from a functional enigma. Blood 1989; 73:625–635.

277. Stimler-Gerard NP. Neutral endopeptidase-like enzyme controls the contractile activity of substance P in Guinea pig lung. J Clin Invest 1987; 79:1819–1825.

278. Nadel JA, Borson DB. Modulation of neurogenic inflammation by neutral endopeptidase. Am Rev Respir Dis 1991; 143(suppl):S33–S36.

279. Chipkin RE, Berger JG, Billard W, Iorio LC, Chapman R, Barnett A. Pharmacology of SCH 34826, an orally active enkephalinase inhibitor analgesic. J Pharmacol Exp Ther 1988; 245:829–838.

280. Miller YE. Pulmonary neuroendocrine cells and lung development: dim outlines emerge. J Clin Invest 1993; 91:1861.

281. Asokananthan N, Cake MH. Stimulation of surfactant lipid secretion from fetal type II pneumocytes by gastrin-releasing peptide. Am J Physiol 1996; 270:L331–337.

282. Li K, Nagalla SR, Spindel ER. A rhesus monkey model to characterize the role of gastrin-releasing peptide (GRP) in lung development. J Clin Invest 1994; 94:1605–1615.

283. Rozengurt E. Early signals in the mitogenic response. Science 1986; 234:161–166.

284. Wang D, Yeger H, Cutz E. Expression of gastrin releasing peptide receptor gene in developing lung. Am J Respir Cell Mol Biol 1996; 14:409–416.

285. Wada E, Battey J, Wray S. Bombesin receptor gene expression in rat embryos: transient GRP-R gene expression in the posterior pituitary. Mol Cell Neurosci 1993; 4:13–24.

286. King KA, Torday JS, Sunday ME. Bombesin and [leu8]phyllolitorin promote fetal murine lung branching morphogenesis via a receptor-mediated mechanism. Proc Natl Acad Sci USA 1995; 92:4357–4361.

287. Plopper CG, St. George JA, Read LC, et al. Acceleration of alveolar type II cell differentiation in fetal rhesus monkey lung by administration of EGF. Am J Physiol 1992; 262:L313–L321.

288. Nilsson R. The artificially ventilated preterm rabbit neonate as experimental model of hyaline membrane disease. Acta Anaesth Scand 1982; 26:89–103.

289. Lorenzo AV. The preterm rabbit: a model for the study of acute and chronic effects of premature birth. Pediatr Res 1985; 19:201–205.

290. deLemos R, Wolfsdorf J, Nachman R, et al. Lung injury from oxygen in lambs: the role of artificial ventilation. Anesthesiology 1969; 30:610–618.
291. Kessler DL, Truog WE, Murphy JH, et al. Experimental hyaline membrane disease in the premature monkey: effects of antenatal dexamethasone. Am Rev Respir Dis 1982; 126:62–69.
292. Prueitt JL, Palmer S, Standaert TA, Luchtel DL, Murphy JH, Hodson WA. Lung development in the fetal primate *Macaca nemestrina*. III. HMD. Pediatr Res 1979; 13:654–659.
293. Prueitt JL, Palmer S, Standaert TA, Luchtel DL, Murphy JH, Hodson WA. Lung development in the fetal primate macaca nemestrina. Pediatr Res 1979; 13:654–659.
294. Meredith KS, Delemos RA, Coalson JJ, et al. Role of lung injury in the pathogenesis of hyaline membrane disease in premature baboons. J Appl Physiol 1989; 66:2150–2158.
295. Escobedo MB, Hilliard JL, Smith F, et al. A baboon model of bronchopulmonary dysplasia: I. Clinical features. Exp Mol Pathol 1982; 37:323–334.
296. Coalson JJ, Kuehl TJ, Escobedo MB, et al. A baboon model of bronchopulmonary dysplasia: II. Pathologic features. Exp Mol Pathol 1982; 37:335–350.
297. Coalson JJ, Winter VT, Gerstmann DR, Idell S, King RJ, Delemos RA. Pathophysiologic, morphometric, and biochemical studies of the premature baboon with bronchopulmonary dysplasia. Am Rev Respir Dis 1992; 145:872–881.
298. Delemos RA, Coalson JJ. The contribution of experimental models to our understanding of the pathogenesis and treatment of bronchopulmonary dysplasia. Clin Perinatol 1992; 19:521–539.
299. Hodson WA, Luchtel DL, Kessler DL, Murphy J, Palmer S, Truog WE. The immature monkey as a model for studies of bronchopulmonary dysplasia. J Pediatr 1979; 95:895–904.
300. Aguayo SM, Schuyler WE, Murtagh JJ, Roman J. Regulation of lung branching morphogenesis by bombesin-like peptides and neutral endopeptidase. Am J Respir Cell Mol Biol 1994; 10:635–642.
301. Bernfield M, Sanderson RD. Syndecan, a developmentally regulated cell surface proteoglycan that binds extracellular matrix and growth factors. Phil Trans R Soc Lond B 1990; 327:171–186.
302. Klagsbrun M, D'Amore PA. Regulators of angiogenesis. Annu Rev Physiol 1991; 53:217–239.
303. Sunderkotter C, Goebeler M, Schulze-Osthoff K, Bhardwaj R, Sorg C. Macrophage-derived angiogenesis factors. Pharmacol Ther 1991; 51:195–216.
304. Warburton D. Epigenetic autocrine and paracrine factors regulating lung morphogenesis. Chest 1991; 99(suppl):15S–18S.
305. Goldin GV, Opperman LA. Induction of supernumerary tracheal buds and the stimulation of DNA synthesis in the embryonic chick lung and trachea by epidermal growth factor. J Embryol Exp Morphol 1980; 60:235–243.
306. Hilfer SR, Rayner RM, Brown JW. Mesenchymal control of branching pattern in the fetal murine lung. Tissue Cell 1985; 17:523–538.
307. Montesano R, Matsumoto K, Nakamura T, Orci L. Identification of a fibroblast-derived epithelial morphogen as hepatocyte growth factor. Cell 1991; 67:901–908.

308. Hirai Y, Takebe K, Takashina M, Kobayashi S, Takeichi M. Epimorphin: a mesenchymal protein essential for epithelial morphogenesis. Cell 1992; 69:471–481.

309. Infeld MD, Brennan JA, Davis PB. Human fetal lung fibroblasts promote invasion of extracellular matrix by normal tracheobronchial epithelial cells *in vitro*: a model of early airway gland development. Am J Respir Cell Mol Biol 1993; 8:69–76.

310. Heine UI, Munoz EF, Flanders KC, Roberts AB, Sporn MB. Colocalization of TGF-$\beta_1$ and collagen I and III, fibronectin and glycosaminoglycans during lung branching morphogenesis. Development 1990; 109:29–36.

311. Roman J, McDonald JA. Expression of fibronectin, the integrin a5, and a smooth muscle actin in heart and lung development. Am J Respir Cell Mol Biol 1992; 6: 472–480.

312. Roman J, Little CW, McDonald JA. Potential role of RGD-binding integrins in mammalian lung branching morphogenesis. Development 1991; 112:551–558.

313. Brauker JH, Trautman MS, Bernfield M. Syndecan, a cell surface proteoglycan, exhibits a molecular polymorphism during lung development. Dev Biol 1991; 147: 285–292.

314. Souza P, Sedlackova L, Kuliszewski M, Tanswell AK, Post M. Effect of PDGF-BB on growth and branching morphogenesis of embryonic rat lung. Am Rev Respir Dis 1993; 147:A511.

315. Ruff M, Schiffmann E, Terranova V, Pert CB. Neuropeptides are chemoattractants for human tumor cells and monocytes: a possible mechanism for metastasis. Clin Immunol Immunopathol 1985; 37:387–396.

316. Ruiz i Altaba A, Melton DA. Interaction between peptide growth factors and homeobox genes in the establishment of antero-posterior polarity in frog embryos. Nature 1989; 341:33–38.

317. Shimosegawa T, Said SI. Pulmonary calcitonin gene–related peptide immunoreactivity: nerve-endocrine cell interrelationships. Am J Respir Cell Mol Biol 1991; 4: 126–134.

318. Baluk P, Nadel JA, McDonald DM. Calcitonin gene-related peptide in secretory granules of serous cells in the rat tracheal epithelium. Am J Respir Cell Mol Biol 1993; 8:446–453.

319. Wada C, Hashimoto C, Kameya T, Yamaguchi K, Ono M. Developmentally regulated expression of the calcitonin gene related peptide (CGRP) in rat lung endocrine cells. Virchows Archiv B Cell Pathol 1988; 55:217–223.

320. Amara SG, Jonas V, Rosenfeld MG, Ong ES, Evans RM. Alternative RNA processing in calcitonin gene expression generates mRNAs encoding different polypeptide products. Nature 1982; 298:240–244.

321. Hoyt RF, McNelly NA, Sorokin SP. Calcitonin gene-related peptide (CGRP) as regional mitogen for tracheobronchial epithelium of organ cultured fetal rat lungs. Am Rev Respir Dis 1973; 157:A498.

322. Hoyt RF Jr, Sorokin SP, McDowell EM, McNelly NA. Neuroepithelial bodies and growth of the airway epithelium in developing hamster lung. Anat Rec 1993; 236: 15–22.

323. Cadieux A, Lanoue C, Sirois P, Barabe J. Carbamylcholine- and 5-hydroxytryp-

tamine–induced contraction in rat isolated airways: inhibition by calcitonin gene-related peptide. Br J Pharmacol 1990; 101:193–199.

324. Gatto C, Lussky RC, Erickson LW, Berg KJ, Wobken JD, Johnson DE. Calcitonin and CGRP block bombesin- and substance P–induced increases in airway tone. J Appl Physiol 1989; 66:573–577.

325. Brownstein MJ. A brief history of opiates, opioid peptides, and opioid receptors. Proc Natl Acad Sci USA 1993; 90:5391–5393.

326. Zetler G. Antagonism of the gut-contracting effects of bombesin and neurotensin by opioid peptides, morphine, atropine or tetrodotoxin. Pharmacology 1980; 21:348–354.

327. Maneckjee R, Minna JD. Opioid and nicotine receptors affect growth regulation of human lung cancer cell lines. Proc Natl Acad Sci USA 1990; 87:3294–3298.

328. Maneckjee R, Minna JD. Nonconventional opioid binding sites mediate growth inhibitory effects of methadone on human lung cancer cells. Proc Natl Acad Sci 1992; 89:1169–1173.

329. DeBold CR, Nicholson WE, Orth DN. Immunoreactive proopiomelanocortin (POMC) peptides and POMC-like messenger ribonucleic acid are present in many rat nonpituitary tissues. Endocrinology 1988; 122:2648–2657.

330. Texier PL, de Keyzer Y, Lacave R, et al. Proopiomelanocortin gene expression in normal and tumoral human lung. J Clin Endocrinol Metab 1991; 73:414–420.

331. Schteingart DE. Ectopic secretion of peptides of the proopiomelanocortin family. Endocrinol Metab Clin North Am 1991; 20:453–471.

332. Tsuchihashi T, Yamaguchi K, Abe K, Yanaihara N, Saito S. Production of immunoreactive corticotropin-releasing hormone in various neuroendocrine tumors. Jpn J Clin Oncol 1992; 22:232–237.

333. Murakami O, Takahashi K, Sone M, et al. An ACTH-secreting bronchial carcinoid: presence of corticotropin-releasing hormone, neuropeptide Y and endothelin-1 in the tumor tissue. Acta Endocrinol 1993; 128:192–196.

334. Suda T, Tozawa F, Dobashi I, et al. Corticotropin-releasing hormone, proopiomelanocortin, and glucocorticoid receptor gene expression in adrenocorticotropin-producing tumors *in vitro*. J Clin Invest 1993; 92:2790–2795.

335. Kirkland SC, Ellison ML. Secretion of corticotrophin releasing factor-like activity by a human bronchial carcinoid cell line. J Endocrinol 1984; 103:85–90.

336. Dieterich KD, Grigoriadis DE, De Souza EB. Corticotropin-releasing factor receptors in human small cell lung carcinoma cells: radioligand binding, second messenger, and Northern blot analysis data. Endocrinology 1994; 135:1551–1558.

337. Moody TW, Zia F, Venugopal R, Korman LY, Goldstein AL, Fagarasan M. Corticotropin-releasing factor stimulates cyclic AMP, arachidonic acid release, and growth of lung cancer cells. Peptides 1994; 15:281–285.

338. Strand FL, Rose KJ, Zuccarelli LA, et al. Neuropeptide hormones as neurotrophic factors. Physiol Rev 1991; 71:1017–1046.

339. Keegan CE, Herman JP, Karolyi IJ, O'Shea KS, Camper SA, Seasholtz AF. Differential expression of corticotropin-releasing hormone in developing mouse embryos and adult brain. Endocrinology 1994; 134:2547–2555.

340. Muglia L, Jacobson L, Dikkes P, Majzoub J. Corticotropin-releasing hormone deficiency reveals major fetal but not adult glucocorticoid need. Nature 1995; 373: 427–432.

341. Delemos RA, Shermeta DW, Knelson JH, Kotas R, Avert ME. Acceleration of appearance of pulmonary surfactant in the fetal lamb by administration of cortico-steroids. Am Rev Respir Dis 1970; 102:459–461.

342. Liggins GC, Schellenberg JC, Manzai M, Kitterman JA, Lee CC. Synergism of cortisol and thyrotropin-releasing hormone in lung maturation in fetal sheep. J Appl Physiol 1988; 65:1880–1884.

343. Gonzales LW, Ballard PL, Ertsey R, Williams MC. Glucocorticoids and thyroid hormones stimulate biochemical and morphological differentiation of human fetal lung in organ culture. J Clin Endocrinol Metab 1986; 62:678–691.

344. Wang Y, Cutz E. Localization of cholecystokinin-like peptide in neuroendocrine cells of mamalian lungs: a light and electron microscopic immunohistochemical study. Anat Rec 1993; 236:198–205.

345. Dockray GJ. Cholecystokinin. In: Krieger DT, Brownstein MJ, Martin JB, eds. Brain Peptides. New York: Wiley, 1983:851–869.

346. Lee MC, Schiffman SS, Pappas TN. Role of neuropeptides in the regulation of feeding behavior: a review of cholecystokinin, bombesin, neuropeptide Y, and galanin. Neurosci Biobehav Rev 1994; 18:313–323.

347. Younes M, Wank SA, Vinayek R, Jensen RT, Gardner JD. Regulation of bombesin receptors on pancreatic acini by cholecystokinin. Am J Physiol 1989; 256:G291–298.

348. Kovacs GL, Szabo G, Penke B, Telegdy G. Effects of cholecystokinin octapeptide on striatal dopamine metabolism and on apomorphine-induced stereotyped cage-climbing in mice. Eur J Pharmacol 1981; 69:313–319.

349. Fuxe K, Agnati LF, Benfenati F, et al. Modulation by cholecystokinin of $^3$H-spiroperidol bing in rat striatum: Evidence for increased affinity and reduction in the number of binding sites. Acta Physiol Scand 1981; 113:567–569.

350. McQueen DS, Ribeiro JA. Effects of beta-endorphin, vasoactive intestinal polypep-tide and cholecystokinin octapeptide on cat carotid chemoreceptor activity. Q J Exp Physiol 1981; 66:273–284.

351. Bunn PA, Chan D, Stewart J, et al. Effects of neuropeptide analogues on calcium flux and proliferation in lung cancer cell lines. Cancer Res 1994; 54:3602–3610.

352. Seldeslagh KA, Lauweryns JM. Endothelin in normal lung tissue of newborn mammals: immunocytochemical distribution and colocalization with serotonin and calcitonin gene-related peptide. J Histochem Cytochem 1993; 41:1495–1502.

353. Uchida Y, Ninomiya H, Saotome M, et al. Endothelin, a novel vasoconstrictor peptide, as potent bronchoconstrictor. Eur J Pharmacol 1988; 154:227.

354. Secrest R, Cohen M. Endothelin:differential effects in vascular and nonvascular smooth muscle. Life Sci 1989; 45:1365.

355. Simonson MS, Dunn MJ. Cellular signaling by peptides of the endothelin gene family. FASEB J 1990; 4:2989–3000.

356. Takuwa N, Takuwa Y, Yanagisawa M, Yamashita K, Masaki T. A novel vasoactive peptide endothelin stimulates mitogenesis through inositol lipid turnover in Swiss 3T3 fibroblasts. J Biol Chem 1989; 264:7856–7861.

357. Gallego R, Garcia-Caballero T, Roson E, Beiras A. Neuroendocrine cells of the human lung express substance-P-like immunoreactivity. Acta Anat 1990; 139:278–282.

358. Paus R, Heinzelmann T, Schultz KD, Furkert J, Fechner K, Czarnetzki BM. Hair growth induction by substance P. Lab Invest 1994; 71:134.

359. Nilsson J, von Euler AM, Dalsgaard CJ. Stimulation of connective tissue cell growth by substance P and substance K. Nature 1985; 315:61.

360. Payan DG. Neuropeptides and inflammation: the role of substance P. Annu Rev Med 1989; 40:341–352.

361. Rozengurt E. Neuropeptides as cellular growth factors: role of multiple signalling pathways. Eur J Clin Invest 1991; 21:123–134.

362. Buckley TL, Brain SD, Rampart M, Williams TJ. Time-dependent synergistic interactions between the vasodilator neuropeptide, calcitonin gene-related peptide (CGRP) and mediators of inflammation. Br J Pharmacol 1991; 103:1515–1519.

363. Bartfai T, Fisone G, Langel U. Galanin and galanin antagonists: molecular and biochemical perspectives. Trends Pharmacol Sci 1992; 13:312–317.

364. Cella SG, Locatelli V, De Gennaro V, et al. Epinephrine mediates the growth hormone–releasing effect of galanin in infant rats. Endocrinology 1988; 122: 855–859.

365. Dunning BE, Taborsky GJ. Neural control of islet function by norepinephrine and sympathetic neuropeptides. Adv Exp Med Biol 1991; 291:107–127.

366. Sethi T, Rozengurt E. Galanin stimulates $Ca^{2+}$ mobilization, inositol phosphate accumulation, and clonal growth in small cell lung cancer cells. Cancer Res 1991; 51:1674–1679.

367. Gressens P, Hill JM, Gozes I, Fridkin M, Brenneman DE. Growth factor function of vasoactive intestinal peptide in whole cultured mouse embryos. Nature 1993; 362:155.

368. Moody TW, Zia F, Draoui M, et al. A vasoactive intestinal peptide antagonist inhibits non–small cell lung cancer growth. Proc Natl Acad Sci USA 1993; 90:4345–4349.

369. Korman LY, Carney DN, Citron ML, Moody TW. Secretin/vasoactive intestinal peptide–stimulated secretion of bombesin/gastrin releasing peptide from human small cell carcinoma of the lung. Cancer Res 1986; 46:1214–1218.

370. Hokfelt T, Tsuruo Y, Ulfhake B, et al. Distribution of TRH-like immunoreactivity with special reference to coexistence with other neuroactive compounds. Ann NY Acad Sci 1989; 553:76–105.

371. Rodriguez MP, Sosenko IRS, Antigua MC, Frank L. Prenatal hormone treatment with thyrotropin releasing hormone and with thyrotropin releasing hormone plus dexamethasone delays antioxidant exzyme maturation but does not inhibit a protective antioxidant enzyme response to hyperoxia in newborn rat lung. Pediatr Res 1991; 30:522–527.

372. Devaskar UP, deMello DE, Ackerman J. Effect of maternal administration of thyrotropin-releasing hormone or DN1417 on functional and morphologic fetal rabbit lung maturation and duration of survival after premature delivery. Biol Neonate 1991; 59:346–351.

373. Warburton D, Parton L, Buckley S, Cosko L, Enns G, Saluna T. Combined effects of

corticosteroid, thyroid hormones, and β-agonist on surfactant, pulmonary mechanics and β-receptor binding in fetal lamb lung. Pediatr Res 1984; 24:166–170.

374. Liggins GC, Schellenberg JC, Manzai M, Kitterman JA, Lee CH. Synergism of cortisol and thyrotropin releasing hormone in lung maturation in fetal sheep. J Appl Physiol 1988; 65:1880–1884.

375. O'Brien WF. Use of TRH in the fetus to advance lung maturity. Adv Exp Med Biol 1991; 299:243–250.

376. Ballard PL, Ballard RA, Creasy RK, et al. Plasma thyroid hormones and prolactin in premature infants and their mothers after prenatal treatment with thyrotropin-releasing hormone. Pediatr Res 1992; 32:673–678.

377. Tache Y, Stephens RL, Ishikawa T. Central nervous system action of TRH to influence gastrointestinal function and ulceration. Ann NY Acad Sci 1989; 553: 269–285.

378. Morley JE. Extrahypothalamic thyrotropin releasing hormone (TRH)—its distribution and its functions. Life Sci 1979; 25:1539–1550.

379. Fox HE, Badalian SS. Ultrasound prediction of fetal pulmonary hypoplasia in pregnancies complicated by oligohydramnios and in cases of congenital diaphragmatic hernia. Am J Perinatol 1994; 11:104–108.

380. Sherer DM, Davis JM, Woods JR. Pulmonary hypoplasia. Obstet Gynecol Surv 1990; 45:792–803.

381. Gillan JE, Cutz E. Abnormal pulmonary bombesin immunoreactive cells in Wilson-Mikity syndrome (pulmonary dysmaturity) and bronchopulmonary dysplasia. Pediatr Pathol 1993; 13:165–180.

382. Avery ME, Mead J. Surface properties in relation to atelectasis and hyaline membrane disease. J Dis Child 1959; 97:517–523.

383. Hansen T, Corbet A. Disorders of the transition. In: Taeusch HW, Ballard RA, Avery ME, eds. Schaffer and Avery's Diseases of the Newborn. 6th ed. Philadelphia, Saunders, 1991:498–514.

384. Johnson DE, Anderson WR, Burke BA. Pulmonary neuroendocrine cells in pediatric lung disease: alterations in airway structure in infants with bronchopulmonary dysplasia. Anat Rec 1993; 236:115–119.

385. Johnson DE, Lock JE, Elde RP, Thompson TR. Pulmonary neuroendocrine cells in hyaline membrane disease and bronchopulmonary dysplasia. Pediatr Res 1982; 16: 446–454.

386. Ghatei MA, Sheppard MN, Henzen-Logman S, Blank MA, Polak JM, Bloom SR. Bombesin and vasoactive intestinal polypeptide in the developing lung: marked changes in acute respiratory distress syndrome. J Clin Endocrinol Metab 1983; 57: 1226–1232.

387. Lauweryns JM, Cokelaere M, Lerut T. Cross-circulation studies on the influence of hypoxia and hypoxaemia in neuro-epithelial bodies in young rabbits. Cell Tiss Res 1978; 193:373–386.

388. de la Monte SM, Hutchins GM, Moore GW. Respiratory epithelial cell necrosis is the earliest lesion of hyaline membrane disease of the newborn. Am J Pathol 1986; 123: 155–160.

389. Willey JC, Lechner JF, Harris CC. Bombesin and the C-terminal tetradecapeptide of gastrin-releasing peptide are growth factors for normal human bronchial epithelial cells. Exp Cell Res 1984; 153:245–248.

390. Johnson DE, Georgieff MK. Pulmonary neuroendocrine cells, their secretory products and their potential roles in health and chronic lung disease in infancy. Am Rev Respir Dis 1989; 140:1807–1812.

391. Aguayo SM, Miller YE, Waldron JA, Sunday ME, Staton GW, King TE. Brief report: idiopathic diffuse hyperplasia of pulmonary neuroendocrine cells and airways disease. N Engl J Med 1992; 327:1285–1288.

392. Bousbaa H, Fleury-Feith J. Effects of a long-standing challenge on pulmonary neuroendocrine cells of actively sensitized guinea pigs. Am Rev Respir Dis 1991; 144:714–717.

393. Severi C, Jensen RT, Erspamer V, et al. Different receptors mediate the action of bombesin-related peptides on gastric smooth muscle cells. Am J Physiol Gastrointest Liver Physiol 1991; 260:G683–G690.

394. Erspamer GF, Mazzanti G, Farruggia G, Nakajima T, Yanaihara N. Parallel bioassay of litorin and phyllolitorins on smooth muscle preparations. Peptides 1984; 5:765–768.

395. Gosney J, Heath D, Smith P, Harris P, Yacoub M. Pulmonary endocrine cells in pulmonary arterial disease. Arch Pathol Lab Med 1989; 113:337–341.

396. Johnson DE, Wobken JD, Landrum BG. Changes in bombesin, calcitonin and serotonin immunoreactive pulmonary neuroendocrine cells in cystic fibrosis and following prolonged mechanical ventilation. Am Rev Respir Dis 1988; 137:123–131.

397. Aguayo SM, Miller YE, Waldron JA, et al. Idiopathic diffuse hyperplasia of pulmonary neuroendocrine cells and airways disease. N Engl J Med 1992; 327:1285–1288.

398. Stephens NL, Jiang H, Halayko A. Role of airway smooth muscle in asthma: possible relation to the neuroendocrine system. Anat Rec 1993; 236:152–163.

399. Pauwels R, Joos G, Van Der Straeten M. Bronchial hyperresponsiveness is not bronchial hyperresponsiveness is not bronchial asthma. Clin Allergy 1988; 18:317–321.

400. Marchevsky AM, Keller S, Fogel JR, Kleinerman J. Quantitative studies of argyrophilic APUD cells in airways. Am Rev Respir Dis 1984; 129:477–480.

401. Bousbaa H, Fleury-Feith J. Effects of a long-standing challenge on pulmonary neuroendocrine cells of actively sensitized guinea pigs. Am Rev Respir Dis 1991; 144:714–717.

402. Chen MF, Kimizuka G, Wang NS. Human fetal lung changes associated with maternal smoking during pregnancy. Pediatr Pulmonol 1987; 3:51–58.

403. Chen MF, Lewis SJ, Jagoe R, et al. Gastrin-releasing peptide gene products in midtrimester human fetal lung with and without maternal smoking history during pregnancy. Pediatr Pulmonol 1991; 10:30–35.

404. Weitzman M, Gortmaker S, Walker DK, Sobol A. Maternal smoking and childhood asthma. Pediatrics 1990; 85:505–511.

405. Martinez FD, Cline M, Burrows B. Increased incidence of asthma in children of smoking mothers. Pediatrics 1992; 89:21–26.

406.  Hanrahan JP, Tager IB, Segal MR, et al. The effect of maternal smoking during pregnancy on early infant lung function. Am Rev Respir Dis 1992; 145:1129–1135.

407.  Chen MF, Diotallevi MJ, Kimizuka G, King M, Wang NS. Nicotine-induced neuro-epithelial cell changes in young rabbits: a preliminary communication. Pediatr Pulmonol 1985; 1:303–308.

408.  McBride JT, Springall DR, Winter RJD, Polak JM. Quantitative immunocyto-chemistry shows calcitonin gene–related peptide-like immunoreactivity in lung neuroendocrine cells is increased by chronic hypoxia in the rat. Am J of Respir Cell Mol Biol 1990; 3:587–593.

409.  Suzuki K, Minei LJ, Johnson EE. Effect of nicotine upon uterine blood flow in the pregnant rhesus monkey. Am J Obstet Gynecol 1980; 136:1009–1013.

410.  Bousbaa H, Poron F, Fleury-Feith J. Changes in chromogranin A-immunoreactive guinea-pig pulmonary neuroendocrine cells after sensitization and challenge with ovalbumin. Cell Tissue Res 1994; 275:195–199.

411.  Manley HC, Haynes LW. Eosinophil chemotactic response to rat CGRP-1 is in-creased after exposure to trypsin or guinea-pig lung particulate fraction. Neuropep-tides 1989; 13:29–34.

412.  DeLellis RA. Basic techniques of immunohistochemistry. In: DeLellis RA, ed. Diagnostic Immunohistochemistry. New York: Masson, 1981:7–16.

413.  Peters SP, Dvorak AM, Schulman ES. Mast cells. In: Massaro D, ed. Lung Cell Biology. 41st ed. New York: Dekker, 1989:345–387.

414.  Impicciatore M, Bertaccini G. The bronchoconstrictor action of the tetradecapeptide bombesin in the guinea-pig. J Pharm Pharmacol 1973; 25:872–875.

415.  Aguayo SM, Kane MA, King TE, Schwarz MI, Grauer L, Miller YE. Increased levels of bombesin-like peptides in the lower respiratory tract of asymptomatic cigarette smokers. J Clin Invest 1989; 84:1105–1113.

416.  Palmer JBD, Cuss FMC, Mulderry PK, et al. Calcitonin gene–related peptide is localised to human airway nerves and potently constricts human airway smooth muscle. Br J Pharmacol 1987; 91:95–101.

417.  Hamel R, Ford-Hutchinson AW. Contractile activity of calcitonin gene–related peptide on pulmonary tissues. J Pharm Pharmacol 1988; 40:210–211.

418.  Tschirhart E, Bertrand C, Theodorsson E, Landry Y. Evidence for the involvement of calcitonin gene–related peptide in the epithelium-dependent contraction of guinea-pig trachea in response to capsaicin. Naunyn Schmiedebergs Arch Pharmacol 1990; 342:177–181.

419.  Cadieux A, Springall DR, Mulderry PK, et al. Occurrence, distribution and ontogeny of CGRP immunoreactivity in the rat lower respiratory tract: effect of capsaicin treatment and surgical denervations. Neuroscience 1986; 19:605–627.

420.  Kroll F, Karlsson JA, Lundberg JM, Persson CGA. Capsaicin-induced bron-choconstriction and neuropeptide release in guinea pig perfused lungs. J Appl Physiol 1990; 68:1679–1687.

421.  Salonen RO, Webber SE, Widdicombe JG. Effects of neuropeptides and capsaicin on the canine tracheal vasculature in vivo. Br J Pharmacol 1988; 95:1262–1270.

422.  Janerich DT, Thompson WD, Varela LR, et al. Lung cancer and exposure to tobacco smoke in the household. N Engl J Med 1990; 323:532–636.

423. Kleinerman J, Marchevsky A. Quantitative studies of argyrophilic APUD cells in airways: II. The effects of diaplacental diethylnitrosamine. Am Rev Respir Dis 1982; 126:152–155.

424. Alexandrov V, Aiello C, Rossi L. Modifying factors in prenatal carcinogenesis (review). In Vivo 1990; 4:327–335.

425. Autrup H. Transplacental transfer of genotoxins and transplacental carcinogenesis. Environ Health Perspect 1993; 2:33–38.

426. Correa E, Joshi PA, Castonguay A, Schuller HM. The tobacco-specific nitrosamine 4-(methylnitrosamino)-1-(3-pyridyl)-1-butanone is an active transplacental carcinogen in Syrian golden hamsters. Cancer Res 1990; 50:3435–3438.

427. Anderson LM, Hecht SS, Dixon DE, et al. Evaluation of the transplacental tumorigenicity of the tobacco-specific carcinogen 4-(methylnitrosamino)-1-(3-pyridyl)-1-butanone in mice. Cancer Res 1989; 49:3770–3775.

428. Rossignol G, Alaoui-Jamali MA, Castonguay A, Schuller HM. Metabolism and DNA damage induced by 4-(methylnitrosamino)-1-(3-pyridyl)-1-butanone in fetal tissues of the Syrian golden hamster. Cancer Res 1989; 49:5671–5676.

429. Hinds PW, Weinberg RA. Tumor suppressor genes. Curr Opin Genet Dev 1994; 4: 435–141.

430. Aguayo SM. Determinants of susceptibility to cigarette smoke. Am J Respir Crit Care Med 1994; 149:1692–1698.

431. Aguayo SM. Pulmonary neuroendocrine cells in tobacco-related lung disorders. Anat Rec 1993; 236:122–127.

432. Aoki Y. Histopathological findings of the lung and trachea in sudden infant death syndrome. Jpn J Legal Med 1994; 48:141–149.

433. Czegledy-Nagy EN, Cutz E, Becker LE. Sudden death in infants under one year of age. Pediatr Pathol 1993; 13:671–684.

434. Perrin DG, Cutz E, Becker LE, Bryan AC, Madapallimatum A, Sole MJ. Sudden infant death syndrome: increased carotid-body dopamine and noradrenaline content. Lancet 1984; September 8:535–537.

435. Cutz E, Wang D, Perrin DG. Bombesin/gastrin releasing peptide and cholecystokinin gene expression in lungs of sudden infant death syndrome victims. Lab Invest 1991; 1:64–107A.

436. Jeffery PK. Pathology of asthma. Br Med J 1992; 48:23–39.

437. Gillan JE, Pape KE, Cutz E. Association of changes in bombesin immunoreactive neuroendocrine cells in lungs of newborn infants with persistent fetal circulation and brainstem damage due to birth asphyxia. Pediatr Res 1986; 20:828–833.

438. Haque AK, Mancuso MG, Hokanson J, Nguyen ND. Bronchiolar wall changes in sudden infant death syndrome: morphometric study of new observation. Pediatr Pathol 1991; 11:551–568.

439. Southall DP, Samuels MP, Talbert DG. Recurrent cyanotic episodes with severe arterial hypoxemia and intrapulmonary shunting. A mechanism for sudden death. Arch Dis Child 1990; 65:953–961.

440. Stocker JT. Neonatal pulmonary pathology. In: Reed GB, Claireaux AE, Bain AD, eds. Diseases of the Fetus and Newborn. St. Louis: Mosby, 1989:247–274.

441. Kharasch VS, Sweeney TD, Fredberg J, Lehr J, Damokosh AI, Avery ME. Pulmon-

ary surfactant as a vehicle for intratracheal delivery of technetium sulfur colloid and pentamidine in hamster lungs. Am Rev Respir Dis 1991; 144:909–913.

442. Zachary I, Sinnett-Smith JW, Rozengurt E. Early events elicited by bombesin and structurally related peptides in quiescent swiss 3T3 cells. I. Activation of protein kinase C and inhibition of epidermal growth factor binding. J Cell Biol 1986; 102: 2211–2222.

443. Singh G, Singh J, Katyal SL, et al. Identification, cellular localization, isolation, and characterization of human Clara cell-specific 10 kD protein. J Histochem Cytochem 1988; 36:73–80.

444. Wert SE, Glasser SW, Korfhagen TR, Whitsett JA. Transcriptional elements from the human SP-C gene direct expression in the primordial respiratory epithelium of transgenic mice. Dev Biol 1993; 156:426–443.

445. Lebacq-Verheyden AM, Krystal G, Sartor O, Way J, Battey JF. The prepro gastrin releasing peptide gene is transcribed from two initiation sites in the brain. Mol Endocrinol 1988; 2:556–563.

446. Lumsden A. Multipotent cells in the avian neural crest. Trends Neurosci 1989; 12: 81–83.

# 15

## Developmental and Hormonal Regulation of the Surfactant System

**MICHAEL W. ODOM**

The University of Texas Health Science
  Center at San Antonio
San Antonio, Texas

**PHILIP L. BALLARD**

University of Pennsylvania School of
  Medicine
The Children's Hospital of Philadelphia
Philadelphia, Pennsylvania

## I. Introduction

Mammalian lung development entails a number of complex processes that prepare the developing organism for an extrauterine environment. Among these, the synthesis, secretion, and metabolism of pulmonary surface active material is of fundamental importance. Pulmonary surfactant is produced by type II cells, or granular pneumonocytes, and stored in unique organelles known as lamellar bodies. Besides synthesis, secretion, and metabolism of surfactant, type II cells play an important role in transepithelial ion transport and in maintaining the cellular integrity of the alveolus by proliferating and differentiating into type I cells in response to injury. A variety of factors, including hormones, cytokines, growth factors, and other agents, have been shown to regulate lung development, alveolar epithelial cell differentiation, and the surfactant system (reviewed in refs. 1–3). In this chapter, we will describe the components of the surfactant system and review the developmental and hormonal regulation of surfactant synthesis, focusing particularly on recent advances in cellular and molecular regulatory mechanisms. This review includes studies published up to June 1995. Other aspects of surfactant physiology and metabolism are addressed in other chapters.

## II.  Components of Surfactant

### A.  Lipid Composition

Pulmonary surfactant is a complex mixture of lipids and proteins that acts to lower surface tension at the alveolar air-liquid interface, thereby stabilizing alveoli on deflation and preventing alveolar collapse. Surfactant can be isolated by differential centrifugation of material from either tracheobronchial lavage or whole lung homogenate followed by extraction of the lipoprotein mixture into an organic solvent. The composition of human surfactant is shown in Figure 1. Phosphatidylcholine (PC) is the most abundant component and makes up over two thirds of surfactant by weight in all mammalian species; the proportion varies from 67% in human (4) to 88% in dog surfactant (5). Most PC in mammalian surfactant (from 53 to 85%) is present in the disaturated form as dipalmitoyl phosphatidylcholine (DPPC), and this component is responsible for surfactant's high surface activity. Phosphatidylglycerol (PG) makes up 10% of human surfactant, accounting for the much greater content of this phospholipid in lung than in other tissues. After 30–32 weeks of gestation in the human, when surfactant secretion begins, the content of DPPC and PG in amniotic fluid increases substantially, and this increasing content of surfactant phospholipids relative to structural lipids can be used as a marker of fetal lung maturity. Despite its high abundance in surfac-

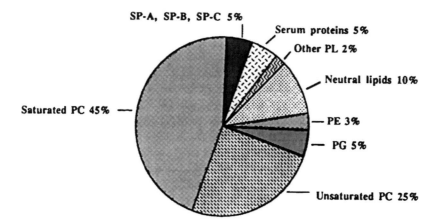

**Figure 1**  Composition of surfactant isolated from bronchoalveolar lavage fluid. The major components contributing to establishment of the surface active film in air spaces are disaturated phosphatidylcholine, phosphatidylglycerol, and the surfactant associated proteins. PC, phosphatidylcholine; PL, phospholipid; PE, phosphatidylethanolamine; PG, phosphatidylglycerol; SP, surfactant protein.

tant, the exact functional role of PG is unclear. Several mammalian species produce a surfactant that contains relatively little PG without any apparent adverse effect on the physical properties of surfactant or lung function (6,7). Most studies to examine the developmental or hormonal regulation of surfactant phospholipid synthesis have determined either the content or rate of incorporation of radio-labeled precursors into PC, DPPC, or PG. However, because these phospholipids are not unique to surfactant but are also present in nonsurfactant fractions particularly cell membranes, these methods are inexact. Surfactant also contains small amounts of other phospholipids such as phosphatidylinositol, phosphatidyl-ethanolamine, and phosphatidylserine and neutral lipids such as cholesterol but their function is uncertain. Secretion of surfactant is an energy-dependent, highly regulated process that involves movement of lamellar bodies to the apical surface of the type II cell via interactions with the cytoskeleton and exocytosis of the phospholipid bilayers into the alveolar space. The transformation of surfactant phospholipid bilayers into the monolayer present at the air-liquid interface is an incompletely understood process that involves a unique intermediary structure known as tubular myelin. This membrane lattice can be formed in vitro from DPPC, PG, surfactant-associated proteins, and calcium. Non-DPPC components of surfactant appear to be eventually excluded as the secreted material forms the surface-active monolayer. Surfactant synthesis results from de novo reactions as well as recycling of components that are reclaimed by type II cells through endocytosis of lipids and proteins at the apical surface.

## B. Biosynthesis of Surfactant Phospholipids

The major pathway for the synthesis of PC is by the transfer of CDP-choline to carbon 3 of diacylglycerol, as shown in Figure 2 (reviewed in refs. 1 and 8–10). Cholinephosphate cytidylyltransferase, which catalyzes the formation of CDP-choline from choline-phosphate, is a key regulatory enzyme in this process, and this reaction appears to be rate limiting. Diacylglycerol is produced by the removal of inorganic phosphate from phosphatidic acid, which occupies a central position in these pathways and is the common lipid precursor of all glycero-phospholipids. Fatty acids used by the fetal lung for the synthesis of phosphatidic acid appear to arise principally through de novo synthesis from glucose which can originate from the fetal bloodstream or by breakdown of intracellular glycogen stores. Morphological and biochemical evidence indicate that intracellular gly-cogen plays a major role in this process. The development of the alveolar epithe-lium is characterized by a gradual change from glycogen-rich immature epithelial cells to differentiated type II cells which contain an abundance of lamellar bodies and a paucity of intracellular glycogen. Biochemically, a developmental increase in glycogen content and in the activity of glycogen synthase is followed by a

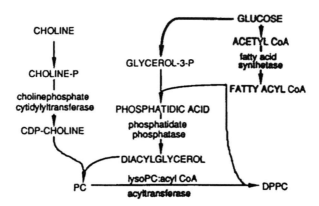

**Figure 2**   Pathways for synthesis of surfactant lipids. Key enzymes are indicated in each of the pathways leading to synthesis of phosphatidylcholine (PC) and remodeling to dipalmitoylphosphatidylcholine (DPPC). (From ref. 188.)

decrease in glycogen content, a decline in the activities of the enzymes of glycogenolysis, and a surge in the synthesis of surfactant phospholipids, suggesting a causal relationship between these events (10). Acetyl-CoA carboxylase and fatty acid synthetase catalyze reactions of de novo fatty acid synthesis. After birth, preformed fatty acids from dietary sources predominate and the de novo pathway is less active. DPPC, or disaturated PC, may be synthesized de novo or by remodeling mechanisms. For remodeling, 1-saturated–2-unsaturated PC is first deacylated to 1-acyl-2-lyso PC and then reacylated by reaction with saturated acyl-CoA. A transacylation reaction is also possible but appears to be inconsequential. Although earlier studies indicated that DPPC synthesis occurred almost exclusively by the remodeling pathway, more recent evidence suggests that de novo synthesis occurs in the lung as well (11,12).

### C.   Surfactant-Associated Proteins

Proteins make up about 5–10% of surfactant preparations and include serum proteins as well as four species of surfactant-associated proteins. Serum proteins have no known functional role in surfactant and can inhibit surfactant activity. They may represent an artifact of isolation procedures, or they may normally be present in air spaces in association with surfactant lipids. Specific, surfactant-associated proteins have important roles in the structural organization, function, and metabolism of surfactant and have been designated surfactant proteins (SPs) A, B, and C (SP-A, SP-B, and SP-C). These three proteins are expressed only in lung tissue. A fourth surfactant-associated protein, SP-D, has recently been identified. SP-A and SP-D are water-soluble glycoproteins, whereas SP-B and SP-C are hydrophobic proteolipids. Several detailed reviews of the structure and function of surfactant-associated proteins have recently been published (13–17). Structural features of these proteins and their genes are summarized in Table 1.

### SP-A

SP-A, the most abundant of the surfactant proteins, is a water-soluble glycoprotein that undergoes extensive posttranslational modification and assembly to form a large multimeric structure. Genes encoding SP-A have been cloned and partially characterized in a variety of mammalian species (18–23). These genes consist of five or six exons, four of which contain coding sequence, and span ~4.5–5.0 kb. A single gene encodes SP-A in the rat, mouse, and rabbit, whereas in the human two genes, designated SP-A1 and SP-A2, as well as a pseudogene have been identified (24–26), all of which appear to be located on the long arm of chromosome 10 (27). The human SP-A1 and SP-A2 genes are 94% identical; the major difference is an additional exon (exon II of VI) in SP-A2 that encodes 5' untranslated sequence. Using primer extension analysis and polymerase chain reaction rapid amplification of 5'-cDNA ends, McCormick and associates (25) characterized a minimum of nine different alternatively spliced transcripts, including one major SP-A1 and two major SP-A2 transcripts. Two SP-A cDNAs, 6A and 1A, described by Floros et al. (28), appear to originate from SP-A1 and SP-A2, respectively. Overall, the coding portions of mammalian SP-A genes exhibit a high degree of homology (~75%), but the noncoding portions are less similar. The predominant SP-A messenger RNA (mRNA) in the human is ~2.2 kb in size and includes a 1300-bp 3' untranslated region. In other mammalian species, alternate sites of poly-

**Table 1**  Surfactant Associated Proteins in Human Lung

|      | Chromosomal location | No. of genes | No. of exons | Primary translation product (aa) | Mature protein (kDa) |
|------|----------------------|--------------|--------------|----------------------------------|----------------------|
| SP-A | 10                   | 2 (+ pseudogene) | 5–6      | 248                              | 28–36 reduced ~650 native |
| SP-B | 2                    | 1            | 10           | 381                              | ~8 reduced           |
| SP-C | 8                    | 2            | 6            | 197                              | ~4 reduced           |
| SP-D | 10                   | 1            | 7            | 375                              | 43 reduced ~620 native |

References are cited in the text.

adenylation result in mRNA species ranging in size from 0.9 kb in the rat to 3.0 kb in the mouse.

The primary translation product of human SP-A is made up of 248 amino acids that form four structural domains. As in other secretory proteins, SP-A contains a 20–amino acid N-terminal signal peptide followed by 7 amino acids to complete this N-terminal domain. A cysteine residue within this 7–amino acid portion forms an intermolecular disulfide bond that is invariant in the four species examined to date. A collagen-like domain flanks the N-terminal region and consists of 24 repeating Gly-X-Y triplets in which Y is hydroxyproline in 13 of the 24 triplets. Next, a 24–amino acid segment of noncollagenous sequence is found which may play a role in phospholipid binding (29). The C-terminal region forms a globular, carbohydrate-recognition domain of 130 amino acids. Eighteen amino acids within this region are highly conserved, including four cysteine residues which form intrachain disulfide bonds important for carbohydrate binding (30). In addition to the formation of intra- and interchain disulfide bonds, SP-A undergoes posttranslational modifications, including hydroxylation of proline residues in the collagen-like domain, carboxylation of glutamic acid, acetylation, and variable glycosylation at an asaparagine residue. These modifications result in a series of glycoprotein monomers with a $M_r$ of 28–36 kDa and pI of 4.6–5.2. Studies using circular dichroism and rotary shadowing electron microscopy have shown that in vivo SP-A is assembled into an octadecamer composed of six groups of three monomers with the collagen-like domain of each trimer forming a triple helix stalk and the carbohydrate-recognition domain extending out as a globular, spherical structure (30–32). The SP-A multimer is similar structurally and in many ways functionally to C1q and the mannose binding protein.

The complex structure of SP-A facilitates a number of diverse functions. SP-A binds lipids and promotes aggregation of phospholipid vesicles in the presence of $Ca^{+2}$ ions. Lipid binding is dependent on an intact collagen-like domain and may be mediated through the 21-residue portion of the peptide just beyond the collagen-like domain. Interactions between SP-A, surfactant lipids, SP-B, and $Ca^{+2}$ ions are required for the formation of tubular myelin (33,34). SP-A appears also to be involved in the regulation of surfactant secretion and recycling, since SP-A inhibits surfactant secretion and stimulates reuptake of phospholipids by type II cells in primary culture presumably through a receptor-mediated process (35). In addition to interactions with lipids, SP-A also binds carbohydrates through its C-terminal domain and, like SP-D, is a C-type lectin. This characteristic along with structural similarities to C1q suggest a role for SP-A in pulmonary defenses against infection, possibly by binding polysaccharides on bacterial surfaces and promoting phagocytosis by alveolar macrophages. SP-A has been shown in recent studies to bind a variety of bacterial and viral pathogens and to enhance alveolar macrophage chemotaxis, phagocytosis, and chemiluminescence responses (36–41).

### SP-D

Like SP-A, SP-D is a water-soluble collagenous C-type lectin that is secreted into the alveolus by type II cells, but its role as a surfactant-associated protein is tentative, because no property directly relevant to surfactant function has as yet been defined (42–46). The human SP-D gene has recently been cloned and partially characterized. It consists of seven exons spanning over 11 kb from 10q22.2 to q23.1. This region of chromosome 10 contains a cluster of homologous genes, including the two SP-A genes and the mannose binding protein. The seven exons of the SP-D gene encode the same structural domains as SP-A with exon 1 coding for a signal peptide, an aminoterminal noncollagen domain, and the first portion of the collagen domain; exons 2–5 coding for the remainder of the collagen domain; exon 6 coding for an α-helical linking sequence and exon 7 coding for the C-type carbohydrate-recognition domain. Posttranslational modifications include glycosylation by the attachment of a sialylated oligosaccharide to an asparagine residue and hydroxylation of proline and lysine residues in the collagen domain (43) and result in a mature protein with a $M_r$ of 43 kDa under reducing conditions (45). The collagenous portion of SP-D is homologous to that of SP-A but is longer, consisting of 59 rather than 24 Gly-X-Y repeats. SP-D subunits are assembled into disulfide-linked trimers, and rotary shadowing electron microscopy has suggested that four trimers then form a cruciform structure with the collagen domains extending inward (47).

The role of SP-D in surfactant physiology is currently unclear. SP-D is more loosely associated with other surfactant components than is SP-A, and this association appears to be mediated principally through carbohydrate-dependent interactions (45). One recent study found that SP-D was not localized in lamellar bodies (48). SP-D may play a role in surfactant secretion by countering the inhibitory effects of SP-A (49). Although the functional importance of SP-D in surfactant is unclear, SP-D, like SP-A, appears to play an important role in pulmonary defense mechanisms. SP-D causes agglutination of gram-negative organisms and facilitates phagocytosis by alveolar macrophages (50,51). The carbohydrate binding domain of SP-D has also been shown recently to mediate an inhibitory effect on the hemagglutination activity of several strains of influenza A and to enhance neutrophil binding and intracellular killing of this virus (52).

### SP-B and SP-C

SP-B and SP-C are small hydrophobic proteins that coisolate with surfactant lipids and facilitate their spreading at the air-liquid interface. SP-B is encoded by 11 exons of a gene that encompasses ~9.5 kb on chromosome 2 (53,54). Southern analysis of restriction digests of human genomic DNA indicates a single SP-B gene (55). In the human, transcription of this gene gives rise to a 2.0 kb mRNA that encodes a 381–amino acid precursor protein (56,57). A 20- to 23-amino acid signal peptide along with N- and C-terminal peptides are removed during intra-cellular processing and result in the formation of the 79–amino acid active airway peptide that has a $M_r$ of 8 kDa under reducing conditions. The active SP-B peptide exhibits greater than 80% homology across mammalian species examined to date and is rich in cysteine and basic and hydrophobic residues. Structurally, the mature SP-B peptide contains sequences that predict three amphipathic helices, each interrupted by a proline residue, and an extremely hydrophobic region that may be closely associated with surfactant lipids (58).

The human SP-C gene spans 2.7 kb on the short arm of chromosome 8 and contains six exons. Restriction analysis of human genomic DNA suggests the presence of two very similar SP-C genes, both of which appear to be transcribed (59,60). In the rabbit, similar studies have indicated the presence of a single gene (61). Alternate splice sites result in a heterogeneous group of mRNAs; the major transcript is 0.9 kb in size. The primary translation product consists of 197 amino acids, but interestingly, it does not include an N-terminal signal peptide. Like SP-B, the mature SP-C protein of 35 amino acids is released after cleavage of N- and C-terminal peptides and exhibits greater than 80% homology across mammalian species. The SP-B and SP-C precursor proteins are presumably necessary to maintain the proteins in a soluble state within the cell prior to secretion. Mature SP-C is one of the most hydrophobic proteins found in nature and has a $M_r$ of 3.5 kDa. The region from amino acids 13–33 is rich in valine and leucine or isoleucine and is predicted to form a rigid $\alpha$-helix capable of spanning a lipid bilayer. This predicted structure has recently been confirmed by infrared spectroscopy (62). Unlike other surfactant proteins, mature human SP-C contains two covalently bound palmitic acid residues near its amino terminus. Most palmitylated proteins are plasma membrane-associated, further strengthening the notion that at least at some point during its life cycle SP-C is membrane-bound.

The hydrophobicity of SP-B and SP-C allows for several important interac-tions with surfactant lipids. When combined with liposomes made of DPPC and PG, both SP-B and SP-C enhance lipid spreading and the formation of a mono-layer (58). SP-B appears to be somewhat more effective in this process than SP-C. Studies using surfactant phospholipids indicate that SP-B along with SP-A, but not SP-C, are necessary for the formation of tubular myelin (34,63). Both SP-B and SP-C also tend to inhibit the inactivation of surfactant phospholipids by serum proteins.

## III.  Ontogeny of Surfactant Phospholipids and Proteins

### A.  Phospholipids

Although the time of initiation of surfactant phospholipid synthesis varies some-what, the rate of synthesis increases substantially during the last 15% of gestation

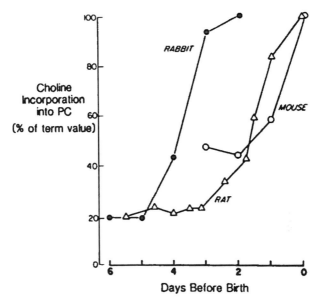

**Figure 3** Developmental pattern of phosphatidylcholine (PC) synthesis as assessed by choline incorporation in three species. Rate of synthesis increases before birth resulting in increased content of PC in lung tissue and air spaces. (From ref. 1.)

in all mammalian species (Fig. 3). In the human, surfactant synthesis begins as the second trimester ends and increases during the third trimester in preparation for the onset of air breathing at birth. Recognizable type II cells containing lamellar bodies appear at about 20–24 weeks in the human and surfactant secretion begins at about 30 weeks (64). In other mammalian species, surfactant synthesis begins at a somewhat later stage of development. For example, lamellar body–containing type II cells are not seen in fetal lambs and rodents until gestation is ~80 and 95% complete, respectively (65). Concentrations of DPPC and other surfactant phospholipids in lung tissue, lung lavage, and amniotic fluid increase during the latter portion of gestation in all mammalian species. In rabbit lung lavage, the proportion of PC increases from less than 30% of the total phospholipid at 27 days' gestation to almost 70% at term (31 days). Concomitantly, sphingomyelin decreases from about 40% to less than 10% of the total at term. Changes in the content of the acidic phospholipids PG and phosphatidylinositol also reflect surfactant synthesis and secretion; as PG increases, phosphatidylinositol decreases (66). Thus, the ratio of PC (lecithin) to sphingomyelin and the presence of PG in amniotic fluid have been used as clinical indicators of lung maturity. In addition to developmental increases in the content of surfactant phospholipids, precursor incorporation into PC and activities of enzymes involved in fetal lung PC and DPPC biosynthesis increase near the end of gestation (reviewed in ref. 10).

### B. Surfactant Proteins

Although SP-A, SP-B, and SP-C are each developmentally regulated, these processes are not coordinate and, at least in some respects, are species specific. In the human, SP-A gene expression and protein synthesis tend to parallel the synthesis of surfactant phospholipids. In second-trimester human fetal lung, both SP-A mRNA and protein content by immunoassay are undetectable or are present at very low levels (67–69). SP-A protein in amniotic fluid is generally not detectable until 28–30 weeks, after which its concentration increases exponentially to term (64,70). Fetal gender does not appear to greatly alter SP-A content in human amniotic fluid (70,71). McCormick et al. (72) recently examined the proportion of SP-A1 and SP-A2 transcripts in tissue from a 28-week infant and four adult samples. Only SP-A1 transcripts were found in the 28-week lung, whereas adult lung tissue contained 75% SP-A2 and 25% SP-A1 transcripts. Further studies are required to determine if this finding represents a general change in SP-A gene expression during lung development. In the rabbit, SP-A gene expression begins several days prior to the synthesis of surfactant phospholipids. SP-A gene transcription is evident on days 21–22 of the 31-day gestation, and low levels of SP-A mRNA can be detected by days 24–26 just prior to augmented synthesis of surfactant phospholipids (73–75). Subsequently, the rate of SP-A gene transcription and mRNA levels increase substantially and are at a maximum by 28 and 31 days, respectively, before declining slightly after birth. Chen et al. (23) have recently identified a DNase I hypersensitive site ~80–180 bp upstream from the transcription initiation site in DNA isolated from 21- and 28-day fetal and adult rabbit lung nuclei but not in DNA from kidney, liver, or heart nuclei, suggesting that the altered chromatin structure in this region could play a role in the transcriptional activation of this gene. SP-A protein and mRNA are first found in rat lung tissue on day 18 (term is 22 days) when recognizable type II cells are also first apparent (76). Levels increase substantially by day 21 to ~50% of those found in the adult, then decline during the first week of life, and finally increase to near adult levels by 28 days' postnatal age.

Only limited data on the ontogeny of SP-D is available to date. Two groups have used a sandwich ELISA assay to examine levels of SP-D in human amniotic fluid from a relatively small number of third-trimester pregnancies (77,78). SP-D was detected as early as 26 weeks and increased moderately by term. SP-A levels examined simultaneously showed similar levels to SP-D initially, but by term SP-A was on average 5.5-fold higher than SP-D. Ogasawara et al. (79) used an ELISA assay to examine SP-D levels in rat lung homogenate and have found SP-D to be present at very low levels on day 18 of gestation. As in human amniotic fluid, SP-D increased moderately to near adult levels by the time of birth and was about one fourth of the level of SP-A. In this study, SP-D content did not decline significantly after birth, as has been described for SP-A in this species, but remained near adult levels throughout the first 5 days of life. Consistent with the developmental pattern reported for the SP-D protein in the rat, Deterding et al. (80) first detected SP-D mRNA on days 18–19 of gestation during the canalicular period of lung development. Levels increased through the first several days of postnatal life, declined slightly on neonatal day 7 and then increased to adult levels. In another study, Crouch et al. (81) did not detect SP-D mRNA until day 21 of gestation. In this study, a degenerate oligomeric cDNA was used, whereas Deterding and coworkers used a full-length cDNA, which might be somewhat more sensitive and explain detection of message at an earlier point in gestation. In a later report from this laboratory using a full-length cDNA, SP-D message was detected on days 19–20 of gestation (82).

Studies in a number of species have shown that SP-B and SP-C gene expression begins at an earlier stage of lung development than does SP-A or SP-D. In human fetal lung tissue, SP-B and SP-C mRNAs are present as early as 13 weeks and increase to ~50 and 15% of adult levels by 24 weeks (83). However, tissue levels of both proteins are very low at 24 weeks (M. Beers and P. Ballard, unpublished data), and a recent study of amniotic fluid from over 400 pregnancies of 19–42 weeks' gestation found that the mature SP-B protein was not present prior to 31 weeks' gestation (70). SP-B levels increased exponentially thereafter. Studies using Northern analysis of rabbit fetal lung have detected SP-C and SP-B mRNAs as early as days 19 and 26 of gestation, respectively (61,75,84,85). Levels for both mRNAs increased rapidly to term and then declined somewhat in the adult. Transcription of both the SP-B and SP-C genes, as assessed by nuclear elongation assay, was detected on day 22 of gestation and increased to term. In the rat, SP-C, but not SP-B or SP-A, mRNA was detected in day 17 glandular lung tissue (76). SP-B message was present at 18 days, and then both SP-B and SP-C mRNAs increased to near adult levels by day 21. In the mouse, both SP-B and SP-C mRNAs are present at low levels in glandular lungs on day 15 of gestation and increase severalfold to near adult levels by birth (86,87). A chimeric gene containing 3.7 kb of 5′ sequence from the human SP-C gene used to drive the chloramphenicol acetyl transferase (CAT) reporter gene has been shown to confer tissue-specific and developmentally regulated expression in a transgenic mouse model as early as day 10 of gestation (87–89). Expression of CAT was detected in epithelial cells of the primordial lung buds of transgenic animals as early as day 10 of gestation and increased rapidly thereafter resulting in high levels of CAT expression in the distal epithelial elements of the branching bronchial tubules throughout organogenesis. Developmentally regulated expression of the endogenous murine SP-C gene differed from that of the transgene in that expression increased later on day 15 of gestation, coincident with the differentiation of primitive acinar tubules. Differences in expression of the transgene and the murine SP-C gene may be due to the heterologous nature of this system; that is, expression of a human transgene in a mouse model. Information on the ontogeny of the mature SP-C protein has been limited by difficulties in generating antibodies to this peptide due to its extreme hydrophobicity.

A developmental deficiency of pulmonary surfactant has long been recognized as the cause of infantile respiratory distress syndrome, a leading contributor to neonatal morbidity and mortality (90). Recently, an isolated deficiency of SP-B has been shown to be responsible for an uncommon but uniformly fatal disorder producing respiratory failure in full-term neonates. This disease is characterized clinically by the rapid onset of respiratory distress leading to inexorable respiratory failure and histopathologically by the accumulation of granular, eosinophilic, lipid- and protein-rich material in the alveoli (alveolar proteinosis) (91,92). Nogee et al. (93) used Western blots and immunohistochemical techniques to show that the SP-B protein was absent from lung tissue of three siblings with a diagnosis of congenital alveolar proteinosis. Northern analysis failed to identify the SP-B mRNA, suggesting a pretranslational mechanism. Further studies characterized the molecular defect in the index case. Although substantially reduced, SP-B cDNA was detected by the reverse transcriptase–polymerase chain reaction (RT-PCR), and sequence analysis identified a three-base substitution for a single nucleotide in codon 121 of exon 4 that resulted in premature termination and aberrant splicing of the SP-B mRNA and an absence of SP-B protein (94). In addition to deficiency of SP-B, extensive abnormalities of surfactant metabolism have been documented in affected individuals, including an immature phospholipid profile of amniotic fluid, increased amounts of SP-A and SP-C, and an absence of tubular myelin in the alveolar lumen, abnormal lamellar bodies, and increased SP-C and decreased SP-A in the alveolar epithelium (95). Results from this initial family have been extended to include 10 patients from seven families and have indicated that this familial SP-B deficiency may be more common than previously recognized (96). These studies combined with work in rabbits and rats in which an antibody to SP-B produced respiratory failure and comparable impairments in pulmonary physiology and alveolar morphology indicate that SP-B is essential for normal lung function (97,98). Moreover, these studies, confirm that SP-B is required for the formation of tubular myelin and suggest that SP-B may be important in the metabolism and intracellular trafficking of other surfactant components.

## IV.  Hormonal Effects on the Surfactant System

### A.  Overview

Although a variety of hormones, growth factors, cytokines, and other agents have been shown to affect certain aspects of lung development, glucocorticoids appear to have particularly wide-ranging effects and have been extensively studied.

Glucocorticoid, thyroid, and β-adrenergic receptors have been well characterized in fetal lung from several species, and evidence strongly supports receptor mediation of in vitro effects. Rising glucocorticoid and thyroid hormone levels during the last 10–20% of gestation are coincident with a surge in surfactant synthesis in most mammalian species, and ablation studies support their relevance as regulators of lung development in vivo. In addition to glucocorticoids, cAMP agonists also are strong positive regulators of the surfactant system both in vivo and in vitro. Thus, available evidence strongly supports a physiological role for these three hormones in the regulation of lung development.

Liggins was the first to recognize the accelerated synthesis of surfactant in response to glucocorticoid treatment when in 1969 he reported that dexamethasone treatment of sheep prior to delivery at 117–123 days of gestation (term is 148 days) resulted in partial lung aeration and survival of lambs for several hours at a point in gestation when survival would not otherwise have been possible (99). He reasoned that persistence of lung expansion in these immature animals indicated the accelerated appearance of surfactant, possibly as a result of increased biosynthesis. Glucocorticoids have since been shown in a number of different model systems, both in vivo and in vitro, to accelerate physiological, morphological, biochemical, and molecular indices of lung maturation and to induce all components of the surfactant system. For example, Seidner et al. (100) have shown in a premature rabbit model that antenatal glucocorticoid treatment improved maximal lung volumes, dynamic compliance, and hysteresis. Synergistic effects were observed when antenatal corticosteroids were combined with postnatal surfactant treatment. Similar improvements in lung mechanics have been reported in other species (101,102). At the level of light microscopy, antenatal glucocorticoid treatment produced larger air spaces, thinning of the alveolar septa, and increased invasion of capillaries into air spaces (1,103,104). The ultrastructure of the alveolar epithelium has also shown precocious maturation following glucocorticoid treatment. Kikkawa et al. (103) injected cortisol into the peritoneal cavity of fetal rabbits from 19–25 days' gestation (term is 31 days) and delivered the animals 2 or 3 days later. Treated animals were compared with a control group that received either injections of saline or no injections. Alveolar epithelial cells of treated animals delivered on day 21 were more cuboidal than columnar and had less cytoplasmic glycogen than control animals. By day 26, treatment resulted in complete maturation of type II cells that contained numerous lamellar inclusions. Overall, glucocorticoid treatment resulted in an acceleration of normal developmental events by approximately 1.5 days in this species. Gonzales et al. (105) examined the effects of hormonal treatment on the morphology of human fetal lung in organ culture. Second-trimester explants were cultured either in a control media, 2 nM triiodothyronine ($T_3$), 10 nM dexamethasone, or $T_3$ plus dexamethasone. Although explants cultured for 4 days in a control media showed some maturation of epithelial cells, including a few early lamellar bodies, dexamethasone produced a much more pronounced acceleration of maturation. Epithelial cells had the appearance of mature type II cells with numerous well-developed lamellar bodies, apical microvilli, and a paucity of cytoplasmic glycogen. Dexamethasone plus $T_3$ produced somewhat greater effects on cellular morphology than dexamethasone alone. This acceleration of normal developmental processes resulting from glucocorticoid treatment has proven to be useful for premature infants. A large number of controlled trials beginning in 1972 have shown that antenatal glucocorticoid treatment prior to premature birth consistently reduces the incidence of respiratory distress syndrome and results in lower neonatal mortality and morbidity (reviewed in ref. 106).

In addition to the maturational effects of exogenous glucocorticoids, experimental data in a number of species supports a physiological role for endogenous glucocorticoids (reviewed in ref. 1). In the sheep, free cortisol increases twofold from 135 to 139 days and an additional sevenfold by the day preceding birth (107,108). Surfactant phospholipids are first detectable in tracheal fluid at about 130 days of gestation and increase exponentially until term, suggesting that endogenous cortisol regulates but does not initiate surfactant synthesis. In the rat, mouse, and nonhuman primate, free corticosteroid concentrations also rise substantially during the last 10% of gestation when surfactant synthesis and accumulation surge. Adrenal glucocorticoid blockade by metyrapone in fetal rats has been shown to retard development of the surfactant system (109). Hypophysectomy has been used to abolish adrenocortical function and impairs the synthesis and release of surfactant as well as the structural development of the lung in fetal sheep (110–112). Cortisol treatment of hypophysectomized animals prevented morphological abnormalities but did not enhance lung distensibility or phospholipid content. In contrast, adrenocorticotropin (ACTH) treatment improved all of these indices of maturation, suggesting that the lung is subject to multihormonal regulation. In the human, the developmental pattern of amniotic fluid corticoid conjugates, reflecting fetal cortisol levels, parallels the lecithin/sphingomyelin ratio, which is an indicator of lung maturity (Fig. 4).

## B.  Receptors

### Glucocorticoid Receptor

Since the role of receptors in the fetal lung was last reviewed in this series (113), molecular studies have provided considerable new insights into mechanisms of gene regulation by hormones and their receptors. Receptors for steroid hormones are members of a superfamily of ligand-dependent transcription factors that contain several homologous functional domains and regions (Fig. 5). In addition to receptors for steroid hormones, receptors for vitamins A and D, peroxisomal activators, and a number of so-called orphan receptors whose ligands and function are unknown are members of this family of proteins (114–117). Members of this

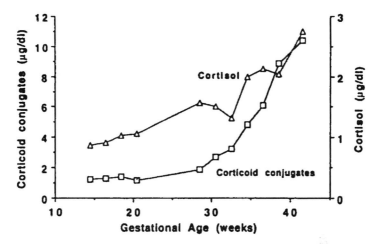

**Figure 4** Developmental patterns for cortisol and corticoid conjugates in human amniotic fluid during the last two trimesters of pregnancy. Cortisol, which is primarily of maternal origin, increases in a linear fashion. Corticoid conjugates, which include both cortisol and corticosterone and are mainly of fetal origin, increase slowly until ~30 weeks gestation when concentrations increase similar to the profile for lipid indices of lung maturity. (From Ballard PL, Ballard RA. Scientific basis and therapeutic regimens for use of antenatal glucocorticoids. Am J Obstet Gynecol 1995; 153:254–262.)

group contain three major consensus domains identified by nucleotide and amino acid homologies. The centrally located DNA binding domain contains the greatest sequence homology; 66–68 amino acids within this region are highly conserved and 36, including nine cysteines, are invariant among human receptors. This region forms two zinc finger motifs analogous to the structures formed by transcription factor IIIA. Four cysteine residues are tetrahedrally arranged around the zinc ion in each finger and are required for proper folding and DNA binding. The first finger determines response element specificity within a region known as the P box and the second finger appears to be involved in protein-protein interactions, such as receptor dimerization, through a region termed the D box. Two additional conserved domains of 42 and 22 amino acids are found in the carboxyl-terminal portions of receptors and are likely important in ligand binding. The amino-terminal region is hypervariable both in size and sequence and is less well characterized. Sometimes referred to as the immunodomain, since epitopes for many hormonal antibodies have been directed here, this region may in many instances have a modulatory effect on *trans*-activation.

The glucocorticoid receptor (GR), unlike other steroid hormone receptors which are nuclear regardless of hormonal state, appears to be localized to the cytoplasm when unbound by hormone (Fig. 6). In the absence of hormone, the GR

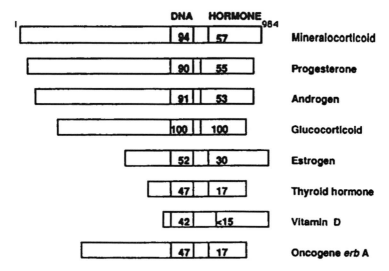

**Figure 5** Schematic comparison of amino acid sequences for the steroid receptor super family. Homologies are shown for both the DNA and hormone binding domains compared with the glucocorticoid receptor as 100%. The amino-terminal end which contributes to ligand binding activity has less than 15% homology among the family. Relative lengths of the receptors are shown compared with the mineralocorticoid receptor which contains 984 amino acids. Oncogene *erbA* is identical to thyroid hormone receptor. (From Rudolph A. Pediatrics. 18th ed. Norwalk, CT: Appleton & Lange, 1996.)

exists in an inactive form but is maintained in a conformation that has a high binding affinity for hormone. Studies using cell extracts indicate that the unbound receptor forms oligomeric complexes with the 90-kDa heat shock protein (HSP90), and disruption of this complex prior to hormone binding yields a receptor incapable of binding hormone (118,119). One model has proposed that two molecules of HSP90 are bound to each molecule of the C-terminal portion of GR protein and on binding of hormone, the HSP90 molecules are released, giving rise to an activated receptor-hormone complex which is then translocated to the nucleus (115). The human GR has been cloned (120,121), and sequences highly homologous to the nuclear translocation signal of the SV40 T antigen have been identified (120).

Following nuclear translocation, the receptor-hormone complex binds to specific DNA elements known as glucocorticoid response elements (GREs) to enhance or repress transcription of target genes. The DNA binding domain of the GR consists of 110 amino acids, and nuclear magnetic resonance spectroscopy has

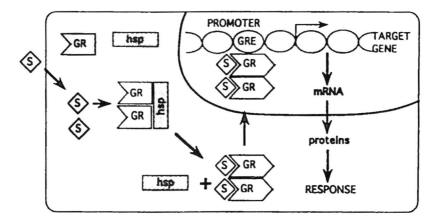

**Figure 6** Model of glucocorticoid-receptor interaction. Glucocorticoids bind to GR in the cell cytoplasm, causing activation and disassociation from heat shock protein. The activated GR translocates to the nucleus where it binds to GRE of steroid-responsive genes to influence gene expression. S, steroid; GR, glucocorticoid receptor; GRE, glucocorticoid response element; HSP, 90-kDa heat shock protein. (From Venkatesh VC, Ballard PL. Glucocorticoids and gene expression. Am J Respir Cell Mol Biol 1991; 4:301–303.)

confirmed that the region consists of a globular body from which extend two zinc fingers each made up of 12–13 amino acids that are separated by a linker region of 15–17 amino acids (122). The consensus GRE, GGTACAnnnTGTTCT where n is any nucleotide, is an imperfect palindrome whose diad symmetry is consistent with experimental data suggesting that the receptor dimerizes prior to or concurrent with DNA binding (123,124). GREs may be closely linked to promoters or may be several kilobases upstream or even downstream from genes they regulate. Moreover, GREs frequently exist in multiple copies or in combination with binding sites for other transcription factors and produce synergistic effects in combination with these agents (125,126). Binding to nonconsensus sequences can occur, but the magnitude of effect may be altered. A number of examples of repression resulting from glucocorticoid binding to DNA sequences have been described but sequences bound are diverse (116). The GR-hormone complex appears to modulate transcription by altering the formation of a productive transcription complex at the promoter either by interaction with general transcription factors (127) or by inducing changes in chromatin structure (128). A major site of *trans*-activation activity, referred to as tau1, resides within the N-terminal portion of the receptor from residues 77–262 in the human GR.

Consistent with its relatively ubiquitous distribution in mammalian tissues, GR has been detected in adult and fetal lung of a variety of species (1,113). The concentration of GR sites in lung is relatively high compared to other tissues and ranges from 0.24–0.82 pmol/mg protein. Although data on the distribution of receptor among the approximately 40 different pulmonary cell types is sparse, one study using autoradiography identified GR in alveolar epithelial cells (including type II cells), endothelial cells, airway smooth muscle cells, and fibroblasts of the lamina propria underlying bronchiolar epithelium (129). Binding studies using various corticosteroids have confirmed specific binding with a $K_d$ for dexamethasone that is similar for type II cells, fibroblasts, and whole lung tissue (~2–10 nM), suggesting that receptor in different pulmonary cell types is functionally identical. The number of binding sites identified has ranged from 5700 to 15,000 sites per cell in freshly isolated cells to 57,000 sites per cell in established cell lines.

The ontogeny of the pulmonary GR has been examined in five species: rat, rabbit, sheep, pig, and human. In rat lung (Fig. 7), receptor number has been shown to increase ~100% during the last 4–6 days of gestation (130) and another two to threefold in the early postnatal period (131,132). In rabbit lung, dexamethasone binding capacity increased 47% from 23 to 30 days of gestation (130). GR increased nearly sevenfold in ovine lung tissue during the second trimester

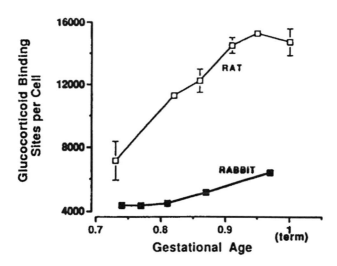

**Figure 7** Ontogeny of glucocorticoid binding capacity in fetal lung of rat and rabbit. Total binding capacity (nuclear and cytoplasmic dexamethasone binding sites) was determined in explants of tissue obtained at various times during the third trimester. Binding sites increased ~50 and 100% for rabbit and rat, respectively, during the last quarter of gestation. (Data from ref. 130.)

and then declined somewhat during the third trimester (133). In the porcine lung, GR concentration was high (1.44 pmol/mg protein) from day 82 to 100 of gestation (term is 114 days) and then declined through the remainder of gestation and the first 2 weeks of postnatal life (134). This rise in GR concentration during late gestation may be a major mechanism by which glucocorticoids modulate lung maturation, since a key factor determining the magnitude of response in most systems is the number of receptor molecules expressed in the target cell (135,136).

GR gene expression is subject to regulation by a number of factors at several different levels of control. Autoregulation of GR occurs following exposure to glucocorticoid (reviewed in ref. 137). In most tissues and cell lines, exposure to the cognate ligand downregulates GR concentration; however, examples of up-regulation also exist. In adult rat liver, exposure to dexamethasone produced a 60–80% decrease in GR mRNA which was maximal at 18–24 hr; content of receptor protein declined but was not as pronounced as the fall in mRNA content (138). Downregulation was mediated both by a decrease in rate of transcription and an increase in rate of degradation of GR protein. In fetal rat lung, maternal beta-methasone treatment 24 hr prior to delivery at 16–21 days' gestation caused a consistent drop in GR mRNA to 50–65% of control levels (132). However, GR protein content was unchanged by hormonal treatment from 16–19 days and then decreased in 21-day and adult lung. Agents which increase intracellular cAMP increase GR binding capacity in some systems, and this process could represent a mechanism for additive or synergistic effects by these two classes of hormones (139). To examine the mechanism of this effect, Dong et al. (140) treated a rat hepatoma cell line with forskolin and found a rapid (within 4 hr) increase in GR ligand binding activity, GR protein, and GR mRNA levels. Experiments with actinomycin D showed that this induction was at least in part due to an enhancement in stability of GR mRNA. Combined treatment with forskolin and dexamethasone resulted in an approximately twofold higher GR protein level than in cells treated with dexamethasone alone. The products of two glucocorticoid-responsive genes increased 11- to 16-fold following combined treatment as compared with an approximately sixfold increase following treatment with dexamethasone alone and no increase following treatment with forskolin alone.

### Thyroid Hormone Receptors

Although initially characterized biochemically as a single protein with a $M_r$ of ~50 kDa, more recent molecular studies have shown the existence of multiple thyroid hormone receptor (TR) isoforms which are expressed in a developmentally regulated and tissue-specific fashion. Two TR genes, designated $\alpha$ and $\beta$ and localized to chromosomes 17 and 3, respectively, in the human, have been cloned in a variety of species (reviewed in ref. 141). TR-$\alpha$ isoforms are similar to c-*erbA*, the cellular homologoue of the viral oncogene v-*erbA*, which has also been shown to be a functional TR. TR-α1 and TR-α2 arise from alternate splicing during mRNA synthesis. However, TR-α2 is unable to bind $T_3$, because it lacks a highly conserved 40–amino acid segment in its C-terminal domain. It may therefore act as a negative modulator of thyroid hormone action. A third TR-α isoform, Rev-erbAα, results from transcription of the opposite strand of the α gene and also does not bind $T_3$. Two TR-β isoforms, TR-β1 and TR-β2, exist in most mammalian species and differ from α isoforms predominantly in the $NH_2$-terminal domain. Most mammalian cells contain between 2000 and 10,000 TR molecules per cell with the various isoforms expressed in a tissue-specific manner. For example, TR-α1 is found predominantly in brain, cardiac, and skeletal muscle, whereas TR-β1 is most abundant in kidney and liver. Differences in isoform expression may also occur during various stages of development. At present, there is no information on TR isoform distribution in mammalian fetal lung. Diversity of receptor proteins includes differing affinities for $T_3$ and likely contributes significantly to tissue-specific variations in thyroid hormone responsiveness.

TRs possess the same structural domains as the glucocorticoid receptor and other members of the steroid hormone receptor superfamily, including the highly conserved DNA binding domain (reviewed in ref. 141). TR binds to genes containing two copies of the sequence AGGTCA arranged either as an inverted repeat (TREp) or as a direct repeat with a 4-bp gap (DR4). Positive cooperativity appears to favor binding of homodimers, although TR binds DNA much more stably as a heterodimer with other nuclear proteins. Major partners for heterodimerization are isoforms of the retinoid X receptor and to a lesser extent the retinoic acid receptor. Even in the absence of hormonal ligand, TRs are located in the cell nucleus bound to target genes and inhibit basal transcription. Binding of $T_3$ can activate or repress TR-mediated gene transcription. TREp and DR4 are both positive TREs, but the exact receptor form (monomer, homodimer, or heterodimer) involved in positive or negative regulation remains unknown. The preferred binding of TR heterodimers and the ubiquitous distribution of retinoid X receptor isoforms suggests that TR heterodimers play a major role in $T_3$ action. Mechanisms of negative regulation of transcription by TRs are poorly understood. In some cases, negative TREs contain only a single half-site (142), and in others specific orientation and spacing of two half-sites may mediate negative regulation (143). Negative regulation may occur by interfering with the assembly of the basal transcription complex or by inhibition of DNA binding by transcriptional enhancers such as c-*Jun* and c-*Fos*.

$T_3$ binds with high affinity to nuclei isolated from rat and rabbit lung ($K_d = 0.01$ nM) and with slightly higher affinity to nuclei from human fetal lung ($K_d = 0.04–0.06$ nM) (144). Scatchard plots of dose-response data from fetal lung suggest 900–2500 binding sites per cell depending on the species; lung contained the highest receptor concentration (1980 sites per cell) of four tissues examined in the human fetus (145). The distribution of TRs among various pulmonary cell types has not been studied in detail, and as noted above, there is no information on the type(s) of TR isoforms present in fetal lung. In the adult rat, immuno-cytochemical studies using a monoclonal antibody directed against a TR antigen from liver found receptor only in type II cells and alveolar macrophages (146).

Increases in TR binding capacity and occupancy by thyroid hormone during lung development suggest a physiological role for thyroid hormone (Fig. 8). In the fetal rabbit, $T_3$ binding capacity increases 44% from days 21 to 28 of gestation and then decreases by term (147). During this period, lung development in the rabbit is characterized by increasing numbers of differentiated type II cells and increased surfactant synthesis. Similarly, occupancy of TR by endogenous thyroid hormone increases during development. In the rabbit, occupancy increased from 11.3% of total sites at 21 days to ~23% at 28–31 days. In the rat, receptor occupancy increased from 26% in the newborn to 60% at 21 days' postnatal age and then decreased to 48% in the adult (148). Further evidence for a physiological role of TR-mediated responses in lung development comes from a recent study in which 2,4-dichlorophenyl-p-nitrophenyl ether (Nitrofen), a teratogen that is stereo-chemically very similar to $T_3$ and capable of producing pulmonary hypoplasia in rats, was shown to inhibit $T_3$ binding to TR-$\alpha$1 and TR-$\beta$1 in a noncompetitive fashion (149).

### β-Adrenergic Receptors

β-adrenergic receptors (β-ARs) are members of a diverse superfamily of G protein–coupled cell surface receptors that share a common pathway of signal

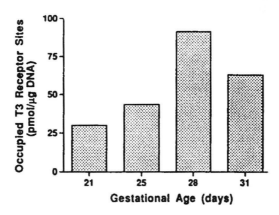

**Figure 8** Occupancy of $T_3$ receptor sites in rabbit fetal lung by endogenous $T_3$. During the last trimester of gestation, both receptor capacity and percentage occupancy increase resulting in an approximately threefold increase in number of nuclear $T_3$ receptor sites occupied by endogenous hormone. (From data in ref. 147.)

transduction (reviewed in refs. 150 and 151). This functionally diverse super-family includes receptors that bind biogenic amines such as catecholamines and histamine, retinals, peptides such as substance P and bradykinin, and large gly-coproteins such as luteinizing hormone and parathyroid hormone. These receptors are characterized by a signaling pathway in which an agonist binding to its specific cell surface receptor produces a high-affinity, agonist-receptor–G protein com-plex that activates an effector protein and thereby modulates levels of intracellular second messengers that carry out the response. Adrenergic receptors mediate a variety of physiological processes via their interactions with catecholamines. Initial studies based on pharmacological properties suggested two classes of adrenergic receptors, $\alpha$ and $\beta$, each containing two subtypes of receptors $\alpha 1AR$, $\alpha 2AR$, $\beta 1AR$, and $\beta 2AR$ (152,153). More recent work has shown the existence of at least nine subtypes, including a third $\beta$-AR, $\beta 3AR$ (154). The $\beta 2AR$ appears to be the predominant form in lung tissue. $\beta$-ARs mediate stimulation of adenylyl cyclase which leads to an increase in intracellular cyclic AMP levels, activation of cAMP-dependent protein kinase A, and subsequent phosphorylation of a variety of intracellular effector proteins. The initial step in $\beta$-AR activation is the forma-tion of a complex consisting of an agonist, a receptor, and a heterotrimeric G protein which includes $\alpha$, $\beta$, and $\gamma$ subunits. Formation of this complex promotes the release of guanosine diphosphate and subsequent binding of guanosine tri-phosphate (GTP) to the $\alpha$ subunit. The $\alpha_s$-GTP complex then dissociates from the $\beta$ and $\gamma$ subunits and directly activates adenylyl cyclase. Recent evidence suggests that $\beta$-ARs may be capable of regulating effector molecules, such as $Na^+$-$H^+$ exchange and L-type $Ca^{2+}$ and $Na^+$ channels, independently of the adenylyl cyclase system.

Despite their diverse group of agonists and effector molecules, G protein–coupled receptors share a common structure within the plasma membrane charac-terized by seven stretches of 20–28 hydrophobic amino acids which form trans-membrane $\alpha$-helices connected by three extracellular loops, an extracellular am-ino terminus, three intracellular loops, and an intracellular carboxyl terminus (151). The transmembrane domains exhibit the greatest degree of homology with a 55% amino acid identity between the human $\beta 1AR$, $\beta 2AR$, and $\beta 3AR$. Addi-tional regions of conservation include the first and second intracellular loops, the proximal and distal ends of the third intracellular loop, and the proximal portion of the carboxyl tail. $\beta$-ARs, like other members of this superfamily, undergo exten-sive posttranslational modifications, including the formation of several important disulfide bonds between cysteine residues, asparagine-linked glycosylation in the aminoterminus of the receptor, palmitylation of a cysteine residue on the carboxyl tail, and phosphorylation, which plays an important role in desensitization of receptor molecules (reviewed in ref. 150).

A major mechanism by which $\beta$-adrenergic agonists modulate gene expres-sion is through the activation of protein kinase A and subsequent phosphorylation of a group of transcription factors that interact with specific DNA control elements (reviewed in refs. 155 and 156). These cAMP-responsive *trans*-activators are part of the so-called bZIP subgroup of the leucine zipper superfamily of transcription factors, the prototype being the cAMP response element binding protein (CREB). bZIP proteins share a special structural motif that is characterized by a basic region containing a high concentration of positively charged amino acids such as lysine and arginine next to a series of amino acids in which leucine occupies every seventh position (heptad repeats). This bZIP domain is essential for binding to specific enhancer sequences of DNA. Residues of the leucine zipper region form an amphipathic $\alpha$-helix that resembles a coiled-coil and promotes dimerization with other bZIP proteins. The dimerized helix is then positioned in the major groove of the DNA helix so that the positively charged basic residues are able to bind the negatively charged bases of their target DNA sequences (157). cAMP-responsive bZIP proteins bind to variations of the consensus palindromic cAMP response element (CRE) TGACGTCA and, in addition to CREB, include the CREB homologues cAMP response element modulator (CREM) and activating transcription factor-1 (ATF-1). CREB readily forms homodimers with itself and heteodimers with CREM and ATF-1, and each of these combinations binds with high affinity to the consensus CRE. Binding to other CREs can occur but binding affinity may be altered. Alternative splicing of exons of CREB and CREM in certain tissues provides greatly expanded combinations for dimerization, changes the *trans*-activational potency of CREB and CREM, and, along with the large number of potential DNA-recognition sequences dimers may bind, provides a further mechanism to diversify greatly cAMP-mediated transcriptional control. In addition to CREB, CREM, and ATF-1, two other classes of bZIP proteins, the Fos/Jun early response proteins and the C/EBP proteins that are expressed near the time of terminal cellular differentiation, may bind CREs, although usually with lesser affinity.

Although a number of bZIP proteins and other DNA binding proteins can form dimers that bind CREs, only CREB, CREM, and ATF-1 have been shown to be activated on phosphorylation by PKA. A consensus serine, located within a 50–amino acid region that contains multiple potential sites of phosphorylation by a variety of other kinases and is known as a phosphorylation box (P box) or kinase-inducible domain (KID), has been shown to be the site of PKA phosphorylation. Phosphorylation by PKA is usually necessary but not sufficient for *trans*-activation, and it may trigger a cascade of phosphorylations within this region. The exact mechanism by which phosphorylation promotes *trans*-activation is incompletely understood, but the phosphorylated sites and other numerous negatively charged residues within the P box have been proposed to stabilize components of the basal transcription complex, including transcription factor IID, in a manner analogous to the yeast transcription factors GAL4 and GCN4 (158). Dephosphorylation by phosphatases has been shown to attenuate the *trans*-

activational activity of CREB. Recently, examples of *trans*-activation by CREB independent of phosphorylation by PKA have also been described (159).

cAMP-responsive bZIP proteins, like many other transcription factors, have a relatively ubiquitous distribution across diverse cellular phenotypes, so specificity of cAMP-regulated changes in gene expression must be mediated by other mechanisms. Although a large number of bZIP proteins and even other transcription factors may bind CREs, binding affinity of various dimers varies considerably and changes in the relative concentrations of bZIP or other proteins available to form dimers is one potential mechanism for specificity. This process may be regulated at several different levels of control. For example, CREM has been shown to either inhibit or stimulate CRE-mediated transcription depending on which exons are spliced in or out (160). Subtle differences in nucleotide sequences of CREs may favor binding by substantially different combinations of *trans*-activators and can provide a further mechanism for specificity of cAMP effects on transcription.

Within the lung, β-ARs have been identified in airway epithelium, submucosal glands, smooth muscle, and alveolar epithelium and have been characterized by a variety of techniques (reviewed in refs. 1, 113, and 161). β-ARs are present in fetal lung from a variety of species but receptor concentration is severalfold less than in adult lung. Autoradiography of fetal rabbit lung using the β-adrenergic antagonists [$^3$H]dihydroalprenolol (DHA) and $^{125}$I-iodocyanopidolol (ICYP) identified β-ARs in airway and alveolar epithelium; receptor density was greater in airways but increased to a much greater extent in alveoli as gestation progressed to term (162,163). In contrast, receptor concentration did not change significantly in fetal myocardium and brain. A similar increase in β-AR concentration has been reported during lung development in rat and guinea pig (1,164). Agonist affinity and antagonist competition studies using second-trimester human fetal lung showed a predominance of β2 receptors (60–75%) capable of generating cAMP in response to isoproteronol (165). Receptor concentration increased from 23 fmol/mg protein at 15 weeks, to 110 fmol/mg protein at 23 weeks, to 223 fmol/mg protein in one lung from a 39-week stillborn infant. Ewing et al. (166) characterized β-ARs from enriched populations of type II cells (~80% purity) and fibroblasts isolated from human fetal lung explants after 5 days of control culture. ICYP bound to a single class of saturable, high-affinity sites on type II cells and the specific β2 antagonist ICI 118551 identified only β2AR, suggesting that the 25–40% of β1AR found in preparations from fetal lung explants were from cell types other than type II cells. Receptor concentration was ~80 fmol/mg protein corresponding to a total of ~960 receptor sites per type II cell. Receptors were also identified on fibroblasts but density was lower (~400 receptors per cell).

β-ARs are subject to complex regulation at several different levels of gene expression (reviewed in refs. 150, 167, and 168). Genes encoding β-ARs have been cloned in a variety of species and, like genes encoding other members of the G protein–coupled receptor superfamily, they do not contain introns in their coding regions (169–172). Both the human and hamster β2AR genes contain consensus GRE and CRE upstream from the transcription initiation site, and these agents have been shown to alter expression of β2AR genes in a variety of tissues and cell types. In the $DDT_1$-MF2 hamster smooth muscle cell line, which contains both GR and β2AR, glucocorticoid treatment increased β2AR number with a maximal effect between 6 and 12 hr. Steady-state levels of β2AR mRNA increased within 1 hr of treatment, and nuclear elongation assays and assessment of mRNA half-life indicated that this effect was due to an increase in gene transcription (173,174). Glucocorticoid treatment both in vivo and in vitro has been shown to increase β-AR concentration by 60–120% in rat and rabbit fetal lung (1). Davis et al. (175) examined β-AR concentration during explant culture of human fetal lung and found an approximately threefold increase by day 3 of culture to ~185 fmol/mg protein. The $K_d$ of receptor for ICYP did not change during culture, but cAMP generation in response to isoproterenol increased significantly. Surprisingly, receptor concentration, cAMP content, and cAMP generation in response to agonists were all reduced by dexamethasone (10 nM) treatment. Agonist-stimulated cAMP production was time dependent and only present by day 5 of culture. The mechanism of inhibition by glucocorticoids appeared to be at a postreceptor level, since basal cAMP generation and cAMP generation in response to forskolin, an agonist which acts at a site distal to the β-AR, were both reduced by treatment. The complexity of the glucocorticoid effect is highlighted by a recent report in which treatment of adult human lung pieces (predominantly bronchioles and small blood vessels) with 1 μM dexamethasone increased β2AR number, mRNA content, and gene transcription (176). mRNA levels peaked at 2 hr and then decreased to control levels by 17 hr of treatment. Dose-response analysis showed that lower concentrations (1 or 10 nM) of dexamethasone produced less of an increase in mRNA content. mRNA stability was unchanged by treatment and the induction was blocked by the glucocorticoid receptor antagonist RU486.

Changes in β-ARs in response to cAMP agonists are also complex and appear to be either tissue-specific or different between adult and fetal tissues. Collins et al. (177) have reported that brief periods (30 min) of exposure to cAMP agonists stimulated transcription of the β2AR gene in $DDT_1$-MF2 cells but did not alter receptor number. In contrast, longer periods of exposure (24 hr) substantially reduced receptor number and β2AR mRNA levels. Desensitization of β-ARs can occur in response to homologous or heterologous stimuli and may involve a number of different mechanisms. Receptor responsiveness is rapidly reduced by phosphorylation, uncoupling of receptor to $G_s$, and sequestration of the receptor protein inside the cell, whereas receptor downregulation is a much slower process due at least in part to a reduction in mRNA stability (178). In human fetal lung explants, cAMP content increases during culture in response to endogenous prostanoids (179), and as noted above, β-AR content also increases spontaneously during culture in this system. Duffy et al. (180) have reported that treatment with either 8-bromo-cAMP or isobutylmethylxanthine (IBMX) further augments receptor concentration over that in control tissue. Addition of H-8, a potent inhibitor of protein kinase A, but not meclofenamate, an inhibitor of prostaglandin synthesis, blocked the spontaneous rise in βAR content that occurred during culture.

A number of other hormones besides glucocorticoids and cAMP agonists have been reported to regulate pulmonary β-ARs. In adult rat lung, thyroidectomy reduced β2AR mRNA levels, and thyroxine replacement reversed this effect within 20 hr (181). Similarly, $T_3$ treatment of fetal rabbits on day 27 of gestation increased β-AR number and cAMP content (182). Male gender has been reported to retard fetal lung development, and along these lines, estrogen and dihydrotestosterone treatment increased and decreased, respectively, β-AR content in fetal rabbit lung (183,184). Also, Warburton et al. (185) found an ~1.5-fold greater content of β-ARs in lungs from female than male lambs at ~90% of gestation. Insulin has been shown to inhibit the β-AR system in two species. Hyperinsulinemia induced by chronic glucose infusion to fetal lambs significantly blunted the usual increase in β-AR content from 130 days to term (186). Davis et al. (187) reported that insulin treatment of explants from fetal rabbit lung did not change β-AR concentration but did reduce cAMP generation by isoproteronol.

### C. Surfactant Phospholipids

*Glucocorticoids*

A number of hormones have been shown to affect surfactant phospholipids in a variety of experimental systems both in vivo and in vitro (reviewed in refs. 1,10,113,188). Glucocorticoids have been studied most extensively, and in general the induction of surfactant lipids by glucocorticoids has been characterized by (1) a similarity of response in different species, (2) dose dependency for natural and synthetic glucocorticoids, (3) a requirement for de novo RNA and protein synthesis, (4) a pattern of response that suggests an acceleration of normal developmental events, and (5) a synergistic response when glucocorticoids are combined with other agents, particularly thyroid hormone and cAMP agonists. Glucocorticoid treatment prior to birth in a number of species produces biochemical effects consistent with an increase in synthesis of surfactant phospholipids. In the fetal rabbit, treatment of either the fetus with cortisol or the doe with betamethasone on day 24 or 25 of gestation followed by delivery 2 days later produced a 50–100% increase in the PC content of lung lavage and increased incorporation of choline into PC by 90% (189,190). Similar effects have been reported in fetal sheep, rats, and monkeys (101,191,192). Although the bulk of experimental evidence indicates that glucocorticoid treatment increases the synthesis of surfactant phospholipids, some studies have been unable to demonstrate an increase in overall pool sizes of surfactant phospholipids. For example, Elkady et al. (193) treated pregnant rabbit does with 0.1 mg/kg of betamethasone on days 24 and 25 of gestation and delivered the litters on days 26 and 27. Glucocorticoid treatment increased both maximal lung volume and decreased the pressure required to produce lung rupture but failed to enhance lung stability on deflation. Content of saturated PC in alveolar wash and lung tissue was not changed by glucocorticoid treatment. Improvements in pulmonary function were believed to be due to changes in lung structure. These investigators have also reported a relatively high incidence of fetal growth retardation and fetal death following a glucocorticoid dose sufficient to induce lung maturation in this preterm rabbit model (194,195). Similar adverse effects have not been reported in large animal or human studies, suggesting possible dose- or species-related problems. Moreover, failure of glucocorticoid treatment to increase total saturated PC content may reflect the relatively large pools of phospholipids in lung tissue from both surfactant and membrane sources and the modest increase in this parameter during normal development.

Glucocorticoid treatment of fetal lung in organ culture has consistently resulted in increases in biochemical indices of surfactant phospholipid synthesis. Treatment of human fetal lung explants with 10 nM dexamethasone increased the incorporation of radiolabeled choline, acetate, and glycerol into PC by ~140, 830, and 80%, respectively, over that in control explants (105). Dexamethasone also increased tissue PC content and the percent saturation of newly synthesized PC. These effects suggest multiple potential sites of glucocorticoid action in the biosynthetic pathways of PC and DPPC. Stimulation was apparent by 24–48 hr of treatment, plateaued by 4–6 days, and was reversible on removal of hormone. The relative effectiveness of steroid hormones in stimulating precursor incorporation into PC paralleled their affinity for the glucocorticoid receptor. Also consistent with receptor mediation, dose-response analyses for choline incorporation showed that half-maximal stimulation occurred at a concentration (2.1 nM for dexamethasone) that was similar to the $K_d$ for receptor binding in this tissue. Dexamethasone has also been reported to increase choline incorporation into PC and the tissue content of DPPC and PG in explant culture of rabbit and rat fetal lung (196–198). Results indicated receptor mediation and the induction was blocked by either actinomycin D or cycloheximide, inhibitors of RNA and protein synthesis, respectively. Thus, glucocorticoid induction of surfactant phospholipids in these experimental systems is consistent with the overall model of glucocorticoid action: hormone binds receptor, and following nuclear translocation, the receptor-hormone complex interacts with specific DNA sequences (GREs) to enhance or repress transcription of target genes and alter the synthesis of specific proteins.

Two-dimensional polyacrylamide gel electrophoresis (2-D PAGE) has been used to obtain an overview of proteins regulated by glucocorticoids in cultured human fetal lung (199). Explants were cultured in the presence or absence of 10 nM dexamethasone, newly synthesized proteins were labeled with $^{35}$S-methionine, and two-dimensional polyacrylamide gel electrophoresis was used to separate proteins by size and isoelectric point. Fluorography showed that ~2% of resolved proteins (20/1000) were regulated by glucocorticoids (summarized in Table 2). The identity of many of these regulated proteins is unknown; however, recent studies have provided insights into some of the genes and proteins that mediate glucocorticoid responses in the developing lung.

Since Liggins' initial study in fetal lambs (99), key enzymes in the biosynthetic pathway of surfactant phospholipids have been suspected targets of glucocorticoid action. Although the catalytic activities of a number of these enzymes are increased by glucocorticoids, many of these effects appear to be indirect and mediated by increased synthesis of cofactors or intracellular translocation of enzyme. Among enzymes of phospholipid biosynthesis, available data are strongest for the induction of the fatty acid synthetase protein. Fatty acids, critical for synthesis of phosphatidic acid and ultimately PC, appear to arise from two major sources in the fetal lung, uptake of circulating free fatty acids, and de novo synthesis from acetyl-CoA. A third potential source, hydrolysis of plasma triglycerides, is probably inactive in the fetus in vivo. De novo synthesis appears to play an important role, since the concentration of fatty acid is lower in fetal than in adult plasma, pulmonary blood flow is low in utero, and undifferentiated epithelial cells contain large glycogen stores which could serve as a potential substrate for fatty acid synthesis. De novo synthesis is controlled by fatty acid synthetase (FAS, EC2.3.1.85), a large multifunctional protein dimer ($M_r$ ~500 kDa), that catalyzes the synthesis of long-chain fatty acids from acetyl-CoA subunits in a multistep enzymatic reaction and is hormonally regulated in liver, adipose, and mammary tissues. De novo fatty acid synthesis increases in parallel with synthesis of PC and DPPC in fetal lung during late gestation in rat and rabbit, then declines during the neonatal period and remains low in the adult (192,200).

**Table 2** Hormonally Regulated Proteins of Human Fetal Lung

| Hormone treatment | No. of proteins | | Type II cellular localization |
|---|---|---|---|
| | induced | repressed | |
| Dexamethasone | 17 | 4 | 6 |
| Forskolin + IBMX | 9 | 0 | 2 |

Proteins of cultured human fetal lungs were analyzed by high-resolution two-dimensional polyacrylamide gel electrophoresis after labeling with radioactive methionine. Treatment with dexamethasone or forskolin/ isobutylmethylxanthine (IBMX), which increases cAMP, regulated a limited number of proteins among the ~1000 resolved proteins, and some were predominantly localized in type II cells. *Source*: Data from ref. 199.

FAS mRNA content also increases during late development of fetal rat lung, peaking on day 21 of gestation coincident with a peak in enzyme activity and de novo synthesis of fatty acids in this species (201). Glucocorticoid treatment of fetal rat lung, either in vivo or in explant culture, has been shown to increase the rate of de novo fatty acid biosynthesis, as measured by incorporation of $^3H_2O$ into total fatty acids (192, 202). In treated explants, the increased FAS activity was apparent by 12 hr, was accompanied by an increase in immunoprecipitable protein, and was abolished by actinomycin D. Maniscalco et al. (203) have also reported that dexamethasone treatment of cultured explants from 20- or 23-day gestation fetal rabbit lung increased incorporation of $^3H_2O$ into total fatty acids by ~50% and increased by ~2.5-fold the proportion of fatty acids used for PC synthesis. In human fetal lung explants, fatty acid synthesis and FAS activity increased spontaneously during culture and were further stimulated by 10 nM dexamethasone (204). FAS activity was greater in type II cells than in fibroblasts, and type II cells from dexamethasone-treated explants exhibited a greater increase in FAS activity than fibroblasts. Moreover, in both rat and human fetal lung explants, dexamethasone treatment rapidly increased FAS mRNA content approximately threefold and treatment with actinomycin D prevented this induction (201, 205,206). In human explants, mRNA content increased progressively through 6 days of glucocorticoid treatment. In contrast, in rat fetal lung, the response was biphasic with an initial rapid increase that peaked at 5 hr, followed by a slight decline until 20 hr, and then a further increase that plateaued between 30 and 48 hr of treatment. More prolonged periods of treatment were not examined in rat explants, and glucocorticoid treatment did not alter mRNA levels of ATP citrate lyase or acetyl-CoA carboxylase, two additional enzymes of fatty acid synthesis in this species. Thus, in both rat and human fetal lung, glucocorticoids act through a receptor-mediated process to increase FAS gene expression via a pretranslational mechanism. Whether glucocorticoids increase the rate of transcription of this gene remains to be determined.

Choline-phosphate cytidylyltransferase (CYT, EC2.7.7.15), which catalyzes the conversion of CDP-choline from choline-phosphate, is the rate-limiting enzyme in the PC synthetic pathway and has long been suspected to be a target of glucocorticoid action in the fetal lung. Although numerous studies have shown that the activity of this enzyme increases during development and in response to glucocorticoid treatment (1,10), results in fetal rat lung indicate that this effect is due in large part to a glucocorticoid-mediated increase in the synthesis of fatty acids and acidic phospholipid cofactors, such as PG, which increase enzyme activity. When fetal rat lung CYT activity was assayed in the presence of PG, its activity was increased and the stimulatory effects of glucocorticoids were substantially reduced (207,208). Xu et al. (209) further elucidated the mechanism of glucocorticoid action in this species by demonstrating that inhibitors of fatty acid synthesis blocked the stimulatory effect of dexamethasone on CYT activity. Moreover, Fraslon and Batenburg (205) used Northern analysis to show that dexamethasone treatment did not change CYT mRNA content. However, a recent study in human fetal lung has produced somewhat different findings and suggested that glucocorticoids may increase the content of CYT protein in this system (210). Treatment of human fetal lung explants with 10 nM dexamethesone for 5 days increased total CYT activity by 115% in the presence of PG and by 77% in the absence of added PG when compared with activities in control cultures. When subcellular fractions were analyzed, the greatest amount of CYT activity was found in the cytosol and glucocorticoid treatment increased the proportion of activity recovered in the cytosolic but not in the microsomal fraction. Although the combined activity of all subcellular fractions failed to fully account for the total activity in the homogenate, this result argues against intracellular translocation of enzyme from soluble to the microsomal or membranous compartment as the mechanism responsible for the observed increase in CYT activity. Although suggestive of possible enzyme induction, further studies are needed to conclusively demonstrate induction of CYT protein and mRNA in this system.

### Thyroid Hormone

Thyroid hormone both in vivo and in vitro has been shown to increase the synthesis of surfactant phospholipids in a number of species and to act in an additive or synergistic fashion when combined with glucocorticoids (1,10,113). For example, injection of pregnant rats on day 18 or 19 of gestation increased choline incorporation into PC by 34%, but whole lung disaturated PC content was unchanged and the percentage of PC that was disaturated was reduced by treatment (207). In this study, maternal $T_3$ injection did not alter fetal levels of corticosterone. Thyroidectomy of fetal lambs has also been shown to lower lecithin/sphingomyelin ratios in tracheal fluid, suggesting a possible physiological role for thyroid hormone in lung maturation. Also, plasma concentrations of thyroid hormone increase in several species during the last trimester as synthesis of surfactant phospholipids is also increasing. In explant cultures of rat (196), rabbit (211), and human fetal lung (105), $T_3$ treatment increased choline incorporation into PC. In these three species, the induction by $T_3$ was less than that for dexamethasone, and combined treatment with dexamethasone produced an additive or synergistic increase (Fig. 9). In human fetal lung, even brief exposures (2 days) to combined treatment produced substantial (more than twofold) increases in choline incorporation. $T_3$ treatment did not alter the rate of incorporation of acetate or glycerol into PC and did not change the percent saturation of PC, suggesting limited sites of thyroid hormone action in the biosynthesis of surfactant phospholipids.

The effect of thyroid hormone on two enzymes of surfactant phospholipid synthesis has been examined recently in rat and human fetal lung. Rooney et al. (208) have reported that $T_3$ administration to pregnant rats 2 days prior to delivery

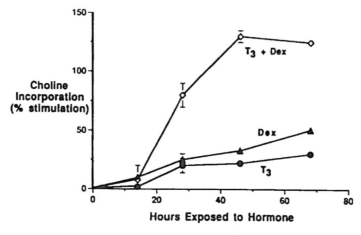

**Figure 9** Time course of hormonal effects on incorporation of choline into PC. Explants of fetal rabbit lung were treated with dexamethasone (Dex, 10 nM), T3 (1 nM), or both hormones for the times shown before assay. The response to combined treatment is synergistic at 28 and 48 hr and additive at 68 hr exposure. (From ref. 188.)

decreased fatty acid synthesis by fetal lung on days 21 and 22 of gestation, and when given in combination with dexamethasone, $T_3$ prevented the increased fatty acid synthesis on day 20 of gestation produced by glucocorticoids alone. $T_3$ also limited the increase in FAS activity produced by dexamethasone in explant culture of 18- and 19-day fetal rat lung but not in human fetal lung (204,212). Treatment with $T_3$ alone did not alter enzyme activity in either species. Similarly, Gonzales et al. (206) have reported no effect of thyroid hormone treatment on FAS mRNA content in human fetal lung explants. In this system, 2 nM $T_3$ increased CYT activity by 40% in the presence of added PG. However, combined treatment with dexamethasone produced a similar increase in CYT activity to that for dexamethasone alone. These results suggest one possible mechanism for increased PC synthesis in response to thyroid hormone treatment, but additive effects by combined treatment with glucocorticoids appear to be mediated through another pathway.

### cAMP Agonists

Although the principle effects of cAMP agonists have traditionally been considered to be stimulation of surfactant secretion and reabsorption of fetal lung fluid just prior to birth, recent evidence suggests that these agents also stimulate the synthesis of several elements of the surfactant system. In one of the first reports of stimulation of surfactant phospholipid synthesis by cAMP agonists, Gross et al.

(196) found that treatment of explants from fetal rat lung with the methylxanthines aminophylline and caffeine increased the rate of choline and acetate incorporation into PC. Additive stimulation occurred when these phosphodiesterase inhibitors were combined with dexamethasone. cAMP agonists (8-Br-cAMP, IBMX, forskolin, and $PGE_1$) have also been shown to increase FAS activity and content of its mRNA in explant culture of human fetal lung (206). The magnitude of the cAMP-induced increase in mRNA content was somewhat less than that for dexamethasone (twofold versus threefold) and was maximal by 24 hr of treatment. Combined treatment with dexamethasone produced a synergistic response such that FAS mRNA levels increased by 24 hr of exposure to dexamethasone, forskolin, and IBMX to ~11-fold levels in control tissue. In contrast to dexamethasone, induction of FAS mRNA by cAMP agonists was not inhibited by actinomycin D, indicating a nontranscriptional mechanism such as increased mRNA stability. cAMP agonists also increased the activity of cytosolic CYT when assayed in the presence of PG, but combined treatment with dexamethasone did not produce an additive effect (210). Thus, the additive stimulation of PC synthesis by glucocorticoids and cAMP agonists may be mediated at least in part through induction of FAS but not by increased cytosolic CYT activity.

Explant culture of fetal lung from a variety of species results in spontaneous maturation of alveolar epithelial cells. Control culture of mid trimester human fetal lung results in morphological maturation and an increased content of PC, activity of FAS, and mRNA levels of SP-A and SP-B but not SP-C (83,105,213). Ballard et al. (179) have recently shown a correlation between these maturational processes and increased tissue cAMP levels, apparently in response to endogenous prostaglandins. Increased production of surfactant components occurred in response to a relatively modest (twofold) elevation in cAMP content. Addition of indomethacin (10 mg/ml) or H-8, an inhibitor of protein kinase A, on day 3 or 4 of culture substantially inhibited subsequent accumulation of cAMP and SP-A mRNA. Lesser degrees of inhibition were noted for SP-B mRNA, FAS activity, and PC content; indomethacin-treated explants also appeared less mature by light microscopy than control tissue. Addition of prostaglandin E1 (PGE1) (from 1 nM to 10 mM) in the presence of indomethacin produced progressive increases in tissue cAMP and SP-A levels and in FAS activity to values greater than that in control tissue. These results suggest that developmental changes in endogenous cAMP content independent of stimulation by $\beta$-agonists or other hormones may influence type II cell differentiation.

## Other Hormones and Growth Factors

### Fibroblast Pneumonocyte Factor

Besides the three classes of hormones discussed above, a number of additional hormones and growth factors have been reported to influence certain aspects of the surfactant system; this topic has been reviewed recently in another volume of this series (113). Fibroblast pneumonocyte factor (FPF) is an 8-kDa protein that has been isolated from the medium of cultured lung fibroblasts and proposed to mediate the glucocorticoid induction of phospholipid synthesis by type II cells (reviewed in ref. 214). Identification of this paracrine factor arose from studies in which fibroblasts were required for initial growth of epithelial cells from human fetal lung. A population of epithelial cells was isolated after several weeks of culture and used to establish a clone of cells which were responsive to conditioned medium from cortisol-treated fibroblasts and which exhibited certain characteristics of type II cells, including lamellar inclusions, an increase in choline incorporation into PC, and a similar phospholipid profile following growth in conditioned medium (215). Lung fibroblasts from a number of species (human, rat, cat, rabbit, monkey, and chicken) showed FPF activity following glucocorticoid treatment. FPF activity was also tentatively identified in human amniotic fluid; however, activity was negatively correlated with other indicators of lung maturation, including gestational age, lecithin/sphingomyelin (L/S) ratio, incidence of respiratory distress syndrome (RDS), and cortisol concentration. Perhaps the strongest evidence for a physiological role for FPF comes from a study showing that monoclonal antibodies against FPF blocked both FPF and cortisol stimulation of DPPC synthesis in cell culture and in chick embryos (216).

The mechanism of FPF action on type II cells and its regulation have been addressed by recent studies. FPF has been shown to increase the cAMP content of cultured cells (mixed fibroblast and type II cells and enriched populations of type II cells) and exposure to $T_3$ further increases cAMP content and choline incorporation into PC. These studies suggested a possible role for cAMP in mediating FPF effects and indicated that $T_3$ may act by increasing type II cell responsiveness to FPF. Further insights into the mechanism of FPF induction have come from a study by Floros et al. (217), who reported that both cycloheximide and actinomycin D inhibited accumulation of FPF. This study also demonstrated that FPF activity could be produced from in vitro translation of polyA RNA isolated from cortisol-treated fibroblasts. Together, these results indicated glucocorticoid induction of FPF via a pretranslational mechanism. Recent studies have reported inhibition of FPF activity by dihydrotestosterone and transforming growth factor-$\beta$ (TGF-$\beta$) and positive regulation by epidermal growth factor (EGF) (218–220). FPF has also been shown to increase CYT activity in organotypic cultures of fetal type II cells (221).

Despite accumulating information on the role of FPF in organotypic cell culture, a number of questions remain. First, what is the physiological relevance of FPF? Although the antibody studies are intriguing, negative correlations with certain parameters of lung maturation in human amniotic fluid and rat lung raise questions about the physiological significance of this factor. Second, do glucocorticoids act only through FPF? The complexity of the glucocorticoid effect on a number of components of the surfactant system, for example SP-A (see below), suggest multiple sites of glucocorticoid action. Third, does FPF act solely through cAMP? Divergent effects of glucocorticoids and cAMP agonists in several areas, for example effects on FAS mRNA content and synergistic stimulation by combined treatment, do not support this proposition. Finally, does $T_3$ stimulate surfactant synthesis only by increasing type II cell responsiveness to FPF? The numerous differences in glucocorticoid and thyroid hormone effects on a variety of surfactant components suggest other mechanisms for thyroid hormone action. In sum then, FPF may be one part of a large and complex system of multihormonal regulation of the fetal lung. Further insights into mechanisms of FPF action and its role in lung development will likely require isolation of the cDNA(s) and gene that encode this factor.

### Epidermal Growth Factor

Epidermal growth factor (EGF) is a small polypeptide ($M_r$ of 6045 Da) that promotes generalized epithelial growth and mitogenesis in a variety of tissues and, at least under certain conditions, can also influence the expression of specific differentiated cell products independent of its effects on cell growth. EGF, originally isolated from the mouse submaxillary gland and implicated in tooth eruption and eyelid opening (222), acts through a specific transmembrane receptor protein which consists of an extracellular ligand-binding domain, a single membrane-spanning region, and a functional intracellular tyrosine-kinase domain (223). Although the exact mechanism of EGF action is unclear, binding of EGF to its receptor is known to activate intracellular kinase activity and result in phosphorylation of both the receptor and exogenous substrate proteins. The receptor-hormone complex is then internalized into lysosomal structures and degraded.

There is accumulating evidence to support a role for EGF in the regulation of lung development and surfactant synthesis. In embryonic mouse lung, EGF mRNA, protein, and receptor can be detected as early as day 11 (term is 19 days) within mesenchymal and epithelial cells of branching terminal airways (224,225). Branching morphogenesis was stimulated by the addition of exogenous EGF to an explant culture of embryonic mouse lung and was inhibited by tyrphostin, a specific EGF receptor-kinase antagonist and by an antisense oligonucleotide directed against the first five codons of the EGF mRNA precursor (226). These data suggest an autocrine or paracrine role for EGF in the induction and regulation of secondary embryonic morphogenesis. EGF has also been detected in type II cells from fetal and adult rat (227,228), and the EGF receptor has been characterized in membrane preparations from fetal rat, rabbit, lamb, and human lung (229–232). Binding of EGF was specific, saturable, and time and temperature dependent with a $K_d$ of ~1-3 nM. Recently, EGF has been measured in human amniotic fluid samples from 186 third-trimester pregnancies. EGF was first detected at 28–30 weeks and increased 10-fold by 40 weeks. Rising EGF concentrations correlated significantly with increasing PC and PG concentrations and with rising L/S ratios, consistent with a physiological role for EGF in lung maturation. Purified mouse EGF (5 μg) has been administered in utero to rabbit fetuses on day 24 of gestation, and following delivery 3 days later, lung distensibility and inflation stability were greater than that in control animals (233). Similarly, EGF treatment of fetal lambs was reported to prevent hyaline membrane disease during the first 6 hr after premature delivery (234). In both of these studies, enhanced morphological maturation of the alveolar epithelium, including an increased proportion of type II cells, was reported. Recently, a rhesus model of RDS was used to test the effects of antenatal EGF on lung maturation (235,236). Recombinant human EGF (40 μg) was administered into the amniotic fluid and peritoneal cavity of rhesus monkeys from 121–127 days' gestation. Animals were delivered on day 128 and compared with saline-injected controls. EGF treatment resulted in reduced ventilator and $Fio_2$ requirements; increased PC, PG, and SP-A levels in amniotic fluid; a threefold increase in lamellar bodies; and a 50% reduction in cytoplasmic glycogen of type II cells. EGF has also been reported to increase the synthesis of surfactant phospholipids in organ culture. In rat fetal lung explants, EGF increased incorporation of choline into PC and DPPC and acetate into PC and PG in a dose-dependent fashion (237). Half-maximal stimulation occurred at a concentration that was similar to the $K_d$ for EGF binding, consistent with receptor mediation. Combined treatment with EGF and $T_3$, but not dexamethasone, resulted in an additive increase in PC synthesis. Studies using isolated preparations of type II cells from fetal rabbit and rat lungs have found that EGF treatment increased choline incorporation into PC and thymidine incorporation into DNA (238,239).

Interactions between other hormones and EGF have been reported. Maternal betamethasone treatment of rabbits on days 25 and 26 of gestation resulted in a threefold increase in EGF receptors (240). However, dexamethasone treatment of an epithelial cell line derived from fetal rat lung produced a 50% reduction in EGF receptor synthesis (241). Also, in rat fetal lung explants, dexamethasone treatment did not alter EGF binding capacity (237). Klein and Nielsen (242) examined sex-specific differences in EGF receptor content of membrane preparations from fetal rabbit lung and found lower receptor density in male than female fetuses. Treatment with exogenous dihydrotestosterone also reduced receptor density in this study. Intra-amniotic administration of thyroxine during the third trimester of 29 human pregnancies accelerated the appearance of EGF in amniotic fluid (243). These results indicate that EGF is a positive regulator of lung maturation and suggest that some hormonal effects on the fetal lung may be mediated through EGF or its receptor.

### Prolactin

Prolactin is present in the fetus and its developmental pattern along with clinical studies showing lower cord prolactin levels in infants with RDS than in comparable infants without RDS (244) suggested a possible role for prolactin in the regulation of lung maturation. However, prolactin levels increase from about 115 to 125 days' gestation in the fetal sheep, well before increased synthesis of surfactant phospholipids begins at about 135 days, whereas glucocorticoids increase later at about 140–145 days (245). The majority of in vivo studies have failed to demonstrate increased surfactant synthesis in response to prolactin administration (reviewed in ref. 1). Although one study using cultured explants of fetal rat lung showed that prolactin increased PC synthesis (246), similar work using rabbit and human explants showed no effect of prolactin on choline incorporation or PC content (213,247). Studies of prolactin binding have also provided inconsistent results. Specific binding was found in membrane preparations from lungs of fetal rhesus monkeys and adult and fetal rabbit lung tissue but not in fetal sheep or human fetal lung (248–250).

Results of studies examining hormonal combinations which include prolactin are also conflicting. For example, Schellenberg et al. (251) administered cortisol, $T_3$, prolactin, and epidermal growth factor either alone or in various combinations to fetal lambs between 124 and 128 days' gestation and found that only the combination of cortisol, $T_3$, and prolactin improved both lung distensibility and stability; however, cortisol and $T_3$ or cortisol, $T_3$, and prolactin produced similar improvements in alveolar DPPC content. In explant culture of human fetal lung, Mendelson et al. (213) found that all combinations of insulin, prolactin, and cortisol increased choline incorporation into PC but none preferentially increased choline incorporation into saturated PC. Also, no single hormone stimulated PC synthesis in this system. Other studies using cultured human, rat, and rabbit fetal lung explants found that dexamethasone alone stimulated precursor incorporation into PC and combined treatment with prolactin offered no additional advantage (105,113). Thus, increased synthesis of surfactant phospholipids in response to prolactin alone has not been conclusively demonstrated; however, the in vivo data are consistent with a permissive role for prolactin in responsiveness to glucocorticoid plus $T_3$.

## Estrogen

Maternal estrogen levels rise throughout gestation and low concentrations of estriol in cord blood have been associated with RDS in some clinical studies, suggesting a possible role for estrogen in lung maturation. Administration of 17β-estradiol to pregnant rabbits has been shown to increase surfactant phospholipid content of lung lavage, choline incorporation into PC by lung slices, and activities of regulatory enzymes of PC synthesis (252,253). Treatment also accelerated morphologic maturation of fetal rabbit and rat lung. However, estradiol treatment had no effect on lung PC content or morphology in 127-day fetal sheep. In organ culture of fetal rat and rabbit lung, 17β-estradiol (10 μM) treatment increased PC synthesis and CYT activity, but the magnitude of effect was less than that observed in vivo (254,255). One additional study using fetal rabbit lung explants failed to show stimulation of these same indices (197). Moreover, even in studies that were able to demonstrate increased synthesis of surfactant phospholipids, the mechanism of this effect is uncertain, and mediation by the classic estrogen receptor appears to be unlikely (1,10).

### Androgens

Both clinical and experimental data indicate that androgens may have an inhibitory effect on both endogenous and glucocorticoid-stimulated synthesis of surfactant phospholipids. Epidemiological studies have reported a higher incidence of respiratory distress syndrome in premature male infants than in females of comparable gestational age (256). Analysis of amniotic fluid from nearly 150 pregnancies between 28 and 40 weeks' gestation showed that male fetuses exhibited a delayed (by 1.2–2.5 weeks) increase in lecithin/sphingomyelin ratio and DPPC content as compared to female fetuses. A similar delay in the synthesis of surfactant phospholipids exists in male rats but not rabbits. Nielsen et al. (257) recently investigated one possible mechanism for this maturational delay by injecting pregnant rats with dihydrotestosterone and found significant elevations in several parameters of lung growth, including lung weight, DNA and protein concentrations, and numbers of type II cells and fibroblasts isolated from treated lungs. When type II cells from untreated animals were cultured and exposed to dihydrotestosterone, cell number and DNA synthesis were increased but synthesis of DPPC was reduced, suggesting that androgens promote lung growth at the expense of type II cell differentiation and surfactant phospholipid synthesis.

In addition to inhibition of endogenous surfactant synthesis, androgens appear to inhibit glucocorticoid-stimulated synthesis of surfactant phospholipids. Clinical trials of antenatal glucocorticoid treatment for the prevention of RDS have reported reduced efficacy in males (258), and one possible mechanism for this lack of response is the inhibitory effect of androgens on glucocorticoid-induced stimulation of FPF activity described above. Torday (259) has recently reported that the addition of dihydrotestosterone or fetal adrenal androgens to cultured explants of human fetal lung inhibited the spontaneous and dexamethasone-stimulated increase in choline incorporation into DPPC. The effects of dihydrotestosterone were dose-dependent and inhibited by flutamide, an agent that antagonizes binding to the androgen receptor, consistent with receptor mediation.

### Insulin

An association between milder forms of maternal diabetes and delayed fetal lung maturation has long been suspected, and in 1976, Robert et al. (260) clearly established an increased risk for respiratory distress in infants of diabetic women independent of other risk factors. Consistent with this observation, several studies have documented abnormalities in the phospholipid profile of amniotic fluid from diabetic pregnancies indicating delayed appearance of surfactant. Although the Pederson hypothesis of maternal hyperglycemia producing fetal hyperglycemia and consequent hypertrophy of the pancreatic islets and fetal hyperinsulinemia is widely accepted, development of valid animal models for this condition has proven to be problematic and in vitro studies have produced inconsistent results.

Animal models have used a variety of approaches to mimic the diabetic condition. Two agents, alloxan and streptozotocin, have been used to produce chemical pancreatectomy; however, these studies have in many cases not resulted in fetal hyperinsulinemia or macrosomia (reviewed in ref. 1). In fact, treatment frequently lowered body weight and organ weight of diabetic fetuses, and produced inconsistent alterations in surfactant phospholipids. For example, alloxan treatment of pregnant rabbits reduced saturated PC content of lavage fluid in one study but had no effect on this or any other parameter of surfactant phospholipid content or synthesis in another study (261,262). Both groups reported reduced surface activity and deflation stability of lungs from alloxan-treated pregnancies. Streptozotocin treatment of pregnant rats has produced similarly confusing results. Difficulties with these models may be due at least in part to dosages of alloxan and streptozotocin used, which tended to produce effects more similar to severe forms of diabetes in the human rather than the milder conditions which result in fetal macrosomia, hyperinsulinemia, and delayed lung maturation. In the human, more severe forms of maternal diabetes (White's classes D, F, and R) often result in accelerated lung maturation. Lower dosages of these two agents (67 mg/ kg of alloxan and 30 mg/kg of streptozotocin) have been more successful in producing fetal hyperinsulinemia and macrosomia. Given the problems of chemical pancreatectomy, some investigators have used glucose infusions to produce secondary hyperinsulinemia. Warburton used this approach in fetal sheep and reported delayed appearance of surfactant, but this study was complicated by a relatively high fetal death rate (263). In a subsequent study, this investigator noted that hyperglycemia prevented the cortisol-induced increase in surface-active material of tracheal fluid and DPPC content of lung tissue (264).

Insulin treatment of fetal lung in explant culture has in general had no apparent effect by itself on choline incorporation into saturated PC, although in one study, insulin appeared to delay the morphological maturation of type II cells and the appearance of lamellar bodies (213,265). Insulin treatment has been shown to inhibit the stimulatory effect of glucocorticoids on choline incorporation into PC and activity of CYT (266,267). The mechanism of insulin effects on the fetal lung has not been clearly elucidated. Carlson et al. (268) reported that insulin treatment blocked the induction of FPF activity by cortisol. Although insulin receptors have been demonstrated in rat, rabbit, and human fetal lung, further study is necessary to confirm that insulin effects are receptor-mediated.

### D. Surfactant Proteins A and D

*Glucocorticoids*

Although glucocorticoids have been shown to stimulate increased synthesis of all elements of the surfactant system including SP-A, glucocorticoid effects on SP-A gene expression are complex and depend, at least in some systems, on dose and duration of exposure. Effects of glucocorticoids in vivo on SP-A synthesis have been reported in the developing rat and fetal rabbit. Phelps et al. (269) treated pregnant and neonatal rats with 200 μg/kg of dexamethasone 24 hr prior to sacrifice, labeled newly synthesized proteins from minced lung tissue with $^{35}$S-methionine, and performed 2-D PAGE to identify immunoprecipitable SP-A. Dexamethasone treatment increased SP-A on days 19 and 22 of gestation and on neonatal days 1 and 6. Shimizu et al. (270) also treated pregnant and neonatal rats with 200 μg/kg of dexamethasone 24 hr prior to sacrifice and used a sandwich ELISA assay to examine SP-A levels. Treatment increased SP-A content by ~60 and ~20% on days 19 and 21 of gestation, respectively, and by ~30% on neonatal day 5; increases on neonatal days 1 and 3 were not statistically significant. However, in another study in which 1 mg/kg of dexamethasone was administered 24 hr prior to sacrifice, SP-A content was increased at all time points from fetal day 19 to postnatal day 5 (271). Schelhase et al. (272) reported that dexamethasone treatment (1 mg/kg) for 1 or 3 days prior to delivery on day 17 of gestation increased SP-A protein and mRNA levels. Maternal treatment for 3 or 5 days, but not 1 day, increased SP-A content on day 19 of gestation, but mRNA levels were not significantly changed. Floros et al. (273) provided additional information regarding glucocorticoid effects on SP-A during later stages of lung development by treating rats during the first 2 months of life with 200 μg/kg of dexamethasone 24 hr prior to sacrifice. Newly synthesized intracellular and newly secreted SP-A protein and SP-A mRNA were all increased by dexamethasone treatment at all time points examined. The mean ratios for treated to control values were 2.2 for intracellular SP-A, 4.5 for secreted SP-A, and 1.4 for SP-A mRNA. Although newly synthesized SP-A was increased by dexamethasone in animals of all ages, total SP-A as measured by ELISA was increased in younger (day 16) but not older (day 35) animals, perhaps because of the already high levels of SP-A present in these older animals. Dose-response analysis in 16-day animals showed stimulation of total SP-A protein and mRNA by all concentrations of dexamethasone from 2 to 20 mg/kg. In the rabbit, antenatal betamethasone (200 μg/kg) on days 25 and 26 of gestation increased SP-A protein and mRNA levels on day 27 of gestation by approximately two- and threefold over those in saline-injected and uninjected controls, respectively (274). Despite minor discrepancies in some studies, it is apparent that glucocorticoid treatment in vivo increases SP-A protein and mRNA in the rat and rabbit across a relatively broad period of lung development.

Results using cultured fetal lung explants have, in some respects, been species-specific and have highlighted the complex nature of the glucocorticoid regulation of SP-A. Although the hormonal response has varied, all studies have shown an accumulation of SP-A and its mRNA with increasing time in control culture. Initial reports using second-trimester human fetal lung explants to examine the effects of glucocorticoids on SP-A were conflicting, with one group reporting induction (67) and another group reporting inhibition (275). Subsequent studies have clarified this discrepancy and shown that glucocorticoids exert biphasic effects on the synthesis of SP-A (Fig. 10). The content of SP-A and its mRNA are increased by exposure to low concentrations of hormone (0.1–10.0 nM dexamethasone) for brief periods (24–48 hr), whereas stimulation is lost and inhibition predominates with exposure to higher concentrations of hormone (⩾100 nM dexamethasone) or longer periods of treatment (3–7 days) (276,277). For example, maximal induction of SP-A mRNA (fivefold greater than control) occurred after 2 days of treatment with 3 nM dexamethasone, but higher hormone concentrations produced less of an effect and stimulation was lost at a concentration of 100 nM. After 4 days of treatment, 0.1 and 1.0 nM dexamethasone increased SP-A mRNA levels 3.2- and 2.1-fold greater than control, respectively, but higher concentrations of hormone produced marked reductions in mRNA levels. Inhibition was reversible on removal of hormone and was characteristic of a receptor-mediated process. The magnitude of response was similar for SP-A and its mRNA suggesting predominantly pretranslational effects.

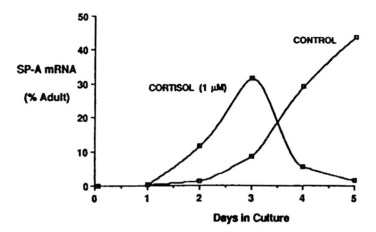

**Figure 10**  Biphasic effect of cortisol on content of SP-A mRNA in cultured human fetal lung. Cortisol added to explants on day 1 stimulates accumulation of SP-A mRNA on days 2 and 3 of culture but is inhibitory with continued exposure. (From ref. 188.)

Recent work has provided insights into mechanisms underlying glucocorticoid regulation of SP-A gene expression in human fetal lung. First, several studies have shown that positive and negative glucocorticoid effects on SP-A and its mRNA are not due to generalized changes in protein or RNA synthesis (67,199,278). Two groups have examined the level of glucocorticoid control of SP-A gene expression by analyzing the half-life of SP-A mRNA and rate of SP-A gene transcription. Boggaram et al. (279) estimated half-life by incubating explants with actinomycin D to block transcription and compared the rate of decay of SP-A mRNA in dexamethasone-treated explants to that in tissue treated with actinomycin D alone. Treatment with 100 nM dexamethasone reduced half-life by 60% from 11.4 hr in control explants to 5.0 hr in treated explants. These investigators also reported that dexamethasone treatment did not cause premature termination of nascent SP-A mRNA transcripts as a mechanism for increased decay of the message (279). Dexamethasone treatment for 5 days produced a dose-dependent increase in rate of SP-A gene transcription, as measured by nuclear elongation assay, with maximal effect at a concentration of 100 nM (278). Addition of 100 nM dexamethasone following 5 days of control culture produced a 1.4-fold increase in SP-A transcription after 48 hr of treatment, but activity was reported to be unchanged during the first 24 hr of treatment. Ianuzzi et al. (280) also examined the stability of the SP-A message and the effects of dexamethasone on SP-A mRNA half-life and gene transcription. In the presence of cycloheximide (2.5 μg/ml), an inhibitor of peptidyltransferase, added after 4 days of control culture, the SP-A message was found to be labile, decreasing to 15% of control levels by 24 hr, and inhibition by dexamethasone was completely blocked by cycloheximide. Cycloheximide also inhibited the accumulation of SP-A mRNA during control culture of rabbit fetal lung explants (21). These results indicate that either stabilization of the SP-A message or basal transcription of the SP-A gene requires synthesis of a labile protein. The half-life of SP-A mRNA was examined by treatment with actinomycin D and label-chase experiments using [³H]uridine. Treatment with dexamethasone (100 nM) after 4 days of control culture produced a log-linear pattern of decay with a rapid phase between ~4 and 7 hr and subsequently a slower rate comparable to that in control tissue. Both methods showed that dexamethasone produced an ~65% reduction in SP-A mRNA half-life. In contrast to the results of Boggaram et al., Iannuzzi found a 60% reduction in SP-A gene transcription following exposure to dexamethasone for 4–8 hr. Additional studies will be necessary to resolve this discrepancy.

Effects of dexamethasone on synthesis of SP-A in fetal rabbit and rat lung in organ culture have differed in some respects from that in human fetal lung. Mendelson et al. (73) reported that treatment of 21-day fetal rabbit lung explants with cortisol for 48 and 72 hr increased SP-A protein and mRNA in a dose-dependent manner with maximum induction by 100 nM cortisol. Further studies showed that glucocorticoids produced biphasic effects on SP-A mRNA and gene transcription in this species. Cortisol treatment for <24 hr reduced SP-A mRNA levels and rates of SP-A gene transcription such that by 12 hr the rate of transcription in treated explants was 50% of that in control tissue (74). Inhibition of SP-A gene transcription in response to brief periods of treatment is consistent with the results of Iannuzzi et al. (280) in human fetal lung. However, by 48 hr, the rate of transcription in treated rabbit tissue was 1.5-fold greater than that in control explants. In lung explants from 18-day fetal rats, exposure to dexamethasone for 48 hr at concentrations of 1–200 nM increased SP-A mRNA content approximately threefold greater than that in control tissue (281). Inhibition was not observed in this species and half-maximal stimulation occurred at 2.7 nM. Thus, in fetal rabbit and rat lung, glucocorticoids appear to produce a predominantly stimulatory effect on SP-A synthesis, whereas in human fetal lung, the dominant effect is inhibition. Whether longer periods of treatment would ultimately lead to inhibition of SP-A gene expression in these two species, as in the human, is unknown. Studies of GREs in the human SP-A gene are underway and should provide insights into mechanisms that underlie this unique biphasic response.

Initial reports in developing rat lung indicate that glucocorticoid treatment both in vivo and in vitro increases the expression of SP-D. Ogasawara et al. (271) treated pregnant rats on days 18 and 20 of gestation and neonatal rats on days 0, 2, and 4 with 1 mg/kg of dexamethasone 24 hr prior to sacrifice. Levels of SP-D in lung homogenate were increased at all points during the perinatal period with a maximum increase (2.7-fold greater than saline injected controls) on postnatal day 1. These investigators also examined levels of SP-A, DPPC, and PG in lung homogenate from treated and control animals and found similar increases in response to dexamethasone. SP-A levels were higher in treated than in control animals at all time points, but the greatest increase (2.1-fold) occurred on postnatal day 5. Deterding et al. (80) found that antenatal treatment with 1 mg/kg of dexamethasone for 1 and 3 days prior to sacrifice on fetal day 18 increased SP-D mRNA levels 7.9- and 12.4-fold greater than saline-injected controls, respectively. SP-D mRNA levels in glucocorticoid-treated animals after either regimen equaled or exceeded adult levels. Mariencheck and Crouch (82) also performed nuclear elongation assays on fetal lung tissue following 3 days of maternal treatment with 1 mg/kg of dexamethasone and reported enhanced SP-D transcriptional activity on day 19 but not on days 20 or 21 of gestation.

Induction of SP-D by glucocorticoids has also been demonstrated recently in cultured fetal rat lung explants from the glandular and canalicular periods of development. In 15- and 18-day explants, SP-D mRNA levels increased spontaneously after 3 days of control culture, as did SP-B and SP-C but not SP-A (80). Treatment of 15-day explants with hydrocortisone for 3 days produced dose-dependent increases in SP-D mRNA levels; concentrations from 1 nM to 10 μM were stimulatory. Immunohistochemical analysis indicated that SP-D protein was increased in bronchiolar and prealveolar epithelial cells of treated explants. The content of SP-D mRNA in 18-day explants was also stimulated by treatment with 1 μM hydrocortisone. Dexamethasone treatment of explants from 19-day fetal rat lung augmented the accumulation of SP-D protein and mRNA in a time- and dose-dependent fashion (82). Higher concentrations (10 and 100 nM) of hormone produced greater degrees of stimulation than did lower concentrations (0.1 and 1 nM). Following 24 hr of treatment with 100 nM dexamethasone, SP-D mRNA levels were increased by approximately fivefold and stimulation was sustained through 72 hr of treatment. Further studies in other systems will be needed to confirm glucocorticoid induction of SP-D in the developing lung.

### cAMP Agonists

In contrast to the disparate results for glucocorticoids depending on species, dose, and duration of treatment, a variety of cAMP agonists have produced consistent and sustained increases in the synthesis of SP-A in human, rabbit, and rat fetal lung. In explants from mid trimester human fetal lung, dibromo–cAMP, dibutyryl cAMP (Bt$_2$cAMP), terbutaline, forskolin, and IBMX all increased SP-A protein and mRNA content (275,277,278). In one study, the magnitude of induction for these agents (approximately fourfold greater than control) was similar to that produced by treatment with 10 nM dexamethasone for 2 days (277). Under these conditions, combined treatment with forskolin and dexamethasone produced an approximately additive increase in both SP-A protein and mRNA. When higher doses of glucocorticoid or more prolonged treatment periods have been used, however, combined treatment did not alter inhibition by the glucocorticoid (277,278,280). McCormick et al. (72) recently reported differential regulation of the SP-A1 and SP-A2 genes by cAMP agonists. Primer extension analysis of RNA from explants cultured in a control media for 5 days showed ~65% of transcripts to be from SP-A1 and 35% to be from SP-A2. Treatment with 1 mM Bt$_2$cAMP for 5 days produced a fivefold increase in SP-A mRNA of which 33% was from SP-A1 and 67% was from SP-A2, which is similar to the pattern observed in adult lung (see Section III.B). Combined treatment with Bt$_2$cAMP and 100 nM dexamethasone for 5 days reduced SP-A mRNA content to 40% of that for Bt$_2$cAMP alone and changed the ratio of transcripts to 76% SP-A1 and 24% SP-A2.

In explants from 21-day gestation fetal rabbits, treatment with Bt$_2$cAMP (1 mM) for 3 days produced an approximately fivefold increase in SP-A protein and translatable mRNA as compared with that in control tissue, and this increase was consistently greater than the two- to threefold increase produced by 3 days of treatment with 100 nM cortisol (73). Combined treatment with cortisol and Bt$_2$cAMP was additive, producing an ~10-fold increase in SP-A protein over that in control tissue. In rat fetal lung explants, 8-bromo–cAMP (200 μM) increased SP-A mRNA content by ~75% over control levels and combined treatment with 100 nM dexamethasone produced a synergistic increase to 7.3-fold that of control tissue (281). Interestingly, in this study, 200 μM Bt₂cAMP produced a slight decrease in SP-A mRNA levels and significantly reduced the stimulatory effect of dexamethasone.

Boggaram et al. (74,278) have reported that Bt₂cAMP increases the rate of transcription of the human and rabbit SP-A gene. In fetal rabbit lung explants, treatment with 1 mM Bt₂cAMP increased the rate of transcription of the SP-A gene by ~4.7-fold over that in control tissue within 12 hr of treatment; longer periods of treatment produced lesser degrees of stimulation. Cycloheximide treatment was shown to act at a transcriptional level to inhibit the induction of SP-A mRNA in Bt₂cAMP-treated explants, suggesting that cAMP-induced transcription of the rabbit SP-A gene requires ongoing synthesis of a protein with a relatively short half-life (74). Combined treatment of rabbit fetal lung explants with 100 nM dexamethasone and 1 mM Bt₂cAMP for 12 hr reduced the rate of transcription to 50% of that in explants treated with Bt₂cAMP alone. In contrast, these investigators reported that combined treatment of human fetal lung explants for 5–6 days with these two agents produced a synergistic increase in rate of SP-A gene transcription to 8.2-fold greater than that in control explants.

### Other Hormones

A variety of other hormones, growth factors, and cytokines act as positive or negative regulators of SP-A gene expression, but in general, these agents have not been studied as extensively as glucocorticoids or cAMP agonists. Thyroid hormone increases the synthesis of surfactant phospholipids alone and acts in an additive fashion when combined with a glucocorticoid; however, data regarding the effects of $T_3$ on SP-A gene expression are conflicting. $T_3$ at concentrations of 2 nM and 1–100 nM had no effect on SP-A protein or mRNA in two studies using human and rat fetal lung (67,281). In rat fetal lung, there was a slight reduction in SP-A mRNA caused by 10–100 nM $T_3$. In contrast, Whitsett et al. (282) found that 5 nM $T_3$ produced a threefold increase in SP-A content. EGF, which appears to increase synthesis of surfactant phospholipids and accelerate physiological indices of lung maturation, has been reported to produce a dose-dependent increase in the content of SP-A protein and mRNA in human fetal lung explants (282). Concentrations of 0.01–100.0 ng/ml were stimulatory and half-maximal stimulation occurred at a concentration of 1 ng/ml. The magnitude of induction (fivefold greater than control) was comparable to that of cAMP agonists, and high concentrations of dexamethasone completely blocked this response. Administration of EGF in vivo to fetal rhesus monkeys prior to delivery also increased SP-A concentrations in amniotic fluid and in cuboidal alveolar epithelial cells, consistent with a stimulatory role for this agent (235). 17β-Estradiol (2.2 μg/kg) treatment of pregnant rabbits on day 26 of gestation followed by delivery 24 hr later produced a 12-fold increase in fetal SP-A levels (84). When examined by sex, the increase in SP-A levels of female pups was not significant. In this study, estradiol also increased choline incorporation into total PC and DPPC by lung slices. Interferon-γ (IFN-γ) produced a dose-dependent increase in SP-A and its mRNA in human fetal lung with a maximal effect at ≥30 ng/ml but did not alter the synthesis of any other component of the surfactant system (283). Combined treatment for 3 days with 10 nM dexamethasone and interferon-γ produced a synergistic increase in content of SP-A. Induction of SP-A by this cytokine may play a role in the pulmonary inflammatory or immune response against microbial invasion.

Four agents, insulin, transforming growth factor-β (TGF-β), tumor necrosis factor-α, and phorbol esters, have been proposed to inhibit the synthesis of SP-A. In human fetal lung explants, concentrations of insulin from 2.5 to 250.0 ng/ml inhibited the accumulation of SP-A and its mRNA (284,285). The physiological relevance of this observation is supported by studies that have shown reduced concentrations of SP-A in amniotic fluid samples from diabetic pregnancies (71,286). Two laboratories using cultured human fetal lung reported that TGF-β at concentrations of 1–10 ng/ml reduced the content of SP-A and its mRNA significantly below that in control tissue (188,282). The stimulatory effects of other agents (EGF, 8-bromo-cAMP) were reduced by combined treatment with this growth factor. The response to TGF-β appeared to be relatively specific for SP-A, since the overall rate of protein synthesis was unchanged and other components of the surfactant system were not affected.

Tumor necrosis factor-α (TNF-α) and the phorbol ester 12-O-tetradecanoyl-phorbol-13-acetate (TPA) have been observed to decrease SP-A gene expression in the H441-4 pulmonary adenocarcinoma cell line (287,288). H441-4 cells express SP-A and SP-B but not SP-C. Morphologically, these cells resemble bronchiolar epithelial cells, containing numerous dense cytoplasmic granules but few lamellated lipid inclusions. In this system, both agents reduced SP-A mRNA and gene transcription within 6 hr of exposure and by 24 hr both parameters were reduced to 20% of that in control cells (287,288). Pretreatment with actinomycin D completely blocked the inhibitory effect of TPA and TNF-α on SP-A mRNA, suggesting a possible role for posttranscriptional processes. Recently, similar inhibitory effects by these agents have been observed in cultured human fetal lung (P. Ballard, unpublished data), suggesting that these results may have relevance in vivo.

The regulation of SP-A gene expression has been the subject of extensive recent investigation. Glucocorticoids exert biphasic effects on both SP-A and its mRNA in human fetal lung, and both transcriptional and posttranscriptional mechanisms appear to be responsible for this unique regulatory pattern. In fetal rabbit and rat lung, glucocorticoids appear to be mostly inducers of SP-A gene expression, whereas in human fetal lung, the dominant effect is inhibition. In human fetal lung, inhibition is reversible, receptor-mediated, and involves a reduction in the half half-life of the SP-A mRNA that appears to require ongoing protein synthesis. Results in most systems have shown that cAMP agonists strongly stimulate the synthesis of SP-A and its mRNA. In rabbit fetal lung, cAMP appears to act in large part by increasing SP-A gene transcription. Other positive regulators of SP-A gene expression include IFN-γ and EGF; treatment with combinations of these positive regulators has generally yielded synergistic or additive results. Negative regulation of SP-A gene expression has been suggested for insulin, TGF-β, TNF-α, and TPA.

### E.  Surfactant Proteins B and C

*Glucocorticoids*

Studies both in vivo and in vitro in several species have examined the effects of glucocorticoids on SP-B and SP-C gene expression and have confirmed that components of the surfactant system are independently regulated. The effects of in vivo glucocorticoid treatment on the developing lung have been reported in the rat and rabbit. Shimizu et al. (270) injected pregnant or neonatal rats with 200 μg/kg of dexamethasone 1 day prior to sacrifice and found that treatment significantly increased SP-B content only on day 19 of gestation. Small increases were also observed on day 21, during the first week after birth, and in adult animals but these changes were not significant. SP-A content was increased on fetal days 19 and 21 and on neonatal day 5; DPPC content was also increased on fetal day 21 and neonatal day 5. SP-C was not examined in this study. Because of the hydro-phobicity of SP-B and particularly SP-C, the development of antibodies has been difficult and most other studies have examined the hormonal effects on content of SP-B and SP-C mRNA. Schelhase et al. (272) found that 1 mg/kg of dexa-methasone administered to pregnant rats for 1 or 3 days prior to delivery on day 17 of gestation during the glandular period of lung development resulted in the precocious appearance of SP-A and SP-B mRNA and increased levels of SP-C mRNA over those of a saline-injected control group. This same dose of dexa-methasone administered for 1, 3, or 5 days prior to delivery on day 19 of gestation during the canalicular period also increased SP-B and SP-C but not SP-A mRNA levels. Three or 5 days of treatment produced more pronounced effects than treatment for 1 day and resulted in SP-B and SP-C mRNA levels that were similar to or exceeded those of adult animals. Phelps and Floros (289) injected pregnant rats with dexamethasone 24 hr prior to sacrifice and found a dose-dependent increase in SP-B mRNA levels on day 19 of gestation. A dose of 2 mg/kg produced significant increases in SP-B mRNA content in fetal animals from day 18 of gestation to term (22 days) and in postnatal animals from day 15 to day 45. Although the overall pattern of response was similar for SP-A and SP-B, the magnitude of glucocorticoid effect was greater during fetal life for SP-B than for SP-A. The ratio of treated to control mRNA levels for all fetal animals was 8.4 for

SP-B versus 2.2 for SP-A. Since SP-B is normally expressed in nonciliated bronchiolar epithelial cells as well as in type II cells, these investigators examined the cellular sites of glucocorticoid action by in situ hybridization and showed that antenatal as well as postnatal treatment increased SP-B mRNA levels in both cell types.

Two groups have examined the effects of glucocorticoid treatment in vivo on SP-B and SP-C mRNA in the fetal rabbit. Connelly et al. (84) treated pregnant does on day 26 of gestation (canalicular lung) with two doses of 0.15 mg/kg of betamethasone administered 4 hr apart and sacrificed the animals 24 hr after the first dose. SP-A and SP-B mRNAs and choline incorporation into PC and DPPC were all significantly increased. In contrast to results in the rat, the magnitude of increase was considerably greater for SP-A mRNA than for SP-B mRNA (eight-fold versus twofold greater than control). SP-C mRNA levels were reduced to approximately 50% of that in control animals. Durham et al. (274) treated pregnant does on days 25 and 26 of gestation with 0.2 mg/kg of betamethasone and sacrificed the animals on day 27. Treatment produced fourfold and twofold increases in SP-B and SP-C mRNAs, respectively, as compared with an uninjected control group. However, saline injection also produced a twofold increase in SP-C mRNA, perhaps because of stress-related increases in maternal corticosteroids. Neither study examined the effects of treatment at earlier times in gestation. Whereas in the rat, SP-B mRNA was evident in both type II cells and nonciliated bronchiolar epithelial cells, in the rabbit, SP-B and SP-C mRNA was only apparent in type II cells of treated and control animals. Thus, in the rat during fetal and early postnatal life, glucocorticoid treatment in vivo induces both SP-B and SP-C mRNAs; in the rabbit, SP-B mRNA is increased by treatment during the canalicular period, but effects on SP-C are in question.

Studies using cultured fetal lung explants have consistently found increased SP-B and SP-C gene expression in response to glucocorticoid treatment; however, mechanisms of glucocorticoid action differ somewhat depending on the species studied. Two groups have reported that 10 nM dexamethasone increased the content of SP-B and SP-C mRNA in mid trimester cultured human fetal lung (83,290). The magnitude of increase relative to control tissue was greater for SP-C than for SP-B, in part because, in contrast to SP-A and SP-B mRNA which were both increased by culture, SP-C mRNA levels were reduced after 5 days of control culture to ~20% of that in preculture tissue (83). However, dexamethasone treatment for 4 days still increased SP-C mRNA content to ~4.4-fold greater than that in preculture tissue and to ~30% of that in adult tissue. SP-B mRNA content was increased by dexamethasone to approximately twofold greater than that in adult tissue. The effects of a variety of steroid hormones and dose-response data were consistent with mediation by the glucocorticoid receptor. Half-maximal stimulation occurred at 1 and 5 nM for SP-B and SP-C mRNA, respectively, suggesting possible differences in mechanisms of action. In contrast to SP-A, prolonged treatment periods or high doses of glucocorticoids did not decrease SP-B or SP-C mRNA levels.

Venkatesh et al. (291) recently examined mechanisms underlying the glucocorticoid induction of SP-B and SP-C in human fetal lung. Analysis of the time course of induction by 100 nM dexamethasone showed a more rapid response for SP-B than for SP-C mRNA. Maximal levels were reached in ~12 and 24 hr for SP-B and SP-C mRNAs, respectively (Fig. 11). Cycloheximide (2.5 μg/ml) inhibited the increased accumulation of SP-C mRNA in response to glucocorticoids but SP-B mRNA was not affected. Although exposure to 100 nM dexamethasone for 8 hr increased the rate of transcription of both genes, the magnitude of effect was much greater for SP-C (10- to 30-fold increase) than for SP-B (approximately threefold increase). Glucocorticoids also increased the half-life of SP-B mRNA from ~6 hr

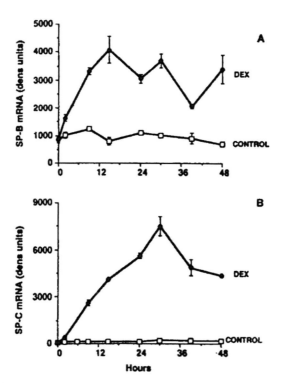

**Figure 11** Time course for dexamethasone induction of SP-B and SP-C mRNA in a representative experiment with cultured human fetal lung. Basal levels of SP-C are low and there is a relatively slow, manyfold induction with dexamethasone. Induction of SP-B occurs more rapidly with a maximal increase of ~3-fold. (From ref. 291.)

in control tissue to ~16 hr in dexamethasone-treated tissue; the half-life of SP-C mRNA was unaffected by treatment. These results indicate that glucocorticoids increase SP-B and SP-C gene expression by different mechanisms in human fetal lung. The induction of SP-B is a rapid, primary response that appears to involve transcriptional and posttranscriptional mechanisms. In contrast, the induction of SP-C is slower and appears to involve entirely transcriptional mechanisms. The requirement for ongoing protein synthesis and the lag time preceding the SP-C response suggest that stimulation of the SP-C gene by glucocorticoids may involve either a labile transcription factor or the induction of an intermediary protein that in turn facilitates transcription of the SP-C gene. Consistent with the latter possibility, Pilot-Matias and co-workers (54) have proposed several putative GREs based on sequence analysis of the human SP-B gene, but similar sequences have not been identified in the SP-C gene (60,292).

Glucocorticoids also induce SP-B and SP-C in two cell lines derived from human lung adenocarcinomas. In the H-820 cell line, which contains certain morphological characteristics of type II cells, including multilamellar inclusions, 10 nM dexamethasone increased the synthesis of both proteins and mRNAs (293). Dexamethasone treatment of this cell line also led to substantial reductions (35–45% of control) in the overall rate of protein synthesis as measured by incorporation of $^{35}$S-methionine into total protein; similar effects were not found in studies with human fetal lung explants (199,275). Treatment of the H441-4 cell line, which is derived from bronchiolar epithelial cells and produces SP-A and SP-B but not SP-C, with 50 nM dexamethasone for 48 hr produced an ~100-fold increase in SP-B mRNA levels but only a 4-fold increase in the rate of SP-B gene transcription (294). Experiments with actinomycin D suggested that glucocorticoids acted to stabilize the SP-B message.

Similar to results with human lung tissue, glucocorticoid treatment of explants from fetal rat and rabbit lung has, for the most part, resulted in increases in the content of SP-B and SP-C mRNAs. Dexamethasone treatment of explants from fetal rat lung on day 18 of gestation produced dose-dependent increases in SP-B and SP-C mRNA levels (295,296). Effects on SP-B mRNA were maximal at 15 hr and were sustained for up to 50 hr, whereas the enhancement of SP-C mRNA was maximal at 24–30 hr and declined thereafter. A more rapid induction of SP-B than SP-C mRNA in rat fetal lung is consistent with the results of Venkatesh et al. (291) in cultured human fetal lung. Dose-response analysis in rat fetal lung showed that concentrations of dexamethasone from 1–200 nM were stimulatory. Exposure to 100 nM dexamethasone for 48 hr produced an ~18-fold and ~2- to 3-fold increases in SP-B and SP-C mRNAs, respectively, over levels in control tissue. Nuclear elongation assays showed an increase in rate of transcription of the SP-C gene in response to treatment with 100 nM dexamethasone for 14–48 hr. Since transcriptional rate and mRNA content increased to a similar extent, the investigators suggested that the major site of glucocorticoid action was on SP-C gene transcription rather than on the stability of the SP-C message. Recently, another laboratory used explants from 15- and 18-day fetal rat lung to examine the effects of treatment with 1 μM hydrocortisone for 72 hr on the mRNAs for all four surfactant proteins (80). In 15-day explants, this regimen produced substantial increases in the abundance of all four mRNAs relative to control tissue. Similar increases in SP-A, SP-B, and SP-D but not SP-C mRNA levels were noted in 18-day treated explants; SP-C mRNA levels increased to a similar extent in treated and control tissue. Shorter periods of treatment were not examined in this study.

In cultured rabbit fetal lung, glucocorticoid effects on SP-B and SP-C gene expression have differed depending on the developmental stage of the tissue. Boggaram and Margana (61,297) reported that dexamethasone treatment of lung explants from 21-day gestation fetal rabbits (glandular lung) produced dose-dependent increases in the content of SP-B and SP-C mRNAs to a maximum of 6.4-fold and 4-fold greater than control values, respectively, at a concentration of 100 nM. These investigators identified two very similar SP-C mRNA species that appeared to arise from alternative splicing and found that both were coordinately increased by glucocorticoid treatment. Analysis of the time course of SP-C induction showed that stimulation was maximal by 24 hr and was lost by 96 hr of treatment. In contrast to results reported for human and rat fetal lung, the mechanism of glucocorticoid induction of SP-C appeared to be entirely posttranscriptional, since treatment with 100 nM dexamethasone for 24 hr produced an increase in the half-life of SP-C mRNA from 11.4 hr to 30.0 hr and no change in the rate of SP-C gene transcription (298). The rate of transcription was actually reduced somewhat by treatment with 100 nM dexamethasone for 48–72 hr. In contrast, 100 nM dexamethasone increased both the rate of SP-B transcription (2.4-fold greater than control) and the half-life of its mRNA from 9 to 25 hr, consistent with results in human fetal lung. Xu et al. (85) treated explants from 26-day fetal lung (canalicular stage of development) for 2 days with dexamethasone and found a dose-dependent increase in SP-B mRNA levels with a maximal effect (sixfold greater than control and sevenfold greater than adult levels) at a concentration of 10 nM. Glucocorticoids also increased SP-C mRNA levels to approximately five- to sixfold greater than control, and maximal induction occurred at a concentration of 1 nM (75). Control culture for up to 7 days produced a sustained increase in SP-B and SP-C mRNA content to levels that were five- and threefold greater than in the adult, respectively. This result differs from that for human fetal lung in which control culture produced a reduction in SP-C mRNA content (83). Explants from 30-day fetal rabbit lungs (saccular stage of development) were less responsive to glucocorticoid, but treatment for 2 days with 100 nM and 1 μM dexamethasone still produced three- to fourfold greater SP-B mRNA levels than those in control tissue. SP-C mRNA content was unchanged by treatment. Nuclear elongation assays using either 26- or 30-day explants showed no change in rate of SP-B or SP-C gene transcription during control culture. The rate of SP-B gene transcription was also unchanged in response to dexamethasone concentrations from 0.1 nM to 1 $\mu$M. SP-C transcription rates were increased modestly by treatment (1.7-fold greater than control) of 26-day explants for 48 hr with higher concentrations (100 nM and 1 $\mu$M) of hormone. Glucocorticoid treatment of 30-day explants did not alter the rate of SP-C transcription at any concentration tested.

Thus, results in the fetal rabbit suggest different mechanisms of SP-B and SP-C induction depending on the developmental stage of the tissue. In cultured explants from glandular lung, glucocorticoids act by transcriptional and post-transcriptional mechanisms to increase SP-B gene expression and by post-transcriptional mechanisms to increase SP-C mRNA levels. In canalicular and saccular lung, the glucocorticoid induction of SP-B and SP-C appears to be primarily a posttranscriptional process. These differences are likely due to sub-stantial increases in basal levels of SP-B and SP-C gene expression that occur during this relatively broad period of lung development. For example, by 26 days of gestation, significant transcriptional activity for both genes is apparent and mRNA levels are increasing. By 30 days, further increases in rates of transcription are evident, and mRNA levels are equal to or greater than those in adult animals.

### cAMP Agonists

Although studied in less detail than glucocorticoids, cAMP agonists have been reported to increase SP-B gene expression in human, rat, and rabbit explant culture but effects on SP-C have been more modest and inconsistent. In mid trimester human fetal lung, Whitsett et al. (290) reported enhancement of SP-B and SP-C mRNAs after 2–4 days of exposure to 100 $\mu$M 3-bromo-cAMP. The magnitude of effect was less than that produced by 10 nM dexamethasone. Liley et al. (83) noted that treatment for 2 days with forskolin (10 $\mu$M) or terbutaline (10 $\mu$M) increased SP-B mRNA levels to ~2.5-fold greater than levels in control tissue but SP-C mRNA was not affected. Combined treatment with 10 nM dexamethasone produced no greater increase in SP-B mRNA than did dex-amethasone alone. Using explants from fetal rat lungs of 18 days' gestation, Floros and co-workers (295,296) found that both 8-bromo-cAMP and Bt$_2$cAMP produced dose-dependent increases in SP-B and SP-C mRNAs. Maximal stimula-tion by both agents occurred at a concentration of 200 $\mu$M; higher concentrations were inhibitory. SP-B responded more rapidly to cAMP agonists than did SP-C; maximal stimulation was reached at ~15 hr for SP-B mRNA and 24–30 hr for SP-C. Interestingly, Bt$_2$cAMP produced a greater degree of stimulation of both SP-B and SP-C mRNAs than did 8-bromo-cAMP. These investigators found previously that only 8-bromo-cAMP enhanced accumulation of SP-A mRNA and Bt$_2$cAMP was inhibitory (281). The enhancement in SP-B mRNA produced by cAMP agonists was considerably less than that produced by treatment with dexa-methasone (18-fold versus 2-fold), whereas the SP-C response was comparable.

Combined treatment with dexamethasone (100 nM) and $Bt_2cAMP$ (200 $\mu M$) produced an additive increase in SP-B mRNA.

Studies with rabbit fetal lung explants from 21 days of gestation have found increased SP-B and SP-C gene expression in response to cAMP agonists and have begun to examine mechanisms underlying this effect. In this system, treatment with $Bt_2cAMP$ (1 mM) increased SP-B and SP-C mRNAs 2.9- and 2.0-fold greater than that in control tissue, and the magnitude of this induction was less than that produced by dexamethasone (61,297). Induction of SP-C mRNA by $Bt_2cAMP$ was also slower in that stimulation was maximal after 48 hr of exposure, whereas dexamethasone produced maximal stimulation by 24 hr. Combined treatment with dexamethasone produced additive or supra-additive induction of both mRNAs by 48 hr. Nuclear elongation assays showed that $Bt_2cAMP$ increased SP-B gene transcription 3.1-fold greater than that of control tissue after 48 hr but had no effect on the half-life of SP-B mRNA ($t_{1/2}$ ~10 hr for both control and treated explants). The rate of SP-C gene transcription was also increased by $Bt_2cAMP$, and the magnitude of increase was comparable to the observed increase in mRNA levels, suggesting little or no posttranscriptional effects. These investigators concluded that $Bt_2cAMP$ stimulated SP-B and SP-C gene expression primarily at a transcriptional level. Thus, in cultured fetal rat and rabbit lung a variety of agents that increase intracellular cAMP have been shown to stimulate SP-B and SP-C gene expression, although the degree of induction is less than that produced by glucocorticoids. In human fetal lung, SP-B mRNA is induced by cAMP agonists, but discrepant effects on SP-C mRNA have been reported.

### Other Hormones and Growth Factors

Relatively few hormones besides glucocorticoids and cAMP agonists have been found to regulate SP-B and SP-C gene expression. Connely et al. (84) treated pregnant rabbits with 2.2 $\mu g/kg$ of 17$\beta$-estradiol 24 hr prior to delivery on day 27 of gestation and found an approximately twofold increase in SP-B mRNA relative to carrier-injected controls. The degree of SP-B induction by estradiol was comparable to that produced by betamethasone. Estradiol reduced SP-C mRNA levels, but its effects were not significant. In explant culture of human fetal lung, exposure to estradiol (1 $\mu M$) for 48 hr did not significantly alter the content of SP-B or SP-C mRNAs (83). Similarly, in human fetal lung, SP-B and SP-C mRNAs are not affected by $T_3$ or IFN-$\gamma$. However, $T_3$ (100 nM) treatment of rat fetal lung explants tended to inhibit accumulation of SP-B mRNA and combined treatment with dexamethasone resulted in a lesser degree of stimulation than that produced by dexamethasone alone (295). $T_3$ did not change SP-C mRNA levels either alone or in combination with dexamethasone (296). TNF-$\alpha$ and TPA have been reported to reduce SP-A and SP-B mRNA levels in H441-4 cells by different mechanisms

(299). SP-A gene transcription was reduced by both agents, whereas the rate of transcription of the SP-B gene was unaffected.

Recent studies have attempted to define the effects of diabetes and insulin on surfactant protein gene expression. Guttentag et al. (300,301) used high-dose streptozotocin treatment (50 mg/kg) to induce chemical pancreatectomy in rats prior to mating and reported reduced levels of SP-A and SP-B proteins and mRNAs in the lungs of fetuses from days 18 through 21 of gestation. SP-C mRNA was also reduced on all of these days except for day 19 when the reduction was not significant. Differences were no longer apparent on neonatal days 1 and 2. The underlying cause of this inhibition remains to be elucidated, and because of significant differences between this model and the human infant of a diabetic mother (discussed above in Section IV.C), its relevance to the human situation is unclear. Dekowski and Snyder (285) treated explants from mid trimester human fetal lung with insulin and found modest reductions (~30% less than control) in SP-B and SP-C mRNA levels only at the highest dose of insulin tested (2500 ng/ml). Insulin inhibition of SP-B but not SP-C mRNA was significant. SP-A protein and mRNA were also reduced by insulin, but the effects were apparent with doses as low as 25 ng/ml and the maximal inhibition of SP-A mRNA (73% reduction) was greater than that for SP-B mRNA.

It is becoming increasingly evident that a variety of different and interacting hormones can influence expression of pulmonary surfactant, either stimulating or inhibiting synthesis of different components (summarized in Table 3). Except for glucocorticoids and possibly thyroid hormones, the physiological/pathological role of this multihormonal regulation is uncertain.

**Table 3**  Hormonal Regulation of Surfactant Components in Cultured Fetal Lung

|  | GC | cAMP | $T_3$ | EGF | IFN-γ | TPA | TNF-α | TGF-β | Insulin |
|---|---|---|---|---|---|---|---|---|---|
| Total PC | ↑ | ↑ | ↑ | ↑ | — | — | ND | ND | — |
| % DPPC | ↑ | ↑ | — | (↑) | — | — | ND | ND | — |
| SP-A | ↑ & ↓ | ↑ | — | ↑ | ↑ | ↓ | ↓ | ↓ | ↓ |
| SP-B | ↑ | ↑ | — | ND | — | ↓ | ↓ | ND | ND |
| SP-C | ↑ | — | — | ND | — | ND | ND | ND | ND |
| SP-D | ↑ | — | ND | ND | — | — | — | ND | ND |

Summary of hormonal effects on content of mRNA and/or protein for surfactant proteins and rate of precursor incorporation and/or content of lipid. Most data are from human tissue as referenced in the text or are unpublished (P. Ballard). SP-A in human and rat lung is either increased or decreased depending on dose and time of glucocorticoid treatment.

↑, increased; ↓, decreased; —, no effect; ND, not determined; GC, glucocorticoids.

### F.  Molecular Regulatory Mechanisms

*SP-A*

Recently, several different strategies have been applied to begin to characterize *cis*- and *trans*-acting regulatory elements that control the lung-specific and hormonally regulated transcription of the SP-A gene. The 5'-flanking region of SP-A genes examined to date contain the TATAA element located ~30 bp upstream from the transcription start site that is typical of many eukaryotic genes. Recently, two groups have reported further on potential 5'-regulatory sequences of the rat SP-A gene. Kouretas et al. (302) compared the sequences of rat and human genomic SP-A clones which contained ~2.7 kb of 5'-flanking sequence in order to identify evolutionarily conserved regions which might serve as *cis*-acting regulatory elements. A computer-based dot matrix analysis identified a number of homologous regions, and the two longest, from −225 to −16 (~75% homology to the human gene) and −1114 to −1025 (~52% homology) in the rat, were used with lung and liver nuclear extracts from adult rats in electrophoretic mobility shift assays (EMSA) to test for the formation of lung-specific DNA-protein complexes. Sequences from −169 to −16 and from −1114 to −1025 formed a number of lung-specific complexes that were eliminated by competition with excess specific but not nonspecific DNA. The −225 to −170 portion of the proximal region was more homologous to the human gene than the −169 to −16 portion, but it did not form lung-specific complexes in EMSA. Although further experimental characterization of these DNA-protein complexes was not accomplished in this study, potential recognition sequences for known transcription factors were identified. The −169 to −16 fragment in the rat and the corresponding region in the human gene both contained identical IFN-γ response elements in similar positions. Other potential recognition sequences identified include an AP-2 site from −53 to −46 in the rat, a C/EBP site at −196 in the rat, a cAMP response element at −251 in the human 5'-untranslated region, and sequences corresponding to half-sites of the consensus GRE at −612 in the human and −161 in the rat. Lacaze-Masmonteil (303) also cloned and sequenced the 5' region of the rat SP-A gene and proposed a potential GRE (GTTTCTaagTGTTCT) 125 bp upstream from the transcription start site, a sequence (TTTTGTAAA) at −740 almost identical to the C/EBP binding site, a potential SP-1 binding site at −1060, and a putative AP-1 binding site (CTGACTCA) at position +400. DNaseI footprint studies showed several protected regions and a number of specific hypersensitive sites within the first 200 bp of 5' sequence. Moreover, the region from −230 to +9 was able to serve as a functional promoter with lung but not liver nuclear extracts in an in vitro transcription assay, suggesting that this region may contain necessary sequences for tissue specific expression of the rat SP-A gene.

Two recent studies have examined *cis*- and *trans*-acting regulation of the rabbit SP-A gene. Alcorn et al. (304) examined ~2.5 kb of 5' sequence from the rabbit SP-A gene and reported a number of potential regulatory elements, including a putative CRE at $-261$, two AP-1 consensus sequences, and four elements homologous to half of the consensus GRE. To define *cis*-acting regulatory elements, these investigators constructed fusion genes in an adenovirus vector that contained varying amounts of 5'-flanking sequence linked to a human growth hormone (hGH) reporter gene for deletional analysis of *cis*-regulatory elements of the rabbit SP-A gene. The adenovirus vector was used to infect differentiated type II cells which were isolated from $Bt_2cAMP$–treated fetal rat lung explants and plated on dishes coated with extracellular matrix. In contrast to primary cultures of adult and fetal type II cells which rapidly "dedifferentiate" in routine culture (305), these cells were reported to contain numerous osmiophilic lamellar bodies and to actively synthesize SP-A for up to 2 weeks in the presence of $Bt_2cAMP$. Constructs containing 1766, 991, 378, and 47 bp of sequence upstream from the transcription start site were tested in order to determine the amount of 5' sequence necessary for basal and cAMP-induced transcription. The $-1766$ and $-991$ constructs conferred comparable low levels of hGH production under control conditions, and treatment with $Bt_2cAMP$ (1 mM) for 5 days produced a 30- to 40-fold increase in hGH levels in cells infected with both constructs. The $-378$ construct produced substantially lower levels of hGH in control and $Bt_2cAMP$–treated cells than the $-1766$ or $-991$ construct, but $Bt_2cAMP$ treatment still caused an 11-fold increase in hGH over that of control cells. The $-47$ bp construct did not support hGH production by control or hormonally treated cells. These results indicated that sequences between $-47$ and $-378$ were sufficient to confer basal and cAMP-induced expression and sequences between $-378$ and $-991$ were necessary for enhanced levels of expression. A potential CRE (TGAC-CTCA) which differed by one nucleotide from the consensus CRE (TGACGTCA) was identified at $-261$, and mutation studies suggested that it played a role in the induction of gene expression during control culture and treatment with $Bt_2cAMP$. The requirement of an intact CRE for optimal expression of the SP-A gene during control culture is consistent with previous work in human fetal lung explants which indicated that this spontaneous induction is due to increases in endogenous cAMP levels (179). Cells infected with the $-1766$, $-991$, and $-378$ constructs and treated for 5 days with dexamethasone (100 nM) plus $Bt_2cAMP$ (1 mM) exhibited a dose-dependent inhibition of cAMP-stimulated hGH levels. This result is contrary to previous work from this laboratory in which combined treatment for 48 hr or longer increased SP-A gene transcription in rabbit fetal lung explants (74). Constructs were also tested in two pulmonary adenocarcinoma cell lines (H358 and A549) of type II cell origin that do not produce SP-A and in an adrenal and a hepatic cell line. The $-1766$ and the $-991$ constructs produced significantly higher basal hGH levels in these four cell lines than in rat type II cells and the $-991$ construct produced higher hGH levels than the $-1766$ construct in the H358 and A549 but not the nonpulmonary cell lines. Based on these results, the investigators proposed an inhibitory element within the region from −991 to −1766. Responsiveness to cAMP was apparent only in rat type II cells. Although this study provides considerable new information on cis-acting regulatory mechanisms, some questions remain unanswered. Expression of these fusion genes in cell lines that do not normally express SP-A would seem to be somewhat inconsistent and problematic. Although sequences between −47 and −378 and an intact CRE at −261 were shown to be necessary for cAMP-stimulated expression, the minimum sequences required for tissue- and cell-specific transcription remain to be clarified. Potential inconsistencies between this system and studies using explants (e.g., glucocorticoid effects) may be due to the use of rat type II cells to study cis-acting regulation of the rabbit gene, particularly in light of the species-specific nature of many of the properties of SP-A gene expression.

A subsequent study by this group of investigators used a variety of methods to begin to characterize trans-acting factors responsible for the tissue-specific and cAMP-regulated expression of the rabbit SP-A gene (311). ~3.2 kb of 5′ sequence flanking the rabbit SP-A gene was digested by restriction endonucleases and the resulting fragments were tested by EMSA for the ability to bind nuclear proteins from 28-day gestation fetal rabbit lungs. Only two regions bound lung nuclear proteins: a proximal fragment containing sequences from −330 to +18 and a more distal fragment from −991 to −879. Using fragments produced by PCR or synthetic oligonucleotides for EMSA, sites of binding were further defined to seven proximal elements, including the putative CRE at −261, the TATA region, sequences from −87 to −70, and a distal element from −991 to −976. Because nonradiolabeled oligonucleotides from either −87 to −70 or −991 to −976 could effectively compete for binding to the other radiolabelled fragment, the investigators concluded that the same proteins bound both of these fragments. Sequence analysis showed that both elements contained potential binding sites for the helix-loop-helix family of transcription factors. DNaseI footprinting showed the distal binding element to be included within a protected region. Of note, these two regions are in the same general locations as those described by Kouretas et al. (302) in their EMSA studies of the rat SP-A gene. However, binding to these fragments from the rabbit gene was not lung-specific, since nuclear proteins from heart and skeletal muscle but not liver or kidney produced a similar but less intense pattern of binding. Also, binding activity was highest in lung extracts from day 19 of gestation and in preculture lung explants. Advancing gestational age and increasing time in culture produced declines in binding activity. These results differ from previous work by this laboratory and others in which rabbit SP-A gene transcription peaked on day 28 of gestation and increased with increasing time in culture (74). DNA-binding proteins identified by EMSA were isolated and further characterized by a variety of methods and shown to include proteins with $M_r$ of 69, 45, and 22 kDa. The 45-kDa protein had the highest apparent binding activity and, because it appeared to produce the band with the highest $M_r$ by EMSA, the investigators suggested that it bound DNA as a dimer. Transfection of rat type II cells with chimeric genes that contained varying amounts of 5' SP-A sequence to drive the hGH reporter gene but in which either the proximal or distal binding element was deleted or replaced with a plasmid polylinker confirmed the importance of these two regions. Alteration of either of these regions produced a significant reduction in basal and cAMP-stimulated hGH levels. The proximal element appeared to be particularly important for cAMP induction since changes in this region resulted in only modest increases in hGH levels in response to Bt$_2$cAMP.

### SP-B

Recent work has provided important new information on *cis-* and *trans*-acting regulatory elements that control the tissue-specific expression of the human and mouse SP-B genes. As an initial step, Bohinski et al. (306) identified four DNaseI hypersensitive sites within the human SP-B gene of H441 nuclei but not of nuclei from a nonpulmonary cell line. Two of these sites were near the transcription start site and two were within the eighth intron. These results were further examined by deletional analysis of nine fusion genes that contained varying amounts 5' SP-B sequence from −2244 to +436 bp linked to the CAT reporter gene. Transient transfections were performed in H441 cells; A549 cells, a pulmonary adenocarcinoma cell line that does not express SP-B; and HeLa cells. Increased CAT expression was apparent only in H441 cells, and deletions up to −218 did not result in any loss of activity relative to the −2244 construct. Among the eight constructs containing 5' sequence from −218 to −2244, the level of CAT expression showed considerable variability and a construct beginning at −650 bp produced the highest level of CAT activity. However, regulatory elements did not appear to be located within this region. Alteration of the −2244 construct to include intron 8 downstream of the CAT reporter gene did not enhance CAT expression in H441 cells, indicating that, at least in this context, this downstream region which contained two sites of DNaseI hypersensitivity was not functionally active. Deletion of sequence from −218 to −80 resulted in an 82% reduction in CAT activity, suggesting a positive regulatory element between −218 and −80. Removal of 3' sequence from +436 to +41 did not significantly alter CAT activity but a further deletion to +7 reduced CAT expression by 91%. Taken together, these results indicate that basal levels of cell-specific transcription of the human SP-B gene is controlled by sequences from −218 to +41. Further information on *cis*-acting regulatory elements within this region was provided by DNaseI footprint analysis using nuclear extracts from H441 and HeLa cells. Five protected regions were identified, two of which were apparent only with the H441 extracts and were located from −107 to −93 and from −90 to −73 and were designated SPB-f1 and SPB-f2, respectively. SPB-f1, contained no previously identified consensus response elements, whereas SPB-f2, contained a TGT3 motif (TGT-TTGT) known to bind hepatocyte nuclear factor-3 (HNF-3). The most distal of the five protected regions was located entirely within protein coding sequence and contained a consensus AP-1 binding site motif.

A search for *trans*-acting factors controlling the cell-specific expression of the SP-B gene has led to the identification of two previously described transcription factors, thyroid transcription factor 1 (TTF-1) and HNF-3 that appear to control the transcription of several lung-specific genes. Using SPB-f1 and SPB-f2 as probes and nuclear extracts from H441 and MLE-15 cells, EMSA identified four DNA-protein complexes that appeared to be composed of two distinct nuclear factors, since unlabeled excess of each probe did not effectively compete for complexes formed with the other probe (307). The MLE-15 cell line was derived from lung tumors produced in transgenic mice bearing a chimeric gene in which the SP-C gene promoter was used to drive expression of the simian virus 40 large tumor antigen. This cell line produces SP-A, SP-B, and SP-C. The addition of antibodies specific for HNF-3$\alpha$ and HNF-3$\beta$ completely eliminated complexes formed by SPB-f2 and MLE-15 nuclear extracts. Northern analysis detected transcripts for HNF-3$\alpha$ and HNF-3$\beta$ in MLE-15 and HNF-3$\alpha$ in H441 cells.

To further characterize complexes formed by SPB-f1 and nuclear extracts from lung cells, 5' and 3' subfragments were used as probes in EMSA, and results indicated that a single factor bound each end of SPB-f1. Sequence comparison of these two portions of SPB-f1 suggested a possible motif (GCnCTnnAG) that shared some similarities with the consensus TTF-1 binding site (CCACTCA-AGT), and a series of results indicated that TTF-1 did indeed bind SPB-f1. An oligonucleotide from a known TTF-1 binding site within the thyroglobulin gene promoter was shown to be a more efficient competitor for the two complexes than unlabeled SPB-f1. Antisera to TTF-1 eliminated the two complexes and produced a single larger complex. When the purified TTF-1 homeodomain was used in place of nuclear extracts from lung cells, two distinct complexes were formed with SPB-f1. These results indicated that TTF-1 bound two degenerate motifs from ~–110 to –90 bp of the human SP-B gene. Northern analysis confirmed the presence of TTF-1 transcripts within H441 and MLE-15 cells. Additionally, a 2-bp mutation within either of the two putative TTF-1 binding sites of SPB-f1 or the putative HNF-3 binding site within SPB-f2 eliminated the formation of complexes in EMSA and substantially reduced CAT activity in H441 cells transfected with the chimeric CAT gene driven by the basal SP-B promoter (sequences from –218 to +41). Mutations in all three proposed binding sites resulted in 95% lower CAT activity than that of the wild-type construct and was no different from the CAT expression produced by the –80 construct, indicating that these binding sites are necessary for transcription of the SP-B gene by H441 cells. Perhaps the strongest evidence for TTF-1 as a key *trans*-activator in the lung came from experiments in which cotransfection of a cell line (HeLa) that does not normally produce either

TTF-1 or surfactant proteins with the chimeric CAT gene driven by the basal SP-B gene promoter and a TTF-1 expression vector produced a marked increase in CAT activity, indicating that the introduction of TTF-1 into this cell line resulted in the transcription of SP-B. In similar experiments, gene promoters for SP-C, SP-A (308), and a Clara cell protein known to be lung-specific were also shown to be activated by TTF-1, whereas promoters from a liver-specific gene and thymidine kinase, a gene that is constitutively expressed, were unaffected.

A recent study of the human SP-B gene promoter by Venkatesh et al. (309) confirms that the proximal ~200 bp of the promoter is sufficient for lung cell–specific expression, and that a DNA fragment from this region ($-404/-35$) confers cell-specific enhancer activity when linked to a heterologous promoter. Furthermore, this region contains a yet unidentified sequence that appears to mediate the inhibitory effect of phorbol esters on SP-B gene expression. AP-1 sequences are present in the promoter region but are outside the sequence mediating phorbol ester responsiveness.

Deletional analysis of the 5'-flanking region of the murine SP-B gene has revealed some similarities and some differences to the human gene. Based on results for the human gene, nine constructs containing varying amounts of 5' murine SP-B sequence from $-1782$ to $+44$ linked to the CAT reporter were transfected into MLE-15 and H441 cells, which express SP-B, and 3T3, MLE-F6, and HeLa cells, which do not express SP-B (310). CAT expression was cell type-specific and deletion of sequence to $-842$ did not significantly alter CAT activity. However, removal of sequence from $-842$ to $-382$, $-382$ to $-283$, and $-132$ to $-82$ all resulted in progressive reductions in CAT expression, with the greatest reduction being produced by the removal of the sequence from $-382$ to $-283$. These results differ somewhat from those for the human gene and indicate that these three regions of the murine gene are functional enhancer elements. Basal levels of transcription appeared to be conferred by sequences from $-82$ to $+44$ bp. Computer-based comparison of ~1800 bp of sequence upstream of the transcription start sites of the mouse and human SP-B genes showed that SPB-f1 and SPB-f2 each contained a 14-bp stretch of identical sequence and indicated more homology overall for the first 600 bp of 5' sequence than for more distal sequences. Under conditions of higher stringency, the three regions that functioned as enhancers continued to show significant homology.

These studies provide important new information about *trans*-acting factors that control pulmonary-specific gene expression in vitro. Further studies in an in vivo model will be necessary to confirm the importance of these findings and to examine the role of TTF-1 in lung development. An additional major area that remains to be addressed is the molecular basis for induction of SP-B by glucocorticoids and cAMP agonists. Glucocorticoids strongly increase production of SP-B in all systems examined to date and available evidence in H441 cells as well as human and rat fetal lung indicates that this response is mediated in part by an increase in gene transcription. *Cis-* and *trans*-acting regulatory elements that control hormonal induction of the SP-B gene remain to be defined. In this regard, the GR has been shown to interact with a TGT3 element within the tyrosine aminotransferase gene, but whether this element plays a role in the glucocorticoid induction of SP-B remains to be determined.

### SP-C

Currently, only limited information is available on the molecular regulation of the SP-C gene, at least partly because of limitations of currently available in vitro systems. Sequence analysis has yielded limited information on potential regulatory elements. Besides the consensus TATAA basal promoter element located ~30 bp upstream from the predicted transcription initiation site, two putative AP-1 sites have been identified at $-389$ and $-505$ as well as a potential half-site of the consensus GRE (ACANNNTGTTCT) ~1.9 kb upstream from the transcription start site of the human gene (60,88). The two putative AP-1 sites were conserved in the mouse gene (87). Recently, a transgenic model has been used to begin to characterize *cis*-regulation of the human SP-C gene. In these studies, 7–10 founder lines were used to examine the expression of fusion genes consisting of ~3.7 kb of 5' sequence from the human SP-C gene linked to the CAT reporter gene (87–89). CAT activity was found only in lung tissue of transgenic animals. In newborn and adult transgenic mice, CAT mRNA was detected by in situ hybridization in both bronchiolar and alveolar epithelial cells, whereas native murine SP-C mRNA was found only in alveolar epithelial cells. Levels of CAT expression varied considerably among founder lines and was not directly related to gene copy number. Dexamethasone treatment of fetal lung explants from two founder lines of transgenic mice for 48 and 72 hr increased CAT activity and endogenous SP-C mRNA content.

These results in a transgenic model indicate that 3.7 kb of 5' sequence from the human SP-C gene is sufficient to direct lung-specific, developmentally regulated and glucocorticoid-induced expression of the SP-C gene. However, a number of questions remain unanswered. For example, is induction of SP-C gene expression by glucocorticoids in this system a primary or secondary phenomenon? What are the minimum *cis*-acting sequences necessary for lung-specific and type II cell–specific expression of the SP-C gene? Additionally, *trans*-acting factors that control expression of the SP-C gene and the regulatory elements to which they bind remain to be defined.

## V. Summary and Conclusions

Over the past 35 years, considerable progress has been made in the study of pulmonary surfactant, a complex mixture of phospholipids and proteins that lowers surface tension at the alveolar air-liquid interface and stabilizes alveoli on deflation. Surfactant components have been isolated, characterized biochemically, and assigned functional roles. Recent advances in molecular biology have greatly accelerated our understanding of the surfactant system and have led to the isolation of genes encoding the four, lung-specific surfactant-associated proteins. Along with surfactant phospholipids, SP-B, in particular, appears to be essential for normal respiratory function. Recently, the importance of SP-B has been confirmed by the characterization of a mutation in the SP-B gene which leads to an isolated deficiency of the SP-B protein, extensive perturbations in the surfactant system, and a severe familial form of respiratory distress in full-term newborns that is uniformly fatal.

The components of the surfactant system are subject to complex developmental and hormonal regulation. Although in all species examined to date the synthesis of surfactant components surges during the last 10–20% of gestation, developmental regulation of each component is not coordinate. SP-B and SP-C transcripts are detectable in glandular human, rat, and rabbit lung well before the appearance of recognizable type II cells or the synthesis or secretion of surfactant phospholipids. In contrast, the synthesis of SP-A and SP-D tends to parallel that of surfactant phospholipids.

A number of hormones, growth factors, cytokines, and other agents have been shown to exert positive and negative effects on lung development and the surfactant system and have emphasized the importance of a multihormonal milieu in the control of lung development. Glucocorticoid, thyroid hormone, and β-adrenergic receptors are all well characterized in fetal lung from several species and evidence strongly supports receptor mediation of their effects. Moreover, these three classes of hormones likely play a physiological role in the regulation of lung development in vivo. Glucocorticoids and cAMP agonists appear to have the most wideranging effects of the agents studied to date; in most systems, these two hormones induce surfactant phospholipids and proteins.

The molecular mechanisms controlling hormonal responses in the developing lung have begun to be clarified but a number of areas require further study. Glucocorticoids and cAMP agonists act at transcriptional as well as posttranscriptional levels. The regulation of SP-A by glucocorticoids is of particular interest, since a unique biphasic pattern has been described that depends on the hormonal concentration and duration of exposure. Initial reports of glucocorticoid effects on SP-A gene transcription from two laboratories have differed somewhat and require clarification. Decreased stability of the SP-A message appears to be a major mechanism underlying the inhibition of SP-A by glucocorticoids, apparently mediated through changes in the synthesis of a labile protein, but the exact nature of this process requires further study.

The characterization of *cis*- and *trans*-acting regulatory elements that control hormonal effects on the developing lung would seem to be a major area for future investigations. Initial studies have begun to identify potential hormonal response elements, evolutionarily conserved regions of surfactant protein genes and *cis*- and *trans*-acting elements that control the tissue-specific expression of SP-A, SP-B, and SP-C. The only study to date to identify a functional hormonal response element is that of Alcorn et al. (304) in which a CRE was characterized in an in vitro system at −261 bp of the rabbit SP-A gene. Because of certain discrepancies between results in this system and those in explant systems, confirmation of these findings in an in vivo model would be desirable. Recent results suggesting that TTF-1 may be a major regulator of lung development and lung-specific gene expression are of considerable interest and in vivo studies to alter this gene by homologous recombination and study its role during development could confirm the physiological relevance of this transcription factor. A final area that deserves further study is the identification and characterization of hormonally regulated proteins in the lung. Glucocorticoids appear to regulate ~2% of proteins in cultured fetal lung, but only a limited number have been identified to date. These hormonally regulated proteins likely mediate many of the diverse effects of hormones on the developing lung, and a complete understanding of these processes will likely require purification, isolation, and characterization of their cDNAs and genes.

## REFERENCES

1. Ballard PL. Hormones and lung maturation. In: Baxter JD, Rousseau GG, eds. Monographs on Endocrinology, Vol. 28. New York: Springer-Verlag, 1986: 24–341.
2. Mendelson CR, Boggaram V. Hormonal control of the surfactant system in fetal lung. Annu Rev Physiol 1991; 53:415–440.
3. Brody JS, Williams MC. Pulmonary alveolar cell differentiation. Annu Rev Physiol 1992; 54:351–374.
4. Gilfillan AM, Chu AJ, Smart CA, Rooney SA. Single plate separation of lung phospholipids including disaturated phosphatidylcholine. J Lipid Res 1983; 24: 1651–1656.
5. King RJ. Pulmonary surfactant. J Appl Physiol 1982; 53:1–8.
6. Beppu OS, Clements JA, Goerke J. Phosphatidylglycerol-deficient lung surfactant has normal properties. J Appl Physiol 1983; 55:496–502.
7. Hallman M, Gluck L. Phosphatidylglycerol in lung surfactant. III. Possible modifier of surfactant function. J Lipid Res 1976; 17:257–262.
8. Farrel PM. Lung Development: Biological and Clinical Perspectives. Vol. 1. New York: Academic Press, 1982.
9. Van Golde LMG, Batenburg JJ, Robertson B. The pulmonary surfactant system: biochemical aspects and functional significance. Physiol Rev 1988; 68:374–455.
10. Rooney SA. Regulation of surfactant associated phospholipid synthesis and secretion. In: Polin RA, Fox WW, eds. Fetal and Neonatal Physiology. Philadelphia: Saunders, 1992:971–985.

11. Van Heusden GP, Ruestow B, Van der Mast MA, Van den Bosch H. Synthesis of disaturated phosphatidylcholine by cholinephosphotransferase in rat lung microsomes. Biochim Biophys Acta 1981; 666:313–321.

12. Rustow B, Kunze D, Rabe H, Reichmann G. The molecular species of phosphatidic acid, diacylglycerol and phosphatidylcholine synthesized from sn-glycerol 3-phosphate in rat lung microsomes. Biochim Biophys Acta 1985; 835:465–476.

13. Weaver TE, Whitsett JA. Function and regulation of expression of pulmonary surfactant-associated proteins. Biochem J 1991; 273:249–264.

14. Mendelson CR, Acarregui MJ, Odom MJ, Boggaram V. Developmental and hormonal regulation of surfactant protein A (SP-A) gene expresssion in fetal lung. J Dev Physiol 1991; 15:61–69.

15. Hawgood S, Shiffer K. Structures and properties of the surfactant-associated proteins. Annu Rev Physiol 1991; 53:375–394.

16. Beers MF, Fisher AB. Surfactant protein C: A review of its unique properties and metabolism. Am J Physiol 1992; 263:L151–L160.

17. Haagsman HP. Surfactant proteins A and D. Biochem Soc Trans 1994; 22:100–106.

18. Benson B, Hawgood S, Schilling J, Clements J, Damm D, Cordell B, White RT. Structure of canine pulmonary surfactant apoprotein: cDNA and complete amino acid sequence. Proc Natl Acad Sci USA 1985; 82:6379–6383.

19. White RT, Damm D, Miller J, Spratt K, Schilling J, Hawgood S, Benson B, Cordell B. Isolation and characterization of the human pulmonary surfactant apoprotein gene. Nature 1985; 317:361–363.

20. Sano K, Fisher J, Mason RJ, Kuroki Y, Schiling J, Benson B, Voelker D. Isolation and sequence of a cDNA clone for the rat pulmonary surfactant-associated protein (PSP-A). Biochem Biophys Res Commun 1987; 144:367–374.

21. Boggaram V, Qing K, Mendelson CR. The major apoprotein of rabbit pulmonary surfactant: Elucidation of primary sequence and cyclic AMP and developmental regulation. J Biol Chem 1988; 263:2939–2947.

22. Korfhagen TR, Bruno MD, Glasser SW, Ciraolo PJ, Whitsett JA, Latt DL, Wikenheiser KA, Clark JC. Murine pulmonary surfactant protein-A gene: cloning, sequence and transcriptional activity. Am J Physiol 1992; 263:L546–L554.

23. Chen Q, Boggaram V, Mendelson CR. Rabbit lung surfactant protein A gene: identification of a lung-specific DNase I hypersensitive site. Am J Physiol 1992; 262:L662–L671.

24. Katyal SL, Singh G, Locker J. Characterization of a second human pulmonary surfactant-associated protein SP-A gene. Am J Respir Cell Mol Biol 1992; 6:446–452.

25. McCormick SM, Boggaram V, Mendelson CR. Characterization of mRNA transcripts and organization of human SP-A1 and SP-A2 genes. Am J Physiol 1994; 266:L354–L366.

26. Korfhagen TR, Glasser SW, Bruno MD, McMahan MJ, Whitsett JA. A portion of the human surfactant protein A (SP-A) gene locus consists of a pseudogene. Am J Respir Cell Mol Biol 1991; 4:463–469.

27. Bruns G, Stroh H, Veldman GM, Latt SA, Floros J. The 35 kd pulmonary surfactant-associated protein is encoded on chromosome 10. Hum Genet 1987; 76:58–62.

28. Floros J, Steinbrink R, Jacobs K, Phelps D, Kriz R, Reeny M, Sultzman L, Jones S, Taeusch HW, Frank HA, Fritsch EF. Isolation and characterization of cDNA clones for the 35-kDa pulmonary surfactant-associated protein. J Biol Chem 1986: 261: 9029–9033.

29. Ross GF, Notter RH, Meuth J, Whitsett JA. Phospholipid binding and biophysical activity of pulmonary surfactant-associated protein (SAP)-35 and its non-collagenous COOH-terminal domains. J Biol Chem 1986; 261:14283–14291.

30. Haagsman HP, White RT, Schilling J, Lau K, Benson BJ, Golden J, Hawgood S, Clements JA. Studies of the structure of lung surfactant protein SP-A. Am J Physiol 1989; 257:L421–L429.

31. Voss T, Eistetter H, Schafer KP. Macromolecular organization of natural and recombinant lung surfactant protein SP 28–36. Structural homology with the complement factor C1q. J Mol Biol 1988; 201:219–227.

32. King RJ, Simon D, Horowitz PM. Aspects of secondary and quaternary structure of surfactant protein-A from canine lung. Biochim Biophys Acta 1989; 1001:294–301.

33. Williams MC, Benson BJ. Immunocytochemical localization and identification of the major surfactant protein in adult rat lung. J Histochem Cytochem 1981; 29: 291–305.

34. Suzuki Y, Jujita Y, Kogishi K. Reconstitution of tubular myelin from synthetic lipids and proteins associated with pig pulmonary surfactant. Am Rev Respir Dis 1989; 140:75–81.

35. Kuroki Y, Mason RJ, Voelker DR. Alveolar type II cells express a high-affinity receptor for pulmonary surfactant protein A. Proc Natl Acad Sci USA 1988; 85: 5566–5570.

36. Manz-Keinke H, Egenhofer C, Plattner H, Schlepper-Schafer J. Specific interaction of lung surfactant protein-A (SP-A) with rat alveolar macrophages. Exp Cell Res 1991; 192:597–603.

37. Pison U, Wright JR, Hawgood S. Specific binding of surfactant apoprotein SP-A to rat alveolar macrophages. Am J Physiol 1992; 262:L412–L417.

38. Van Iwaarden JF, Welmers B, Verhoef J, Haagsman HP, Van Golde LMG. Pulmonary surfactant protein A enhances the host defense mechanism of rat alveolar macrophages. Am J Respir Cell Mol Biol 1990; 2:91–98.

39. Zimmerman PE, Voelker DR, McCormack FX, Paulsrud JR, Martin WJ. 120-kD surface glycoprotein of Pneumocystis carinii is a ligand for surfactant protein A. J Clin Invest 1992; 89:143–149.

40. van Iwaarden JF, van Strijp JA, Ebskamp MJ, Welmers AC, Verhoef J, van Golde LMG. Surfactant protein A is opsonin in phagocytosis of herpes simplex virus type 1 by rat alveolar macrophages. Am J Physiol 1991; 261:L204–L209.

41. Wright JR, Youmans DC. Pulmonary surfactant protein A stimulates chemotaxis of alveolar macrophage. Am J Physiol 1993; 264:L338–L344.

42. Persson A, Rust K, Chang D, Moxley M, Longmore W, Crouch E. CP4: a pneumocyte-derived collagenous surfactant-associated protein. Biochem 1988; 27: 8576–8584.

43. Persson A, Chang D, Rust K, Moxley M, Longmore W, Crouch E. Purification and

biochemical characterization of CP4 (SP-D), a collagenous sufactant-associated protein. Biochemistry 1989, 28:6361–6367.

44. Rust K, Grosso L, Zhang V, Chang D, Persson A, Longmore W, Cai GZ, Crouch E. Human surfactant protein D: SP-D contains a C-type lectin carbohydrate recognition domain. Arch Biochem Biophys 1991; 290:116–126.

45. Lu J, Willis AC, Reid KBM. Purification, characterization and cDNA cloning of human lung surfactant protein D. Biochem J 1992; 284:795–802.

46. Crouch E, Rust K, Veile R, Donis-Keller H, Grosso L. Genomic organization of human surfactant protein D (SP-D). J Biol Chem 1993; 268:2976–2983.

47. Lu J, Wiedemann H, Holmskov R, Thiel S, Timpl R, Reid KBM. Structural similarity between lung surfactant protein D and conglutinin. Two distinct, C-type lectins containing collagen-like sequences. Eur J Biochem 1993; 215:793–799.

48. Voorhout WF, Teenendaal T, Kuroki Y, Ogasawara Y, Van Golde LMG, Geuze HJ. Immunocytochemical localization of surfactant protein D (SP-D) in type II cells, Clara cells, and alveolar macrophages of rat lung. J Histochem Cytochem 1992; 40:1589–1597.

49. Kuroki Y, Shiratori M, Murata Y, Akino T. Surfactant protein D (SP-D) counteracts the inhibitory effect of surfactant protein A (SP-A) on phospholipid secretion by alveolar type II cells. Biochem J 1991; 279:115–119.

50. Kuan SF, Rust K, Crouch E. Interactions of surfactant protein D with bacterial lipopolysaccharides: surfactant protein D is an Escherichia coli–binding protein in bronchoalveolar lavage. J Clin Invest 1992; 90:97–106.

51. Kuan SF, Persson A, Parghi D, Crouch E. Lectin-mediated interactions of surfactant protein D with alveolar macrophages. Am J Respir Cell Mol Biol 1994; 10:430–436.

52. Hartshorn KL, Crouch EC, White MR, Eggleton P, Tauber AI, Chang D, Sastry K. Evidence for a protective role of pulmonary surfactant protein D (SP-D) against influenza A viruses. J Clin Invest 1994; 94:311–319.

53. Emrie PA, Jones C, Hofmann T, Fisher JH. The coding sequence for the human 18,000 dalton hydrophobic pulmonary surfactant protein is located on chromosome 2 and identifies a restriction fragment length polymorphism. Somat Cell Mol Gen 1988; 14:105–110.

54. Pilot-Matias TJ, Kister SE, Fox JL, Kropp K, Glasser SW, Whitsett JA. Structure and organization of the gene encoding human pulmonary surfactant proteolipid SP-B. DNA 1989; 8:75–86.

55. Emrie PA, Shannon JM, Mason RJ, Fisher JH. cDNA and deduced amino acid sequence for the rat hydrophobic pulmonary surfactant-associated protein, SP-B. Biochim Biophys Acta 1989; 994:215–221.

56. Jacobs KA, Phelps DS, Steinbrink R, J. F, Kriz R, Mitsock L, Dougherty JP, Taeusch HW, Floros J. Isolation of a cDNA clone encoding a high molecular weight precursor to a 6-kDa pulmonary surfactant-associated protein. J Biol Chem 1987; 262: 9808–9811.

57. Glasser SW, Korfhagen TR, Weaver T, Pilot-Matias T, Fox JL, Whitsett JA. cDNA and deduced amino acid sequence of human pulmonary surfactant-associated proteolipid SPL(Phe). Proc Natl Acad Sci USA 1987; 84:4007–4011.

58. Hawgood S, Benson BJ, Schilling J, Damm D. Clements JA, White RT. Nucleotide and amino acid sequences of pulmonary surfactant protein SP18 and evidence for cooperation between SP 18 and SP 28–36 in surfactant lipid adsorption. Proc Natl Acad Sci USA 1987; 84:66–70.

59. Glasser SW, Korfhagen TR, Weaver TE, Clark JC, Pilot-Matias T, Meuth J, Fox JL, Whitsett JA. cDNA, deduced polypeptide structure and chromosomal assignment of human pulmonary surfactant proteolipid SPL (pVal). J Biol Chem 1988; 263: 9–12.

60. Glasser SW, Korfhagen TR, Perme CM, Pilot-Matias TJ, Kister SE, Whitsett JA. Two SP-C genes encoding human pulmonary surfactant proteolipid. J Biol Chem 1988; 263:10326–10331.

61. Boggaram V, Margana R. Rabbit surfactant protein C: cDNA cloning and regulation of alternatively spliced surfactant protein C mRNAs. Am J Physiol 1992; 263:L634–L644.

62. Vandenbussche G, Clerc A, Curstedt T, Johannson J, Jornvall H. Structure and orientation of the surfactant associated protein C in lipid bilayer. Eur J Biochem 1992; 203:201–209.

63. Williams MC, Hawgood S, Hamilton RL. Changes in lipid structure produced by surfactant proteins SP-A, SP-B and SP-C. Am J Respir Cell Mol Biol 1991; 5: 41–50.

64. King RJ, Ruch J, Gikas EG, Platzker ACG, Creasy RK. Appearance of apoproteins of pulmonary surfactant in human amniotic fluid. J Appl Physiol 1975; 39:735–741.

65. Frank L. Preparation for Birth. In: Massoro D, ed. Lung Cell Biology. New York: M Dekker, 1989:1141–1197.

66. Hallman M, Gluck L. Formation of acidic phospholipids in rabbit lung during perinatal development. Pediatr Res 1980; 14:1250–1259.

67. Ballard PL, Hawgood S, Liley HG, Wellenstein G, Gonzales LW, Benson B, Cordell B, White TR. Regulation of pulmonary surfactant apoprotein SP 28–36 gene in fetal human lung. Proc Natl Acad Sci USA 1986; 83:9527–9531.

68. Weaver TE, Ross G, Daugherty C, Whitsett JA. Synthesis of surfactant-associated protein, 35,000 daltons, in fetal lung. J Appl Physiol 1986; 61:694–700.

69. Liley HG, Hawgood S, Wellenstein GA, Benson B, White RT, Ballard PL. Surfactant protein of molecular weight 28,000–36,000 in cultured human fetal lung: Cellular localization and effect of dexamethasone. Mol Endocrinol 1987; 1:205–215.

70. Pryhuber GS, Hull WM, Fink I, McMahan MF, Whitsett JA. Ontogeny of surfactant proteins A and B in human amniotic fluid as indices of fetal lung maturity. Pediatr Res 1991; 30:597–605.

71. Snyder JM, Kwun JE, O'Brien JA, Rosenfeld CR, Odom MJ. The concentration of the 35-kDa surfactant apoprotein in amniotic fluid from normal and diabetic pregnancies. Pediatr Res 1988; 24:728–734.

72. McCormick SM, Mendelson CR. Human SP-A1 and SP-A2 genes are differentially regulated during development and by cAMP and glucocorticoids. Am J Physiol 1994; 266:L367–L374.

73. Mendelson CR, Chen C, Boggaram V, Zacharias C, Snyder JM. Regulation of the

synthesis of the major surfactant apoprotein in fetal rabbit lung tissue. J Biol Chem 1986; 261:9938–9943.

74. Boggaram V, Mendelson CR. Transcriptional regulation of the gene encoding the major surfactant protein (SP-A) in rabbit fetal lung. J Biol Chem 1988; 263:19060–19065.

75. Xu J, Yao L-J, Possmayer F. Regulation of mRNA levels for pulmonary surfactant-associated proteins in developing rabbit lung. Biochim Biophys Acta 1995; 1254: 302–310.

76. Schelhase DE, Emrie PA, Fisher JH, Shannon JM. Ontogeny of surfactant apoproteins in the rat. Pediatr Res 1989; 26:167–174.

77. Miyamura K, Malhotra R, Hoppen H-J, Reid KBM, Phizackerley PJR, Macpherson P, Bernal AL. Surfactant proteins A (SP-A) and D (SP-D): levels in human amniotic fluid and localization in the fetal membranes. Biochim Biophys Acta 1994; 1210: 303–307.

78. Inoue T, Matsuura E, Nagata A, Ogasawara Y, Hattori A, Kuroki Y, Fujimoto S, Akino T. Enzyme-linked immunosorbent assay for human pulmonary surfactant protein D. J Immunol Methods 1994; 173:157–164.

79. Ogasawara Y, Kuroki Y, Shiratori M, Shimizu H, Miamura K, Akino T. Ontogeny of surfactant apoprotein D, SP-D, in the rat lung. Biochim Biophys Acta 1991; 1083: 252–256.

80. Deterding RR, Shimizu H, Fisher JH, Shannon JM. Regulation of surfactant protein D expression by glucocorticoids in vitro and in vivo. Am J Respir Cell Mol Biol 1994; 10:30–47.

81. Crouch E, Rust K, Marienchek W, Parghi D, Chang D, Persson A. Developmental expression of pulmonary surfactant protein D (SP-D). Am J Respir Cell Mol Biol 1991; 5:13–18.

82. Mariencheck W, Crouch E. Modulation of surfactant protein D expression by glucocorticoids in fetal rat lung. Am J Respir Cell Mol Biol 1994; 10:419–429.

83. Liley HG, White TR, Warr RG, Benson BJ, Hawgood S, Ballard PL. Regulation of messenger RNAs for the hydrophobic surfactant proteins in human lung. J Clin Invest 1989; 83:1191–1197.

84. Connelly IH, Hammond GL, Harding PGR, Possmayer F. Levels of surfacant-associated protein messenger ribonucleic acids in rabbit lung during perinatal development and after hormonal treatment. Endocrinology 1991; 129:2583–2591.

85. Xu J, Possmayer F. Exposure of fetal rabbit lung to glucocorticoids in vitro does not enhance transcription of the gene encoding pulmonary surfactant-associated protein-B (SP-B). Biochim Biophys Acta 1993; 1169:146–155.

86. D'Amore-Bruno MA, Wikenheiser KA, Carter JE, Clark JC, Whitsett JA. Sequence, ontogeny and cellular localization of murine surfacant protein B mRNA. Am J Physiol 1991; 262:L40–L47.

87. Glasser SW, Korfhagen TR, Bruno MD, Dey C, Whitsett JA. Structure and expression of the pulmonary surfactant protein SP-C gene in the mouse. J Biol Chem 1990; 265:21986–21991.

88. Glasser SW, Korfhagen TR, Wert SE, Bruno MD, McWilliams KM, Vorbroker DK,

Whitsett JA. Genetic element from human surfactant protein SP-C gene confers bronchiolar-alveolar cell specificity in transgenic mice. Am J Physiol 1991; 261: L349–L356.

89. Wert SE, Glasser SW, Korfhagen TR, Whitsett JA. Transcriptional elements from the human SP-C gene direct expression in the primordial respiratory epithelium of transgenic mice. Dev Biol 1993; 156:426–443.

90. Avery ME, Mead J. Surface properties in relation to atelectasis and hyaline membrane disease. Am J Dis Child 1959; 97:517–523.

91. Coleman M, Dehner LP, Sibley RK, Burke BA, L'Heureux PRL, Thompson TR. Pulmonary alveolar proteinosis: an uncommon cause of chronic neonatal respiratory failure. Am Rev Respir Dis 1980; 121:583–586.

92. Moulton SL, Krous HF, Merritt TA, Odell RM, Gangitano E, Cornish JD. Congenital alveolar proteinosis: failure of treatment with extracorporeal life support. J Pediatr 1992; 120:297–302.

93. Nogee LM, DeMello DE, Dehner L, Colten HR. Brief report: deficiency of pulmonary surfactant protein B in conenital alveolar proteinosis. N Engl J Med 1993; 328: 406–410.

94. Nogee LM, Garnier G, Dietz HC, Singer L, Murphy AM, deMello DE, Colten HR. A mutation in the surfactant protein B gene responsible for fatal neonatal respiratory disease in multiple kindreds. J Clin Invest 1994; 93:1860–1863.

95. Hamvas A, Cole FS, deMello DE, Moxley M, Whitsett JA, Colten HR, Nogee LM. Surfactant protein B deficiency: antenatal diagnosis and prospective treatment with surfactant replacement. J Pediatr 1994; 125:356–361.

96. deMello DE, Nogee LM, Heyman S, Krous HF, Hussain M, Merritt TA, Hsueh W, Haas JE, Heidelbergeer K, Schumacher R, Colten HR. Molecular and phenotypic variability in the congenital alveolar proteinosis syndrome associated with inherited sufactant protein B deficiency. J Pediatr 1994; 125:43–50.

97. Kobayashi T, Nitta K, Takahashi R, Kurashima K, Robertson B, Suzuki Y. Activity of pulmonary surfactant after blocking the associated proteins SP-A and SP-B. J Appl Physiol 1991; 71:530–536.

98. Robertson B, Kobayashi T, Ganzuka M, Grossmann G, Li WZ, Suzuki Y. Experimental neonatal respiratory failure induced by a monoclonal antibody to the hydrophobic surfactant-associated protein SP-B. Pediatr Res 1991; 30:239–243.

99. Liggins GC. Premature delivery of foetal lambs infused with glucocorticoids. J Endocrinology 1969; 45:515–523.

100. Seidner S, Pettenazzo A, Ikegami M, Jobe A. Corticosteroid potentiation of surfactant dose response in preterm rabbits. J Appl Physiol 1988; 64:2366–2371.

101. Platzker ACG, Kitterman JA, Mescher EJ, Clements JA, Tooley WH. Surfactant in the lung and tracheal fluid of the fetal lamb and acceleration of its appearance by dexamethasone. Pediatrics 1975; 56:554–561.

102. Johnson J, Mitzner W, London W, Palmer A, Scott R, Kearney K. Glucocorticoids and the rhesus fetal lung. Am J Obstet Gynecol 1978; 130:906–916.

103. Kikawa Y, Kaibara M, Motoyama EK, Orzalesi MM, Cook CD. Morphologic development of fetal rabbit lung and its acceleration with cortisol. Am J Pathol 1971; 64:423–442.

104. Bunton TE, Plopper CG. Triamcinolone-induced structural alterations in the development of the lung of the fetal rhesus macaque. Am J Obstet Gynecol 1984; 148: 203–215.

105. Gonzales LW, Ballard PL, Ertsey R, Williams MC. Glucocorticoids and thyroid hormones stimulate biochemical and morphological differentiation of human fetal lung in organ culture. J Clin Endocrinol Metab 1986; 62:678–691.

106. Crowley P, Chalmers I, Keirse MJNC. The effects of corticosteroid administration before preterm delivery: an overview of the evidence from controlled trials. Brit J Obstet Gynecol 1990; 97:11–25.

107. Fairclough RJ, Liggins GC. Protein binding of plasma cortisol in the foetal lamb near term. J Endocrinol 1975; 67:333–341.

108. Ballard PL, Kitterman JA, Bland RD, Clyman RI, Gluckman PD, Platzker CG, Kaplan SL, Grumbach MM. Ontogeny and regulation of corticosteroid binding globulin capacity in plasma of fetal and newborn lambs. Endocrinology 1982; 110: 359–366.

109. Hitchcock KR. Hormones and the lung. I. Thyroid hormones and glucocorticoids in lung development. Anat Rec 1979; 195:15–40.

110. Liggins GC, Kitterman JA, Campos GA, Clements JA, Forster CS, Lee CC, Creasy RK. Pulmonary maturation in the hypophysectomized ovine fetus. Differential responses to adrenocorticotrophin and cortisol. J Dev Physiol 1981; 3:1–14.

111. Kitterman JA, Liggins GC, Campos GA, Clements JA, Forster CS, Lee CC, Creasy RK. Prepartum maturation of the lung in fetal sheep: relation to cortisol. J Appl Physiol 1981; 51:384–390.

112. Crone RK, Davies P, Liggins GC, Reid L. The effects of hypophysectomy, throidectomy and postoperative infusion of cortisol or adrenocorticotrophin on the structure of the ovine fetal lung. J Dev Physiol 1983; 5:281–288.

113. Gonzales LW, Ballard PL. Hormones and their receptors. In: Massoro D., ed. Lung Cell Biology. New York: Dekker, 1989:539–589.

114. Beato M. Gene regulation by steroid hormones. Cell 1989; 56:335–344.

115. Carson-Jurica MA, Schrader WT, O'Malley BW. Steroid receptor family: structure and functions. Endocr Rev 1990; 11:201–220.

116. Fuller PJ. The steroid receptor superfamily: mechanisms of diversity. FASEB J 1991; 5:3092–3099.

117. Wright APH, Zilliacus J, McEwan IJ, Dahlman-Wright K, Almof T, Carlstedt-Duke J, Gustafsson J-A. Structure and function of the glucocorticoid receptor. J Steroid Biochem Mol Biol 1993; 47:11–19.

118. Bresnick E, Dalman F, Sanchez E, Pratt W. Evidence that the 90-kDa heat shock protein is necessary for the steroid binding conformation of the L cell glucocorticoid receptor. J Biol Chem 1989; 264:4992–4997.

119. Nemoto T, Ohara NY, Denis M, Gustafsson J-A. The transformed glucocorticoid receptor has a lower steroid-binding affinity than the nontransformed receptor. Biochemistry 1990; 29:1880–1886.

120. Hollenberg S, Weingerger C, Ong E, Cerelli G, Oro A, Lebo R, Thompson E, Rosenfeld M, Evans R. Primary structure and expression of a functional human glucocorticoid receptor cDNA. Nature 1985; 313:635–641.

121. Encio IJ, Detera-Wadleigh SD. The genomic structure of the glucocorticoid receptor. J Biol Chem 1991; 266:7182–7188.

122. Hard T, Kelenbach E, Boelens R, Maler BA, Dahlman K, Freedman LP, Carlstedt-Duke J, Yamamoto KR, Gustafsson J-A, Kaptein R. Solution structure of the glucocorticoid receptor DNA-binding domain. Science 1990; 249:157–160.

123. Tsai SY, Carlstedt-Duke J, Weighel NL, Dahlman K, Gustafsson J-A, Tsai MJ, O'Malley BW. Molecular interactions of steroid hormone receptor with its enhancer element: evidence for receptor dimer formation. Cell 1988; 55:361–369.

124. Wrange O, Eriksson P, Perlmann T. The purified activated glucocorticoid receptor is a homodimer. J Biol Chem 1989; 264:5253–5259.

125. Schule R, Muler M, Kaltschmidt C, Renkawitz R. Many transcription factors interact synergistically with steroid receptors. Science 1988; 242:1418–1420.

126. Lucas PC, Granner DK. Hormone response domains in gene transcription. Annu Rev Biochem 1992; 61:1131–1173.

127. McEwan IJ, Wright APH, Dahlman-Wright K, Carstedt-Duke J, Gustafsson J-A. Direct interaction of the tau1 transactivation domain of the human glucocorticoid receptor with the basal transcriptional machinery. Mol Cell Biol 1993; 13:399–407.

128. Cordingley MG, Riegel AT, Hager GL. Steroid-dependent interaction of transcription factor with the inducible promoter of mouse mammary tumor virus in vivo. Cell 1987; 48:261–270.

129. Beer PG, Cunha GR, Malkinson AM. Autoradiographic demonstration of the specific binding and nuclear localization of $^3$H dexamethasone in adult mouse lung. Lab Invest 1983; 49:725–734.

130. Ballard PL, Ballard RA, Gonzales LK, Wilson CM, Gross I. Corticosteroid binding by fetal rat and rabbit lung in organ culture. J Steroid Biochem Mol Biol 1984; 21:117–126.

131. Granberg JP, Ballard PL. The role of sulfhydryl groups in the binding of glucocorticoids by cytoplasmic receptors of lung and other mamalian tissues. Endocrinology 1977; 100:1160–1168.

132. Bronnegard M, Okret S. Regulation of the glucocorticoid receptor in fetal rat lung during development. J Steroid Biochem Mol Biol 1991; 39:13–17.

133. Flint APF, Burton RD. Properties and ontogeny of the glucocorticoid receptor in the placenta and fetal lung of the sheep. J Endocrinol 1984; 103:31.

134. Yarney TA, Kendall JZ, Randall GCB. Cytosolic glucocorticoid receptors in the porcine lung during development and after hypophysectomy or thyroidectomy. J Endocrinology 1990; 127:341–349.

135. Bourgeois S, Newby RF. Correlation between glucocorticoid receptor and cytolytic response of murine lymphoid cell lines. Cancer Res 1979; 39:4749–4751.

136. Vanderbilt JN, Miesfeld R, Maler BA, Yamamoto KR. Intracellular receptor concentration limits glucocorticoid-dependent enhancer activity. Mol Endocrinol 1987; 1:68–74.

137. Okret S, Dong Y, Bronnegard M, Gustafsson J-A. Regulation of glucocorticoid receptor expression. Biochimie 1991; 73:51–59.

138. Dong Y, Poellinger L, Gustafsson JA, Okret S. Regulation of glucocorticoid receptor expression: evidence for transcriptional and posttranslational mechanisms. Mol Endocrinol 1988; 2:1256–1264.

139. Gruol DJ, Faith CN, Bourgeois S. Cyclic AMP-dependent kinase promotes glucocorticoid receptor function. J Biol Chem 1986; 261:4909–4914.

140. Dong Y, Aronsson M, Gustafsson J-A, Okret S. The mechanism of cAMP-induced glucocorticoid receptor expression. Correlation to cellular glucocorticoid response. J Biol Chem 1989; 264:13679–13683.

141. Lazar MA. Thyroid hormone receptors: multiple forms, multiple possibilities. Endocr Rev 1993; 14:184–193.

142. Hudson LG, Santon JB, Glass CK, Gill GN. Ligand-activated thyroid hormone and retinoid acid receptors inhibit growth factor receptor promoter expression. Cell 1990; 62:1165–1175.

143. Baniahmad A, Steiner C, Kohne AC, Renkawitz R. Modular structure of a chicken lysozyme silencer: involvement of an unusual thyroid hormone receptor binding site. Cell 1990; 61:505–514.

144. Gonzales LW, Ballard PL. Identification and characterization of nuclear 3,5,3′ triiodothyronine receptors in rabbit lung: characterization and developmental changes. J Clin Endocrinol Metab 1981; 53:21–28.

145. Bernal J, Pekonen F. Ontogenesis of the nuclear 3,5,3′-triiodothyronine receptor in the human fetal brain. Endocrinology 1984; 127:278–284.

146. Luo M, Faure R, Tong YA, Dussault JH. Immunocytochemical localization of the nuclear 3,5,3′-triiodothyronine receptor in the adult rat: liver, kidney, heart lung and spleen. Acta Endocrinol 1989; 120:451–458.

147. Gonzales LW, Ballard PL. Nuclear 3,5,3′-triiodothyronine receptors in rabbit lung: characterization and developmental changes. Endocrinology 1982; 111:542–552.

148. Ruel J, Coulombe P, Dussault JH. Characterization of nuclear 3,5,3′-triiodothyronine receptors in the developing rat lung: effects of hypo- and hyperthyroidism. Pediatr Res 1982; 16:238–242.

149. Brandsma AE, Tibboel D, Vulto IM, de Vijlder JJ, Ten Have-Opbroek AA, Wiersinga WM. Inhibition of T3-receptor binding by Nitrofen. Biochim Biophys Acta 1994; 1201:266–270.

150. Gomez J, Benovic JL. Molecular and regulatory properties of the adenylyl cylase-coupled beta-adrenergic receptors. Int Rev Cytol 1992; 137B:1–34.

151. Strader CD, Fong MT, Tota MR, Underwood D. Structure and function of G protein-coupled receptors. Annu Rev Biochem 1994; 63:101–132.

152. Ahlquist R. A study of the adrenotropic receptors. Am J Physiol 1948; 153:586–600.

153. Lands AM, Arnold A, McAuliff JP, Cuduena FP, Brown TG. Differentiation of receptor systems activated by sympathomimetic amines. Nature 1967; 214:597–598.

154. Dohlman HG, Thorner J, Caron MG, Lefkowitz RJ. Model systems for the study of seven-transmembrane-segment receptors. Annu Rev Biochem 1991; 60:653–688.

155. Hoeffler JP, Habener JF. Characterization of a cAMP regulatory element binding protein. Trends Endocrinol Metab 1990; 1:115–158.

156. Meyer TE, Habener JF. Cyclic adenosine 3',5'-monophosphate response element binding protein (CREB) and related transcription-activating deoxyribonucleic acid-binding proteins. Endocr Rev 1993; 14:269–290.

157. O'Shea EK, Klemm JD, Kim PS, Alber T. X-ray structure of the GCN4 leucine zipper, a two-stranded parallel coiled coil. Science 1991; 254:539–544.

158. Horikoshi M, Hai T, Ln YS, Green MR. Roeder RG. Transcription factor ATF interacts with the TATA factor to facilitate establishment of a preinitiation complex. Cell 1988; 54:1033–1042.

159. Leonard J, Serup P, Gonzalez G, Edlund T, Montminy MR. The LIM family transcription factor Isl-1 requires cAMP response element binding protein to promote somatostatin expression in pancreatic islet cells. Proc Natl Acad Sci USA 1992; 89:6247–6251.

160. Foulkes NS, Mellstrom B, Benusiglio E, Sassone-Corsi P. Developmental switch of CREM function during spermatogenesis from antagonist to activator. Nature 1992; 355:80–84.

161. Nijkamp FP. Beta-adrenergic receptors in the lung: an introduction. Life Sci 1993; 52:2073–2082.

162. Barnes P, Jacobs M, Roberts JM. Glucocorticoids preferentially increase fetal alveolar beta-adrenoreceptors: autoradiographic evidence. Pediatr Res 1984; 18:1191–1194.

163. Lewis V, Goldfien AC, Day JP, Roberts JM. Rabbit alveolar beta-adrenergic receptors increase with gestational age. Am J Obstet Gynecol 1990; 162:269–272.

164. Lyon ME, Lefebvre CA, Davis DJ. Characterisation of the beta-adrenergic response cascade in fetal guinea pig lung. Thorax 1994; 49:664–669.

165. Davis DJ, Dattel BJ, Ballard PL, Roberts JM. Beta-adrenergic receptors and cyclic adenosine monophosphate generation in human fetal lung. Pediatr Res 1987; 21:142–147.

166. Ewing CK, Duffy DM, Roberts JM. Characterization of the beta-adrenergic receptor in isolated human fetal lung type II cells. Pediatr Res 1992; 32:350–355.

167. Collins S, Bolanowski MA, Caron MG, Lefkowitz RJ. Genetic regulation of beta-adrenergic receptors. Annu Rev Physiol 1989; 51:203–215.

168. Collins S. Recent perspectives on the molecular structure and regulation of the β2-adrenoceptor. Life Sci 1993; 52:2083–2091.

169. Dixon RA, Kobilka BK, Strader DJ, Benovic JL, Dohlman HG, Frielle T, Bolanowski MA, Bennett CD, Rands E, Diehl RE. Cloning of the gene and cDNA for mammalian beta-adrenergic receptor and homology with rhodopsin. Nature 1986; 321:75–79.

170. Kobilka BK, Frielle T, Dohlman HG, Bolanowski MA, Dixon RA, Keler P, Caron MG, Lefkowitz RJ. Delineation of the intronless nature of the genes for the human and hamster beta 2-adrenergic receptor and their putative promoter regions. J Biol Chem 1987; 262:7321–7327.

171. Frielle T, Collins S, Daniel KW, Caron MG, Lefkowitz RJ, Kobilka BK. Cloning of the cDNA for the human beta 1-adrenergic receptor. Proc Natl Acad Sci USA 1987; 84:7920–7924.

172. Emorine LJ, Marullo S, Delavier-Klutchko C, Kaven SV, Durieu-Trautmann O, Strosberg AD. Structure of the gene for human beta 2-adrenergic receptor: expression and promoter characterization. Proc Natl Acad Sci USA 1987; 84:6995–6999.
173. Hadcock JR, Malbon CC. Regulation of beta-adrenergic receptors by "permissive" hormones: glucocorticoids increase steady-state levels of receptor mRNA. Proc Natl Acad Sci USA 1988; 85:8415–8419.
174. Collins S, Caron MG, Lefkowitz RJ. Beta-adrenergic receptors in hamster smooth muscle cells are transcriptionally regulated by glucocorticoids. J Biol Chem 1988; 263:9067–9070.
175. Davis DJ, Jacobs MM, Ballard PL, Gonzale LK, Roberts JM. β-adrenergic receptors and cAMP response increase during explant culture of human fetal lung: partial inhibition by dexamethasone. Pediatr Res 1990; 28:190–195.
176. Mak JC, Nishikawa M, Barnes PJ. Glucocorticosteroids increase β2-adrenergic receptor transcription in human lung. Am J Physiol 1995; 268:L41–L46.
177. Collins S, Bouvier M, Bolanowski MA, Caron MG, Lefkowitz RJ. cAMP stimulates transcription of the beta 2-adrenergic receptor gene in response to short-term agonist exposure. Proc Natl Acad Sci USA 1989; 86:4853–4857.
178. Hadcock JR, Ros M, Malbon CC. Agonist regulation of beta-adrenergic receptor mRNA. Analysis in S49 mouse lymphoma mutants. J Biol Chem 1989; 264:13956–13961.
179. Ballard PL, Gonzales LG, Williams MC, Roberts JM, Jacobs MM. Differentiation of type II cells during explant culture of human fetal lung is accelerated by endogenous prostanoids and adenosine 3′,5′-monophosphate. Endocrinology 1991; 128:2916–2924.
180. Duffy DM, Ballard PL, Goldfien A, Roberts JM. Cyclic adenosine 3′,5′-monophosphate increase β-adrenergic receptor concentration in cultured human fetal lung explants and type II cells. Endocrinology 1992; 131:841–846.
181. Lazar-Wesley E, Hadcock JR, Malbon CC, Kunos G, Ishac EJ. Tissue-specific regulation of alpha 1B, beta 1 and beta 2-adrenergic receptor mRNAs by thyroid state in the rat. Endocrinology 1991; 129:1116–1118.
182. Das DK, Ayrolmloi J, Bandyopadhyay D, Bandyopadhyay S, Neogi A, Steinberg H. Potentiation of surfactant release in fetal lung by thyroid hormone action. J Appl Physiol 1984; 56:1621–1626.
183. Moawad AH, River LP, Lin C-C. Estrogen increases β-adrenergic binding in the preterm fetal rabbit lung. Am J Obstet Gynecol 1985; 151:514–519.
184. Moawad AH, River LP, River JM. Dihydrotestosterone decreases β-adrenergic receptor binding in the fetal rabbit lung. Am J Perinatol 1988; 5:283–285.
185. Warburton D, Parton L, Buckley S, Cosico L, Saluna T. β-receptors and surface active material flux in fetal lamb lung: female advantage. J Appl Physiol 1987; 63:828–833.
186. Warburton D, Buckley S, Parton L, Saluna T. Chronic glucose infusion inhibits development of β-receptor binding in fetal lamb lung. Pediatr Res 1988; 24:171–174.
187. Davis DJ, Hickman JM, Lefebvre CA, Lyon ME. Insulin inhibits β-adrenergic responses in fetal rabbit lung in explant culture. Am J Physiol 1992; 263:L562–L567.

188. Ballard PL. Hormonal regulation of pulmonary surfactant. Endocr Rev 1989; 10: 165–181.

189. Rooney SA, Gobran L, Gross I, Wai-lee TS, Nardone LL, Motoyama EK. Studies on pulmonary surfactant. Effects of cortisol administration to fetal rabbits on lung phospholipid content, composition and biosynthesis. Biochim Biophys Acta 1976; 450:121–130.

190. Rooney SA, Gobran LI, Marino PA, Maniscalco WM, Gross I. Effects of betamethasone on phospholipid content, composition and biosynthesis in the fetal rabbit lung. Biochim Biophys Acta 1979; 572:64–76.

191. Kessler DL, Truog WE, Murphy JH, Palmer S, Standaert TA, Woodrum DE, Hodson WA. Experimental hyaline membrane disease in the premature monkey. Effects of antenatal dexamethasone. Am Rev Respir Dis 1982; 126:62–69.

192. Rooney SA, Gobran LI, Chu AJ. Thyroid hormone opposes some glucocorticoid effects on glycogen content and lipid synthesis in developing fetal rat lung. Pediatr Res 1986; 20:545–550.

193. Elkady T, Jobe A. Corticosteroids and surfactant increase lung volumes and decrease rupture pressures of preterm rabbit lungs. J Appl Physiol 1987; 63:1616–1621.

194. Sun B, Jobe AH, Rider E, Ikegami A. Single dose versus two doses of betamethasone for lung maturation in preterm rabbits. Pediatr Res 1993; 33:256–260.

195. Tabor BL, Rider ED, Ikegami M, Jobe AH, Lewis JF. Dose effects of antenatal corticosteroids for induction of lung maturation in preterm rabbits. Am J Obstet Gynecol 1993; 164:675–681.

196. Gross I, Wilson CM, Ingleson LD, Brehier A, Rooney SA. Fetal lung in organ culture. III. Comparison of dexamethasone, thyroxine, and methylxanthines. J Appl Physiol 1980; 48:872–877.

197. Gross I, Ballard PL, Ballard RA, Jones CT, Wilson CM. Corticosteroid stimulation of phosphatidylcholine synthesis in cultured fetal rabbit lung: evidence for de novo protein synthesis mediated by glucocorticoid receptors. Endocrinology 1983; 112: 829–837.

198. Xu Z, Rooney SA. Influence of dexamethasone on the lipid distribution of newly synthesized fatty acids in fetal rat lung. Biochim Biophys Acta 1989; 1005:209–216.

199. Odom MW, Ertsey R, Ballard PL. Hormonally regulated proteins in cultured human fetal lung: analysis by two-dimensional polyacrylamide gel electrophoresis. Am J Physiol 1990; 259:L283–L293.

200. Das DK. Fatty acid synthesis in fetal lung. Biochem Biophys Res Commun 1980; 92: 867–875.

201. Xu ZX, Stenzel W, Sasic SM, Smart DA, Rooney SA. Glucocorticoid regulation of fatty acid synthase gene expression in fetal rat lung. Am J Physiol 1993; 264:L140–L147.

202. Pope TS, Smart DA, Rooney SA. Hormonal effects on fatty-acid synthase in cultured fetal rat lung: induction by dexamethasone and inhibition of activity by triiodothyronine. Biochim Biophys Acta 1988; 959:169–177.

203. Maniscalco WM, Finkelstein JN, Parkhurst A. Dexamethasone increases de novo fatty acid synthesis in fetal rabbit lung explants. Pediatr Res 1985; 19:1272–1277.

204. Gonzales LW, Ertsey R, Balllard PL, Froh D, Goerke J, Gonzales J. Glucocorticoid

stimulation of fatty acid synthesis in explants of human fetal lung. Biochim Biophys Acta 1990; 1042:1–12.

205. Fraslon C, Batenbug JJ. Pre-translational regulation of lipid synthesizing enzymes and surfactant proteins in fetal rat lung in explant culture. FEBS Lett 1993; 325: 285–290.

206. Gonzales LW, Ballard PL, Gonzales J. Glucocorticoid and cAMP increase fatty acid synthetase mRNA in human fetal lung explants. Biochim Biophys Acta 1994; 1215: 49–58.

207. Gross I, Dynia DW, Wilson CM, Wilson CM, Ingleson LD, Gewolb IH, Rooney SA. Glucocorticoid-thyroid hormone interactions in fetal rat lung. Pediatr Res 1984; 18:191–196.

208. Rooney SA, Dynia DW, Smart DA, Chu AJ, Ingleson LD, Wilson CM, Gross I. Glucocorticoid stimulation of choline-phosphate cytidylyltransferase activity in fetal rat lung: Receptor response relationships. Biochim Biophys Acta 1986; 888: 208–216.

209. Xu Z, Smart DA, Rooney SA. Glucocorticoid induction of fatty acid synthase mediates the stimulatory effect of the hormone on choline-phosphate cytidylyltransferase activity in fetal rat lung. Biochim Biophys Acta 1990; 1044:70–76.

210. Sharma A, Gonzales LW, Ballard PL. Hormonal regulation of cholinephosphate cytidylyltransferase in human fetal lung. Biochim Biophys Acta 1993; 1170: 237–244.

211. Ballard PL, Hovey ML, Gonzales LK. Thyroid hormone stimulation of phosphatidylcholine synthesis in cultured fetal rabbit lung. J Clin Invest 1984; 74:898–905.

212. Pope TS, Rooney SA. Effects of glucocorticoid and thyroid hormones on regulatory enzymes of fatty acid synthesis and glycogen metabolism in developing fetal rat lung. Biochim Biophys Acta 1987; 918:141–148.

213. Mendelson CR, Johnston JM, MacDonald PC, Snyder JM. Multihormonal regulation of surfactant synthesis by human fetal lung in vitro. J Clin Endocrinol Metab 1981; 53:307–317.

214. Smith BT, Post M. Fibroblast-pneumonocyte factor (review). Am J Physiol 1989; 257:L174–L178.

215. Tanswell AK, Smith BT. Cultured pulmonary epithelial cells: clonal isolation of human fetal alveolar type II cells. Birth defects: original article series: March of Dimes Birth Defects Foundation, 1980:249–259.

216. Post M, Floros J, Smith BT. Inhibition of lung maturation by monoclonal antibodies against fibroblast-pneumonocyte factor. Nature 1984; 308:284–286.

217. Floros J, Post M, Smith BT. Glucocorticoids affect the synthesis of pulmonary fibroblast-pneumonocyte factor at a pretranslational level. J Biol Chem 1985; 260:2265–2267.

218. Torday JS. Dihydrotestosterone inhibits fibroblast-pneumonocyte factor–mediated synthesis of saturated phosphatidylcholine by fetal rat lung cells. Biochim Biophys Acta 1985; 835:23–28.

219. Floros J, Nielsen HC, Torday JS. Dihydrotestosterone blocks fetal lung fibroblast-pneumonocyte factor at a pretranslational level. J Biol Chem 1987; 262:13592–13598.

220. Nielsen HC. Epidermal growth factor influences the developmental clock regulating maturation of the fetal lung fibroblast. Biochim Biophys Acta 1989; 1012:201–206.

221. Post MA, Barsoumian A, Smith BT. The cellular mechanism of glucocorticoid acceleration of fetal lung maturation. Fibroblast-pneumonocyte factor stimulates choline-phosphate cytidylyltransferase activity. J Biol Chem 1986; 261:2179–2184.

222. Cohen S. Isolation of a mouse submaxillary gland protein accelerating incisor eruption and eyelid opening in the newborn animal. J Biol Chem 1963; 237:1555–1562.

223. Campion SR, Niyogi SK. Interaction of epidermal growth factor with its receptor. Prog Nucl Acid Res Mol Biol 1994; 49:353–384.

224. Adamson ED, Meek J. The ontogeny of epidermal growth factor receptors during mouse development. Dev Biol 1984; 103:62–70.

225. Warburton D, Seth R, Shum L, Horcher PG, Hall FL, Werb Z, Slavkin HC. Epigenetic role of epidermal growth factor expression and signalling in embryonic mouse lung morphogenesis. Dev Biol 1992; 149:123–133.

226. Seth R, Shum L, Wu F, Wuenschell C, Hall FL, Slavkin HC, Warburton D. Role of epidermal growth factor expression in early mouse embryo lung branching morphogenesis in culture: antisense oligodeoxynucleotide inhibitory strategy. Dev Biol 1993; 158:555–559.

227. Raaberg L, Nexo E, Poulsen SS. Epidermal growth factor in the rat lung. Histochemistry 1991; 95:471–475.

228. Raaberg L, Nexo E, Buckley S, Luo W, Snead ML, Warburton D. Epidermal growth factor transcription, translation and signal transduction by rat type II pneumocytes in culture. Am J Respir Cell Mol Biol 1992; 6:44–49.

229. Raaberg L, Nexo E, Damsgaard Mikkelsen J, Seier Poulsen S. Immunohistochemical localisation and developmental aspects of epidermal growth factor in the rat. Histochemistry 1988; 89:351–356.

230. Devaskar UP. Epidermal growth factor receptors in fetal and maternal rabbit lung. Biochem Biophys Res Commun 1982; 107:714–720.

231. Johnson MD, Gray ME, Carpenter G, Pepinsky RB, Sundell H, Stahlman MT. Ontogeny of epidermal growth factor receptor/kinase and of lipocortin-1 in the ovine lung. Pediatr Res 1989; 25:535–541.

232. Nexo E, Kryger-Baggesen N. The receptor for epidermal growth factor is present in human fetal kidney, liver and lung. Regul Pept 1989; 26:1–8.

233. Catterton WZ, Escobedo MB, Sexson WR, Gray ME, Sundell HW, Stahlman MT. Effect of epidermal growth factor on lung maturation in fetal rabbits. Pediatr Res 1979; 13:108–118.

234. Sundell HW, Gray ME, Serenius FS, Escobedo MB, Stahlman MT. Effects of epidermal growth factor on lung maturation in fetal lambs. Am J Pathol 1980; 100:707–719.

235. Plopper CG, St. George JA, Read LC, Nishio SJ, Weir AJ, Edwards L, Tarantal AF, Pinkerton KE, Merritt TA, Whitsett JA, George-Nascimento C, Styne D. Acceleration of alveolar type II cell differentiation in fetal rhesus monkey lung by administration of EGF. Am J Physiol 1992; 262:L313–L321.

236. Goetzman BW, Read LC, Plopper CG, Tarantal AF, George-Nasciemento C, Merritt TA, Whitsett JA, Styne D. Prenatal exposure to epidermal growth factor attenuates respiratory distress syndrome in rhesus infants. Pediatr Res 1994; 35:30–36.

237. Gross I, Dynia DW, Roney SA, Smart DA, Warshaw JB, Sissom JF, Hoath SB. Influence of epidermal growth factor on fetal rat lung development in vitro. Pediatr Res 1986; 20:473–477.

238. Haigh RM, Hollingsworth M, Micklewright LA, Boyd RD, D'Souza SW. The effect of human urogastrone on lung phospholipids in fetal rabbits. J Dev Physiol 1988; 10:433–443.

239. Fraslon C, Bourbon JR. Comparison of effects of epidermal and insulin like growth factors, gastrin releasing peptide and retinoic acid on fetal lung cell growth and maturation in vitro. Biochim Biophys Acta 1992; 1123:65–75.

240. Sadiq HF, Uday PD. Glucocorticoids increase pulmonary epidermal growth factor receptors in female and male fetal rabbit. Biochem Biophys Res Commun 1984; 1984:408–414.

241. Oberg KC, Carpenter G. Dexamethasone acts as a negative regulator of epidermal growth factor receptor synthesis in fetal rat lung cells. Mol Endocrinol 1989; 3:915–922.

242. Klein JM, Nielsen HC. Androgen regulation of epidermal growth factor receptor binding activity during fetal rabbit lung development. J Clin Invest 1993; 91: 425–431.

243. Hofmann GE, Romaguera J, Williams RF, Adamsons K, Norfolk VA, San Juan PR. Intra-amniotic thyroxine for acceleration of fetal maturation. Acta Obstet Gynecol Scand 1993; 72:252–257.

244. Gluckman PD, Ballard PL, Kaplan SL, Liggins GC, Grumbach MM. Prolactin in umbilical cord blood and the respiratory distress syndrome. J Pediatr 1978; 93: 1011–1014.

245. Ballard PL, Gluckman PD, Brehier A, Kitterman JA, Kaplan SL, Rudolph AM, Grumbach MM. Failure to detect an effect of prolactin on pulmonary surfactant and adrenal steroids in fetal sheep and rabbits. J Clin Invest 1978; 62:879–883.

246. Mullon DK, Smith YF, Richardson LL, Hamosh M, Hamosh P. Effect of prolactin on phospholipid synthesis in organ cultures of fetal rat lung. Biochim Biophys Acta 1983; 751:166–174.

247. Cox MA, Torday JS. Pituitary oligopeptide regulation of phosphatidylcholine synthesis by fetal rabbit lung cells. Lack of effect with prolactin. Am Rev Respir Dis 1981; 123:181–184.

248. Josimovich JB, Merisko K, Boccella L, Tobon H. Binding of prolactin by fetal Rhesus cell membrane fractions. Endocrinology 1977; 100:557–570.

249. Chan JSD, Robertson HA, Friesen HG. Distribution of binding sites for ovine placental lactogen in the sheep. Endocrinology 1978; 102:632–640.

250. Labbe A, Delcros B, Dechelotte P, Nouailles C, Grizard G. Comparative study of the binding of prolactin and growth hormone by rabbit and human lung cell membrane fractions. Biol Neonate 1992; 61:179–187.

251. Schellenberg JC, Liggins GC, Manzai M, Kitterman JA, Lee CC. Synergistic hormonal effects on lung maturation in fetal sheep. J Appl Physiol 1988; 65:94–100.

252. Khosla SS, Rooney SA. Stimulation of fetal lung surfactant production by administration of 17β-estradiol to the maternal rabbit. Am J Obstet Gynecol 1979; 133: 213–216.

253. Khosla SS, Walker S, G.J., Parks PA, Rooney SA. Effects of estrogen on fetal rabbit lung maturation: morphological and biochemical studies. Pediatr Res 1981; 15: 1274–1981.

254. Gross I, Wilson CM, L.D. I, Brehier A, Rooney SA. The influence of hormones on the biochemical development of fetal rat lung in organ culture. I. Estrogen. Biochim Biophys Acta 1979; 575:375–383.

255. Khosla SS, Brehier A, Eisenfeld AJ, Ingleson LD, Parks PA, Rooney SA. Influence of sex hormones on lung maturation in the fetal rabbit. Biochim Biophys Acta 1983; 750:112–126.

256. Miller HC, Futrakul P. Birth weight, gestational age and sex as determining factors in the incidence of respiratory distress syndrome of prematurely born infants. J Pediatr 1968; 72:628–635.

257. Nielsen HC, Kirk WO, Sweezey N, Torday JS. Coordination of growth and differentiation in the fetal lung. Exp Cell Res 1990; 188:89–96.

258. Collaborative Group on Antenatal Steroid Therapy. Effect of antenatal dexamethasone administration on the prevention of respiratory distress syndrome. Am J Obstet Gynecol 1981; 141:276–287.

259. Torday JS. Androgens delay human fetal lung maturation in vitro. Endocrinology 1990; 126:3240–3244.

260. Robert MF, Neff RK, Hubbell JP, Taeusch HW, Avery ME. Association between maternal diabetes mellitus and the respiratory-distress syndrome in the newborn. N Engl J Med 1976; 294:357–360.

261. Bose CL, Manne DN, D'Ercole AJ, Lawson EE. Delayed fetal pulmonary maturation in a rabbit model of the diabetic pregnancy. J Clin Invest 1980; 66:220–226.

262. Sosenko IR, Lawson EE, Demottaz V, Frantz ID. Functional delay in lung maturation in fetuses of diabetic rabbits. J Appl Physiol 1980; 48:643–647.

263. Warburton D. Chronic hyperglycemia reduces surface active material flux in tracheal fluid of fetal lambs. J Clin Invest 1983; 71:550–555.

264. Warburton D. Chronic hyperglycemia with secondary hyperinsulinemia inhibits the maturational response of fetal lambs to cortisol. J Clin Invest 1983; 72:433–440.

265. Gross I, Smith GJ, Wilson CM, Maniscalco WM, Ingleson LD, Brehier A, Rooney SA. The influence of hormones on the biochemical development of fetal rat lung in organ culture. II. Insulin. Pediatr Res 1980; 14:834–838.

266. Smith BT, Giroud CJP, Robert M, Avery ME. Insulin antagonism of cortisol action on lecithin synthesis by cultured fetal lung cells. J Pediatr 1975; 87:953–955.

267. Rooney SA, Ingleson LD, Wilson CM, Gross I. Insulin antagonism of dexamethasone-induced stimulation of cholinephosphate cytidylyltransferase in fetal rat lung in organ culture. Lung 1980; 158:151–155.

268. Carlson KS, Smith BT, Post M. Insulin acts on the fibroblast to inhibit glucocorticoid stimulation of lung maturation. J Appl Physiol 1984; 57:1577–1579.

269. Phelps DS, Church S, Kourembanas S, Taeusch HW, Floros J. Increases in the 35

kDa surfactant-associated protein and its mRNA following in vivo dexamethasone treatment of fetal and neonatal rats. Electrophoresis 1987; 8:235–238.

270. Shimizu H, Miyamura K, Kuroki Y. Appearance of surfactant proteins, SP-A and SP-B, in developing rat lung and the effects of in vivo dexamethasone treatment. Biochim Biophys Acta 1991; 1081:53–60.

271. Ogasawara Y, Kuroki Y, Tsuzuki A, Ueda S, Misaki H, Akino T. Pre- and postnatal stimulation of pulmonary surfactant protein D by in vivo dexamethasone treatment of rats. Life Sci 1992; 50:1761–1767.

272. Schellhase DE, Shannon JM. Effects of maternal dexamethasone on expression of SP-A, SP-B, and SP-C in the fetal rat lung. Am J Respir Cell Mol Biol 1991; 4: 304–312.

273. Floros J, Phelps DS, Harding HP, Church S, Ware J. Postnatal stimulation of rat surfactant protein A synthesis by dexamethasone. Am J Physiol 1989; 257:L137–L143.

274. Durham PL, Wohlford-Lenane CL, Snyder JM. Glucocorticoid regulation of surfactant-associated proteins in rabbit fetal lung in vivo. Anat Rec 1993; 237: 365–377.

275. Whitsett JA, White T, Clark JC, Weaver TE. Induction of surfactant protein in fetal lung. Effects of cAMP and dexamethasone on SAP-35 RNA and synthesis. J Biol Chem 1987; 262:5256–5261.

276. Odom MJ, Snyder JM, Boggaram V, Mendelson CR. Glucocorticoid regulaton of the major surfactant associated protein (SP-A) and its messenger ribonucleic acid and of morphological development of human fetal lung *in vitro*. Endocrinology 1988; 123: 1712–1720.

277. Liley HG, White TR, Benson BJ, Ballard PL. Glucocorticoids both stimulate and inhibit production of pulmonary surfactant-protein A in fetal human lung. Proc Natl Acad Sci USA 1988; 85:9096–9100.

278. Boggaram V, Smith ME, Mendelson CR. Regulation of expression of the gene encoding the major surfactant protein (SP-A) in human fetal lung in vitro. J Biol Chem 1989; 264:11421–11427.

279. Boggaram V, Smith ME, Mendelson CR. Posttranscriptional regulation of surfactant protein-A mRNA in human fetal lung in vitro by glucocorticoids. Mol Endocrinol 1991; 5:414–423.

280. Iannuzzi DM, Ertsey R, Ballard PL. Biphasic glucocorticoid regulation of pulmonary SP-A: characterization of inhibitory process. Am J Physiol 1993; 264:L236–L244.

281. Nichols KV, Floros J, Dynia DW, Veletza SV, Wilson CM, Gross I. Regulaton of surfactant protein A mRNA by hormones and butyrate in cultured fetal rat lung. Am J Physiol 1990; 259:L488–L495.

282. Whitsett JA, Weaver TE, Lieberman MA, Clark JC, Daugherty C. Differential effects of epidermal growth factor and transforming growth factor-β on synthesis of Mr=35,000 surfactant-associated protein in fetal lung. J Biol Chem 1987; 262:7908–7913.

283. Ballard PL, Liley HG, Gonzales LW, Odom MW, Ammann AJ, Benson B, White

TR, Williams MC. Interferon-gamma and synthesis of surfactant components by cultured human fetal lung. Am J Respir Cell Mol Biol 1990; 2:137–143.

284. Snyder JM, Mendelson CR. Insulin inhibits the accumulation of the major lung surfactant apoprotein in human fetal lung explants maintained in vitro. Endocrinology 1987; 120:1250–1257.

285. Dekowski SA, Snyder JM. Insulin regulation of messenger ribonucleic acid for the surfactant-associated proteins in human fetal lung in vitro. Endocrinology 1992; 131:669–676.

286. Katayal SL, Amenta JS, Singh G, Silverman JA. Deficient lung surfactant apoproteins in amniotic fluid with mature phospholipid profile from diabetic pregnancies. Am J Obstet Gynecol 1984; 148:48–53.

287. Pryhuber GS, OR MA, Clark JC, Hull WM, Fink I, Whitsett JA. Phorbol ester inhibits surfactant protein SP-A and SP-B expression. J Biol Chem 1990; 265: 20822–20828.

288. Wispe JR, Clark JC, Warner BB, Fajardo D, Hull WM, Holtzman RB, Whitsett JA. Tumor necrosis factor-alpha inhibits expression of pulmonary surfactant protein. J Clin Invest 1990; 86:1954–1960.

289. Phelps DS, Floros J. Dexamethasone in vivo raises surfactant protein B mRNA in alveolar and bronchiolar epithelium. Am J Physiol 1991; 260:L146–L152.

290. Whitsett JA, Weaver TE, Clark JC, Sawtell N, Glasser SW, Korfhagen TR, Hull WM. Glucocorticoid enhances surfactant proteolipid Phe and pVal synthesis and RNA in fetal lung. J Biol Chem 1987; 262:15618–15623.

291. Venkatesh VC, Iannuzzi DM, Ertsey R, Ballard PL. Differential glucocorticoid regulation of the pulmonary hydrophobic surfactant proteins SP-B and SP-C. Am J Respir Cell Mol Biol 1993; 8:222–228.

292. Warr RG, Hawgood S, Buckley DI, Crisp TM, Schilling J, Benson BJ, Ballard PL, Clements JA, White RT. Low molecular weight human pulmonary surfactant (SP5): Isolation, characterization and cDNA and amino acid sequences. Proceed Natl Acad Sci USA 1987; 84:7915–7919.

293. O'Reilly MA, Gazdar AF, Clark JC, Pilot-Matias TJ, Wert SE, Hull WM, Whitsett JA. Glucocorticoids regulate surfactant protein synthesis in a pulmonary adenocarcinoma cell line. Am J Physiol 1989; 257:L385–L392.

294. O'Reilly MA, Clark JC, Whitsett JA. Glucocorticoid enhances pulmonary surfactant protein B gene transcription. Am J Physiol 1991; 260:L37–L43.

295. Floros J, Gross I, Nichols KV, Veletza SV, Dynia D, Lu H, Wilson CM, Peterec SM. Hormonal effects on the surfactant protein B (SP-B) mRNA in cultured fetal rat lung. Am J Respir Cell Mol Biol 1991; 4:449–454.

296. Veletza SV, Nichols KV, Gross I, Lu H, Dynia DW, Floros J. Surfactant protein C: hormonal control of SP-C mRNA levels in vitro. Am J Physiol 1992; 262:L684–L687.

297. Margana RK, Boggaram V. Transcription and mRNA stability regulate developmental and hormonal expression of rabbit surfactant protein B gene. Am J Physiol 1995; 268:L481–490.

298. Boggaram V, Margana R. Developmental and hormonal regulation of surfactant protein C (SP-C) gene expression in fetal lung. J Biol Chem 1994; 269:27767–27772.

299. Whitsett JA, Clark JC, Wispe JR, Pryhuber GS. Effects of TNF-α and phorbol ester on human surfactant protein and MnSOD gene transcription in vitro. Am J Physiol 1992; 262:L688–L693.

300. Guttentag SH, Phelps DS, Stenzel W, Warshaw JB, Floros J. Surfactant protein-A expression is delayed in fetuses of streptozotocin-treated rats. Am J Physiol 1992; 262:L489–L494.

301. Guttentag SH, Phelps DS, Warshaw JB, Floros J. Delayed hydrophobic surfactant protein (SP-B, SP-C) expression in fetuses of streptozotocin-treated rats. Am J Respir Cell Mol Biol 1992; 7:190–197.

302. Kouretas D, Karinch AM, Rishi A, Melchers K, Floros J. Conservation analysis of rat and human SP-A gene identifies 5' flanking sequences of rat SP-A that bind rat lung nuclear proteins. Exp Lung Res 1992; 19:485–503.

303. Lacaze-Masmonteil T, Fraslon C, Bourbon J, Raymondjean M, Kahn A. Characterization of the rat pulmonary surfactant protein A promoter. Eur J Biochem 1992; 206:613–623.

304. Alcorn JL, Gao E, Chen Q, Smith ME, Gerard RD, Mendelson CR. Genomic elements involved in transcriptional regulation of the rabbit surfactant protein-A gene. Mol Endocrinol 1993; 7:1072–1085.

305. Liley HG, Hawgood S, Gonzales LW, Benson BJ, Odom MW, Ertsey R, Ballard PL. Synthesis of surfactant components by cultured type II cells from human fetal lung. Biochim Biophys Acta 1988; 961:86–95.

306. Bohinski RJ, Huffman JA, Whitsett JA, Lattier DL. Cis-active elements controlling lung cell-specific expression of human pulmonary surfactant protein B gene. J Biol Chem 1993; 268:1160–1166.

307. Bohinski RJ, Di Lauro R, Whitsett JA. The lung-specific surfactant protein B gene promoter is a target for thyroid transcription factor 1 and hepatocyte nuclear factor 3, indicating common factors for organ-specific gene expression along the foregut axis. Mol Cell Biol 1994; 14:5671–5681.

308. Bruno MD, Bohinski RJ, Huelsman KM, Whitsett JA, Korfhagen TR. Lung cell–specific expression of the murine surfactant protein A (SP-A) gene is mediated by interactions between the SP-A promoter and thyroid transcription factor-1. J Biol Chem 1995; 270:6531–6536.

309. Venkatesh VC, Planer BC, Schwartz M, Vanderbilt JN, White RT Ballard PL. Characterization of the promoter of human pulmonary surfactant protein B gene. Am J Physiol 1995; 268:L674–682.

310. Bruno MA, Bohinski RJ, Carter JE, Foss KA, Whitsett JA. Structure and function of the mouse surfactant protein B gene. Am J Physiol 1995; 268:L381–L389.

311. Gao E, Alcorn JL, Mendelson CR. Identification of enhancers in the 5'-flanking region of the rabbit surfactant protein A (SP-A) gene and characterization of their binding proteins. J Biol Chem 1993; 268:19697–19709.

# 16

## Lung Injury When Development Is Interrupted by Premature Birth

**STUART HOROWITZ and JONATHAN M. DAVIS**

CardioPulmonary Research Institute
Winthrop-University Hospital
State University of New York at Stony Brook School of Medicine
Mineola, New York

## I. Introduction

When infants are born prior to term, the neonatal lung is often quite immature and not yet ready to adapt to an air-breathing environment. The premature lung may be also be exposed to toxins from infection, hyperoxia, and mechanical ventilation, which can disrupt the normal process of lung development. If this disruption is severe and the lung is not able to compensate, then irreversible pulmonary abnormalities may develop. However, significant advances in our understanding of both normal and abnormal lung development have been made in the last 25 years based on comprehensive and interactive basic science and clinical studies. These have enabled us to develop new therapies that markedly reduce mortality and improve the outcome of preterm and term newborns. However, much more needs to be learned if we are to continue to improve the outcome of these critically ill premature infants. The application of modern approaches, including molecular and cellular biology, together with carefully planned animal and human studies, should lead to greater improvements.

In this chapter, we examine the acute and chronic disorders of lung maturation and development that occur primarily in premature neonates. A very brief overview of the clinical manifestations and pathophysiological changes that occur in lung is followed by a review of the mechanisms thought to be involved in the pathogenesis of these disorders in infants. Finally, we review data gathered from a variety of animal models in order to glean new concepts and gain insights into acute and chronic lung disease in prematures.

## II.  Respiratory Distress Syndrome

Beginning at approximately 22–24 weeks' gestation, the cuboidal epithelial cells lining the respiratory bronchioles start to thin out and the capillaries begin to grow closer to the primitive alveoli. Type II epithelial cells, which produce pulmonary surfactant, begin to increase in number. In addition, the amount of surfactant present in these cells (stored in the form of lamellar bodies) starts to increase. When an infant is born prematurely, the lung may be structurally immature with insufficient pulmonary surfactant to stabilize alveoli and permit adequate gas exchange. Severe hypoxia and acidosis can also directly injure type II cells and further reduce the production of surfactant. The function of the limited amount of surfactant present in alveoli can also be inhibited by a variety of molecules such as serum proteins or red blood cells (1). With diminished pulmonary surfactant, the surface tension forces are elevated and the alveoli are unstable and largely atelectatic. Those infants who are surfactant deficient usually develop respiratory distress syndrome (RDS).

RDS affects approximately 30,000 infants born in the United States each year. The incidence is 50–60% in infants born at 24–28 weeks' gestation and decreases with increasing gestational age (2). Infants develop respiratory distress (i.e., tachypnea, retractions, cyanosis) soon after birth and chest radiographs demonstrate low lung volumes, air bronchograms, and reticular-granular infil-trates. Pathological findings include atelectasis, pulmonary edema, congestion, and hemorrhage (3). Injury to epithelial cells in the small airways and alveoli is often seen along with characteristic hyaline membrane formation.

### A.  Prevention and Treatment

The recent reduction in the severity of RDS and the ultimate eradication of this disease process depends heavily on continued improvements in maternal care. Comprehensive antenatal care is critical with particular attention to underlying medical conditions and the prevention of preterm labor. Maternal treatment with tocolytics (i.e., $MgSO_4$, terbutaline), antibiotics, and most importantly glucocor-ticoids is essential in decreasing the incidence and severity of RDS. Steroids appear to accelerate fetal lung maturation and prevent RDS and its associated morbidities. A consensus has developed recommending administration of either betamethasone or dexamethasone to all mothers who are in preterm labor and at risk for delivering a preterm infant between 24 and 34 weeks of gestation.

Thyroid-releasing hormone (TRH) appears in a small number of studies to enhance the effects of antenatal corticosteroids and further accelerate lung maturation and surfactant production (4). A large-scale, multicenter trial is currently underway to determine if TRH therapy should be used routinely in conjunction with antenatal corticosteroids.

Treatment of infants with RDS depends on the severity of the clinical symptoms. Oxygen therapy can be used if RDS is mild. For more significant illness, respiratory support with nasal continuous positive airway pressure or positive pressure mechanical ventilation can be instituted. The use of exogenous surfactant therapy in the treatment of RDS has become routine and widespread. Surfactant treatment has been shown in multiple studies to result in significant improvements in survival, gas exchange, and pulmonary mechanics (2,5,6). This is true despite significant differences in the type of surfactant used (i.e., natural, synthetic, human), study populations and timing of administration. Early use of surfactant therapy appears to be most beneficial, especially when the infant's mother has received antenatal steroids (6). Despite rapid clinical improvements following intratracheal instillation, detailed surfactant distribution studies have shown nonuniform distribution patterns (7). With the development of high-efficiency aerosol-delivery systems, the improvements from surfactant administration might occur in a slower, more controlled manner, perhaps at lower dosages and with more homogeneous distribution.

Many premature infants with RDS recover completely following exogenous surfactant therapy, whereas others go on to develop acute and chronic lung injury such as bronchopulmonary dysplasia (BPD). The reasons for this are not clear and are the subject of intense scientific investigations. Infants who recover appear to experience a biphasic response to injury: acute inflammation followed by repair of epithelium (8), whereas those who do not repair experience a continuum of injury and can develop BPD.

## III. Bronchopulmonary Dysplasia

Bronchopulmonary dysplasia was originally described by Northway as chronic lung changes in a group of 32 premature neonates who survived mechanical ventilation for treatment of RDS (9). This definition included clinical, radiological, and pathological criteria. BPD generally occurred beyond 28 days of age in patients who continued to require respiratory support. Chest radiographs demonstrated cyst formation and hyperexpansion alternating with areas of atelectasis. These infants were distinctly different than the majority of those who now develop BPD, mostly because the care of neonates has become more sophisticated, resulting in the survival of smaller and sicker infants. Many infants who currently develop chronic lung disease neither require prolonged mechanical ventilation nor have as severe radiographic or pathological changes. BPD is currently defined as oxygen ($O_2$) dependency at 28 days of life with appropriate radiographic findings (i.e., lung hyperinflation, emphysema, interstitial densities, and cardiovascular abnormalities) or $O_2$ dependency at 36 weeks' postconceptional age (10–12).

The reported incidence of BPD has varied, largely as a function of the definition used and the patient population studied. The introduction of surfactant replacement therapy has significantly improved survival for premature infants with RDS (13–18). However, the reported incidence of BPD (ranging from 15 to 60%) has been largely unaffected. With the improved survival of many critically ill patients, the prevalence of BPD may actually have increased following the introduction of surfactant therapy. Today, BPD affects approximately 7000 infants each year, many of whom suffer associated mortality and morbidities (i.e., asthma and neurological impairments). The long-term outcome for many of these patients is uncertain, and follow-up studies are currently underway. It is therefore crucial that we better understand this complex disease process.

## A.  Pathophysiology and Pathology

Lung compliance is reduced in infants with BPD (19). The decrease in lung compliance is correlated with atelectasis, edema, and fibrosis. In the early stages, an increase in pulmonary resistance and airway reactivity can be demonstrated (20). The increased resistance may cause increased work of breathing and marked abnormalities in ventilation-perfusion matching. Functional residual capacity can be reduced initially due to atelectasis but can be elevated in later stages of BPD owing to excessive air trapping and hyperinflation. Arterial blood gases can show a combination of hypoxemia, hypercarbia, and acidosis secondary to these abnormalities. As the disease worsens, airway obstruction can become more significant with expiratory flow limitation seen on flow-volume curves (21).

The most prominent pathological changes are usually seen in the terminal bronchioles and alveolar ducts (22). Hyaline membranes that are present with RDS become covered with a dysplastic lining composed mostly of type II pneumocytes. These membranes may then become incorporated into the underlying airway. Edema, inflammation, exudate, and epithelial cell necrosis usually occur next if the process continues. If the damage is severe, necrotizing bronchiolitis can develop. Cellular debris, inflammatory cells, and proteinaceous exudate can obstruct many of the terminal airways. Fibroblast proliferation and activation in response to this insult leads to peribronchial fibrosis and obliterative bronchiolitis. This causes narrowing of some small airways and further obstruction in others. The large upper airways (trachea, main bronchi) of infants with BPD may also be abnormal if the duration of intubation and mechanical ventilation is prolonged. Mucosal edema and necrosis can be focal or diffuse, with some of the necrotic areas breaking down into ulcerations (23). The earliest histological changes in proximal airways include patchy loss of cilia from columnar epithelial cells. These cells may then become dysplastic or necrotic. Necrotic areas can be superficial or extend into the submucosa, and they are usually accompanied by inflammatory cell infiltration. Hyperplastic goblet cells increase their secretion of mucus, which becomes mixed with dense cellular debris. Mucosal cells can regenerate or be replaced by stratified squamous epithelium or metaplastic epithelium if the injury continues.

The earliest indications found and seen in parenchyma are interstitial and alveolar edema. Later, focal areas of atelectasis, inflammation, exudate, and fibroblast proliferation can be seen. When BPD progresses and becomes more severe, areas of atelectasis become more widespread and alternate with areas of marked hyperinflation. These hyperinflated areas can become emphysematous blebs. End-stage BPD is usually characterized by significant fibrosis both in the interstitial and alveolar compartments. Capillary beds can be severely damaged, and together with medial muscle hypertrophy of pulmonary arterioles, can lead to marked pulmonary hypertension.

### B. Pathogenesis

There is no single cause of BPD in all infants. Its origin is multifactorial and appears to depend on the nature of the initial lung injury and the infant's response to it. BPD was first attributed to prolonged hyperoxia in infants with RDS (9). It is now widely accepted that pulmonary $O_2$ toxicity plays a significant role in the etiology of BPD, and many animal studies have been launched in an attempt to improve our understanding of how hyperoxia injures lungs. However, numerous additional etiologies of BPD have been proposed. This section reviews some of the complex factors that are involved in the pathogenesis of BPD.

#### Hyperoxia

Ventilatory support with supraphysiological concentrations of $O_2$ (>21%) is needed for babies with RDS, but hyperoxia is toxic, especially to lungs, probably because they receive direct exposure (24). Even the normal metabolism of atmospheric $O_2$ (21%) requires a family of networked and partially redundant enzymatic and nonenzymatic antioxidants, which have presumably evolved to detoxify highly reactive $O_2$-derived radicals that are natural by-products of aerobic metabolism. That hyperoxia is toxic to cells and organs suggests that evolution has not endowed antioxidants with inducible mechanisms sufficient to cope with this insult. Indeed, animal studies indicate that pulmonary antioxidant enzymes are only somewhat inducible by hyperoxia. Exposure of human volunteers to 100% $O_2$ for up to 15 hr, during which 24 of 33 individuals had evidence of tracheobronchitis, did not result in increased expression of mRNAs for catalase, Cu, Zn–superoxide dismutase (SOD), or Mn-SOD, in bronchial epithelial cells from these patients. This suggests that antioxidant expression might be constitutive in human lung (25). Clinical evidence supports the notion that endogenous antioxidants are overwhelmed by hyperoxia, resulting in the accumulation of reactive $O_2$ species, which damage the lung. Exposure of human volunteers to 50% $O_2$ caused increased fluorescent products of lipid peroxidation and partial oxidation of $\alpha_1$-antitrypsin in BAL fluid. In addition, leukotriene $B_4$ production by lavaged alveolar macrophages was increased, and there was a small but significant increase in lavaged neutrophils (26), suggesting that even a relatively moderate hyperoxic insult is damaging. Premature babies may be at increased risk, since they show evidence of oxidant stress in the levels of reduced glutathione (GSH) and oxidized glutathionine (GSSH) in peripheral blood (27). Antioxidant augmentation, either by nutritional supplements or novel therapies, therefore appears to be a rational approach to potentially mitigating oxy radical injury and preventing BPD (see Prevention below).

### Barotrauma

Although the initial phases of lung injury in BPD are often the eventual result of a primary disease process (e.g., RDS), positive-pressure mechanical ventilation superimposes additional lung injury (28). This acute injury is initially characterized by a complex inflammatory cascade, which ultimately leads to chronic lung disease. The role of barotrauma in BPD depends on several factors, including the structure of the tracheobronchial tree and the pathophysiological effects of surfactant deficiency. With surfactant deficiency and RDS, surface tension forces are elevated and significant atelectasis occurs. As a result, the ventilatory pressures needed to open these collapsed alveoli are high and are transmitted to the terminal bronchioles and alveolar ducts. In the premature neonate, these airways are highly compliant and subject to significant damage.

Since mechanical ventilation and $O_2$ are generally given concurrently to premature infants, it is difficult to distinguish their relative contribution to the lung injury process. The severity of the injury appears to correlate well with the amount of peak inspiratory pressure used. A small number of animal studies have attempted to separate the relative contribution of barotrauma and $O_2$ toxicity. The animal model of BPD most comparable with humans is probably the premature primate (baboon) treated with 100% $O_2$ and mechanical ventilation for up to 4 weeks (29–31). These animals develop pathological changes in the lung, termed diffuse alveolar damage, which appears to be similar to BPD in humans. In addition, Davis et al. demonstrated that the physiological, biochemical, cellular, and histological changes of acute lung injury, which precedes the development of BPD, were minimal in neonatal piglets subjected to positive-pressure ventilation with room air. In contrast, there were more significant changes when 100% $O_2$ was added (32), suggesting that the damaging effects of $O_2$ and mechanical ventilation are additive and possibly synergistic.

### Inflammation

The acute phase of RDS involves the destruction of alveolar epithelium and the initiation of an acute inflammatory response. When this response resolves successfully, the lung is repaired and the alveoli are repopulated with epithelial cells. However, BPD is associated with a persistent and aberrant inflammation in the lung and a failure to repair the epithelium (33). The initial inflammatory response appears to be a major determinant in the pathogenesis of BPD and is secondary to cell damage that results in the attraction and activation of neutrophils. The problem is that this beneficial, acute, and adaptive response transforms into BPD in some infants. Efforts to identify those infants with RDS at particular risk for BPD have led to the finding that such newborns have 100-fold increases in interleukin-6 (IL-6) in their tracheal aspirates relative to infants who recover without BPD (34). IL-6 is a cytokine and major mediator of inflammation, and it may have a role in the large neutrophil influx found in tracheal aspirates at 2–3 days of life prior to the development of significant pathophysiological abnormalities (35,36). Activated neutrophils and macrophages both have the potential for further release of a variety of inflammatory mediators, which can result in persistent inflammation and amplify lung injury (36–38).

Inflammation also involves the release of toxic products, including lipid from plasma membranes which are metabolized to arachidonic acid, platelet-activating factor, eicosanoids, leukotrienes, thromboxane, prostaglandin, and prostacyclin (39). These products have potent vasoactive and inflammatory properties. Leukotriene $B_4$, platelet-activating factor, thromboxane, and prostacyclin have been found in tracheal aspirates of patients with BPD (38,39). Reactive $O_2$ species are also released by activated neutrophils. Altogether, these components wreak havoc in the lung by damaging capillary endothelial integrity, leading to macromolecular leakage into alveolar spaces. Albumin and associated pulmonary edema have been postulated to be major factors in the development of BPD (40).

### Proteinases and Antiproteinases

The release of elastase and collagenase from activated neutrophils directly destroys the elastin and collagen framework of the lung. The breakdown products of collagen (hydroxyproline) and elastin (desmosine) have been recovered in the urine of infants who develop BPD (41). An important defense against the action of elastase activity is $\alpha_1$-antiproteinase, which may also be inactivated by $O_2$ radicals (42). Oxidative cleavage products of $\alpha_1$-antiproteinase that bind to elastase have potent chemotactic activity, fueling the destructive cycle of inflammation and proteolytic destruction of lung tissue. Increased elastase activity and compromised antiproteinase function is a homeostatic imbalance that can result in further lung injury (41). This imbalance has been demonstrated in tracheal aspirates and serum of neonates who develop BPD (36,43). If this cycle continues during a particularly critical period of rapid growth, significant injury to the lung occurs (44).

### Nutrition

The nutritional status of the sick premature infant plays a role in the etiology of BPD in several different ways. If caloric intake and essential nutrients are inadequate during a period of stress and growth, vital components of immunological and antioxidant defenses may be missing. Premature infants have special nutritional requirements owing to increased metabolic needs and rapid growth. Superimposed lung disease can further increase energy expenditures by as much as 25% in infants with very limited nutritional reserves. If energy needs are not met, a catabolic state develops that is believed to be a major contributing factor in the pathogenesis of BPD (45), exacerbating the deleterious effects of $O_2$ and barotrauma. Most antioxidant enzymes utilize trace amounts of transition metals (e.g., Cu, Zn, Se) that are essential to their function. Deficiencies in these metals will reduce enzymatic function, compromise lung defenses, and predispose the lungs (and other organs) to injury (46). It has been reported that supplementation with these metals can provide protection to the lung and reduce hyperoxic lung injury (47). Similarly, enzymes that repair extracellular matrix proteins or DNA can require trace amounts of metals (48,49). Increasing serum levels of vitamin E (tocopherol), a natural antioxidant that prevents peroxidation of lipid membranes, does not appear to influence BPD (50–53). Polyunsaturated fatty acids (PUFAs) have been postulated to provide a sink for free radicals, which could prevent injury in the lung (54). However, clinical trials have been unable to demonstrate that increasing PUFAs in preterm infants mitigates the development of BPD. Concentrations of vitamin A (retinol) may also be low in premature neonates less than 36 weeks' gestation (55–57). Vitamin A levels in serum are reported to be lower at birth and in the first month of life in infants who developed BPD (57,58). Despite adequate supplementation, some infants remain vitamin A deficient, although the reason is as yet unclear (59).

### Genetics

Several investigators have noted that neonates are more likely to develop BPD if there is a strong family history of atopy and asthma. A positive family history of asthma was found in 77% of infants with RDS who subsequently developed BPD compared with only 33% who did not (60). When histocompatibility loci (HLA) were examined, it was found that only infants with $HLA_2$ developed BPD, suggesting that there may be genetic components that contribute to the pathogenesis of BPD (61). To investigate genetic factors affecting the susceptibility to lung injury, some investigators have turned to inbred strains of mice that are differentially sensitive to pulmonary $O_2$ toxicity (62–65). In one case, relative sensitivity to hyperoxia was dependent on the presence of the fifth component of complement, C5. In another case, relative resistance appeared to segregate as a single Mendelian trait, although the precise genetic locus has not yet been identified (66). The relevance of these observations to a predisposition to RDS or BPD is currently unknown.

### C. Prevention Strategies

Given the enormous complexity of BPD it seems that a multimodal approach to the prevention of BPD in infants is needed. To date, no "magic bullet" has been found, although several different therapeutic approaches have significant potential. Administration of antenatal steroids to mothers at high risk of delivering a premature infant (<34 weeks of gestation) appears to reduce the severity and incidence of BPD (67). The use of early exogenous surfactant replacement therapy in premature infants with significant RDS will reduce mortality and appears to reduce the severity of BPD. Management strategies for babies with RDS should encourage the rapid reduction of ventilator pressures and inspired $O_2$ concentrations in order to reduce barotrauma, air leak, and $O_2$ toxicity. Aggressive nutritional support, initially with intravenous supplementation followed by enteral feeds when tolerated, is also critical (68). Supplementation with vitamin A in sufficient quantities to establish normal serum retinol concentrations has also been reported to reduce the incidence and severity of BPD (69).

Steroid therapy can be beneficial, although results in animal models and humans indicate that the timing of steroid administration is crucial and may not be the same among species. In infants, early use of dexamethasone has resulted in a lower incidence and severity of BPD, although steroids may have many significant associated side effects (70,71). In newborn piglets, prophylactic dexamethasone treatment is effective in preventing acute inflammatory changes and lung injury caused by hyperoxia and mechanical ventilation (71). Systemic steroid therapy can, in some instances, increase the risk of morbidity and mortality. Mice pretreated with methylprednisolone for 7 days showed significantly greater mortality from hyperoxia than saline-treated control mice (72). Other animal experiments indicate that later use of steroids can be beneficial, whereas early use can be detrimental (73). The use of inhaled, nonabsorbable steroids such as beclomethasone might improve the efficacy of steroid therapy while minimizing the side effects. The development of improved aerosol-delivery systems could have a major impact on this mode of therapy. Clearly, more research is needed to determine the optimum mode, timing, and dose of steroid treatment.

Since hyperoxia causes the overproduction of oxy radicals and plays such a prominent role in the pathogenesis of BPD, any strategy aimed at reducing oxy radicals in the lung might prevent or reduce the severity of BPD. Since iron ($Fe^{2+}$) is known to exacerbate radical accumulation, its chelation could have therapeutic benefits. Newborn rats treated with the $Fe^{2+}$ chelator deferoxamine have reduced lung injury following hyperoxic exposure when compared with nontreated controls (74). This suggests that $Fe^{2+}$ sequestration, or the chelation of other transition metals could mitigate pulmonary $O_2$ toxicity and potentially affect BPD. However, deferoxamine is highly toxic in nonhuman primates, suggesting it might be inappropriate for use in humans (75). A relatively new compound, the 21-aminosteroid drug U74389F, is a potent iron chelator and inhibitor of lipid peroxidation. When administered to newborn rats exposed to hyperoxia, it was found to reduce the inhibition of septation, increase internal surface area of alveoli, and increase elastin deposition relative to sham-treated pups (76).

A rational and novel therapy for preventing BPD is the supplementation of antioxidant enzymes. Several animal studies show that systemic administration of antioxidants can reduce hyperoxic lung injury (77–80). In a pilot study in humans, Rosenfeld et al. demonstrated that subcutaneous administration of bovine SOD decreased the severity of BPD in treated infants, although total duration of respiratory support was the same for the treated and control groups (81). The development of recombinant human SOD and the ability to effectively deliver this and other recombinant antioxidant enzymes directly to the lung hold great promise for the prevention of BPD. The prophylactic use of a single intratracheal dose of recombinant human Cu, Zn-SOD (rhSOD), is reported to prevent significant inflammatory changes and lung injury from $O_2$ and mechanical ventilation in newborn piglets, with apparently no associated toxicity (82). The rhSOD accumulates inside the cells rapidly (within 30 min of administration) and is found in a variety of epithelial cell types in airways and alveoli. Pharmacological concentrations persisted in the serum and lung tissue for 24 to 48 hr. Interestingly, SOD activity is a component of natural lung surfactant (7 U/mmol phospholipid), yet there is no SOD activity in currently used exogenous surfactant preparations (83). It may be useful to consider the addition of antioxidants to future generations of exogenous pulmonary surfactant.

### Insights From Experimental Animal Models

Examination of the cellular, biochemical, and molecular biological factors associated with the development of RDS and BPD is difficult in humans, because safe sampling is limited primarily to tracheal aspirates, blood, and urine. Thus, although studies of human samples have provided new information, important insights have been gained through experiments on animal models. Of course, the relevance of these data can be questioned on the basis of inherent differences between animals and humans. In addition, only a limited number of animal models involve premature delivery and postnatal intensive care. Furthermore, because investigators tend to be (necessarily) focused on research subjects that are narrowly defined, there are very few instances where interdisciplinary approaches have been applied to this multifactorial problem. Nevertheless, a great deal has been learned by studying hyperoxia, since $O_2$ toxicity appears to be a critically important factor leading to BPD. It is therefore not surprising that much attention has been paid to gaining a greater understanding of the events that accompany hyperoxic lung injury in order to treat or prevent RDS and BPD. The following section reviews our current understanding of the cellular, biochemical, and molecular changes that occur in lung during hyperoxia as studied in animal models. Most of the biological systems we touch on are discussed in greater detail in other chapters of this volume, and we urge the reader to refer to them to gain a broader understanding of the systems themselves and to provide a greater developmental context from which to view the changes induced by hyperoxia. Here the discussion is limited to alterations in these systems occurring both in neonatal and adult models, where much has been learned. For the sake of simplicity, $O_2$ toxicity in (ex vivo) isolated lungs, lung explants, lung slices, or cells not derived from in vivo–exposed animals are not discussed. In addition, only brief descriptions are provided of the complex pathophysiology of hyperoxia, which has been reviewed in much greater detail elsewhere (24,84,85).

### Overall Pathophysiology of Hyperoxic Lung Injury

Studies in a variety of animal models have shown that the first visible signs of lung injury after hyperoxic exposure are a swelling of endothelial cells and an altered appearance of mitochondria and microsomes (86). With time, gross morphological changes of individual cells become apparent. There are shifts of lung cell populations as a result of proliferation and hypertrophy of type II pneumocytes, hyperplasia of interstitial cells, and loss of capillary endothelial cells. An inflammatory response also occurs (87). These alterations make it difficult to distinguish between biochemical changes that may be occurring in a single cell type from overall changes as a result of shifts in lung cell populations (88). Often, both pulmonary endothelium and epithelium are damaged, resulting in the leak of fluid and macromolecules into the air spaces (87,88), attenuating respiratory function, and causing death in the worst cases.

When these events occur in newborns, they have profound impact on postnatal lung growth. At birth, the terminal gas-exchange units of many mammals (including humans) are not fully alveolarized, and they are called saccules. Saccules continue to septate postnatally, forming smaller units that eventually become mature alveoli. This septation is notably inhibited by hyperoxia, resulting in fewer (but larger) alveoli, and consequent failure to increase the surface area of the gas-exchange region. Secondary septation can be inhibited as much as 88% and whole lung DNA reduced to 50% of control (89). This problem can be exacerbated by the development of interstitial and alveolar fibrosis. So not only are septa fewer in number, but alveolar walls are also thicker and the lungs usually less compliant, so that gas exchange is further impaired (90). These effects of hyperoxia on growing lung may be unique to newborns, since they are not observed during compensatory lung growth following lung resection in adult lungs. However, hyperoxia does inhibit other aspects of compensatory lung growth in young adult rats (91). Another effect of hyperoxia that may be related to active lung growth is airway hyperresponsiveness, which is induced by hyperoxia in newborn (92) but not in adult rat lungs (93). Taken together, these observations indicate that early postnatal lung growth involves multiple systems that can be adversely affected by hyperoxia.

The study of nonhuman primates holds great promise for the understanding of human lung disease. Adult baboons ventilated with either 40 or 80% $O_2$ show mild lung injury, with increased numbers of alveolar macrophages in peribronchiolar sites and focal alveolar wall widening. The 100% $O_2$-exposed baboons have diffuse alveolar lesions, and type II cells have aberrant lamellar bodies. There are also increases in the number of type II and interstitial cells and decreases in type I and endothelial cells (94).

Not surprisingly, these complex events have roots in alterations in gene expression at multiple levels. For example, the overall rate of protein synthesis decreases by 30% in hyperoxic lung (95). Technological advances have helped improve our understanding of genes, mRNAs, and proteins that are involved in hyperoxic lung injury. Studies of lung gene expression usually involve one of two approaches. Most typically, cDNA probes encoding proteins of known function or suspected importance have been used to measure changes in specific mRNA abundance. By a second approach, subtractive hybridization cloning or differential screening of cDNA libraries have been used to isolate and identify cDNA clones corresponding to mRNAs that increase in lung injury. In this case, genes can be studied in the absence of any preconceived notion of what systems may be affected.

### Pulmonary Surfactant

In studies of hyperoxic lung injury, both of these approaches converged on the pulmonary surfactant system (96). Lung surfactant is the complex phospholipid-protein complex that reduces surface tension at the air-water interface of alveoli, preventing alveolar collapse during normal breathing. Physiological studies have shown that hyperoxia causes deterioration in lung mechanics (97), which is associated with impaired surfactant function (98). It therefore is of interest to determine whether surfactant protein accumulation and gene regulation are altered by hyperoxia. The genes encoding pulmonary surfactant proteins (SPs) A, B, and C are among the best-characterized lung-specific genes. Antibodies have been raised against them, and cDNA clones have been isolated for the study of changes in the abundance of their mRNAs. Exposure of adult rats to 85% $O_2$ (for up to 7 days) results in increased SP-A, SP-B, and SP-C proteins in bronchoalveolar lavage and lung homogenates, as well as increases in the mRNAs encoding these proteins (99–101). Experiments in adult rabbits exposed to 100% $O_2$ for up to 64 hr, led to the cloning of a cDNA for SP-A by subtractive hybridization (96,102). In this model, SP-A mRNA increases about sevenfold. In term newborn rabbits exposed for 96 hr, increases are three- to fivefold (96). By contrast, preterm baboons exposed to hyperoxia and barotrauma show no increase in the abundance of SP-A mRNA but small increases (twofold or less) in SP-B and SP-C mRNAs (103). Whether this represents a difference in the response of the primate surfactant system to hyperoxia or is a complication of barotrauma or prematurity is not yet known. Surfactant expression in adult hamsters is also changed during exposure to 100% $O_2$, but in a different manner still. SP-A is increased in the first 1 or 2 days but decreased by day 8. During this period, SP-B declines continuously and SP-C is unchanged for the first 2 days and then declines (104). These observations indicate that the components of surfactant are not expressed in a coordinate fashion, and there are differences among species. Investigators have also begun studying very early changes in surfactant expression during hyperoxia prior to overt injury. In rats exposed to 95% $O_2$, SP-A and SP-B mRNAs decrease after 12 hr of hyperoxia, returning to basal levels by 24 hr (R. Auten, personal communication, July 1996).

Because only type II alveolar epithelial cells synthesize and secrete surfactant, increased surfactant mRNAs have generally been interpreted in terms of alveolar surfactant function. However, SP-A (105) and SP-B (106,107) are also expressed in nonciliated airway epithelial cells (Clara cells). Quantitative in situ hybridization assays in hyperoxic adult rabbits show that SP-A and SP-B mRNAs increase dramatically (20-fold or more) in airway epithelial cells but modestly (20% to 30%) in alveolar epithelial cells when the data are analyzed on a per cell basis (107). Immunohistochemistry shows increased SP-A protein in airway cells (antibodies to rabbit SP-B were not available). A similar observation was made in hyperoxic adult mice, which also show an apparent reduction in the number of SP-B mRNA-positive cells in the gas-exchange regions (108). This can be interpreted as a reduction in the number of functional type II cells during acute hyperoxia. SP-C mRNA, which is expressed only in type II cells (107,109), is also expressed in many fewer cells after 64 hr of 100% $O_2$ in adult rabbits (our unpublished observations) at a time when surfactant function is decreased (98). Taken together, these observations suggest that increased SP-A and SP-B expression in hyperoxic lung are probably not directly related to surfactant function per se (i.e., reducing surface tension) but rather may reflect other, nonsurfactant roles for these proteins, such as host defense. It will be interesting to learn if SP-D is also increased during hyperoxia, since, like SP-A and SP-B, it is expressed in Clara cells and, although SP-D is surfactant associated, it appears to have host defense (and not surface tension) function. Moreover, the fate of type II pneumocytes that cease to accumulate hybridizable levels of SP-B and SP-C is a subject of further study.

### Antioxidants

Pulmonary $O_2$ toxicity is thought to be mediated by toxic and highly reactive oxy radicals (110,111). Consequently, much attention has been focused on the effects of pulmonary $O_2$ toxicity on the classic antioxidant enzymes, including superoxide dismutases, catalase, and glutathione peroxidases (GPx). These scavengers of reactive $O_2$ species could play a crucial role in the response to oxidant stress by promoting the catabolism of partially reduced $O_2$ species (88,112,113). In adult animals, pulmonary antioxidant enzyme activities respond differently to hyperoxia in different species. In addition, there is no simple dose response to hyperoxia. For example, rats exposed to 80–85% $O_2$ exhibit modest increases in the activities of SOD (114,115) and GPx (116), whereas exposure to 100% $O_2$ results in decreased catalase in adult rat lungs (117). In adult rabbits, SOD, catalase, and GPx enzyme activities do not increase at all in response to hyperoxia (118), nor are there increases in the mRNAs encoding these enzymes (our unpublished observations). The transcription rate of the Mn-SOD gene increases substantially following hyperoxia in adult mice, and steady-state levels of Mn-SOD mRNA increase similarly (119). By contrast, Cu,Zn–SOD mRNA is constitutive. However, in some instances, increased Mn-SOD mRNA may have little or no biological consequence, since increased protein levels are not tightly correlated, suggesting that induced Mn-SOD transcripts are translationally regulated. It should be pointed out, however, that because of increased lung protein from pulmonary edema and increased lung DNA from inflammatory cell influx and cell hyperplasia, there is some controversy over how protein levels and enzyme activity measurements should be normalized, leading to uncertainty over the biological significance of small but statistically significant increases that are not always consistent when different normalization methods are used (88). Newborn rats exposed to hyperoxia also show increased lung catalase, probably resulting from posttranscriptional regulation (120). Although the cells in which this occurs have not yet been identified, the identification of a redox-sensitive, catalase mRNA binding protein in lung homogenates suggests it may be ubiquitous among the many cell types of lung (121).

   In contrast to adult rabbits, which show no increases in antioxidant enzymes (AOEs) in response to hyperoxia, the activities of SOD, catalase, and cellular GPx are induced by hyperoxia (100% $O_2$) in normal newborn (term) rabbits but not in premature rabbits (122). Similarly, type II cells isolated from term newborn rabbits exposed to (100% $O_2$) secrete increased extracellular GPx (N. Avissar, personal communication, July 1996). These observations provide a possible explanation for the observations that neonates of some species (including rabbits) are relatively resistant to hyperoxia (123,124) when compared with adults of the same species. An attractive hypothesis is that the capacity to induce antioxidant enzymes in response to hyperoxia plays an important adaptive role, perhaps tolerizing the animal (124). Additional support for this notion comes from experiments in rats where tolerance to $O_2$ toxicity is induced by pretreatment with hyperoxia, ozone (125), tumor necrosis factor (126), IL-1 (127,128), diethyldithiocarbamate (129), or intravenous endotoxin, all of which induce AOE activities prior to subsequent exposure to hyperoxia. Although suggestive and highly correlative, these agents are all pleiotropic—inducing myriad systems in addition to antioxidant enzymes (102,130–132). The hypothesis is thus not yet proven, and other observations run counter to it. For example, preexposure to hyperoxia can induce tolerance to hyperoxia in adult rabbits in the absence of increased antioxidant enzymes (118). Also, prematurely weaned newborn rats are more tolerant of hyperoxia than normally weaned littermates, yet their antioxidant enzyme activity levels are indistinguishable (133). Aged rats, which have lower SOD levels than newborns, are more tolerant to hyperoxia than young rats (174,175). Interestingly, GPx levels are slightly higher in the lungs of unexposed aged rats, although none of the antioxidant enzyme activities were induced by hyperoxic exposure (174). Furthermore, transgenic mice that overexpress Cu, Zn-SOD, or cellular GPx in a generalized fashion (via their endogenous promoter or an actin promoter) are not more resistant to normobaric 100% $O_2$ than their nontransgenic counterparts (134,135; Y.-S. Ho, personal communication, July 1996). Thus, the question of whether endogenous increases in any of these enzymes in response to hyperoxia provides any protection from lung injury awaits further experiments. Formal proof might come from the engineering of animals with targeted disruptions (perhaps conditional) of individual AOE genes. Definitive proof that the constitutive level of at least one AOE is important to survival in hyperoxia comes from a study where EC-SOD–null mice were exposed to 100% $O_2$. These knockout mice were rendered sensitive to hyperoxia relative to control diploids (176). These results support the contention that whether or not endogenously increased AOE activities are protective, antioxidant augmentation could still be of great therapeutic value. For example, transgenic mice overexpressing Mn-SOD via the SP-C promoter, which is expressed only in alveolar type II epithelial cells, survive substantially longer in 100% $O_2$ than do nontransgenic mice (136). Thus, the targeted overexpression of Mn-SOD in cells that ordinarily express relatively little Mn-SOD (88) suggests that Mn-SOD, and perhaps the other classic antioxidant enzymes, might be used therapeutically to augment insufficient endogenous enzymes (137).

The lung is estimated to contain up to 60 different cell types (138), and antioxidant levels found in lung homogenates makes interpretation of the data difficult. Surprisingly little is known of the cell-specific nature of antioxidant enzyme expression in control and hyperoxic lungs. In adult rats exposed to 85% $O_2$, Mn-SOD transcripts increase along the pleura, although the use of [35]S-labeled probes in this study precludes the definitive identification of the cell type(s) involved, because [35]S has a relatively long path length. Since hyperoxia-induced increases in Mn-SOD mRNA abundance in whole-lung homogenates is not always associated with a corresponding increase in protein or activity, it was of interest to determine where Mn-SOD increases in lung. Quantitative electron microscopic immunohistochemistry studies show that type II cells are a locus of the Mn-SOD response in hyperoxic lung, and that increases occur via a combination of increased enzyme in mitochondrial matrix, increased mitochondrial volume and type II cell hyperplasia (139).

In addition to the classic antioxidant enzymes, nonclassic, nonenzymatic antioxidants might play an important role in the response to pulmonary $O_2$ toxicity. For example, the inducible form of heme oxygenase (HO-1) may play a role in protection from $O_2$ stress (140). There are at least three means by which HO-1 could play a protective role. First, heme oxygenase is the rate-limiting enzyme of bilirubin synthesis, and bilirubin is a known antioxidant that may protect from hyperoxia (141). Second, HO-1 can sequester heme, a potential prooxidant. Third, HO-1 can induce ferritin, which can sequester iron and might reduce iron-mediated radical production. In rats, HO-1 expression is higher in newborn rat lungs than in adult rats (142). Hyperoxic exposure of newborn rats results in increased HO-1 activity within the first week of life—a period of relative resistance to hyperoxia—but not in older animals.

Ceruloplasmin is a Cu-binding plasma protein that functions as an extracellular antioxidant. In addition to its potential antioxidant function in lung, its Cu-binding function could have an indirect effect on another antioxidant, Cu, Zn-SOD, and on other Cu-dependent enzymes. Ceruloplasmin levels increase during hyperoxic lung injury. The abundance of ceruloplasmin mRNA in total lung homogenates increased five- to sixfold after exposure of rats to 95% $O_2$, or seven- to ninefold after intraperitoneal injection of rats with bacterial endotoxin (143). Nuclear run-on experiments indicate that these increases are the result of de novo transcription. Studies with lavaged macrophages show that ceruloplasmin synthesis and mRNA levels increase markedly in these cells. Ceruloplasmin mRNA levels increase in the lungs of prematurely delivered guinea pigs 12 hr after delivery, but by 72 hr, fall to levels below those seen in term lung (144). Adult lungs have the highest levels. In contrast to rats, there is no observed increase in ceruloplasmin mRNA levels following hyperoxia in guinea pigs.

Another Cu-binding protein whose gene expression has been studied during lung injury is metallothionein (MT). By subtractive hybridization, a metallothionein II (MT-II) cDNA clone was isolated from hyperoxic rabbit lung (102,145). Metallothioneins (MTs) are a family of small (61 amino acids), cysteine-rich (20

Cys residues) proteins (146). In mammals, there are currently four known classes of MT isoforms, called MT-I–IV. MT-I and MT-II are expressed in most mouse tissues, including lung (65). MT-III is brain-specific (147), and expression of MT-IV appears to be limited to cornified epithelium (148). MT binds not only Cu, but also several other transition metals, notably Zn and Cd. A large body of evidence suggests that MT probably has a role in heavy metal detoxification, although its role in normal, healthy cells is not known. MT is primarily an intracellular protein, and is thought to be involved in transition metal homeostasis, perhaps akin to the regulation of calcium by calmodulin. There is evidence that MT is an antioxidant, although the mechanistic basis of this activity is not yet clear (149). Based on in vitro assays, it might be argued that as a chemical (nonenzymatic) antioxidant, MT plays a minor role in cells. On the other hand, there is compelling evidence that MT can substitute for Cu, Zn-SOD in vivo, in the yeast *Saccharomyces cerevisiae* (150).

In whole lung homogenates of hyperoxic newborn and adult rabbits, MT mRNA levels increase an average of 5- and 60-fold, respectively (145). In lungs of hyperoxic adult mice, MT mRNA levels increase an average of about 60-fold and up to 200-fold in some individuals (65). Hyperoxia-induced MT expression is cell type–specific, occurs at the protein and mRNA levels, and MT isoforms in rabbit lung are differentially regulated. Single and dual-label in situ hybridizations indicate that MT is expressed in smooth muscle of arteries, adventitial cells surrounding airways, tracheal chondrocytes, and type II pneumocytes (145; our unpublished data). Independent experiments in hyperoxic rats exposed to 85% $O_2$ show eightfold increases in MT as estimated by metal binding activity (151). The observations that MT induction by hyperoxia is conserved in rabbits, rats, and mice and that the increases are cell type–specific, suggest that MT has an important role in pulmonary $O_2$ toxicity. Preinduction of MT by inhaled Cd confers partial tolerance to hyperoxia in rats (152). However, these animals also had pulmonary inflammation, indicating that inhaled Cd is pleiotropic. A more direct test of the importance of MT in $O_2$ toxicity involves using mouse models with altered complements of MT genes. In preliminary experiments recently completed in our laboratory, male mice with 56 extra copies of a minimally marked MT-1 gene under the control of its own promoter (MT-1* mice) were exposed to 100% $O_2$ together with their nontransgenic littermates. No significant difference in survival was observed, suggesting that additional MT genes do not confer extra protection from toxicity. To determine if endogenous (diploid) MT gene expression is important in hyperoxia, MT-null (double knockout) mice, which have disrupted and nonfunctional MT-I and MT-II genes were exposed. Preliminary data indicate that most MT knockout mice died 1 day sooner than their cohorts, which share the same genetic background but have a normal complement of MT genes. Neither MT-III nor MT-IV were expressed in normal or hyperoxic lung. These preliminary data suggest that expression of MT provides limited protection from hyperoxia and that additional copies of MT-1 may not be sufficient to confer additional protection. The mechanism by which this protection is conferred is under investigation.

### Cytochrome P450

Cytochrome P450 generates the toxic oxy radical superoxide in microsomes. Cytochrome P450 is also induced in lung during hyperoxia, (153,154). This could be a maladaptive response which, if inhibited, might reduce injury from hyperoxia. When the cytokine IL-1 is administered to adult rats, it causes decreased cytochrome P450 and decreased P450 IIB1 mRNA in lungs. At the same time, superoxide production from pulmonary microsomes also decreases. Under the same conditions, IL-1 induces tolerance to hyperoxia, suggesting that reduced superoxide from the cytochrome P450 mono-oxygenase system could be an important mediator of IL-1-induced tolerance to hyperoxia. It should be noted that others have attributed tolerance to hyperoxia induced by IL-1 to increased antioxidant enzymes (127).

### Sodium Channels and Na-K ATPase

As mentioned earlier, significant pulmonary edema accompanies hyperoxic lung injury. Because Na-K ATPase might have a role in keeping the air space free of fluid, it has been hypothesized that it would increase during edema in hyperoxic rat lungs. Indeed, levels of Na-K ATPase mRNA increase by three- to fourfold when lung edema is evident and wet/dry lung weight ratios peak. An increase in Na-K ATPase protein levels follows and persists for several days (155). Immunohistochemical assays by light and electron microscopy indicate that increased Na-K ATPase is found in the basolateral membranes of type II pneumocytes. Sodium channels are also upregulated in alveolar cells, as shown by in situ hybridization (178). Both sodium transport and edema clearance increase in rat lungs during hyperoxia (179). Perhaps increased sodium channels and Na-K ATPase play a protective role by clearing edema. These studies either suggest or demonstrate that type II cells express these proteins. Type II cells are relatively resistant to $O_2$ toxicity and other forms of lung injury and are essential for repopulating injured alveolar epithelium (33).

### Extracellular Matrix and Its Regulation

Because pulmonary fibrosis is a late and particularly severe component of BPD, and a hallmark of fibrosis is the accumulation of extracellular matrix (ECM), some investigators have begun to study the effects of hyperoxia on extracellular matrix components and their regulation. An important ECM protein that is found ubiquitously in lung and is known to have a role in lung repair is fibronectin (FN). FN is not only a structural component of ECM, but it also has several effector functions, such as stimulating fibroblast proliferation and ECM production and enhancing the opsonizing function of macrophages, and it is chemotactic. Because increased FN is a component of other fibrotic lung disease, it was postulated that increased FN during acute hyperoxia might be a harbinger of later fibrosis. FN is known to be synthesized and secreted by alveolar macrophages. To determine if FN expression increases in hyperoxic lung, adult rabbits were exposed to 100% $O_2$ for up to 64 hr, and cells were isolated form bronchoalveolar lavage. A novel quantitative in situ hybridization assay was employed and showed greater than 20-fold increases in FN mRNA levels after 64 hr of hyperoxia (156). These levels increased during 24 hr of subsequent recovery in room air and returned to baseline by 72 hr of recovery. In addition to increased per cell levels of FN transcripts, the number of alveolar macrophages expressing FN increases 10-fold. Although this animal model does not result in the development of fibrosis, these observations suggest that FN plays an important role in hyperoxic lung injury.

Basement membranes in lung contain proteoglycans in ECM. To determine if proteoglycan density and distribution are altered during hyperoxia, newborn rats were exposed to >95% $O_2$ for up to 4 weeks. With increased duration of exposure, alveolar basement membranes progressively thicken, and the normal distribution of proteoglycans is altered. The density of proteoglycans in this region decreases to nearly half of controls by 2 weeks of exposure and remains low throughout (157). Proteoglycans are enzymatically hydrolyzed by metalloproteinases (158), suggesting a role for these enzymes in $O_2$ toxicity of newborn lung. Changes in proteoglycan density and distribution could affect the lung by increasing lung permeability and altering the cell-matrix interactions involved in cell adhesion, migration, and growth.

Elastin is another important ECM protein that has a role in lung integrity and compliance. Tropoelastin (TE) expression is a regulated event in early postnatal lung, and exposure of rats to >95% $O_2$ for up to 14 days results in reduced TE expression and a delay in peak TE mRNA levels (day 16 vs day 11). This peak is sustained during recovery in room air, persisting until day 23, 1 week after TE mRNA levels decrease in controls (159). These observations indicate that the regulation of elastin synthesis that accompanies alveolar septation is altered during hyperoxia. Interestingly, the total length of elastin fibers is greater in hyperoxic rat pups than in newborns reared in air, and pressure-volume curves indicate that this increase correlates with increased lung compliance.

Plasminogen activator inhibitor type 1 (PAI-1) is a single-chain glycoprotein that inhibits plasminogen activators by stoichiometrically binding to them (1:1). It is secreted by endothelial cells and can remain latent in the extracellular environment (160). Northern blots show that PAI-1 mRNA levels increase up to 15-fold in lungs of rats exposed to 100% $O_2$ for up to 50 hr (161). Because PAI-1 regulates proteolysis in the pericellular environment, its expression might be important in the mitigation of further injury during the acute phase of hyperoxia, and it might be important to lung repair.

Although neutrophil elastase has so far been the focus attention in studies in lung proteases, matrix metalloproteinases and their inhibitors have been studied far less among pulmonary researchers (162). This class of enzymes are Zn dependent and digest a broad array of extracellular matrix (ECM) proteins (158). They play a pivotal role in acute and chronic inflammation, and they are also critical to the regulation of ECM accumulation, being capable not only of directly hydrolyzing ECM proteins (e.g., collagens, fibronectin, proteoglycans) but also of activating each other by proteolytic cleavage of proenzymes. Matrix metalloproteinases are regulated by tissue inhibitor of metalloproteinases (TIMPs), which stoichiometrically (1:1) inactive them. TIMP-1 was the first to be isolated and identified, and although there are at least three mammalian TIMPs (163), TIMP-1 is probably the broadest acting, inhibiting the largest number of matrix metalloproteinases identified to date. TIMP-1 is thus a key regulatory protein of ECM turnover, and may have a role in the fibrosis that occurs during the chronic phase of hyperoxic lung injury or in other models of pulmonary fibrosis, since an increase in TIMP-1 can result in the net accumulation of ECM, which is the hallmark of fibrosis. TIMP-1 is also an autocrine growth factor for erythropoiesis (164). By subtractive hybridization of cDNAs from control and hyperoxic rabbit lungs, a cDNA for TIMP-1 was cloned, reflecting increased levels of mRNA during hyperoxia (102). Studies of whole-lung mRNA from hyperoxic and unexposed rabbits indicate that TIMP-1 increase at least sixfold after hyperoxic exposure in both adults and neonates (102,145). In situ hybridizations in adult rabbits and mice (65) indicate that basal levels of TIMP-1 are not detectable over background. However, during hyperoxia, TIMP-1 is expressed in endothelial cells of venules, tracheal chondrocytes, bronchiolar-associated lymphoid tissue, and unidentifiable cells in alveolar septa. Although some of these cells are in the corners of alveoli, dual-label in situ hybridizations (using TIMP-1 and SP-C probe) suggest that in vivo, type II cells do not express TIMP-1 (our unpublished observations). TIMP-1 regulation is more complex in newborn rabbits. Although whole-lung homogenates showed no changes in TIMP-1 mRNA levels during the first week of (normoxic) life, in situ hybridizations reveal that the pattern of cell type–specific expression shifts dramatically in the few days following birth, and that hyperoxia changes this shifting pattern. These preliminary observations suggest that lung injury caused by hyperoxia in newborns is more complicated than in adults and might be different in many instances. Moreover, the in situ data contrast sharply with the observed absence of a net change in TIMP-1 mRNA abundance in whole-lung homogenates, indicating that studies of gene expression in lung that are limited to homogenates yield relatively limited conclusions. TIMP-1 mRNA abundance is relatively low during fetal lung development in baboons, but it increases sharply after term or premature birth (165). Unlike rabbits, TIMP-1 expression does not increase in response to ventilation with 100% $O_2$ (165). The cell-specific expression of TIMP-1 in baboons has not yet been studied.

### Growth Factors

Many aspects of the pathophysiology of hyperoxic lung injury seem likely to be mediated by growth factors and cytokines (these terms are used interchangeably here because of their overlapping functions). For example, a host of cytokines have a role in the initiation and propagation of inflammation, a hallmark of pulmonary $O_2$ toxicity. In addition, cell hyperplasia that occurs during tissue remodeling from hyperoxia is almost certain to involve growth factors. In hyperoxic rats, it was observed that c-sis mRNA, which encodes the B-chain of platelet-derived growth factor (PDGF), increases two- to threefold after 3 days of exposure to 85% $O_2$, and this increase persists up to 7 days. Interestingly, at 7 days, the abundance of actin mRNA (used as a constitutively expressed control message) also increases, suggesting that actin mRNA might not be an appropriate control during prolonged hyperoxia in rat lung. Immunohistochemistry localized PDGF-BB homodimers to pulmonary interstitium, the major site of hyperplasia (166). The PDGF-A chain was not affected by hyperoxia.

Prolonged sublethal hyperoxia induces pulmonary hypertension, which is associated with the appearance of new contractile cells. These cells develop from intermediate cells and interstitial fibroblasts, which proliferate at between 4 and 7 days of hyperoxia. Northern blot hybridization shows the level of mRNA encoding heparin binding EGF-like growth factor (HB-EGF) increased 100-fold by day 7 of hyperoxia (167). In situ hybridization showed induced HB-EGF expression in eosinophils clustered around microvessels. Whether HB-EGF plays a significant role in hyperoxic lung remodeling is a subject of further investigation. A growth factor known to be important in lung remodeling is transforming growth factor-β (TGF-β). We hypothesized that TGF-β, which regulates several aspects of matrix synthesis and accumulation, and induces TIMP-1 expression, might also be induced in lung during hyperoxia. Using immunohistochemistry and in situ hybridization, all three isoforms were found in control tissue, but the relative tissue distribution of each isoform was different. During hyperoxia, the cell-specific patterns of accumulation of TGF-β isoforms were differentially regulated (S. Horowitz, B. Piedboeuf, L. Gold, J. Kazzaz, unpublished observations).

The cytokines known as interleukins are also known to have active roles in lung injury. As discussed earlier, increased IL-6 in extracellular lung fluids appears to be an early marker for the later development of BPD (34). IL-1 is an early inflammatory mediator that is sufficient to elicit many of the responses associated with acute injury. In adult mice exposed to 100% $O_2$, IL-1β mRNA abundance increased 35-fold after 4 days. In situ hybridization and immuno-histochemistry show that basal expression of IL-1β is so low as to be indistinguishable from background. By 3 days of hyperoxia, IL-1β transcripts and protein are detected in interstitial monocytes and in a subset of neutrophils. By 4 days, IL-1β mRNA is present in many areas of lung, but colocalized protein is not always found. These data suggest that IL-1β might function transiently in hyperoxic lung. This could be important because of the pleiotropic effects of this molecule (S. Horowitz, B. Piedboeuf, unpublished data).

### Cellular Adhesion Molecules

A prominent feature of pulmonary $O_2$ toxicity is the influx of neutrophils, yet the mechanisms of neutrophil accumulation have not been extensively investigated. Intercellular adhesion molecule-1 (ICAM-1) is necessary for the tight adhesion of neutrophils to endothelial cells at sites of inflammation. Northern blot hybridizations of mouse lungs indicate that ICAM-1 message abundance increases more than fivefold by 96 hr of >95% $O_2$ (168). Western blots suggest a commensurate increase in ICAM-1 protein (168). Electron microscopic immunohistochemical techniques were used to demonstrate ICAM-1 accumulation at the surface of the boundary between adjoining type I cells of normal mouse lung and relatively less ICAM-1 on endothelial cells and type II pneumocytes. Exposure to 100% $O_2$ resulted in a dramatic increase in ICAM-1 on type II alveolar cell surfaces and a reduction at the junctions between type I cells (169). Dual-label in situ hybridization indicates that type II cells have abundant ICAM-I transcripts in hyperoxic lung but not in controls, indicating (our unpublished results) that type II cells synthesize ICAM-I in response to hyperoxia. The platelet/endothelial cell adhesion molecule 1 (PECAM-1) is a member of the immunoglobulin superfamily that is expressed at the junctions between endothelial cells and is essential for the transendothelial migration of leukocytes (170). In situ hybridization was used to show that PECAM-1 mRNA is rare or undetectable in lung sections of unexposed mice or mice exposed for up to 48 hr of hyperoxia. By 72 hr, however, PECAM-1 mRNA is found in endothelial cells of small pulmonary veins and in alveolar walls. Alveolar and venous hybridization is not uniform but focally localized primarily in lung periphery. These preliminary observations (B. Piedboeuf, S. Horowitz, unpublished data) suggest that cell adhesion molecules have a role hyperoxic lung injury and may be targets of future intervention strategies.

### Nitric Oxide

Nitric oxide (NO) is a toxic, highly reactive, and short-lived radical that is produced naturally in cells and functions to mediate biological function (171). In lungs, it has a role in regulating vascular tone, and it may have other functions as well. Hyperoxia, which is associated with increased superoxide production, can potentially cause NO-mediated cell injury by the reaction of NO and superoxide to form a highly toxic radical called peroxynitrite (172). Because peroxynitrite is so short lived, it can only be detected indirectly. It reacts rapidly with tyrosine-containing proteins to form nitrotyrosine, which is stable and can be detected immunologically. A recent study showed that adult rats exposed to 100% $O_2$ for 60 hr had increased nitrotyrosine in lung tissue, suggesting a role for NO and its metabolites in pulmonary $O_2$ toxicity (173). Clinical trials testing the use of NO for treatment of persistent pulmonary hypertension of the newborn (PPHN) involve critically ill neonates who are also being mechanically ventilated with high levels of $O_2$. However, there are few published studies on the toxicity of these combined therapies. We have recently found that mechanically ventilated newborn piglets receiving concurrent NO have impaired surfactant function (177), suggesting that further studies are warranted. Increased nitrotyrosine is also found in lung tissue of newborn piglets ventilated with 100% $O_2$ either alone or accompanied by inhaled NO (C. Robbins, J. Davis, S. Horowitz, J. Kazzaz, unpublished).

## IV. Summary and Conclusions

When lung development is interrupted by premature birth, many events that were supposed to occur in utero in an aqueous environment at relatively low $O_2$ tensions are adversely affected. To the underdeveloped lungs of the premature infant, breathing even room air is probably an oxidative insult. The side effects of critical care, due largely to hyperoxia and mechanical ventilation, cause cell and tissue injury and wreak additional havoc on the lung during what is normally a crucial period of lung growth and development. Acutely, premature infants who are surfactant deficient suffer from the respiratory distress syndrome. When lung injury is resolved in these infants, they often successfully adapt to breathing air. Surfactant-replacement therapy has made this possible for many. However, in some prematures, especially in smaller infants who now survive because of surfactant, nonresolving lung disease still occurs. This can lead to a failure to adapt and to the chronic lung disorder bronchopulmonary dysplasia, which can be thought of as a metastable intermediate in a continuum of lung injury. The events that accompany and lead up to this disorder appear to be as complex as the lung itself, perhaps involving every conceivable aspect of lung biology. Biomedical investigators have made significant inroads toward a greater understanding of these events, but it is likely that much more must be learned before the picture is complete. Nevertheless, emerging data have already provided the impetus for the development new therapies for the prevention and treatment of RDS and BPD.

**REFERENCES**

1. Ikegami M. Surfactant inactivation. In: Boynton BR, Carlo WA, Jobe Att, eds. New Therapies for Neonatal Respiratory Failure. Cambridge: Cambridge University Press 1994:36–48.
2. Kendig JW, Notter RH, Cox C, Reubens LJ, Davis JM, Maniscalco WM, Sinkin RA, Bartoletti A, Dweck HS, Horgan MJ. A comparison of surfactant as immediate prophylaxis and as rescue therapy in newborns of less than 30 weeks' gestation N Engl J Med 1991; 324:865–871.
3. Whitsett JA, Pryhuber GS, Rice WR, Warner BB, Wert SE. Acute respiratory disorders. Neonatology 1994; 429–452.
4. Ballard RA, Ballard PL, Creasy RK, Padbury J, Polk DH, Bracken M, Moya FR, Gross I. Respiratory disease in very-low-birthweight infants after prenatal thyrotropin-releasing hormone and glucocorticoid. TRH Study Group. Lancet 1992; 339: 510–515.
5. Davis JM, Veness-Meehan K, Notter RH, Bhutani VK, Kendig JW, Shapiro DL. Changes in pulmonary mechanics after the administration of surfactant to infants with respiratory distress syndrome. N Engl J Med 1988; 319:476–479.
6. Soll RF, Merritt TA, Hallman M. Surfactant in the prevention and treatment of respiratory distress syndrome. In: Boynton BR, Carlo WA, Jobe Att, eds. New Therapies for Neonatal Respiratory Failure. Cambridge, UK: Cambridge University Press, 1994:49–80.
7. Jobe AH. Surfactant function and metabolism In: Boynton BR, Carlo WA, Jobe Att, eds. New Therapies for Neonatal Respiratory Failure. Cambridge, UK: Cambridge University Press, 1994; 16–35.
8. Massaro D, Massaro GD. Biochemical and anatomical adaptation of the lung to $O_2$-induced injury. Fed Proc 1978; 37:2485–2488.
9. Northway WH Jr, Rosan RC, Porter DY. Pulmonary disease following respirator therapy of hyaline-membrane disease. Bronchopulmonary dysplasia. N Engl J Med 1967; 276:357–368.
10. Toce SS, Farrell PM, Leavitt LA, Samuels DP, Edwards DK. Clinical and roentgenographic scoring systems for assessing bronchopulmonary dysplasia. Am J Dis Child 1984; 138:581–585.
11. Edwards DK. Radiographic aspects of bronchopulmonary dysplasia. J Pediatr 1979; 95:823–829.
12. Northway WH. Bronchopulmonary dysplasia — 25 years later. Pediatrics 1992; 89: 969–973.
13. Hoekstra RE, Jackson JC, Myers TF, Frantz ID III, Stern ME, Powers WF, Maurer M, Ray JR, Carrier ST, Gunkel JH, et al. Improved neonatal survival following multiple doses of bovine surfactant in very premature neonates at risk for respiratory distress syndrome. Pediatrics 1991; 88:10–18.
14. Merritt TA, Hallman M, Berry C, Pohjavuori M, Edwards DK III, Jaaskelainen J, Grafe MR, Vaucher Y, Wozniak P, Heldt G. Randomized, placebo-controlled trial of human surfactant given at birth versus rescue administration in very low birth weight infants with lung immaturity. J Pediatr 1991; 118:581–594.
15. Soll RF, Hoekstra RE, Fangman JJ, Corbet AJ, Adams JM, James LS, Schulze K, Oh

W, Roberts JD Jr, Dorst JP. Multicenter trial of single-dose modified bovine surfactant extract (Survanta) for prevention of respiratory distress syndrome. Ross Collaborative Surfactant Prevention Study Group. Pediatrics 1990; 85:1092–1102.

16. Bose C, Corbet A, Bose G, Garcia-Prats J, Lombardy L, Wold D, Donlon D, Long W. Improved outcome at 28 days of age for very low birth weight infants treated with a single dose of a synthetic surfactant. J Pediatr 1990; 117:947–953.

17. Long W, Thompson T, Sundell H, Schumacher R, Volberg F, Guthrie R. Effects of two rescue doses of a synthetic surfactant on mortality rate and survival without bronchopulmonary dysplasia in 700- to 1350-gram infants with respiratory distress syndrome. The American Exosurf Neonatal Study Group I. J Pediatr 1991; 118: 595–605.

18. Lang MJ, Hall RT, Reddy NS, Kurth CG, Merritt TA. A controlled trial of human surfactant replacement therapy for severe respiratory distress syndrome in very low birth weight infants. J Pediatr 1990; 116:295–300.

19. McCann EM, Goldman SL, Brady JP. Pulmonary function in the sick newborn infant. Pediatr Res 1987; 21:313–325.

20. Goldman SL, Gerhardt T, Sonni R, Feller R, Hehre D, Tapia JL, Bancalari E. Early prediction of chronic lung disease by pulmonary function testing. J Pediatr 1983; 102:613–617.

21. Tepper RS, Morgan WJ, Cota K, Taussig LM. Expiratory flow limitation in infants with bronchopulmonary dysplasia. J Pediatr 1986; 109:1040–1046.

22. Davis JM, Rosenfeld WR. Chronic lung disease. Neonatology 1994; 453–477.

23. Stocker JT. Pathologic features of long-standing "healed" bronchopulmonary dysplasia: a study of 28 3- to 40-month-old infants. Hum Pathol 1986; 17:943–961.

24. Fracica PJ, Piantadosi CA, Crapo JD. Oxygen toxicity. In: Crystal RG, West JB, eds. Lung Injury. New York: Raven Press, 1992:333–339.

25. Erzurum SC, Danel C, Gillissen A, Chu CS, Trapnell BC, Crystal RG. In vivo antioxidant gene expression in human airway epithelium of normal individuals exposed to 100-percent $O_2$. J Appl Physiol 1993; 75:1256–1262.

26. Griffith DE, Garcia JGN, James HL, Callahan KS, Iriana S, Holiday D. Hyperoxic exposure in humans—effects of 50-percent oxygen on alveolar macrophage leukotriene-B4 synthesis. Chest 1992; 101:392–397.

27. Smith CV, Hansen TN, Martin NE, Mcmicken HW, Elliott SJ. Oxidant stress responses in premature infants during exposure to hyperoxia. Pediatr Res 1993; 34: 360–365.

28. Delemos RA, Coalson JJ, Gerstmann DR, Null DM Jr, Ackerman NB, Escobedo MB, Robotham JL, Kuehl TJ. Ventilatory management of infant baboons with hyaline membrane disease: the use of high frequency ventilation. Pediatr Res 1987; 21:594–602.

29. Delemos RA, Coalson JJ, Gerstmann DR, Kuehl TJ, Null DM Jr. Oxygen toxicity in the premature baboon with hyaline membrane disease. Am Rev Respir Dis 1987; 136:677–682.

30. Coalson JJ, Kuehl TJ, Prihoda TJ, deLemos RA. Diffuse alveolar damage in the evolution of bronchopulmonary dysplasia in the baboon. Pediatr Res 1988; 24:357–366.

31. Coalson JJ, Winter VT, Gerstmann DR, Idell S, King RJ, Delemos RA. Patho-

physiologic, morphometric, and biochemical studies of the premature baboon with bronchopulmonary dysplasia. Am Rev Respir Dis 1992; 145:872–881.

32.   Davis JM, Dickerson B, Metlay L, Penney DP. Differential effects of $O_2$ and barotrauma on lung injury in the neonatal piglet. Pediatr Pulmonol 1991; 10: 157–163.

33.   Finkelstein JN, Horowitz S, Sinkin RA, Ryan RM. Cellular and molecular responses to lung injury in relation to induction of tissue repair and fibrosis (review). Clin Perinatol 1992; 19:603–620.

34.   Bagchi A, Viscardi RM, Taciak V, Ensor JE, McCrea KA, Hasday JD. Increased activity of interleukin-6 but not tumor necrosis factor-alpha in lung lavage of premature infants is associated with the development of bronchopulmonary dysplasia. Pediatr Res 1994; 36:244–252.

35.   Rinaldo JE, English D, Levine J, Stiller R, Henson J. Increased intrapulmonary retention of radiolabeled neutrophils in early $O_2$ toxicity. Am Rev Respir Dis 1988; 137:345–352.

36.   Merritt TA, Cochrane CG, Holcomb K, Bohl B, Hallman M, Strayer D, Edwards DK III, Gluck L. Elastase and alpha 1-proteinase inhibitor activity in tracheal aspirates during respiratory distress syndrome. Role of inflammation in the pathogenesis of bronchopulmonary dysplasia. J Clin Invest 1983; 72:656–666.

37.   Fantone JC, Feltner DE, Brieland JK, Ward PA. Phagocytic cell-derived inflammatory mediators and lung disease. Chest 1987; 91:428–435.

38.   Stenmark KR, Eyzaguirre M, Westcott JY, Henson PM, Murphy RC. Potential role of eicosanoids and PAF in the pathophysiology of bronchopulmonary dysplasia. Am Rev Respir Dis 1987; 136:770–772.

39.   Holtzman MJ. Arachidonic acid metabolism. Implications of biological chemistry for lung function and disease (review). Am Rev Respir Dis 1991; 143:188–203.

40.   O'Brodovich HM, Mellins RB. Bronchopulmonary dysplasia. Unresolved neonatal acute lung injury (review). Am Rev Respir Dis 1985; 132:694–709.

41.   Bruce MC, Wedig KE, Jentoft N, Martin RJ, Cheng PW, Boat TF, Fanaroff AA. Altered urinary excretion of elastin cross-links in premature infants who develop bronchopulmonary dysplasia. Am Rev Respir Dis 1985; 131:568–572.

42.   Ossanna PJ, Test ST, Matheson NR, Regiani S, Weiss SJ. Oxidative regulation of neutrophil elastase-alpha-1-proteinase inhibitor interactions. J Clin Invest 1986; 77:1939–1951.

43.   Rosenfeld W, Concepcion L, Evans H, Jhaveri R, Sahdev S, Zabaleta I. Serial trypsin inhibitory capacity and ceruloplasmin levels in prematures at risk for bronchopulmonary dysplasia. Am Rev Respir Dis 1986; 134:1229–1232.

44.   Koppel R, Han RNN, Cox D, Tanswell AK, Rabinovitch M. Alpha(1)-antitrypsin protects neonatal rats from pulmonary vascular and parenchymal effects of $O_2$ toxicity Pediatr Res 1994; 36:763–770.

45.   Frank L, Groseclose E. Oxygen toxicity in newborn rats: the adverse effects of undernutrition. J Appl Physiol 1982; 53:1248–1255.

46.   Hawker FH, Ward HE, Stewart PM, Wynne LA, Snitch PJ. Selenium deficiency augments the pulmonary toxic effects of oxygen exposure in the rat. Eur Respir J 1993; 6:1317–1323.

47. Forman HJ, Rotman EI, Fisher AB. Roles of selenium and sulfur-containing amino acids in protection against $O_2$ toxicity. Lab Invest 1983; 49:148–153.

48. O'Dell BL, Kilburn KH, McKenzie WN, Thurston RJ. The lung of the copper-deficient rat. A model for developmental pulmonary emphysema. Am J Pathol 1978; 91:413–432.

49. Guzder SN, Sung P, Bailly V, Prakash L, Prakash S. RAD25 is a DNA helicase required for DNA repair and RNA polymerase II transcription. Nature 1994; 369: 578–581.

50. Ehrenkranz RA, Bonta BW, Ablow RC, Warshaw JB. Amelioration of bronchopulmonary dysplasia after vitamin E administration. A preliminary report. N Engl J Med 1978; 299:564–569.

51. Ehrenkranz RA, Ablow RC, Warshaw JB. Effect of vitamin E on the development of $O_2$-induced lung injury in neonates. Ann NY Acad Sci 1982; 393:452–466.

52. Hittner HM, Godio LB, Rudolph AJ, Adams JM, Garcia-Prats JA, Friedman Z, Kautz JA, Monaco WA. Retrolental fibroplasia: efficacy of vitamin E in a double-blind clinical study of preterm infants. N Engl J Med 1981; 305:1365–1371.

53. Saldanha RL, Cepeda EE, Poland RL. The effect of vitamin E prophylaxis on the incidence and severity of bronchopulmonary dysplasia. J Pediatr 1982; 101:89–93.

54. Sosenko IR, Innis SM, Frank L. Polyunsaturated fatty acids and protection of newborn rats from $O_2$ toxicity. J Pediatr 1988; 112:630–637.

55. Brandt RB, Mueller DG, Schroeder JR, Guyer KE, Kirkpatrick BV, Hutcher NE, Ehrlich FE. Serum vitamin A in premature and term neonates. J Pediatr 1978; 92: 101–104.

56. Shenai JP, Rush MG, Stahlman MT, Chytil F. Plasma retinol-binding protein response to vitamin A administration in infants susceptible to bronchopulmonary dysplasia. J Pediatr 1990; 116:607–614.

57. Hustead VA, Gutcher GR, Anderson SA, Zachman RD. Relationship of vitamin A (retinol) status to lung disease in the preterm infant. J Pediatr 1984; 105:610–615.

58. Shenai JP, Chytil F, Stahlman MT. Vitamin A status of neonates with bronchopulmonary dysplasia. Pediatr Res 1985; 19:185–188.

59. Hartline JV, Zachman RD. Vitamin A delivery in total parenteral nutrition solution. Pediatrics 1976; 58:448–451.

60. Nickerson BG, Taussig LM. Family history of asthma in infants with bronchopulmonary dysplasia. Pediatrics 1980; 65:1140–1144.

61. Clark DA, Pincus LG, Oliphant M., Hubbell C, Oates RP, Davey FR. HLA-A2 and chronic lung disease in neonates. JAMA 1982; 248:1868–1869.

62. Gonder JC, Proctor RA, Will JA. Genetic differences in $O_2$ toxicity are correlated with cytochrome P-450 inducibility. Proc Natl Acad Sci USA 1985; 82:6415–6319.

63. Mansour H, Levacher M, Azoulay Dupuis E, Moreau J, Marquetty C, Gougerot Pocidalo MA. Genetic differences in response to pulmonary cytochrome P-450 inducers and $O_2$ toxicity. J Appl Physiol 1988; 64:1376–1381.

64. Parrish DA, Mitchell BC, Henson PM, Larsen GL. Pulmonary response of fifth component of complement-sufficient and -deficient mice to hyperoxia. J Clin Invest 1984; 74:956–965.

65. Piedboeuf B, Johnston CJ, Watkins RH, Hudak BB, Lazo JS, Cherian MG, Horowitz

S. Increased expression of tissue inhibitor of metalloproteinases (TIMP-1) and metallothionein in murine lungs after hyperoxic exposure. Am J Respir Cell Mol Biol 1994; 10:123–132.

66. Hudak BB, Zhang LY, Kleeberger SR. Inter-strain variation in susceptibility to hyperoxic injury of murine airways. Pharmacogenetics 1993; 3:135–143.

67. Van Marter LJ, Leviton A, Kuban KC, Pagano M, Allred EN. Maternal glucocorticoid therapy and reduced risk of bronchopulmonary dysplasia. Pediatrics 1990; 86:331–336.

68. Frank L, Sosenko IR. Undernutrition as a major contributing factor in the pathogenesis of bronchopulmonary dysplasia. Am Rev Respir Dis 1988; 138:725–729.

69. Shenai JP, Kennedy KA, Chytil F, Stahlman MT. Clinical trial of vitamin A supplementation in infants susceptible to bronchopulmonary dysplasia. J Pediatr 1987; 111:269–277.

70. Cummings JJ, D'Eugenio DB, Gross SJ. A controlled trial of dexamethasone in preterm infants at high risk for bronchopulmonary dysplasia. N Engl J Med 1989; 320:1505–1510.

71. Davis JM, Whitin J. Prophylactic effects of dexamethasone in lung injury caused by hyperoxia and hyperventilation. J Appl Physiol 1992; 72:1320–1325.

72. Gross NJ, Smith DM. Methylprednisolone increases the toxicity of $O_2$ in adult mice. Mechanical and biochemical effects on the surfactant system. Am Rev Respir Dis 1984; 129:805–810.

73. Koizumi M, Frank L, Massaro D. Oxygen toxicity in rats. Varied effect of dexamethasone treatment depending on duration of hyperoxia. Am Rev Respir Dis 1985; 131:907–911.

74. Frank L. Hyperoxic inhibition of newborn rat lung development—protection by deferoxamine. Free Radic Biol Med 1991; 11:341–348.

75. deLemos RA, Roberts RJ, Coalson JJ, delemos JA, Null DM Jr, Gerstmann DR. Toxic effects associated with the administration of deferoxamine in the premature baboon with hyaline membrane disease. Am J Dis Child 1990; 144:915–919.

76. Frank L, Mclaughlin GE. Protection against acute and chronic hyperoxic inhibition of neonatal rat lung development with the 21-aminosteroid drug-U74389F. Pediatr Res 1993; 33:632–638.

77. Heffner JE, Repine JE. Antioxidants and the lung. In: Crystal RG, West JB, eds. Lung Injury. New York: Raven Press, 1992:51–60.

78. Jacobson JM, Michael JR, Jafri MH Jr, Gurtner GH. Antioxidants and antioxidant enzymes protect against pulmonary $O_2$ toxicity in the rabbit. J Appl Physiol 1990; 68:1252–1259.

79. Tanswell AK, Freeman BA. Liposome-entrapped antioxidant enzymes prevent lethal $O_2$ toxicity in the newborn rat. J Appl Physiol 1987; 63:347–352.

80. Walther FJ, Gidding CE, Kuipers IM, Willebrand D, Bevers EM, Abuchowski A, Viau AT. Prevention of $O_2$ toxicity with superoxide dismutase and catalase in premature lambs. J Free Radic Biol Med 1986; 2:289–293.

81. Rosenfeld W, Evans H, Concepcion L, Jhaveri R, Schaeffer H, Friedman A. Prevention of bronchopulmonary dysplasia by administration of bovine superoxide dis-

mutase in preterm infants with respiratory distress syndrome. J Pediatr 1984; 105: 781–785.

82. Davis JM, Rosenfeld WN, Sanders RJ, Gonenne A. Prophylactic effects of recombinant human superoxide dismutase in neonatal lung injury. J Appl Physiol 1993; 74: 2234–2241.

83. Matalon S, Holm BA, Baker RR, Whitfield MK, Freeman BA. Characterization of antioxidant activities of pulmonary surfactant mixtures. Biochim Biophys Acta 1990; 1035:121–127.

84. Curran SF, Amoruso MA, Goldstein BD, Berg RA. Degradation of soluble collagen by ozone or hydroxyl radicals. FEBS Lett 1984; 176:155–160.

85. Durr RA, Dubaybo BA, Thet LA. Repair of chronic hyperoxic lung injury: changes in lung ultrastructure and matrix. Exp Mol Pathol 1987; 47:219–240.

86. Crapo JD, Peters-Golden M, Marsh Salin J, Shelburne JS. Pathologic changes in the lungs of $O_2$-adapted rats: a morphometric analysis. Lab Invest 1978; 39:640–653.

87. Crapo JD, Barry BE, Foscue HA, Shelburne J. Structural and biochemical changes in rat lungs occurring during exposures to lethal and adaptive doses of $O_2$. Am Rev Respir Dis 1980; 122:123–143.

88. Freeman BA, Mason RJ, Williams MC, Crapo JD. Antioxidant enzyme activity in alveolar type II cells after exposure of rats to hyperoxia. Exp Lung Res 1986; 10: 203–222.

89. Bucher JR, Roberts RJ. The development of the newborn rat lung in hyperoxia: a dose-response study of lung growth, maturation, and changes in antioxidant enzyme activities. Pediatr Res 1981; 15:999–1008.

90. Blanco LN, Frank L. The formation of alveoli in rat lung during the third and fourth postnatal weeks — effect of hyperoxia, dexamethasone, and deferoxamine. Pediatr Res 1993; 34:334–340.

91. Sekhon HS, Smith C, Thurlbeck WM. Effect of hypoxia and hyperoxia on postpneumonectomy compensatory lung growth. Exp Lung Res 1993; 19:519–532.

92. Hershenson MB, Aghili S, Punjabi N, Hernandez C, Ray DW, Garland A, Glagov S, Solway J. Hyperoxia-induced airway hyperresponsiveness and remodeling in immature rats. Am J Physiol 1992; 262:L263–L269.

93. Murchie P, Johnston PW, Ross JAS, Godden DJ. Effects of hyperoxia on bronchial wall dimensions and lung mechanics in rats. Acta Physiol Scand 1993; 148: 363–370.

94. Coalson JJ, King RJ, Winter VT, Prihoda TJ, Anzueto AR, Peters JI, Johanson WG Jr. $O_2$- and pneumonia-induced lung injury. I. Pathological and morphometric studies. J Appl Physiol 1989; 67:346–356.

95. Kelly FJ. Effect of hyperoxic exposure on protein synthesis in the rat (published erratum appears in Biochem J 1988 Jun 15; 252:935). Biochem J 1988; 249: 609–612.

96. Horowitz S, Shapiro DL, Finkelstein JN, Notter RH, Johnston CJ, Quible DJ. Changes in gene expression in hyperoxia-induced neonatal lung injury. Am J Physiol 1990; 258:L107–L111.

97. Gacad G, Massaro D. Hyperoxia: influence on lung mechanics and protein synthesis. J Clin Invest 1973; 52:559–565.

98.   Holm BA, Notter RH, Siegle J, Matalon S. Pulmonary physiological and surfactant changes during injury and recovery from hyperoxia. J Appl Physiol 1985: 59:1402–1409.

99.   Nogee LM, Wispe JR. Effects of pulmonary $O_2$ injury on airway content of surfactant-associated protein A. Pediatr Res 1988; 24:568–573.

100.  Nogee LM, Wispe JR, Clark JC, Weaver TE, Whitsett JA. Increased expression of pulmonary surfactant proteins in $O_2$-exposed rats. Am J Respir Cell Mol Biol 1991; 4:102–107.

101.  Nogee LM, Wispe JR, Clark JC, Whitsett JA. Increased synthesis and mRNA of surfactant protein A in $O_2$-exposed rats. Am J Respir Cell Mol Biol 1989; 1:119–125.

102.  Horowitz S, Dafni N, Shapiro DL, Holm BA, Notter RH, Quible DJ. Hyperoxic exposure alters gene expression in the lung. Induction of the tissue inhibitor of metalloproteinases mRNA and other mRNAs. J Biol Chem 1989; 264:7092–7095.

103.  Minoo P, Segura L, Coalson JJ, King RJ, Delemos RA. Alterations in surfactant protein gene expression associated with premature birth and exposure to hyperoxia. Am J Physiol 1991; 26:L386–L392.

104.  Minoo P, King RJ, Coalson JJ. Surfactant proteins and lipids are regulated independently during hyperoxia. Am J Physiol 1992; 3:491–496.

105.  Auten RL, Watkins RH, Shapiro DL, Horowitz S. Surfactant apoprotein A is synthesized in airway cells. Am J Respir Cell Mol Biol 1990; 3:491–496.

106.  Phelps DS, Floros J. Localization of surfactant protein synthesis in human lung by *in situ* hybridization. Am Rev Respir Dis 1988; 137:939–942.

107.  Horowitz S, Watkins RH, Auten RL Jr, Mercier CE, Cheng ER. Differential accumulation of surfactant protein A, B, And C mRNAs in two epithelial cell types of hyperoxic lung. Am J Respir Cell Mol Biol 1991; 5:511–515.

108.  Wikenheiser KA, Wert SE, Wispe JR, Stahlman M, Damorebruno M, Singh G, Katyal SL, Whitsett JA. Distinct effects of oxygen on surfactant protein-B expression in bronchiolar and alveolar epithelium. Am J Physiol 1992; 262:L32–L39.

109.  Kalina M, Mason RJ, Shannon JM. Surfactant protein C is expressed in alveolar type II cells but not in Clara cells of rat lung. Am J Respir Cell Mol Biol 1992; 6:594–600.

110.  Freeman BA, Crapo JD. Hyperoxia increases $O_2$ radical production in rat lungs and lung mitochondria. J Biol Chem 1981; 256:10986–10992.

111.  Freeman BA, Topolosky MK, Crapo JD. Hyperoxia increases $O_2$ radical production in rat lung homogenates. Arch Biochem Biophys 1982; 216:477–484.

112.  Pappas CT, Obara H, Bensch KG, Northway WH Jr. Effect of prolonged exposure to 80% $O_2$ on the lung of the newborn mouse. Lab Invest 1983; 48:735–748.

113.  McCord JM. Human disease, free radicals, and the oxidant/antioxidant balance. Clin Biochem 1993; 26:351–357.

114.  Crapo JD, McCord JM. Oxygen-induced changes in pulmonary superoxide dismutase assayed by antibody titrations. Am J Physiol 1976; 231:1196–1203.

115.  Vincent R, Chang LY, Slot JW, Crapo JD. Quantitative immunocytochemical analysis of Mn-SOD in alveolar type II cells of the hyperoxic rat. Am J Physiol Lung Cell Mol Physiol 1994; 11:L475–L481.

116. Keeney SE, Cress SE, Brown SE, Bidani A. The effect of hyperoxic exposure on antioxidant enzyme activities of alveolar type-II cells in neonatal and adult rats. Pediatr Res 1992; 31:441–444.

117. Ahotupa M, Mantyla E, Peltola V, Puntala A, Toivonen H. Pro-oxidant effects of normobaric hyperoxia in rat tissues. Acta Physiol Scand 1992; 145:151–157.

118. Baker RR, Holm BA, Panus PC, Matalon S. Development of $O_2$ tolerance in rabbits with no increase in antioxidant enzymes. J Appl Physiol 1989; 66:1679–1684.

119. Ho YS, Howard AJ, Crapo JD. Molecular structure of a functional rat gene for manganese-containing superoxide dismutase. Am J Respir Cell Mol Biol 1991; 4: 278–286.

120. Clerch LB, Iqbal J, Massaro D. Perinatal rat lung catalase gene expression: influence of corticosteroid and hyperoxia. Am J Physiol 1991; 260:L428–L433.

121. Clerch LB, Massaro D. Oxidation-reduction–sensitive binding of lung protein to rat catalase messenger RNA. J Biol Chem 1992; 267:2853–2855.

122. Frank L, Sosenko IR. Failure of premature rabbits to increase antioxidant enzymes during hyperoxic exposure: increased susceptibility to pulmonary $O_2$ toxicity compared with term rabbits. Pediatr Res 1991; 29:292–296.

123. Fini ME, Karmilowicz MJ, Ruby PL, Beeman AM, Borges KA, Brinckerhoff CE. Cloning of a complementary DNA for rabbit proactivator. A metalloproteinase that activates synovial cell collagenase, shares homology with stromelysin and transin, and is coordinately regulated with collagenase. Arthritis Rheum 1987; 30:1254–1264.

124. Yam J, Frank L, Roberts RJ. Oxygen toxicity: comparison of lung biochemical responses in neonatal and adult rats. Pediatr Res 1978; 12:115–119.

125. Jackson RM, Frank L. Ozone-induced tolerance to hyperoxia in rats. Am Rev Respir Dis 1984; 129:425–429.

126. Jensen JC, Pogrebniak HW, Pass HI, Buresh C, Merino MJ, Kauffman D, Venzon D, Langstein HN, Norton JA. Role of tumor necrosis factor in $O_2$ toxicity. J Appl Physiol 1992; 72:1902–1907.

127. Lewis-Molock Y, Suzuki K, Taniguchi N, Nguyen DH, Mason RJ, White CW. Lung manganese superoxide dismutase increases during cytokine-mediated protection against pulmonary $O_2$ toxicity in rats. Am J Respir Cell Mol Biol 1994; 10:133–141.

128. Tsan MF, Lee CY, White JE. Interleukin-1 protects rats against oxygen toxicity. J Appl Physiol 1991; 71:688–697.

129. Mansour H, Levacher M, Gougerot Pocidalo MA, Rouveix B, Pocidalo JJ. Diethyldithiocarbamate provides partial protection against pulmonary and lymphoid $O_2$ toxicity. J Pharmacol Exp Ther 1986; 236:476–480.

130. Hamburg DC, Tonoki H, Welty SE, Geske RS, Montgomery CA, Hansen TN. Endotoxin induces glutathione reductase activity in lungs of mice. Pediatr Res 1994; 35:311–315.

131. Hass MA, Massaro D. Mitogenic response of rat lung to endotoxin exposure. Biochem Pharmacol 1987; 36:3841–3846.

132. Kikkawa Y, Yano S, Skoza L. Protective effect of interferon inducers against hyperoxic pulmonary damage. Lab Invest 1984; 50:62–71.

133. Frank L. Premature weaning of rat pups results in prolongation of neonatal tolerance to hyperoxia. Pediatr Res 1991; 29:376–380.

134. White CW, Avraham KB, Shanley PF, Groner Y. Transgenic mice with expression of elevated levels of copper-zinc superoxide dismutase in the lungs are resistant to pulmonary $O_2$ toxicity. J Clin Invest 1991; 87:621–628.

135. Oberley TD, Coursin DB, Cihla HP, Oberley LW, el-Sayyad N, Ho YS. Immuno-localization of manganese superoxide dismutase in normal and transgenic mice expressing the human enzyme. Histochem J 1993; 25:267–279.

136. Wispe JR, Warner BB, Clark JC, Dey CR, Neuman J, Glasser SW, Crapo JD, Chang LY, Whitsett JA. Human Mn–superoxide dismutase in pulmonary epithelial cells of transgenic mice confers protection from $O_2$ injury. J Biol Chem 1992; 267:23937–23941.

137. Turrens JF. The potential of antioxidant enzymes as pharmacological agents in vivo Rev Xenobiot 1991; 21:1033–1040.

138. Mercer RR, Russell ML, Roggli VL, Crapo JD. Cell number and distribution in human and rat airways. Am J Respir Cell Mol Biol 1994; 10:613–624.

139. Vincent R, Chang LY, Slot JW, Crapo JD. Quantitative immunocytochemical analysis of Mn-SOD in alveolar type II cells of the hyperoxic rat. Am J Physiol 1994; 267:L475–L481.

140. Applegate LA, Luscher P, Tyrrell RM. Induction of heme oxygenase: a general response to oxidant stress in cultured mammalian cells. Cancer Res 1991; 51: 974–978.

141. Dennery PA, McDonagh AF, Spits DR, Rodgers PA, Stevenson DK. Hyper-bilirubinemia results in reduced oxidative injury in neonatal Gunn rats exposed to hyperoxia. Free Radic Biol Med 1995; 19:395–404.

142. Rodgers PA, Lee CS, Stevenson DK, Dennery PA. Ontogeny of lung heme oxygenase in the neonatal Wistar rat (abstr). Pediatr Res 1995; 37:234.

143. Fleming RE, Whitman IP, Gitlin JD. Induction of ceruloplasmin gene expression in rat lung during inflammation and hyperoxia (published erratum appears in Am J Physiol 1991; 260:following Table of Contents). Am J Physiol 1991; 260:L68–L74.

144. Bingle CD, Kelly F, Epstein O, Srai SK. Induction of hepatic and pulmonary caeruloplasmin gene expression in developing guinea pigs following premature delivery. Biochim Biophys Acta 1992; 1139:217–221.

145. Veness-Meehan KA, Cheng ERY, Mercier CE, Blixt SL, Johnston CJ, Watkins RH, Horowitz S. Cell-specific alterations in expression of hyperoxia-induced messenger RNAs of lung. Am J Respir Cell Mol Biol 1991; 5:516–521.

146. Hamer DH. Metallothionein. Ann Rev Biochem 1986; 55:913–951.

147. Palmiter RD, Findley SD, Whitmore TE, Durnam DM. MT-III, a brain-specific member of the metallothionein gene family. Proc Natl Acad Sci USA 1992; 89: 6333–6337.

148. Quaife CJ, Findley SD, Erickson JC, Froelick GJ, Kelly EJ, Zambrowicz BP, Palmiter RD. Induction of a new metallothionein isoform (MT-IV) occurs during differentiation of stratified squamous epithelia. Biochemistry 1994; 33:7250–7259.

149. Sato M, Bremner I. Oxygen free radicals and metallothionein (review). Free Radic Biol Med 1993; 14:325–337.

150. Tamai KT, Gralla EB, Ellerby LM, Valentine JS, Thiele DJ. Yeast and mammalian metallothioneins functionally substitute for yeast copper-zinc superoxide dismutase. Proc Natl Acad Sci USA 1993; 90:8013–8017.

151. Hart BA, Voss GW, Garvey JS. Induction of pulmonary metallothionein following $O_2$ exposure. Environ Res 1989; 50:269–278.

152. Hart BA, Voss GW, Shatos MA, Doherty J. Cross-tolerance to hyperoxia following cadmium aerosol pretreatment. Toxicol Appl Pharmacol 1990; 103:255–270.

153. Okamoto T, Mitsuhashi M, Fujita I, Sindhu RK, Kikkawa Y. Induction of cytochrome P450 1A1 and 1A2 by hyperoxia. Biochem Biophys Res Commun 1993; 197:878–885.

154. Tindberg N, Ingelman-Sundberg M. Cytochrome P-450 and $O_2$ toxicity. Oxygen-dependent induction of ethanol-inducible cytochrome P-450 (IIE1) in rat liver and lung. Biochemistry 1989; 28:4499–4504.

155. Nici L, Dowin R, Gilmore-Hebert M, Jamieson JD, Ingbar DH. Upregulation of rat lung Na-K-ATPase during hyperoxic injury. Am J Physiol 1991; 261:L307–L314.

156. Sinkin RA, LoMonaco MB, Finkelstein JN, Watkins RH, Cox C, Horowitz S. Increased fibronectin mRNA in alveolar macrophages following *in vivo* hyperoxia. Am J Respir Cell Mol Biol 1992; 7:548–555.

157. Ferrara TB, Fox RB. Effects of oxygen toxicity on cuprolinic blue-stained proteoglycans in alveolar basement membranes. Am J Respir Cell Mol Biol 1992; 6:219–224.

158. Matrisian LM. Metalloproteinases and their inhibitors in matrix remodeling. Trends Genet 1990; 6121–6125.

159. Bruce MC, Bruce EN, Janiga K, Chetty A. Hyperoxic exposure of developing rat lung decreases tropoelastin mRNA levels that rebound postexposure. Am J Physiol 1993; 265:L293–L300.

160. Ge M, Ryan TJ, Malik AB. Pulmonary endothelium and coagulation In: Crystal RG, West JB, eds. Lung Injury. New York: Raven Press, 1992:329–336.

161. White JE, Ryan MP, Tsan MF, Higgins PJ. Hyperoxic stress elevates p52(PAI-1) messenger RNA abundance in cultured cells and adult rat pulmonary tissue. Am J Physiol 1993; 265:L121–L126.

162. Senior RM, Shapiro SD. Introduction: the matrix metalloproteinase family. Am J Respir Cell Mol Biol 1992; 7:119.

163. Apte SS, Hayashi K, Seldin MF, Mattei MG, Hayashi M, Olsen BR. Gene encoding a novel murine tissue inhibitor of metalloproteinases (TIMP), TIMP-3, is expressed in developing mouse epithelia, cartilage, and muscle, and is located on mouse chromosome 10. Dev Dyn 1994; 200:177–197.

164. Avalos BR, Kaufman SE, Tomonaga M, Williams RE, Golde DW, Gasson JC. K562 cells produce and respond to human erythroid-potentiating activity. Blood 1988; 71:1720–1725.

165. Minoo P, Penn R, Delemos DM, Coalson JJ, Delemos RA. Tissue inhibitor of metalloproteinase-1 messenger RNA is specifically induced in lung tissue after birth. Pediatr Res 1993; 34:729–734.

166. Han RNN, Buch S, Freeman BA, Post M, Tanswell AK. Platelet-derived growth factor and growth-related genes in rat lung. 2. Effect of exposure to 85-percent $O_2$. Am J Physiol 1992; 262:L140–L146.

167. Powell PP, Klagsbrun M, Abraham JA, Jones RC. Eosinophils expressing heparin-binding EGF-like growth factor mRNA localize around lung microvessels in pulmonary hypertension. Am J Pathol 1993; 143:784–794.

168. Welty SE, Rivera JL, Elliston JF, Smith CV, Zeb T, Ballantyne CM, Montgomery CA, Hansen TN. Increases in lung tissue expression of intercellular adhesion molecule-1 are associated with hyperoxic lung injury and inflammation in mice. Am J Respir Cell Mol Biol 1993; 9:393–400.

169. Kang BH, Crapo JD, Wegner CD, Letts LG, Chang LY. Intercellular adhesion molecule-1 expression on the alveolar epithelium and its modification by hyperoxia. Am J Respir Cell Mol Biol 1993; 9:350–355.

170. Albelda SM. Endothelial and epithelial cell adhesion molecules (review). Am J Respir Cell Mol Biol 1991; 4:195–203.

171. Jorens PG, Vermeire PA, Herman AG. L-arginine-dependent nitric oxide synthase: a new metabolic pathway in the lung and airways (review). Eur Respir J 1993; 6: 258–266.

172. Haddad IY, Crow JP, Hu P, Ye Y, Beckman J, Matalon S. Concurrent generation of nitric oxide and superoxide damages surfactant protein A. Am J Physiol 1994; 267: L242–L249.

173. Haddad IY, Pataki G, Hu P, Galliani C, Beckman JS, Matalon S. Quantitation of nitrotyrosine levels in lung sections of patients and animals with acute lung injury J Clin Invest 1994; 94:2407–2413.

174. Canada AT, Herman LA, Young SL. An age-related difference in hyperoxia lethality: role of lung antioxidant defense mechanisms. Am J Physiol 1995; 268:L539–L545.

175. Choi AM, Sylvester S, Otterbein L, Holbrook NJ. Molecular responses to hyperoxia in vivo: relationship to increased tolerance in aged rats. Am J Respir Cell Mol Biol 1995; 13:74–82.

176. Carlsson LM, Jonsson J, Edlund T, Marklund SL. Mice lacking extracellular superoxide dismutase are more sensitive to hyperoxia. Proc Natl Acad Sci USA. 1995; 92: 6264–6268.

177. Robbins CG, Davis JM, Merritt TA, Amirkhanian J, Sahgal N, Morin FC III, Horowitz S. Combined effects of nitric oxide and hyperoxia on surfactant function and pulmonary inflammation. Am J Physiol 1995; 13:L545–L550.

178. Yue G, Russell WJ, Benos DJ, Jackson RM, Olman MA, Matalon S. Increased expression and activity of sodium channels in alveolar type II cells of hyperoxic rats. Proc Natl Acad Sci USA 1995; 92:8418–8422.

179. Sznajder JI, Olivera WG, Ridge KM, Rutschman DH. Mechanisms of lung liquid clearance during hyperoxia in isolated rat lungs. Am J Respir Crit Care Med 1995; 151:1519–1525.

# 17

# In Vitro Models of Lung Development and Cytodifferentiation

**S. ROBERT HILFER and ROBERT L. SEARLS**

Temple University
Philadelphia, Pennsylvania

## I. Introduction

### A. Background

Much of the current understanding of lung morphogenesis and cytodifferentiation is based on studies which have been done in vitro. This chapter concentrates on work done in organ culture, because this approach preserves the three-dimensional organization of the tissues. The goal of this chapter is to describe the types of studies which have been done on (1) lung branching and (2) the establishment of respiratory cell types (cytodifferentiation). In doing so, we will provide some examples of the questions which have been addressed and the questions which remain unanswered. More detailed coverage of some of these topics will be found in the chapters which follow.

Culture methods have changed greatly over the years since the technique was developed. The original methods relied heavily on animal proteins from sources such as serum and extracts of embryonic tissue to support survival. It was realized early that these fluids contain both toxic components (such as antibodies in sera) and undefined and variable growth factors, and they may vary in their content of essential nutrients. The development of methods to promote growth from dissociated cell populations and from single isolated cells resulted in improvements in the composition of culture media (e.g., see ref. 1). Currently, it is customary to use culture media which are low or lacking in animal fluids and high in amino acids, vitamins, hormones, and growth factors. These media (2–5) are known as serum-free or defined media. Some of the differences in results from different laboratories, discussed in the following sections, could result from variations in media formulations.

### B. Summary of Lung Development

The lung forms from endoderm in the floor of the posterior pharynx. In the mouse, the primordium consists of two lateral buds which elongate as primary bronchi and branch continuously to form successive generations of the respiratory tree (6). At the same time, the trachea is formed by horizontal partitioning of the pharyngeal floor. Lung development in mammals usually is divided into four stages based on morphological criteria (7,8). During the pseudoglandular phase, the basic branching pattern is established in the early embryo. This is followed in the early fetus by a canalicular phase of continued branching characterized by columnar epithelial tubules having narrow lumina. During the third, or saccular, phase, the respiratory endings expand to form saccules. The final, or alveolar, phase completes the formation of the adult morphology and takes place after birth in most mammals. Except for the branching pattern, development is similar in birds.

During the pseudoglandular stage, the lobular pattern of the lung is established by the formation of different numbers of buds at each branch point. The simple columnar epithelium forms bronchi as the buds branch and grow out. The epithelial tubules are surrounded by densely packed mesenchyme which forms the lung capsule. These tubules frequently have a lumen too narrow to be easily visible by light microscopy. Both the respiratory epithelium and the mesenchyme begin to assume their adult morphologies during the transition from the canalicular stage to the saccular stage (7,8). By the saccular stage, the epithelial tubules have swelled to form saccules with enlarged lumina, and the dense mesenchyme has thinned to form narrow partitions. Some of the epithelial cells become flattened (approaching the morphology of type I pneumocytes), and others become almost cuboidal and contain lamellar bodies (approaching the morphology of type II pneumocytes).

The above description implies that both the epithelium and the mesenchyme are required to obtain morphologically recognizable differentiation. The differentiation of type II pneumocytes can be obtained in cell culture (e.g., see ref. 5), but one can not describe with confidence the differentiation of the mesenchyme or of type I pneumocytes except in organ culture.

## II. Branching Morphogenesis

### A. Extracellular Matrix and Branching

A major area of investigation is directed at learning what causes the early lung primordium to undergo repeated branching. It was recognized as early as 1933 (9) that the mesenchymal capsule surrounding the lung bud plays a role in this process. Early experiments showing an effect of mesenchyme on branching (10–12) led to examination of the components of the extracellular matrix as possible sources of developmental cues.

### Role for Mesenchyme in Branching
#### Background

The general interest during the 1950s and 1960s in an interaction between epithelium and mesenchyme during the development of organs led to examination of such a relationship in the lung. Alescio and Cassini showed that pulmonary mesenchyme can cause the trachea to branch (10). The response is relatively specific for lung mesenchyme; replacement of lung mesenchyme with mesenchyme of other endodermal organ primordia results in an unbranched bud (11). Tracheal mesenchyme, in contrast, suppresses branching of bronchial buds (10,11). The effect of mesenchyme on branching is quantitative; the number of branches which bronchial buds can form is proportional to the amount of mesenchyme that is provided (12). Salivary mesenchyme causes branching reminiscent of the salivary, and chick lung mesenchyme causes formation of tubular structures in mouse respiratory epithelium characteristic of chick bronchi rather than mammalian saccular endings (13). There is some evidence that the specificity of the mesenchymal response depends on the inability of foreign mesenchyme to support proliferation of the bronchial epithelium (14) (see discussion of control of cell proliferation in Section II.B). These observations raise the question of whether the mesenchyme acts to promote cell division, to place physical constraints on epithelial growth, or to provide signals which direct epithelial differentiation.

#### Organization of the Mesenchymal Capsule

The most obvious feature of a connective tissue is the organization of its matrix. Mesenchyme, as an embryonic connective tissue, tends to be watery and relatively cellular. Capsules which surround developing organs have a more defined structure with a higher collagen content, often organized as bundles or lattices. The lung capsule is no exception. Formation of bronchial tubes is accompanied by the formation of a collagenous sheath consisting of bundles lying parallel to the tracheal and bronchial axes (11). The bronchial buds are covered with a loose meshwork of thinner collagen fibrils. A basal lamina covers epithelial cell bases and separates the epithelium from the extracellular matrix of the capsule. This layer is thin and patchy at bronchial buds, so that filopodia of mesenchymal cells make contact with the epithelial surface (15–17).

The extracellular matrix contains a variety of macromolecules in addition to soluble components which are supplied by the vascular system. The major classes are collagens, proteoglycans, and glycoproteins. The capsular matrix contains types I, III, and V collagens, hyaluronan, several different proteoglycans, and the glycoprotein fibronectin. Basal lamina is characterized by its content of type IV collagen, distinctive heparan sulfate and chondroitin sulfate proteoglycans, and glycoproteins such as laminin, entactin (nidogen), and tenascin (cytotactin, hexabrachion). The extracellular components are anchored to the epithelial surface by integral membrane proteins which serve as receptors for one or more of these macromolecules. Receptor classes include integrins, the heparan sulfate proteoglycan syndecan, and cell adhesion molecule families of CAMs and cadherins.

Components of the extracellular matrix could affect branching by several mechanisms. They could be differentially deposited or removed from surfaces at specific developmental stages and act as a physical barrier. They could bind growth factors or other soluble molecules which affect either cell proliferation or establishment of a branch point. They could occupy binding sites on epithelial membranes and either exclude cell contacts by steric hindrance or could change the volume of extracellular space according to the species which are present. Most of these molecules are relatively large; they differ in the amount of water they bind and could thereby change the permeability of the extracellular space.

### Roles of Extracellular Matrix in Branching

With a few exceptions, branching of bronchial buds has not been studied with the same thoroughness as branching of the salivary primordium. The elegant studies on the salivary by Bernfield, Nakanishi, and others (e.g., see refs. 18–20) has shown that branching is controlled by coordinated secretions by cells of the epithelium and capsule. In the salivary, the first step in forming a bud is the formation of an indentation in the basal surface of the epithelium by activity within the epithelial cells. Mesenchyme cells stabilize this cleft by depositing a small bundle of type III collagen within it. The tip of the bud is accessible to mesenchyme cells, which expose the surface by secreting enzymes to degrade proteoglycans and collagen. The duct system becomes stabilized by the deposition first of a continuous basal lamina and secondarily by deposition of oriented bundles of collagen I. The limited data on lung branching at the present time do not permit comparisons to be made with this suggested scheme for salivary branching.

### Collagen

There is little experimental information on the role of collagen in branching of bronchial buds. Collagen bundles become oriented along the airways as they are formed (11), and the basal lamina is thin and discontinuous at the bud tips (15,16). Collagens I and III are present at the earliest stages of bud formation and become localized primarily to the airways as branching continues (21,22). In contrast, type IV (basal lamina) collagen is distributed along the buds as well as along the airways (23); the collagen α1(IV) gene is expressed by both epithelium and mesenchyme (24). Collagen must be involved in branching, since addition to the medium of inhibitors of collagen synthesis (such as L-azetidine-3-carboxylic acid or α,α' dipyridyl) inhibit branching (25,26). However, a detailed analysis of localization and temporal appearance of each collagen type of the sort which was done for salivary branching has not been done for the lung.

### Proteoglycans

Histochemical techniques have shown that acidic particles, presumably proteoglycans, are distributed along the basal surfaces of the epithelial branches from the earliest stages of development (16,22). Treatment of lung cultures with β-xyloside, an inhibitor of chondroitin sulfate proteoglycan (CSPG) synthesis, inhibits branching (27). However, the α-anomer, which does not inhibit CSPG synthesis, also inhibits branching at high doses.

### Glycoproteins

Of the structural glycoproteins, laminin has been studied most extensively relative to lung branching (28–30). The A and B chains are produced by epithelial and mesenchymal cells from the beginning of lung development (31). The two different B chains are produced by both cell types, but the A chain is expressed by mesenchyme in the bronchial regions, whereas the epithelium expresses the A chain in the buds. Nidogen is expressed only by mesenchymal cells; by interacting with laminin A chain, it may control the kind of basal lamina which is produced at bud tips (24). Incubation of embryonic lung primordia with polyclonal antibody to laminin results in a reduced number of branches and dilation of end buds (32). Incubation with a panel of monoclonal antibodies against different parts of the laminin complex suggests that the inhibitory effects of the polyclonal antibodies is due to the binding of domains in the terminal knob of the A chain and the cell receptor at the cross (33).

Fibronectin also is distributed along bronchial surfaces at early stages of branching and is accompanied by the appearance of integrin receptors (30). Blocking RGD receptors inhibits branching (34), but these sites also bind laminin.

Tenascin is expressed in the basal lamina region of lung buds and to a lesser degree along bronchial branches (21,35). It also is found in groups of mesoderm cells adjacent to bud tips (21). However, it localizes to thin collagen fibrils external to the basal lamina rather than within the basal lamina itself (36). The mRNA is synthesized in the epithelial cells of the buds (35). Addition of a polyclonal antibody to tenascin-C inhibits branching of lung cultures (36). Bacterial expression proteins containing the fibronectin-like domains also block branching, presumably by competing with tenascin for tenascin receptors, whereas branching continues in the presence of the terminal fibrinogen domain. However, lung buds continue to branch normally when antibodies against the bacterial expression proteins containing the fibronectin-like domains are added to the medium (36). The interpretation of this result is not clear.

## B. Growth Factors, Cell Proliferation, and Branching

The work on macromolecules of the extracellular matrix suggests that they may control branching by providing a structural environment which differs at buds as compared with the bronchial tree. The extracellular matrix also may affect branching by controlling the access of molecules which control cell proliferation. Early work on branching in organ culture shows a correlation between cell division and bud formation (37). Incorporation of [$^3$H]thymidine into DNA is high in all areas of the early primordium but decreases in the trachea and bronchi as they are formed. In the buds, 95% of the cells continue to incorporate [$^3$H]thymidine, whereas the percentage drops to 70% in the established branches.

### Growth Factors

The major role of growth factors is to control cell proliferation. Addition of epithelial growth factor (EGF) to culture medium stimulates thymidine incorporation, and a pellet of EGF placed next to the trachea stimulates the formation of a supernumerary lung bud in chicks (38). Mouse lung epithelium expresses both EGF mRNA and EGF receptor. Incubation of lung primordia with EGF stimulates DNA synthesis and branching, whereas an inhibitor of EGF receptor tyrosine kinase has the reverse effect (39). Antisense EGF oligodeoxynucleotide inhibits branching, EGF mRNA, its peptide, and DNA synthesis (40). Treatment of lung primordia with retinoic acid stimulates branching with a concomitant increase in EGF receptors (41). In contrast, transforming growth factor -β1 (TGF-β1) localizes to proximal airways and branch points rather than bud tips (22), and the addition of TGF-β1 to the culture medium inhibits branching (42). Platelet-derived growth factor (PDGF) appears to be involved solely in growth; treatment with either antibody against PDGF homologue B or antisense oligonucleotide decreases DNA synthesis and lung size but does not affect the number of buds which are formed (43).

### Control of Cell Proliferation

The effects of growth factors may be to control cell division. Thus, one role of mesenchyme may be to provide a stimulus for cell poliferation at buds and to suppress it within the bronchial tree. The specific effect of lung mesenchyme on branching may depend on the production of a balance of stimulatory and inhibitory factors which controls mitosis. The difference between homologous and foreign mesenchymes could be the kind of factor(s) or the quantity which is produced. For instance, cultures formed by recombining bronchial buds with salivary mesenchyme do not branch. However, if fresh salivary mesenchyme is supplied at daily intervals, branching continues (14). Possible interpretations are that salivary mesenchyme either does not produce enough of a factor which stimulates proliferation or that its production is not maintained by lung epithelium. Similarly, the ability of bronchial mesenchyme to allow the trachea to form a bud may depend on reestablishment of the original higher rate of cell proliferation (37,38).

Recent work on growth factors has shown that many of the effects are on gene activation. These genes primarily are proto-oncogenes which produce transcription factors regulating the expression of other genes or groups of genes. Of these regulatory genes, a connection has been established between TGF-β1 and N-*myc* expression. Normal N-*myc* expression is necessary for lung branching; mutations of the gene produce embryos in which only the first bronchial branches are formed (44). Concentrations of TGF-β1 which inhibit branching substantially reduce N-*myc* expression (42). The reduced expression occurs before inhibition of branching is detectable and expression returns when TGF-β1 is removed from the medium. This result correlates with absence of branching along established bronchi, where TGF-β1 expression is high. It would be interesting to know if N-*myc* expression is turned off in bud tips under other conditions where branching is inhibited and turned on by agents, such as EGF, which stimulate branching.

### C. Conclusions

Collagens, proteoglycan, and a variety of structural glycoproteins have been implicated in branching of the embryonic bronchial tree. However, the ways in which most of these macromolecules influence branching has not been investigated systematically and the causes are not well understood. In addition to a structural role, the extracellular matrix may act as a filter to limit access of soluble factors to the tips of branches where budding continues. The implication is that a different environment is established at buds as compared with the previously formed proximal branches. Current analyses suggest that growth factors are differentially expressed in these two regions, EGF at bud tips and TGF-β1 at ducts. The effects of these growth factors may be to control cell proliferation, maintaining a high division rate at the buds and suppressing division proximally. The action of the growth factors may be through expression of transcription factors, such as N-*myc*, which regulate gene expression.

## III. Cytodifferentiation

Cytodifferentiation is the process by which unspecialized or embryonic cells become committed to express their specialized characteristics. A number of cell types have been described in the airways. This section will be limited to the major intrinsic cell types of the respiratory region: type I and II pneumocytes of the epithelium and fibroblasts of the connective tissue.

### A. Requirement for Mesenchyme in Cytodifferentiation

*Influence of Mesenchyme on Epithelium*

The differentiation of respiratory epithelium requires the presence of homologous mesenchyme (45). Mouse respiratory epithelium from the canalicular phase does not branch and forms few type II pneumocytes when combined with mouse tracheal mesenchyme or nonrespiratory air sac mesenchyme from chick embryos. Chick air sacs, which normally form nonbranching structures, will form buds in combination with mouse mesenchyme from respiratory regions. However, the chick air sac epithelial cells do not differentiate into pneumocytes. Thus, the branching pattern is controlled by mesenchyme even during fetal development, but formation of pneumocytes occurs only in respiratory epithelium. The expression of the differentiated phenotype is at least partly controlled by the mesenchyme.

Much effort has been dedicated to discovering the nature of the influence mesenchyme exerts on the respiratory epithelium. This influence could be through either extracellular matrix materials produced by the mesenchyme, or through soluble factors, or both.

*Extracellular Matrix*

Proteoglycan

Inhibition of proteoglycan synthesis using $\beta$-xyloside causes abnormal development of the respiratory region of the lung. Saccules do not form, the tubules remain so narrow that the lumen is difficult to visualize in light micrographs, and the mesenchymal partitions between branches remain thick and cellular (46). The percentage of columnar (embryonic) cells is higher than in cultures incubated with the inactive $\alpha$ anomer and is accompanied by a decrease in the percentage of type II cells while the percentage of type I cells remains unchanged. This decrease in percentage of type II cells is accompanied by a 74% reduction in surfactant content as compared with neonatal lungs. The β-xyloside causes essentially no change in heparan sulfate and heparin but chondroitin sulfate in proteoglycan decreases by 70% (47).

The lung has been demonstrated to contain PG-M/versican (48), PG-I/biglycan, and PG-II/decorin (49). Each of these chondroitin sulfate proteoglycans is a major component of the extracellular matrix. The distribution of these proteoglycans within different compartments of the lung, and particularly at the respiratory endings, has not been reported. It must be assumed that β-xyloside would affect all of these proteoglycans equally. Therefore, it can not be suggested which proteoglycan(s) is(are) involved in the maturation of the lung and the differentiation of type II pneumocytes.

### Glycoprotein

Tunicamycin, an inhibitor of N-glycosylation, interferes with maturation of the mouse lung. Organ culture in tunicamycin of respiratory regions at the canalicular stage (50) results in only partial expansion of the epithelial tubules, whereas the septa remain thick and highly cellular and the epithelial cells lining the lumina are primarily columnar to cuboidal. On the basis of examination by transmission electron microscopy, these cultures are seen to have more columnar cells without lamellar bodies, a normal number of type II pneumocytes, and fewer type I pneumocytes than normal control lungs. This demonstrates that glycoprotein(s) is(are) required for the differentiation of type I pneumocytes. Since synthesis of all N-linked glycoproteins are inhibited by tunicamycin, it is not possible to identify which glycoprotein(s) might be responsible for the inhibitory effects. Blocking antibodies have not been used on fetal lungs to study the involvement of individual glycoproteins in cytodifferentiation the way they have been used to study branching.

### Collagen

Growth of lungs in the presence of inhibitors of collagen synthesis (*cis*-hydroxyproline or L-azetidine-2-carboxylic acid) inhibits saccule formation (51) and the differentiation of type II cells (52,53). The lung contains collagens types I, III, IV, and V (23,54,55). The lung also contains elastin, the synthesis of which should be inhibited by the same compounds (56). The abnormalities are unlikely to result from interference with type I collagen, however, since lungs develop almost normally in mutant mice which do not synthesize type I collagen (54). Collagen synthesis is rapid from the beginning to the end of the saccular phase (57). Almost half of this new collagen is degraded rapidly. During this time, a high level of type IV collagenase activity but little type I collagenase activity can be detected. These results support the suggestion that rapid synthesis and turnover of type IV collagen plays a role during the maturation to the saccule phase of lung development. Thus, it is possible, but not proven, that interference with maturation by the inhibitors of collagen synthesis may be exerted through effects on assembly of the basal laminae.

### B. Hormones, Growth Factors, and Cytodifferentiation

A large number of growth substances have been tested for their influence on maturation of the lung. It is well established that corticosteroids and thyroxine accelerate the maturation of the fetal lung in utero judged by morphogenesis of the alveoli and differentiation of the respiratory epithelium (58,59). In addition, convincing evidence has been found for the activity of fibroblast pneumocyte factor (FPF), epidermal growth factor (EGF), and transforming growth factor-$\beta$ (TGF-$\beta$). All of these substances stimulate or inhibit the production of surfactant by differentiating type II cells.

#### Corticosteroids and Thyroxine

Portions of a late canalicular lung placed in culture with serum-free medium will show considerable development without added growth factors, corticosteroid, or thyroxine (e.g., see ref. 4). However, the addition of defined growth suplements to serum-free medium without hormones permits survival without necrosis but does not permit maturation beyond one additional day (2). Addition of physiological levels of dexamethasone and thyroxine in addition to growth factors permits normal maturation of the respiratory regions. Thyroxine acts synergistically with corticosteroid, so that thyroxine at physiological concentration plus corticosteroid at a very low concentration can produce near normal development. (3,60).

#### Fibroblast Pneumocyte Factor

FPF is produced by lung fibroblasts and causes enhanced differentiation of type II pneumocytes (61; reviewed in ref. 62). Fibroblasts from the canalicular stage do not produce FPF activity. At the beginning of the saccular stage, the fetal fibroblasts produce FPF activity in culture in response to stimulation by glucocorticoids. It has been suggested that FPF activity is required for type II cell differentiation (63). Production of FPF activity becomes constitutive during maturation of the lung and then stops in the mature lung. FPF is a protein of 5–15 kDa synthesized on an mRNA of about 400 bases. The protein has been purified and anti-FPF monoclonal antibodies have been prepared (62). However, the gene has not been cloned and sequenced. Therefore, it is not known if FPF is a member of one of the families of growth factors, and FPF is not available except in the form of fibroblast-conditioned medium prepared in the individual laboratory.

### Androgens

In utero, lungs from females become responsive to glucocorticoids at an earlier stage than lungs from males (64,65). If lung fibroblasts from female fetuses are treated with androgen and glucocorticoid, the conditioned medium has no FPF activity, whereas fibroblasts from mutant males lacking androgen receptors produce FPF at levels similar to female fibroblasts (66). The effect of corticosteroids is on the fibroblasts and not epithelial cells; if type II cells are treated with both androgen and FPF-conditioned medium, normal maturation occurs (67).

### Epidermal Growth Factor

EGF has been demonstrated to enhance the maturation of type II cells both in vivo and in organ cultures (68,69). However, EGF does not enhance the synthesis of surfactant by type II cells in cell culture (70,71). EGF is synthesized by lung mesenchyme cells (72), and EGF receptors are found on the mesenchyme rather than on the respiratory epithelium (70,73). Medium conditioned by fibroblasts from lungs at the canalicular stage does not have FPF activity unless the fibroblasts are grown in the presence of EGF and then in EGF plus cortisol. Thus, EGF seems to stimulate lung fibroblasts to mature more quickly and to become capable of synthesizing FPF in response to glucocorticoids.

### TGF-β

Exogenous TGF-β inhibits the action of FPF (69); if lungs are treated with both TGF-β and FPF-conditioned medium, normal maturation does not occur (67). Messenger RNA for TGF-β is present in rat lungs from 17 to 21 days of development through the period of lung maturation (74).

### C. Conclusions

It is clear that the mesenchyme controls the morphogenesis and differentiation of the alveoli. This control appears to be exerted partially through control of the extracellular matrix and partially through the action of growth factors. Inhibition of the synthesis of any of the three general classes of extracellular matrix macromolecules inhibits the formation of saccules and the thinning of the septa. Inhibition of the synthesis of proteoglycan or of collagen inhibits the formation of type II pneumocytes as well. The mesenchyme also synthesizes FPF in response to glucocorticoids. Thyroxine potentiates the activity of glucocorticoids. FPF appears to be required for the differentiation and maturation of type II cells. EGF stimulates the differentiation of fibroblasts to become responsive to glucocorticoids and produce FPF. Androgens inhibit the synthesis of FPF by the mesenchyme. TGF-β inhibits the responsiveness of the alveolar epithelial cells to FPF.

Inhibition of glycoprotein synthesis inhibits the differention of only type I pneumocytes, so the action of tunicamycin can not be explained by an inhibition of the synthesis of FPF. The differentiation of a normal percentage of type I pneumocytes under conditions where saccules do not form suggests that the formation of type I pneumocytes is not simply a response to the stretching of the surface. The lack of markers for type I cells has made investigation of cytodifferentiation difficult. Some progress is currently being made (75).

## REFERENCES

1.  Ambesi-Impiombato FS, Parks LA, Coon HG. Culture of hormone-dependent functional epithelial cells from rat thyroids. Proc Natl Acad Sci USA 1980; 77:3455–3459.

2.  Hilfer SR, Schneck SL, Brown JW. The effect of culture conditions on cytodifferentiation of fetal mouse lung respiratory passageways. Exp Lung Res 1986; 115–136.

3.  Smith CI, Searls RL, Hilfer SR. Effects of hormones on functional differentiation of mouse respiratory epithelium. Exp Lung Res 1990; 16:191–209.

4.  Jaskoll TF, Don-Wheeler G, Johnson R, Slavkin HC. Embryonic mouse lung morphogenesis and type II cytodifferentiation in serumless, chemically defined medium using prolonged in vitro culture. Cell Differ 1988; 24:105–118.

5.  Kawada H, Shannon JM, Mason RJ. Maintenance of differentiation of adult rat alveolar type II cells under low serum and serum free conditions (abstr). Am Rev Respir Dis 1988; 137(suppl.):277.

6.  Spooner BS, Wessells NK. Mammalian lung development interactions in primordium formation and bronchial morphogenesis. J Exp Zool 1972; 175:445–454.

7.  Ten Have-Opbroek A AW. Lung development in the mouse embryo. Exp Lung Res 1991; 17:111–130.

8.  Hilfer SR. Development of terminal buds in the fetal mouse lung. SEM 1983; III:1387–1401.

9.  Rudnick D. Developmental capacities of the chick lung in chorioallantoic grafts. J Exp Zool 1933; 66:125–154.

10. Alescio T, Cassini A. Induction in vitro of tracheal buds by pulmonary mesenchyme grafted on tracheal epithelium. J Exp Zool 1962; 150:83–94.

11. Wessells NK. Mammalian lung development: interactions in formation and morphogenesis of tracheal buds. J Exp Zool 1970; 175:455–466.

12. Masters JRW. Epithelial-mesenchymal interaction during lung development: the effect of mesenchymal mass. Dev Biol 1976; 51:98–108.

13. Taderera JV. Control of lung differentiation in vitro. Dev Biol 1967; 16:489–512.

14. Lawson KA. Stage specificity in the mesenchyme requirement of rodent lung epithelium in vitro: a matter of growth control? J Embryol Exp Morphol 1983; 74:183–206.

15. Bluemink JG, Maurik PV, Lawson KA. Intimate cell contacts at the epithelial/mesenchymal interface in embryonic mouse lung. J Ultrastruc Res 1976; 55:257–270.

16. Grant MM, Cutts NR, Brody JS. Alterations in lung basement membrane during fetal growth and type 2 cell development. Dev Biol 1983; 97:173–183.

17. Gallagher BC. Basal laminar thinning in branching morphogenesis of the chick lung as demonstrated by lectin probes. J Embryol Exp Morphol 1986; 94:173–188.

18. Fukuda Y, Masuda Y, Kishi J-I, Hasimoto Y, Hayakawa T, Nogawa H, Nakanishi Y. The role of interstitial collagens in cleft formation of mouse embryonic submandibular gland during initial branching. Development 1988; 103:259–267.

19. Nakanishi Y, Nogawa H, Hashimoto Y, Kishi J-I, Hayakawa T. Accumulation of collagen III at the cleft points of developing mouse submandibular epithelium. Development 1988; 104:51–59.

20. Spooner BS, Thompson-Pletscher HA. Matrix Accumulation and the development of form: proteoglycans and branching morphogenesis. In: Regulation of Matrix Accumulation. New York: Academic Press, 1986:399–444.

21. Abbott LA, Lester SM, Erickson CA. Changes in mesenchymal cell-shape, matrix collagen and tenascin accompany bud formation in the early chick lung. Anat Embryol (Berl) 1991; 183:299–311.

22. Heine UI, Munoz EF, Flanders KC, Roberts AB, Sporn MB. Colocalization of TGF-beta 1 and collagen I and III, fibronectin and glycosaminoglycans during lung branching morphogenesis. Development 1990; 109:29–36.

23. Chen JM, Little CD. Cellular events associated with lung branching morphogenesis including the deposition of collagen type IV. Dev Biol 1987; 120:311–321.

24. Thomas T, Dziadek M. Expression of collagen-1(IV), laminin and nidogen genes in the embryonic mouse lung: Implications for branching morphogenesis. Mech Dev 1994; 45:193–201.

25. Alescio T. Effect of a proline analogue, azetidine-2-carboxylic acid, on the morphogenesis of mouse embryonic lung. J Embryol Exp Morphol 1973; 29:439–451.

26. Spooner BS, Faubion JM. Collagen involvement in branching morphogenesis of embryonic lung and salivary gland. Dev Biol 1980; 77:84–102.

27. Spooner B, Basset K, Spooner Jr. Sulfated GAG anf lung development (abstr). J Cell Biol 1988; 107:59a.

28. Wu T-C, Wan Y-J, Chung A, Damjanov I. Immunohistochemical localization of entactin and laminin in mouse embryos and fetuses. Dev Biol 1983; 100:496–505.

29. Jaskoll TF, Slavkin HC. Ultrastructural and immunofluorescence studies of basal-lamina alterations during mouse-lung morphogenesis. Differentiation 1984; 28:36–48.

30. Chen W-T, Chen J-M, Mueller SC. Coupled expression and colocalization of 140K cell adhesion molecules, fibronectin, and laminin during morphogenesis and cytodifferentiation of chick lung cells. J Cell Biol 1986; 103:1073–1090.

31. Schuger L, Varani J, Killen PD, Skubitz APN, Gilbride K. Laminin expression in the mouse lung increases with development and stimulates spontaneous organotypic rearrangement of mixed lung cells. Dev Dyn 1992; 195:43–54.

32. Schuger L, O'Shea S, Rheinheimer J, Varani J. Laminin in lung development: effects of anti-laminin antibody in murine lung morphogenesis. Dev Biol 1990; 137:26–32.

33. Schuger L, Skubitz APN, O'Shea KS, Chang JF, Varani J. Identification of laminin domains involved in branching morphogenesis: Effects of anti-laminin monoclonal antibodies on mouse embryonic lung development. Dev Biol 1991; 146:531–541.

34. Roman J, Little CW, McDonald JA. Potential role of RGD-binding integrins in mammalian lung branching morphogenesis. Development 1991; 112:551–558.
35. Koch M, Wehrle-Haller B, Baumgartner S, Spring J, Brubacher D, Chiquet M. Epithelial synthesis of tenascin at tips of growing bronchi and graded accumulation in basement membrane and mesenchyme. Exp Cell Res 1991; 194:297–300.
36. Young SL, Chang L-Y, Erickson HP. Tenascin-C in rat lung: Distribution, ontogeny and role in branching morphogenesis. Dev Biol 1994; 161:615–625.
37. Goldin GV, Wessells NK. Mammalian lung development: the possible role of cell proliferation in the formation of supernumerary tracheal buds and in branching morphogenesis. J Exp Zool 1979; 208:337–346.
38. Goldin GV, Opperman LA. Induction of supernumerary tracheal buds and the stimulation of DNA synthesis in the embryonic chick lung and trachea by epidermal growth factor. J Embryol Exp Morphol 1980; 60:235–243.
39. Warburton D, Seth R, Shum L, Horcher PG, Hall FL, Werb Z, Slavkin HC. Epigenetic role of epidermal growth factor expression and signalling in embryonic mouse lung morphogenesis. Dev Biol 1992; 149:123–133.
40. Seth R, Shum L, Wu F, Wuenschell C, Hall FL, Slavkin HC, Warburton D. Role of epidermal growth factor expression in early mouse embryo lung branching morphogenesis in culture: Antisense oligodeoxynucleotide inhibitory strategy. Dev Biol 1993; 158:555–559.
41. Schuger L, Varani J, Mitra R Jr., Gilbride K. Retinoic acid stimulates mouse lung development by a mechanism involving epithelial-mesenchymal interaction and regulation of epidermal growth factor receptors. Dev Biol 1993; 159:462–473.
42. Serra R, Pelton RW, Moses HL. TGF$\beta$1 inhibits branching morphogenesis and N-myc expression in lung bud organ cultures. Development 1994; 120:2153–2161.
43. Souza P, Sedlackova L, Kuliszewski M, Wang J, Liu J, Tseu I, Liu M, Tanswell AK, Post M. Antisense oligodeoxynucleotides targeting PDGF-B mRNA inhibit cell proliferation during embryonic rat lung development. Development 1994; 120:2163–2173.
44. Moens CB, Stanton BR, Parada LF, Rossant J. Defects in heart and lung development in compound heterozygotes for two different targeted mutations at the N-myc locus. Development 1993; 119:485–499.
45. Hilfer SR, Rayner R, Brown JW. Mesenchymal control of branching pattern in the fetal mouse lung. Tissue Cell 1985; 17:523–538.
46. Smith CI, Hilfer SR, Searls RL, Nathanson MA, Allodoli MD. Effects of $\beta$-D-xyloside on differentiation of the respiratory epithelium in the fetal mouse lung. Dev Biol 1990; 138:42–52.
47. Smith CI, Webster EH, Nathanson MA, Searls RL, Hilfer SR. Altered patterns of proteoglycan deposition during maturation of the fetal mouse lung. Cell Differ Dev 1990; 32:83–96.
48. Yamagata M, Shinomura T, Kimata K. Tissue variation of two large chondroitin sulfate proteoglycans (PG-M/versican and PG-H/aggrecan) in chick embryos. Anat Embryol 1993; 187:433–444.
49. Romaris M, Heredia A, Molist A, Bassols A. Differential effect of transforming

growth factor β on proteoglycan synthesis in human embryonic lung fiboblasts. Biochim Biophys Acta 1991; 1093:229–233.

50. Webster EH, Hilfer SR, Searls RL. The effect of Tunicamycin on maturation of the fetal mouse lung. Am J Respir Cell Mol Biol 1993; 265:L250–L259.

51. Hilfer SR, Allodoli MD, Searls RL. Involvement of extracellular matrix in branching and cytodifferentiation of the fetal mouse lung (abstr). J Cell Biol 1984; 99:158.

52. Adamson IY, King GM. L-azetidine-2-carboxylic acid retards lung growth and surfactant synthesis in fetal rats. Lab Invest 1987; 57:439–445.

53. King GM, Adamson IY. Effects of cis-hydroxyproline on type II cell development in fetal rat lung. Exp Lung Res 1987; 12:347–362.

54. Kratochwil K, Dziadek M, Lohler J, Harbers K, Jaenisch R. Normal epithelial branching morphogenesis in the absence of collagen I. Dev Biol 1986; 117:596–606.

55. DiMari SJ, Howe AM, Haralson MA. Effects of transforming growth factor-beta on collagen sysnthesis by fetal rat lung epithelial cells. Am J Respir Cell Mol Biol 1991; 4:455–462.

56. Schellenberg JC, Liggins GC. Elastin and collagen in the fetal sheep lung. I. Ontogenesis. Pediatr Res 1987; 22:335–338.

57. Arden MG, Spearman MA, Adamson IY. Degradation of type IV collagen during the development of fetal rat lung. Am J Respir Cell Mol Biol 1993; 9:99–105.

58. Ballard PL. Hormonal aspects of fetal lung development. In: Farrell PM, ed. Lung Development: Biological and Clinical Perspectives. New York: Academic Press, 1982; 2:205–253.

59. Post M, Barsoumian A, Smith BT. The cellular mechanisms of glucocorticoid acceleration of fetal lung maturation. J Biol Chem 1986; 261:2179–2184.

60. Smith BT, Sabry K. Glucocorticoid-thyroid synergism in in lung maturation: a mechanism involving epithelial-mesenchymal interaction. Proc Natl Acad Sci USA 1983; 80:1951–1954.

61. Smith BT. Lung maturation in the fetal rat: acceleration by the injection of fibroblast pneumocyte factor. Science 1979; 20:1094–1095.

62. Smith BT, Post M. Fibroblast-pneumocyte factor. Am J Phys 1989; 257:L174–L178.

63. Post M, Floros J, Smith BT. Inhibition of lung maturation by monoclonal antibodies against fibroblast-pneumocyte factor. Nature 1984; 308:284–286.

64. Kotas RV, Avery ME. The influence of sex on fetal rabbit lung maturation and on the response to glucocorticoid. Am Rev Respir Dis 1981; 121:377–380.

65. Nielsen HC, Torday JS. Sex differences in fetal rabbit pulmonary surfactant production. Pediatr Res 1981; 15:1245–1247.

66. Floros J, Nielsen HC, Torday JS. Dihydrotestosterone blocks fetal lung fibroblast-pneumocyte factor at a pretranslational level. J Biol Chem 1987; 262:13592–13598.

67. Nielsen HC, Kellogg CK, Doyle CA. Development of fibroblast-type-II cell communications in fetal rabbit lung organ culture. Biochim Biophys Acta 1992; 1175:95–99.

68. Catterton WZ, Escobedo MB, Sexson WR, Gray ME, Sndell HW, Stahlman MT. Effect of epidermal growth factor on lung maturation in fetal rabbits. Pediatr Res 1979; 13:104–108.

69. Whitsett JA, Weaver TE, Lieberman MA, Clark JC, Daugherty C. Differential effects of

epidermal growth factor and transforming growth factor-β on synthesis of $M_r$=35,000 surfactant-associated protein in fetal lung. J Biol Chem 1987; 262:7908–7913.

70.  Keller GH, Ladda RL. Correlation between phosphatidylcholine labeling and hormone receptor levels in alveolar type II epithelial cells: effects of dexamethasone and epidermal growth factor. Arch Biochem Biophys 1981; 211:321–326.

71.  Nielsen HC. Epidermal growth factor influences the developmental clockregulating maturation of the fetal lung fibroblast. Biochem Biophys Acta 1989; 1012:201–206.

72.  Snead ML, Luo W, Oliver P, Nakamura M, Don-Wheeler G, Bessem C, Bell GI, Rall LB, Slavkin HC. Localization of epidermal growth factor precursor in tooth and lung during embryonic mouse development. Dev Biol 1989; 134:420–429.

73.  Partanen A-M, Thesleff I. Localization and quantitation of [125]I epidermal growth factor binding in mouse embryonic tooth and other embryonic tissues at different developmental stages. Dev Biol 1987; 120:186–197.

74.  Torday JS, Kourembanas S. Fetal rat lung fibroblasts produce a TGF-β homolog that blocks alveolar type II cell maturation. Dev Biol 1990; 139:35–41.

75.  Joyce-Brady MF, Brody JS. Ontogeny of pulmonary alveolar epithelial markers of differentiation. Dev Biol 1990; 137:331–348.

# 18

## Hormonal Control of Compensatory Lung Growth

**KIRK A. GILBERT, LIDIJA PETROVIC-DOVAT,
and D. EUGENE RANNELS**

Pennsylvania State University College of Medicine
Hershey, Pennsylvania

## I. Introduction

In a variety of mammalian species, partial resection of the lung results in rapid compensatory growth of the remaining lobes to restore normal total lung mass, volume, and function. Although this phenomenon was first described more than 100 years ago (1), it was the classic studies of Cohn in 1939 (2) which stimulated investigations of the mechanisms by which compensatory lung growth is initiated and controlled. Numerous laboratories have contributed to the latter work in providing a description of the general characteristics of compensatory growth, of the time course over which it occurs, and of the resulting changes in tissue structure and function. These results show that the detailed aspects of compensatory lung growth reflect not only the species in which the surgery is performed but also the age, sex, and hormonal status of the animal. Several investigators have previously reviewed the considerable body of data which describes the compensatory growth response (3–6). In spite of this extensive descriptive information, regulation of the response at both the cellular and subcellular levels remains poorly understood (7), and almost no information is available concerning the impact which lung injury may have on compensatory growth of the organ.

This chapter is focused primarily on the regulation of compensatory lung growth, particularly by hormones. There is evidence that function of the pituitary, adrenal, and possibly other endocrine glands modulates the compensatory growth response. In addition, a number of observations suggest a role for paracrine and/or autocrine mediators in progression of the response. These aspects will be discussed in detail. Evidence as to hormonal regulation of the response will be placed in context by presentation of the general characteristics of compensatory lung growth and by consideration of the variety of mechanisms by which compensation may be initiated or controlled. The goal of this chapter is to stimulate interest in compensatory growth of the lung and to lead new investigators to initiate research in this interesting and novel aspect of lung biology.

## II. Characteristics of Compensatory Lung Growth Following Pneumonectomy

### A. Tissue and Organ Level

A variety of species exhibit compensatory growth of the remaining lung tissue following removal of one or several lobes. Growth of the alveolar region of the organ is rapid and complete, providing full replacement of the resected tissue. The course of postoperative change in lung mass is shown in Figure 1, which was derived from experiments using rats of approximately 200 g body weight at the time of surgery. The figure shows the effect of left pneumonectomy to increase right lung mass over a 28-day interval. Solid lines show the course of growth of the right lung (R) and both lungs (R+L) in control animals. The dashed line illustrates the time course of growth of the right lung following resection of the single lobe of the left lung on experimental day 0. Following removal of the left lung, which accounts for 35% of total lung mass (8), there is a short lag after which the rate of growth of the remaining right lung increases eightfold relative to the control value (9). Accelerated right lung growth continues in a linear fashion until normal total lung mass is achieved at day 14. Subsequently, right lung growth continues at a rate appropriate to the ongoing growth of both lungs of control animals.

Compensatory lung growth has been studied most extensively in rats, but there is sufficient data to indicate that it occurs in a wide variety of small mammals, generally resulting in complete restoration of normal total lung mass (4,5). In the case of the experiment above, where approximately one third of total lung mass was removed at surgery, the compensatory response involves a 50% increase in right lung mass. In cases where more tissue has been resected by removal of either the entire (10) or several lobes of the right lung (11,12), restoration of normal total lung mass remains complete. For example, resection of the right lung results in at least a twofold increase in left lung mass (10).

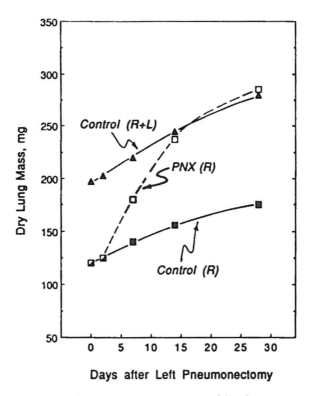

**Figure 1** Time course of compensatory lung growth following pneumonectomy. The time course of compensatory growth of the right lung (R) of rats (300 g body weight) subjected to left pneumonectomy on day 0 (PNX, open squares) is compared with that of the right lung (R, solid squares) or both lungs (R+L, solid triangles) of control animals. Data are mean values for selected time points from Rannels et al., 1984 (9).

Although the compensatory growth response is common to many species (3), the bulk of published evidence suggests that it occurs only in cases where lung growth is ongoing at the time of surgery. In most strains of rats, somatic growth proceeds throughout life, and in the adult rat, a stable ratio of lung to body weight is maintained (8). Thus, lung growth also continues in the adult animal (see Fig. 1, solid curves). In contrast, compensatory growth of the lung appears to be abolished in species which undergo sexual maturation accompanied by stabilization of body mass. The growth response which is present in kittens and puppies is absent in mature cats and dogs (13–16). There may be exceptions to the latter observations, however, in that rapid compensatory growth of the right lung has been documented following left pneumonectomy in adult female mice in which somatic growth was not detected (S. R. Rannels, personal communication, December 1994).

Data derived from the rat model in this laboratory (8,9,17) and others (18–20) indicate that complete restoration of lung mass is more rapid in young than in older animals. For example, rats of 85 g body weight at the time of left pneumonectomy require 7 days to reach normal total lung mass (9) in contrast to the 14-day time course shown in Figure 1. It is of interest, however, that these results do not reflect differences in the net rate of increase in tissue mass, which is equal in the two groups of animals. As rates of accumulation of right lung protein do not differ in these animals when expressed per lung (9), the contrasting time courses in young and older rats could be interpreted to reflect the greater mass of tissue removed at surgery in the latter animals. These observations suggest a consistency in the character of the response which may be pertinent to understanding its regulation.

The change in the net rate of right lung growth following left pneumonectomy is dramatic but transient, as shown in Figure 2. In the rats, between 4 and 10 weeks of age, the rate of right lung growth declines sixfold, from about 30 to 5 mg/day (solid curve, filled symbols). Following pneumonectomy at 5 or 7 weeks, the basal rate of growth accelerates six- to eightfold to more than 100 mg/day. This transient increase in growth is more prolonged in the older animals, resulting in greater accumulation of tissue mass.

The case in humans also appears to be complex. Most of the clinical observations recently have been reviewed by Cagle and Thurlbeck (4), and the reader is referred to this review for studies prior to 1988. Although no direct experiments have been performed, clinical observations suggest that compensatory lung growth may occur in infants and young children. In older individuals, hyperplastic compensatory growth appears to be replaced by enlargement of existing alveoli. There is no consensus as to when the critical period occurs. Infants have about 50 million alveoli at birth and multiplication is rapid during the first few years of life. Most alveoli are formed in the first 2 years, but a small increase occurs between 2 and 8 years of age (reviewed in ref. 21). Thus, if compensatory lung growth can occur in humans, it would appear most likely to be in this age group. In contrast, lobectomy typically is followed in adult humans by increased inflation of the surrounding parenchymal regions, which results in overinflated alveoli with thin walls (4).

In a 30-year study, Laros and Westermann followed 98 patients in whom pneumonectomy was performed at ages ranging from 2–40 years (22). Based on results of pulmonary function tests, it was shown that patients 5 years and younger had total lung capacities (TLCs) and ratios of tidal volume to functional residual capacity similar to the predicted values for both lungs of normal age-matched individuals. Patients 6–20 years old had TLCs 85% of predicted values, whereas patients older than 20 years had TLCs 70–78% of predicted. These results were

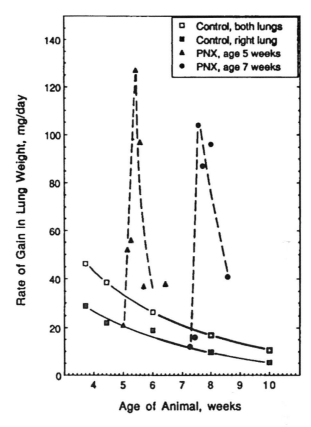

**Figure 2** Effect of pneumonectomy on rate of gain in right lung weight. The solid lines show the decline in the rate of growth of the right lung (solid squares) or both lungs (open squares) of rats between 3.5 and 10 weeks of age. The broken curves show the rate of gain in right lung weight following left pneumonectomy in animals of 5 weeks (solid triangles) or 7 weeks (solid circles) of age. Rates of gain in lung weight were calculated based on the difference between multiple sets of two data points in a growth curve (not shown) and are plotted at the mid point of the respective interval. Mean values were calculated from data in Rannels et al., 1984 (9).

interpreted to suggest that compensatory lung growth in individuals fewer than 5 years old occurs primarily by cell division ("hyperplasia") with minor alveolar enlargement ("hypertrophy"). It is not possible, however, to confirm cell growth and division based solely on pulmonary function tests.

Werner et al. followed 14 patients for 3–20 years following partial lung resections performed at ages 1 week to 30 months (23). In addition to lung volume, pulmonary ventilation-perfusion characteristics also were evaluated. Follow-up showed good functional performance; most lung volumes were close to normal. These results were interpreted to indicate hyperplastic growth combined with hypertrophy. Radiographic evidence, however, suggested an abnormal distribution of alveolar perfusion. Altered ventilation-perfusion relationships were interpreted to indicate dysplastic growth of alveolar tissue and the vascular bed. The latter characteristic may be related to the dysanaptic compensatory growth observed in animals discussed below.

These results and others (reviewed in ref. 4) suggest the following conclusions regarding the sequelae of pneumonectomy in humans: (1) the adaptive mechanisms in response to lung resection generally lead to a good clinical outcome; (2) in younger individuals, compensation may involve tissue growth as well as increased inflation, whereas in older individuals, adaptation is achieved mainly through alveolar distention; (3) many factors, including age, the site and volume of resected lung, the type of primary illness, and/or the existence of residual lung disease may influence the mechanism and extent of compensatory lung growth.

## B. Cellular and Subcellular Levels

After restoration of right lung mass is complete following left pneumonectomy, alveolar function appears to be essentially normal with respect to gas exchange (19) and to tissue compliance (24,25). These conclusions are supported by more detailed investigations at the cellular and subcellular levels which indicate a normal tissue structure and organization consistent with normal physiological function. At the biochemical level, the time course of postoperative change in right lung protein and RNA and DNA content largely parallels the increase in right lung mass. Although in some experiments there appeared to be a transient disproportionate increase in RNA concentration during the early phase of the growth response (8), for the most part, these parameters appear to change in parallel, suggesting coordinated cell growth and division.

On completion of the response, it appears that cells of the alveolar region are present in proportions and total numbers equivalent to those in control tissue (11,26–28). Both capillary and alveolar surface areas and volumes are restored, along with the arithmetic mean thickness and harmonic mean thickness of the alveolar wall (26,28). These observations suggest a normal barrier to gas exchange; they are consistent with physiological observations of normal oxygenation and carbon dioxide elimination (19).

In contrast, there has been a standing controversy as to whether the compensatory growth response involves increases in alveolar number as opposed to enlargement of existing alveoli (18,20,29–31). Conflicting data have been published concerning this aspect of the response; these results have been discussed elsewhere (4). Much of the historic data were obtained using morphometric methods which require assumptions regarding alveolar shape (32). Recent studies using methods where these assumptions have not been required (33) indicate that postpneumonectomy lung growth in the rat results in an increase in alveolar number, without a significant increase in mean alveolar volume (28).

Although the completed compensatory growth response following pneumonectomy in the rat appears to result in essentially normal tissue with physiological gas-exchange function, much remains to be learned regarding the extent and fidelity of the compensatory growth process in other species and under abnormal conditions. In this context, there is evidence to indicate changes in tissue structure and function during the course of compensatory lung growth. The most evident of these differences is that between growth of the proximal airways and the gas-exchange region. Studies based on morphometry (26), airway casting (34), and functional measurements of airway resistance (35) indicate that the overall growth response is dysanaptic, in that larger more proximal airways do not grow in proportion to the tissue of the distal lung. These measurements are consistent with results which show that total lung mass increases more rapidly than does lung volume during the course of the response (20,25,36,37). These and other observations led Berger and Burri (11) to suggest that compensatory growth of the lung involves a four-step process including extension of the air spaces, proliferation of cells in the parenchymal region, remodeling of the tissue, and finally restoration of normal tissue architecture.

A number of investigators have focused on delineation of the time course of cell growth and proliferation in the alveolar region during the postoperative interval (reviewed in refs. 4 and 6). In spite of these efforts, surprisingly little is known concerning the sequence of alveolar cell growth and division nor regarding which cell populations, if any, may be most sensitive to the signals which initiate and sustain the compensatory growth response (27,28,38). These issues have been approached using biochemical, morphometric, and, most recently, cell culture techniques.

Biochemical studies indicate that right lung DNA increases over a postpneumonectomy time course which parallels that of increased right lung mass. The time course and extent of increase in right lung protein is similar. Taking the ratio of protein to DNA as an index of cell size and total DNA as an index of cell number, these observations suggest that compensatory lung growth involves cellular hyperplasia with, on average, minimal cellular hypertrophy (8,17). These general conclusions are supported by the morphometric results cited above, which indicate few changes in cellular composition of the alveolar region upon completion of compensatory growth (27,28,38).

There are only limited data, however, from morphometric observations made during the course of the compensatory response (11,27,28,38). These suggest highly synchronized growth and division of the major parenchymal cell populations, with the possible exception of the type II alveolar epithelial cell (27).

Although peak DNA synthesis in the type II cell appears to be synchronized with that in other cell populations of the alveolar region (38), disproportionate changes in type II cells have been observed by a number of investigators during the early phase of growth (27,28,39). For example, Thet and Law (27) observed disproportionate elevations in type II cell surface area and volume during the course of the compensatory response in rats. Similarly, flow cytometric analysis of type II cells isolated from the lungs of pneumonectomized animals demonstrated the presence of an enlarged subpopulation of the pneumocytes (40,41). Additional data suggests "activation" of the type II cell population during the compensatory growth response (39,40,42); these observations are consistent with the established role of the type II cell in the response of the lung to injury (43,44). Nevertheless, the role of the type II cell or other alveolar cells to determine the extent or nature of compensatory lung growth is not known. These possible roles have been discussed elsewhere (28).

## III. Regulation of Compensatory Lung Growth

### A. Evidence for Regulation

There is considerable information regarding the nature and extent of compensatory lung growth following pneumonectomy, but the physiological factors which regulate the compensatory process are not well understood. Nevertheless, available data demonstrate that the compensatory growth is highly controlled and synchronized, in that pneumonectomy is followed by rapid and orderly restoration of normal pulmonary structure and function (4,5). The latter conclusion is supported by evidence drawn at the physiological, biochemical, molecular, and ultrastructural levels. Details of the time course, extent, and character of compensatory lung growth suggest close physiological regulation. A variety of potential regulatory processes or factors have been proposed, largely based on circumstantial or indirect evidence.

Most hypotheses concerning regulation of the response have been drawn from experiments conducted in vivo, but few have been tested in well-defined in vitro model systems. There is little understanding of the cellular or molecular mechanisms which underlie compensatory growth nor of whether these regulatory processes are unique to the lung. Progress in this area has been hampered somewhat by the restricted number of approaches for isolation and culture of purified lung cell populations in vitro and by limited application of sensitive molecular techniques to resolution of compensatory changes at the cellular or molecular levels. Sufficient information is available, however, to allow formulation of several testable hypotheses concerning pathways by which compensatory lung growth may be regulated. Consideration of these possibilities provides insight as to the focus and design of future experiments to investigate further the factors which may initiate or control compensatory growth.

### B. Proposed Signals for Compensatory Lung Growth

Factors which have been proposed to regulate the onset, progression, or extent of compensatory lung growth following partial pneumonectomy include (1) postoperative changes in tissue inflation, (2) elevated blood flow in the residual pulmonary vasculature, (3) intraoperative or perioperative hypoxemia, and (4) circulating or soluble factors acting by endocrine, paracrine, or autocrine mechanisms.

#### Altered Inflation of the Remaining Lung

The normal balance of pressures across the alveolar wall dictates that following resolution of pneumothorax after pneumonectomy, the remaining lobes will inflate to fill the available space. Clinical evidence, cited above, reveals increased inflation of the surrounding parenchyma following lobectomy in humans (4). Both x-ray (37) and morphometric (11) data confirm similar changes following partial pneumonectomy in the rat. In the animal model, these transitions are accompanied by increases in the depth and rate of ventilation during the immediate postoperative interval, providing further evidence that the gradient of pressure across the alveolar wall is altered acutely. In addition, clinical data support the premise that the lung grows to fill the space available in the thoracic cavity (3). The fact that space-filling lesions can severely restrict normal developmental lung growth supports this premise. In the context of postpneumonectomy growth, the key issue is to identify the pathway(s) by which increased inflation may initiate hyperplastic changes in the tissue.

A number of lines of experimentation, beginning with the work of Cohn (2), provide evidence to suggest a role for altered lung inflation in regulating compensatory growth of the tissue. Cohn conducted a number of experiments where increased or reduced inflation resulted, respectively, in elevated or decreased lung mass. Cohn hypothesized that the postpneumonectomy increase in lung mass "is due solely to the mechanical stimulus of the change in the pull exerted by the alteration in size of the thoracic cage which the lung must fill" (2). This premise is supported by the observation that replacement of resected lobes by inert exogenous material (plombage) reduces compensatory growth (2,45,46), but the potential for compensation is retained (47). These and related observations prompted investigators to consider increased inflation or "stretch" of the remaining lung as the initiating signal to compensatory lung growth. Additional evidence which supports a role for mechanical or physical forces in compensatory growth of the lung has been reviewed recently (7). A number of pertinent considerations are highlighted below.

The classic experiment taken to indicate a role for increased inflation in initiation of compensatory lung growth centers on the observation that when inert material is placed in the thorax to replace the tissue removed at pneumonectomy, compensatory growth of the remaining lung is reduced or prevented (2,45,46).

This type of manipulation has been achieved by placing wax (2,46), plastic sponge (45), or a balloon modeled to mimic the lobes removed at surgery (47) into the thorax or by injecting air into the peritoneum (2). Reversibility of the effects of this procedure was demonstrated (47). Although these studies provide observations consistent with the premise that inflation governs growth, their interpretation is not straightforward. Evidence that lungs grow to fill the space available suggests that if the resected lobe is replaced by inert material, growth will not occur. Furthermore, it is reasonable to assume that signals which stop growth (no available space) would override those which initiate or maintain the process. Imposition of the "off" signal by placement of inert material into the thorax may override an independent initiating signal that is not linked to lung inflation (e.g., the activity of a circulating factor). Thus, the hypothesis that changes in lung inflation and, presumably, consequent changes in physical parameters of the remaining tissue, may signal compensatory growth of the lung requires confirmation independent of studies using thoracic plombage in vivo. This issue has been raised and discussed in more detail elsewhere (7).

Independent of these issues, it is of interest to consider whether altered lung inflation is a plausible regulator of tissue growth. In nonpulmonary systems, there is strong and extensive evidence that application of mechanical force to tissues and cells can result in changes in metabolism, growth, and differentiation (7). The events which lead to cardiac hypertrophy provide a well-known example. Increased afterload on the left ventricle and the associated elevated end-diastolic pressure lead to increased ventricular work and to hypertrophy of ventricular myocytes (48) associated with elevations in ribosome formation (49) and in the synthesis of contractile proteins (50). As the ventricular muscle undergoes hypertrophy, cells of the ventricular connective tissue divide (51). Thus, cell-specific signals to hypertrophy and hyperplasia are delivered simultaneously within the same tissue, affecting cardiac myocytes and fibroblasts, respectively. Extension of these observations to in vitro models suggest that growth is elicited in response to mechanical signals through associated mechanochemical signal transduction pathways (52,53). Similar observations have been made in other tissues including the gut (54), urinary bladder (55), and uterus (56).

These observations are consistent with a large body of evidence to indicate that cell shape is an important determinate of growth and differentiation. Changes in shape at the cellular level may be mediated directly, for example, through shear stress on the vascular endothelium (57), or indirectly on cellular components of tissues exposed to external force in vivo or in vitro, as discussed above. A second indirect pathway to modulate cell shape involves interaction with the extracellular matrix. In this case, specific extracellular matrix components act through membrane receptors known as integrins to modulate not only general cellular characteristics such as growth and differentiation (58) but also to elicit specific changes in gene expression (59). In the classic model system, Bissell and co-workers demonstrated that cultured mammary epithelial cells maintain differentiated function and specialized gene expression only when in association with appropriate elements of the extracellular matrix (60). More recently, work from this and other laboratories (reviewed in ref. 61) has confirmed that similar considerations of cell-matrix interaction impinge on differentiation of cells of the alveolar region, particularly the type II epithelium.

Thus, although the premise that mechanical signals initiate or modulate compensatory growth of the lung following pneumonectomy is plausible, considerable additional evidence is required to link observations in the animal, in isolated organs, and in cultured cells. Based on these and additional considerations (7), it appears that postoperative changes in mechanical forces acting on the remaining lung following partial pneumonectomy are likely to play a significant role in initiation of compensatory growth of the tissue. As discussed below, the overall outcome of the effects of these mechanical signals appears to be modulated by the condition of the animal, particularly by its hormonal status.

### Changes in Blood Flow to the Remaining Lung

If it is assumed that cardiac output is not changed following pneumonectomy, resection of the left lung (35% of total lung mass) would increase blood flow to the lobes of the right lung by 50%. Evidence obtained both in vivo (62) and in vitro (63) indicates that acute changes in pulmonary flow of this magnitude are accommodated rapidly in the pulmonary circulation and result in little or no increase in vascular pressure. Although chronic accommodation of flow may result in structural remodeling of the vasculature in some species (64), there appears to be no such effect of pneumonectomy on the pulmonary vasculature of the rat (11,28).

The possibility that postoperative changes in pulmonary capillary blood flow may influence lung growth was evaluated by Tartter and Goss (10), who ligated the right mainstem pulmonary artery. Modest growth of the left lung consequent to the ligation was consistent with a role for elevated pulmonary flow in the compensatory growth response, presumably mediated by "stretch" or distention of the pulmonary endothelium or of other components of the vasculature. This effect is not likely to be accounted for by the proposed washout of putative growth-inhibitory chalones from the tissue (65). It must be noted, however, that reduced blood flow to the right lung over the 4-week interval of these studies (10) would have resulted in right lung deflation and a consequent increase in the space available to be occupied by the left lung. Thus, stimulatory signals initiated through increased left lung inflation, rather than increased blood flow, could account for the modest growth response obtained.

More recent work provides a strong indication that elevated blood flow in the contralateral lung does not account for compensatory growth of the tissue. In the ferret, McBride and co-workers (66) placed a band around a segment of pulmonary artery leading to the caudal lobe of the left lung. The band was calibrated such that following right pneumonectomy, increased flow to that lobe was prevented, while the cranial lobe of the left lung accommodated the remainder of cardiac output. Subsequent compensatory growth was evident in all lobes including the lobe that did not receive increased blood flow during the post-pneumonectomy interval. Therefore, although changes in vascular pressures and flow with associated elevations in shear stress at the vascular endothelium (67,68) can modulate cellular growth and differentiation, current evidence suggests that elevated flow to the remaining lung following pneumonectomy is not necessary for compensatory growth and thus is not likely to be the sole regulator of the response.

### Perioperative Changes in Oxygenation

When rats are housed chronically under hypoxic conditions, both tidal volume and diffusion capacity are increased (69,70). In newborn animals exposed to low oxygen, body growth is reduced, while both lung weight and lung-weight-to-body-weight ratio increase (71). These results are consistent with the fact that humans who live at high altitude exhibit large lung volumes in proportion to body mass (72), and that mice raised at altitude exhibit characteristic changes in lung volume and alveolar structure (69). These observations led to speculation that hypoxemia may be a stimulus to postpneumonectomy lung growth (19), based on the premise that lung size may reflect the demand for oxygen delivery. Most published evidence suggests, however, that hypoxemia is not a probable mediator of compensatory lung growth.

Surgical procedures for left pneumonectomy are accompanied by transient deficits in oxygenation that can result in acute hypoxemia. In routine procedures, hemoglobin saturation may drop below 50%, and both hypercapnea and acidosis may be evident (19). These transient changes are not consistent with the chronic changes above that were proposed to initiate the compensatory response. In addition, when animals are intubated and ventilated to improve intraoperative oxygenation, there appears to be no consequent effect on subsequent compensatory increases in right lung mass, protein, RNA, or DNA (73). These results suggest that acute and transient deficiencies in oxygenation during or following surgical thoracotomy do not modulate the extent or nature of compensatory lung growth.

It is evident, however, that the response to pneumonectomy is altered by changes in ambient oxygen. The postoperative increase in total lung volume is modified when ambient oxygen is varied over a range from 14 to 35% during the first postoperative week (36). In addition, exposure of animals to normobaric hypoxia elevates the postoperative gain in total lung volume, whereas high oxygen reduces the resulting total lung volume. These and other observations suggest that although hypoxia may not be involved in the initiation of the compensatory growth response, the nature of the response apparently is oxygen sensitive. In a study where normobaric hyperoxia appeared to have little effect on overall compensatory lung growth, it did alter the resulting volume densities of alveolar type II and interstitial cells (12). These results are consistent with the above cited observations that normal lung growth is sensitive to chronic changes in oxygen availability.

### Soluble Factors

There is evidence to indicate that soluble or circulating factors could play a role in regulating compensatory growth of the lung. These factors, which may be stimulatory or inhibitory, could act by endocrine, paracrine, or autocrine pathways. Control of compensatory lung growth by soluble factors is the main topic of this chapter and is discussed below.

## IV. Role of Soluble Factors in Compensatory Lung Growth

A variety of hormones can modify normal growth and development of the lung (3,21,74). Few studies exist, however, concerning hormonal regulation of compensatory lung growth following partial pneumonectomy. To date, contributions of pituitary and adrenal hormones and to a lesser extent thyroid and parathyroid hormones have been investigated to determine their roles in regulation of compensatory lung growth. Additional soluble growth factors produced within the lung may contribute to the control of compensatory lung growth by autocrine or paracrine mechanisms. Table 1 summarizes those studies which examined the role of specific soluble factors on the compensatory response to pneumonectomy.

### A. Endocrine Factors

#### Pituitary Hormones

The anterior lobe of the mammalian pituitary gland secretes nine or more hormonally active substances. With the exception of growth hormone and prolactin, most known roles of these products are to regulate the function of other endocrine organs. Several studies have examined the potential role of growth hormone in lung growth and development from the prenatal and perinatal periods to adulthood. Low levels or lack of growth hormone typically result in reduced body mass with proportionate reduction in lung to body weight ratio (75). Excess growth hormone produces the opposite effect (76–78). Thus, growth hormone effects on normal lung growth appear to be indirect, in that the degree of lung growth remains proportional to overall somatic growth.

**Table 1** Soluble Factors and Compensatory Lung Growth

| Authors | Surgery | Factor(s) | Effect on Growth | Conclusion |
|---|---|---|---|---|
| Brody and Buhain, 1973 (77) | Left PNX; growth hormone–secreting tumor implantation | Growth hormone, prolactin, ACTH | Increased lung volume | Mixture of hyperplasia and hypertrophy in compensatory growth |
| Khadempour et al., 1992 (84) | Left PNX | Growth hormone | Not determined | Circulating levels of growth hormone increased after PNX |
| Brody and Buhain 1973 (77) | Left PNX; HPX | Pituitary hormones | None | Compensatory response conserved in the absence of pituitary hormones |
| Bennett et al., 1985 (101) | Left PNX; bilateral ADX | Adrenal hormones | Increased rate of growth; increased right lung mass | Accentuation of compensatory response beyond that observed by PNX alone |
| Rannels et al., 1987 (103); Bennett et al., 1987 (25) | Left PNX; bilateral ADX | Adrenal hormones; hydrocortisone acetate replacement | Reversed ADX effects | Steroid treatment slows rapid growth in ADX animals; lung volumes return later than lung mass |
| Rannels et al., 1991 (28) | Left PNX; bilateral ADX | Adrenal hormones | Increased rate and extent of growth | Increased thickness of interstitial and epithelial cell compartments in ADX/PNX animals |
| Khadempour et al., 1992 (84) | Left PNX | IGF-1 | Not determined | IGF-1 increased after PNX |

| Reference | Procedure | Factor | BAL fluid / effect | Conclusion |
|---|---|---|---|---|
| McAnulty et al., 1992 (130) | Left PNX | IGF-1 | BAL fluid from PNX animals stimulated in vitro fibroblast replication; IGF-1 levels increased in BAL fluid after PNX | BAL fluid stimulation blocked by antibodies to IGF-1 |
| Sekhon and Thurlbeck, 1992 (124) | Left PNX | Sex hormones | None | Compensatory growth is not gender dependent |
| Faridy et al., 1988 (125) | Left PNX | Hormones of pregnancy | None | Compensatory growth conserved in altered hormonal state of pregnancy |
| Khadempour et al., 1992 (84) | Left PNX | Hormones of pregnancy | None | Compensatory growth conserved in altered hormonal state of pregnancy |
| McAnulty et al., 1992 (130) | Left PNX | PDGF | Not determined | BAL fluid stimulatory activity not blocked by antibodies to PDGF |
| Khadempour et al., 1992 (84) | Left PNX | Bombesin | Not determined | No change in lung bombesin-like immunoreactivity |

Summary of studies which have examined effects of or levels of specific soluble factors during compensatory growth response to partial pneumonectomy. Abbreviations: ACTH, adrenocorticotropic hormone; ADX, adrenalectomy; BAL, bronchoalveolar lavage; HPX, hypophysectomy; IGF-1, insulin-like growth factor 1; PDGF, platelet-derived growth factor; PNX, pneumonectomy.

Conflicting results have been reported concerning the presence of growth hormone receptors in the lung, partly due to the ability of growth hormone to bind to prolactin and lactogen receptors (79). Growth hormone receptors have been localized to adult and fetal rabbit lungs (80,91) but have not been detected in lungs of human (81). Prolactin receptors, however, have been localized in lungs of both rabbit (80) and rat (82). Lack of growth hormone receptors in the lung of some species is consistent with the view that growth hormone actions on the lung may be indirect.

Aside from normal lung growth, it has been suggested that growth hormone may regulate compensatory growth of the lung following pneumonectomy (83,84). Elevations in serum levels of growth hormone have been reported in rats at 3 days postpneumonectomy (84); this corresponds to the time when changes in lung mass are detected (8). Implantation of a growth hormone–secreting tumor into rats 2 weeks prior to pneumonectomy resulted in a 35% increase in total lung capacity compared with pneumonectomized rats not bearing tumors (83). The compensatory increase in lung mass was comparable with control animals, but rats with tumor implants had less total lung DNA than tumor-free controls. Thus, the growth hormone–secreting implants apparently inhibited lung cell division following pneumonectomy and concurrently caused an increase in average cell size, resulting in a mixture of hypertrophic and hyperplastic responses. Indeed, implantation of the growth hormone–secreting tumor into normal adult rats caused hypertrophic growth of the lung, resulting in increased lung mass and volume compared with age-matched controls (77).

Interpretation of these studies is complicated by the fact that the growth hormone–secreting tumor also secreted large amounts of prolactin and adrenocorticotropic hormone (ACTH). As mentioned above, prolactin receptors have been localized to the lung (80,81), and prolactin has been shown to modulate fetal lung production of pulmonary surfactant in vitro (85). In addition, large amounts of ACTH secreted by the implanted tumor might be expected to elevate levels of circulating glucocorticoids by direct action of ACTH on the adrenal glands. Strong evidence exists for a potential regulatory role for adrenal hormones in lung growth and maturation and in compensatory lung growth. This evidence is discussed below.

The effects of growth hormone deficiency contrast to those of growth hormone excess. In hypophysectomized rats which were subsequently pneumonectomized, the compensatory increase in lung mass was greater than that in either control rats or in rats subjected only to hypophysectomy (83). Thus, the compensatory response to pneumonectomy is not blocked by removal of pituitary hormones. Total lung capacity of hypophysectomized rats subjected to pneumonectomy was identical to that of the hypophysectomized animal, but both were significantly below unoperated controls (83). Unfortunately, rats subjected only to pneumonectomy were not examined in this study. Thus, direct comparisons of the effects of hypophysectomy combined with pneumonectomy against the effects of pneumonectomy alone could not be made. Interpretation of these results is also complicated by the fact that hypophysectomy obviously resulted in removal of all pituitary hormones. It thus remains to be determined what role, if any, each of the pituitary hormones contribute to both normal and compensatory growth of the lung.

### Adrenal Hormones

Growth of fetal and early postnatal lung is characterized by a rapid increase in cell number, protein, RNA, and DNA (3). Adrenal steroid hormones can influence fetal lung development, largely by accelerating lung maturation (reviewed in ref. 86; 87). Normal hyperplastic lung growth in developing animals can be inhibited by increasing the level of corticosteroids through direct exogenous administration to the fetus during late gestation (88,89). Steroid-induced lung hypoplasia quickly rebounds postnatally in the absence of excess steroid, and the lungs become structurally normal (90,91). Administration of glucocorticoids to pregnant animals slows the rate of cellular proliferation and growth in the fetal lung, yet accelerates lung maturation by advancing production of surfactant (87,92–95). Postnatal administration of high doses of corticosteroids during an interval of rapid lung growth in ferrets results in reduced lung volumes and decreased airway conductance (96). In adult animals, when lung growth is reduced or absent, steroid administration does not cause any significant changes in lung mass or in the mechanical properties of the lung (97,98).

Although enhancement of lung maturation by excess corticosteroids is well documented, there is some disagreement concerning the effects of removing adrenal hormones by adrenalectomy in adult animals. Liebowitz et al. (99) reported a significant increase in lung mass following adrenalectomy; this was reversed with steroid treatment. In contrast, Nijjar and Chaudhary (100) reported that adrenalectomy did not effect lung to body weight ratios, protein, DNA or protein/DNA ratios to any significant degree. These differences may be due in part to the use of different surgical procedures and different strains of rats. In general, it appears that adrenalectomy in adult animals has little effect on lung mass.

There is evidence to support a modulatory role of adrenal hormones in postpneumonectomy compensatory lung growth. Bennett et al. (101) demonstrated that the compensatory response could be modified by prior adrenalectomy. Figure 3 shows the effect of adrenalectomy on the increase in right lung mass following left pneumonectomy. Values are expressed as a percentage of right lung mass in control rats at day 0, the time of pneumonectomy. Arrows with each set of bars indicate the mass of both lungs of unoperated controls at the times specified. The open bars show the time-dependent growth of the right lung in unoperated control animals. The left bars show that adrenalectomy 5 days prior to pneumonectomy (ADX/PNX; dark bars) resulted in restoration of normal lung mass by day 7. In animals subjected to pneumonectomy alone (PNX, shaded bars), normal lung mass was only partly restored at the same interval. After 14 days, right lung

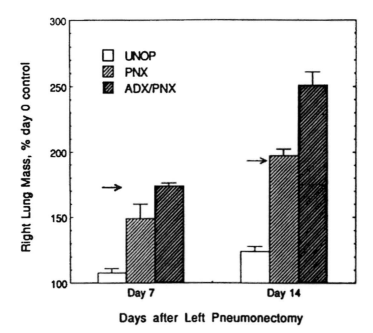

**Figure 3**   Effect of adrenalectomy on changes in right lung mass due to pneumonectomy. Right lung mass is shown on postoperative day 7 and day 14 in animals subjected to pneumonectomy alone (PNX) or to adrenalectomy followed after 5 days by pneumonectomy (ADX/PNX) as compared with unoperated controls (UNOP). Bars indicate mean and SEM of right lung mass expressed as a percentage of control right lung mass on the day of pneumonectomy (day 0). Arrows indicate total lung mass at day 7 and day 14, respectively. Data are calculated from Bennett et al., 1985 (101).

mass of pneumonectomized rats (shaded bar) reached the control value for both lungs (arrow) (101), whereas that of adrenalectomized pneumonectomized animals exceeded both the control and pneumonectomy values. Thus as compared with pneumonectomy alone, compensatory lung growth in adrenalectomized animals was accelerated and resulted in a total lung mass greater than that required to restore the tissue resected at pneumonectomy.

In addition to increased lung mass, adrenalectomized pneumonectomized rats had increased thickening of both the interstitial and endothelial cell compartments and increased volume of the type II epithelial and interstitial fibroblast populations on day 14 (28). The stimulatory effects of adrenalectomy were evident only in rats which subsequently were subjected to pneumonectomy, as adrenalectomy alone had no effect on right lung mass in the same studies (28,101). As mentioned above, the effect of adrenalectomy alone on lung growth is somewhat controversial. Interestingly, lung mass and volume are not restored at the same rate following pneumonectomy (25). Adrenalectomy further accentuates the lag in restoration of volume associated with dysanaptic growth, such that lung volumes in adrenalectomized pneumonectomized animals remain 35% below those predicted 4 weeks after pneumonectomy (25,37). The results of these studies suggest that compensatory lung growth following pneumonectomy in adrenalectomized animals is not coordinated to the same degree as that during normal growth or that following pneumonectomy alone (11).

Adrenalectomy results in loss of mineralocorticoids, as well as glucocorticoids. A change in salt balance, particularly sodium deficiency, slows the rate of compensatory lung growth (102). Adrenalectomized animals thus were allowed free access to a solution of 0.15 M NaCl in order to minimize the possible effects of mineralocorticoid deficit. The observation that compensatory lung growth is not altered by adrenalectomy alone under these conditions suggests that these animals are not in abnormal salt balance (102).

Adrenalectomy-induced changes in compensatory lung growth were prevented or reversed in a time-dependent manner when a replacement dose of the glucocorticoid hydrocortisone acetate was administered to adrenalectomized pneumonectomized animals (25,103). Steroid replacement, however, did not alter lung growth in unoperated control animals. Based on these observations, it appears that glucocorticoid excess or deficit in the adult rat alters lung growth under conditions in which growth is rapid, but is without influence under normal conditions.

In the context of studies to define the role of adrenal corticosteroid hormones in compensatory lung growth, an important issue has not been addressed experimentally. It is well known that adrenalectomy, which increases the response to pneumonectomy (25), results in elevated circulating levels of ACTH, and that ACTH levels are reduced by steroid administration. It is also notable that in the experiments where Brody and Buhain (83) investigated the effect of a growth hormone–secreting tumor to alter compensatory lung growth (discussed above), the effect of pneumonectomy was enhanced. That tumor also produced ACTH. Thus an elevated response to pneumonectomy presumably was associated with increased circulating ACTH both following adrenalectomy and in the presence of the tumor. Although some specific characteristics of the resulting growth responses appeared to differ in these cases, these observations raise a possible role for ACTH in modulation of compensatory lung growth. This possibility has not been investigated.

### Thyroid and Parathyroid Hormones

The thyroid gland secretes thyroxine $(T_4)$ and triiodothyronine $(T_3)$, which are known to affect whole body oxygen consumption. The parathyroid gland secretes parathyroid hormone, which is important in calcium and phosphate homeostasis. In addition, calcitonin is associated with the thyroid/parathyroid glands and plays an antagonistic role in calcium metabolism by effectively reducing blood calcium ion concentration. Thus, the thyroid/parathyroid axis acts to maintain overall metabolic rate and calcium homeostasis. The presence of $T_3$ receptors in rabbit (104) and rat (105) lung suggests that thyroid hormones may have direct effects on lung tissue.

To examine the effect of altered metabolic oxygen demand on lung mass, volume, and structure, hypothyroidism was induced in rapidly growing young hamsters by administration of the antithyroid drug methimazole. Hypothyroidism significantly reduced oxygen consumption without altering dry lung mass, total lung volume or total alveolar surface area, number, and size (106). In the same study, hyperthyroidism induced by daily injections of $T_3$ resulted in a significant increase in oxygen consumption with a concomitant increase in dry lung mass, total alveolar surface area, and alveolar number. Increased oxygen consumption, lung mass, and lung volume also were evident in a third group of animals exposed to cold temperatures for extended intervals. Bartlett (107) performed a similar study in young rats and found no differences in lung mass and volume or in alveolar surface area and number between hypothyroid and hyperthyroid animals.

There is evidence that thyroid hormones are involved in some aspects of lung maturation, namely, in surfactant production (reviewed in ref. 108) and in the development of antioxidant enzyme systems (109). For example, direct $T_4$ administration to fetal rabbits accelerates lung maturation by thinning alveolar septa, widening existing air spaces, and increasing the number of lamellar bodies in type II pneumocytes with no effect on overall lung mass (110). Fetal $T_3$ administration in the rat increases disaturated phosphatidylcholine and total phospholipid content with a concomitant decrease in antioxidant enzyme concentrations (109). In contrast, other studies showed that thyroid hormones alone have little effect on surfactant synthesis (111,112), yet when in combination with glucocorticoids, thyroid hormones or thyrotropin-releasing hormone can enhance surfactant production and lung function (111,113–115). Thus, it appears that thyroid hormones act synergistically with glucocorticoids to accelerate lung maturation. Modulation of lung growth by thyroid hormones may be partially indirect, however, in that observed changes in mass and volume appear to reflect changes in whole body oxygen demand.

Parathyroid hormone receptors and their messenger RNAs have been localized to many tissues, including the lung (116,117). The parathyroid hormone receptor has been demonstrated to bind the recently identified parathyroid hormone–related peptide (118). Parathyroid hormone and parathyroid hormone–related peptide act to increase extracellular calcium concentration, the latter being associated with humoral hypercalcemia of malignancy (118). The mechanisms of action of these compounds have recently been reviewed (119). Parathyroid hormone and parathyroid hormone–related peptide can stimulate phosphatidylcholine synthesis both in fetal lung explants and in coculture of pulmonary fibroblasts with type II pneumocytes (120). These observations provide evidence that parathyroid hormone can act directly on lung tissue and may be involved in control of lung maturation.

The compensatory response to pneumonectomy does not appear to be dependent on either thyroid or parathyroid hormones. In 300-g male rats, pneumonectomy was performed 2 days after thyroparathyroidectomy (121). The success of thyroparathyroidectomy was determined by a 40% decrease in blood levels of ionized calcium measured on postthyroparathyroidectomy day 2; circulating calcium levels remained significantly below the level of control animals during a postpneumonectomy interval of 7 days. Although this interval corresponds to the phase of hyperplastic compensatory growth, increase in right lung mass, protein, or DNA was not blocked by prior thyroparathyroidectomy. Thus, the compensatory growth response to pneumonectomy is preserved under hypocalcemic conditions in the absence of thyroid and parathyroid hormones. Interestingly, during compensatory hypertrophy of the liver, experimentally induced changes in circulating $T_3$ had no effect on the rate of liver regeneration (122), whereas the compensatory response to partial hepatectomy was compromised in the absence of parathyroid hormone (123).

### Other Hormones

In addition to those discussed above, several other hormones have been proposed to modify normal lung growth and development, but few studies have addressed the specific effects of other hormones on compensatory lung growth (see Table 1). Sekhon and Thurlbeck (124) investigated the effects of sex differences in postpneumonectomy lung growth. Animals were examined 3 weeks after pneumonectomy, when compensation was complete. The end result of compensatory lung growth was similar for male and female animals, with some small differences attributed mainly to differences in somatic growth, the females being smaller. When lung mass, lung volume, and alveolar surface area and number were expressed as a percentage of change from controls, no differences were found between males and females. The time course of events was not examined in this study to determine whether gender influences the well-characterized sequence of events in postpneumonectomy lung growth, but it appears that the final compensatory response to pneumonectomy is similar in both sexes.

Little data exist concerning the effect of pregnancy on compensatory lung growth. Faridy et al. (125) found no difference in the rate of compensatory growth between pregnant and nonpregnant rats subjected to pneumonectomy. Lung mass, volume, DNA content, and pressure-volume characteristics were not altered by pregnancy. Khadempour et al. (84) examined the compensatory response to pneumonectomy in pregnant rats using pregnant unoperated and pregnant sham controls. Right lung mass was significantly higher on day 3 through day 7 in animals subjected to pneumonectomy compared with control groups, which is consistent with the previously reported time course of compensation (4). These studies suggest that hormonal changes during pregnancy do not effect the time course of the compensatory response.

### B. Autocrine and Paracrine Factors

The earliest line of evidence to indicate a role for soluble factors in mediating the effect of pneumonectomy on lung growth was based on speculation that changes in blood flow to the remaining tissue may dilute or "wash out" local factors which exert tonic inhibitory effects on cellular proliferation and growth (65). Although water-soluble components of lung extracts were demonstrated to inhibit mitotic activity in alveolar cells in vitro (65), a specific role for such inhibitory factors, or chalones, now appears improbable.

In contrast, the presence of stimulatory factors in serum derived from pneumonectomized animals has been reported by several investigators. DNA synthesis by cultured human alveolar type II cells, but not by fibroblasts, was stimulated by rabbit serum collected 9 days following pneumonectomy (126). Although this activity was originally attributed to a somatomedin-like molecule, the significance of this pathway remains unresolved (127). In addition, serum from pneumonectomized animals was reported to stimulate DNA synthesis and uptake of exogenous polyamines, both of which are growth-related processes, by rat type II epithelial cells in primary culture (5,42). Type II cells isolated from the lungs of pneumonectomized animals exhibit increased sensitivity to these unidentified factors. Although the role of these factors in initiation or progress of compensatory lung growth is not defined, the observations are of interest in the context of more recent evidence which indicates that cultured fibroblasts subjected to mechanical stimuli in vitro release growth-promoting factors (128).

The effect of lung-specific growth factors was investigated by Faridy et al. (125), who measured fetal lung growth after maternal pneumonectomy in rats. This work was based in part on the observation that pregnant rats with large litter sizes had larger maternal lungs than rats with small litter sizes and that larger maternal lungs correlated with larger fetal lungs (129). In pneumonectomized pregnant animals, fetal lung growth increased relative to the fetuses of sham-operated controls. The ratio of lung DNA to body weight was increased in fetal rats only when maternal pneumonectomy was performed during the first 2 weeks of pregnancy. No structural differences were evident between fetal lungs of pneumonectomized or sham mothers at any time. Thus, it appears plausible that factors released as a consequence of maternal pneumonectomy can influence fetal lung growth.

Two studies have addressed the role of specific growth factors in the compensatory response to pneumonectomy. McAnulty et al. (130) reported that bronchoalveolar lavage (BAL) fluid concentrates collected at 2 and 6 days post-pneumonectomy stimulated fibroblast replication in vitro to a greater extent than BAL fluid collected from sham or unoperated controls. BAL fluid collected at day 14 postpneumonectomy, when lung growth rates return to normal, had no effect on fibroblast replication. The stimulatory effect of BAL fluid from day 2 was blocked partially by antibodies to insulin-like growth factor-1 (IGF-1) but not by antibodies to platelet-derived growth factor. Levels of IGF-1 in BAL fluid concentrates were elevated in both the sham and pneumonectomized animals; however, BAL IGF-1 concentrations from pneumonectomized animals were significantly greater than those from shams. This study suggests a potential role for IGF-1 in the compensatory response to pneumonectomy, possibly confirming the observations of Smith et al. (126).

Khadempour et al. (84) showed that IGF-1 lung concentration was elevated above pregnant sham and unoperated controls in pregnant rats at day 2 and day 5 postpneumonectomy; IGF-1 concentrations dropped below control values by day 7, even though compensatory lung growth was ongoing. Interpretation of the physiological significance of these results is complicated further by the fact that control lung IGF-1 concentrations rose steadily to day 7, when the highest levels were observed. Although this phenomenon has been associated with pregnancy (131), it was not evident in pneumonectomized pregnant rats. Bombesin-like immunoreactivity was also measured and did not change as the result of pneumonectomy (84). At present, neither a direct association of changes in these or similar factors with compensatory lung growth nor a role for their production or release prior or consequent to pneumonectomy has been established.

More recent studies examined some aspects of second-messenger signal transduction pathways during compensatory lung growth. Calmodulin, a calcium-dependent intracellular regulatory protein (132), is known to participate in the control of cellular proliferation and growth (133) and may play a role in postnatal lung growth and development (134). Increased lung calmodulin concentration was observed prior to increased tissue mass during compensatory lung growth following pneumonectomy (135). It appeared that this trend also occurred in sham-operated rats, but the increase lagged behind that in the pneumonectomy group by approximately 2 days. In addition, daily treatment with a calmodulin antagonist reduced the compensatory increase in lung mass and DNA content normally observed following lung resection (135). These results were interpreted to suggest that calmodulin may contribute to the initiation of compensatory lung growth.

It has been demonstrated that calmodulin can regulate the activities of adenosine 3',5'-cyclic monophosphate (cAMP)–related enzymes in the lung (136). Changes in lung activities of cAMP-related enzymes during the early postpneumonectomy interval (137) suggest that cAMP may be involved in a cascade of events that results in lung growth. Lung levels of cAMP have been demonstrated to increase within 1 day after pneumonectomy and to remain elevated until at least day 3 (138). Similar increases in lung cAMP production can be elicited in vitro in normal animals by increasing positive airway pressure, thereby overdistending or "stretching" the lungs (138). As cited above, hyper-inflation of the remaining lung after pneumonectomy may be a triggering factor for initiation and progression of compensatory lung growth.

## V. Current Status of the Field

### A. Clinical Implications

Compensatory growth of the lung after pneumonectomy in experimental animals ultimately results in tissue with normal function in gas exchange and with normal structure and mass. Much less is known about the nature of lung growth after lobectomy or pneumonectomy in human subjects. Understanding the cellular mechanisms involved in initiation and termination of compensatory lung growth in laboratory animals may provide knowledge which can be applied in a clinical context. For example, the prospect for newborns with congenital lung abnor-malities or for adult patients subjected to lobectomy as a consequence of lung disease would be improved if normal lung growth could be manipulated.

Understanding of mechanisms of compensatory lung growth also is relevant to lung transplantation in humans. In a recent case report (139), the left upper lung lobe from a 2-year-old donor was transplanted into 4-week-old recipient with a good outcome and growth of the airways was reported. Successful transplantation of lobes from a mother into her 12-year-old daughter has also been reported (140), but the long-term outcome of these cases is not yet known. Whether a transplanted lung lobe will grow sufficiently to fulfill the functional requirement of the adult or growing recipient or whether there will be an increase in alveolar number, alveolar volume, or lung mass probably is crucial to long-term restoration of normal lung function.

Because adequate lung donors for pediatric patients are scarce, an important question to be answered is whether adult lung lobes can be used efficiently as transplants for children. In order to address this question and to examine the growth of the transplanted lung in general, several animal models have been developed. A porcine model has been used to study the feasibility of lung transplantation from adult to neonate or between neonates (141–144). For adult-to-neonate lung transplantation, lung mass and volume appeared to increase in the transplanted lung but without a significant increase in alveolar number (144).

Studies of transplanted lungs between immature pigs have been complicated by the adverse effects of immunosuppressive therapy on the overall body growth, such that pigs receiving transplants took twice as long to double their body weight as did controls (141,142). Pulmonary vasculature and bronchial tree measures revealed similarities to nontransplanted lungs of weight-matched controls; however, no measurements of lung mass or volume were reported (141,142). The use of immunosuppressive and steroid therapy to prevent rejection is an underlying concern in organ transplantation. Aggressive drug therapy may compromise the growth of the transplanted lung, as it is known that compensatory lung growth is slowed in the presence of corticosteroids (25,103). Auto transplantation of the immature lung has been performed in a primate model without immunosuppression, and lung volumes after 7 months of growth were similar to sham and unoperated controls (145). Morphometric measures of alveolar multiplication in the primate model, however, have not yet been performed to determine whether hyperplastic growth can occur.

Understanding of compensatory lung growth may provide insight concerning the coordinated pathways which lead to the complex cellular architecture and physiological function of the lung. Whether compensatory growth is simply an accelerated version of normal growth is not known, although it is likely that the mechanisms which govern the response are similar to those which operate in nonpulmonary systems.

### B. Areas of Future Research

The general characteristics of rapid lung growth following pneumonectomy, including relative changes in tissue mass, structural reorganization, and establishment of normal lung function have been reported in animal models (reviewed in refs. 4 and 5). With regard to changes at the cellular level and the molecular mechanisms which underlie the compensatory response, important issues remain unresolved. For instance, although increased tissue mass is not observed until 3 days following pneumonectomy, earlier changes must occur in order to prepare the lung cell populations for a rapid increases in DNA synthesis and for cellular growth and division. The cell populations involved in the early aspect of the response and mitogenic stimuli which trigger cellular growth and division remain to be identified. Additional soluble factors produced by nonpulmonary tissues which act on the lung in an endocrine fashion have not been fully defined. Both the transduction mechanisms that signal the beginning and end of accelerated growth and the mechanisms of cell-cell communication that lead to its coordination are not understood. The influence of factors such as age, species, gender, and hormonal status in the modulation and regulation of the normal compensatory response is not completely known. Regulatory pathways which act through transcriptional and translational regulation to alter expression of specific gene products involved in the initiation, progression, and termination of the response need to be identified. Thus, although it is evident that a great deal of basic knowledge has accumulated to describe the response to pneumonectomy, specific understanding of the response at the mechanistic level is lacking. In recent years, the techniques of cell biology and molecular biology have been used with increasing frequency to resolve issues in lung biology at the basic and clinical levels. These approaches must now be applied in a more extensive and critical examination of the regulatory mechanisms which underlie compensatory growth of the lung. The reward may be great not only in terms of gaining a better understanding of normal lung growth and development but also with regard to the more practical goals such as those to accelerate lung growth in premature infants or to improve lung capacity following transplant.

## VI. Conclusions

Compensatory growth of the lung is a highly complex process. The rate of growth and overall completion of the response can be modified by manipulation of the specific hormonal systems. Among the factors proposed to regulate compensatory growth, increased inflation of the remaining lung tissue following pneumonectomy appears to be a likely candidate for the focus of further investigative efforts. It is plausible that a chronic stimulus such as increased inflation could in turn cause the release of mitogenic soluble factors, which could aid in progression and coordination of the response. Thus, the combination of these pathways may provide the mechanism whereby accelerated lung growth can occur. Despite the fact that it was demonstrated over 100 years ago that the lung is capable of growth to replace lost tissue (1), surprisingly little is known about how the response is regulated nor concerning approaches which could be taken to exploit the phenomenon in the clinical arena.

### Acknowledgments

This work is supported by HL08954 (KAG) and HL20344 (DER) from the National Heart, Lung and Blood Institute of the National Institutes of Health. We thank Suzzanne P. Sass-Kuhn for her help in preparation of this chapter.

### REFERENCES

1. Haasler F. Ueber compensatorische Hypertrophie der Lunge. Virchows Arch Pathol Anat Physiol 1892; 128:527–536.
2. Cohn R. Factors affecting the postnatal growth of the lung. Anat Rec 1939; 75: 195–205.
3. Thurlbeck WM. Postnatal growth and development of the lung. Am Rev Respir Dis 1975; 111:803–844.

4. Cagle PT, Thurlbeck WM. Postpneumonectomy compensatory lung growth. Am Rev Respir Dis 1988; 138:1314–1326.

5. Rannels DE, Rannels SR. Compensatory growth of the lung following partial pneumonectomy. Exp Lung Res 1988: 14:157–182.

6. Rannels DE, Russo LA. Compensatory Growth. In: Crystal RG, West JB, eds. The Lung. New York: Raven Press, 1991:699–709.

7. Rannels DE. Role of physical forces in compensatory growth of the lung. Am J Physiol 1989; 257:L179–L189.

8. Rannels DE, White DM, Watkins CA. Rapidity of compensatory lung growth following pneumonectomy in adult rats. J Appl Physiol 1979; 46:326–333.

9. Rannels DE, Burkhart LR, Watkins CA. Effect of age on the accumulation of lung protein following unilateral pneumonectomy in rats. Growth 1984; 48:297–308.

10. Tartter PI, Goss RJ. Compensatory pulmonary hypertrophy after incapacitation of one lung in the rat. J Thorac Cardiovasc Surg 1973; 66:147–152.

11. Berger LC, Burri PH. Timing and quantitative recovery in the regenerating rat lung. Am Rev Respir Dis 1985; 132:777–783.

12. Cui D, Jafri A, Thet LA. Effect of 70% oxygen on postresectional lung growth in rats. J Toxicol Environ Health 1988; 1:71–86.

13. Bremer JL. The fate of the remaining lung tissue after lobectomy or pneumonectomy. J Thorac Surg 1937; 6:336–343.

14. Wilcox BR, Murray GF, Friedman M, Pimmel RL. The effects of early pneumonectomy on the remaining pulmonary parenchyma. Surgery 1979; 86:294–300.

15. Thurlbeck WM, Galaugher W, Mathers J. Adaptive response to pneumonectomy in puppies. Thorax 1981; 36:424–427.

16. Johnson RLJ, Cassidy SS, Grover R, Ramanathan M, Estrera A, Reynolds RC, Epstein R, Schutte J. Effect of pneumonectomy on the remaining lung in dogs. J Appl Physiol 1991; 70:849–858.

17. Watkins CA, Burkhart LR, Rannels DE. Lung growth in response to unilateral pneumonectomy in rapidly growing rats. Am J Physiol 1985; 248:E162–E169.

18. Buhain WJ, Brody JS. Compensatory growth of the lung following pneumonectomy. J Appl Physiol 1973; 35:898–902.

19. Nattie EE, Wiley CW, Bartlett Jr D. Adaptive growth of the lung following pneumonectomy in rats. J Appl Physiol 1974; 37:491–495.

20. Holmes C, Thurlbeck WM. Normal lung growth and response after pneumonectomy in rats of various ages. Am Rev Respir Dis 1979; 120:1125–1136.

21. Brody JS, Thurlbeck WM. Development, growth, and aging of the lung. In: Fishman AP, ed. Handbook of Physiology, the Respiratory System. Bethesda, MD: American Physiological Society, 1986:355–386.

22. Laros CD, Westermann CJJ. Dilatation, compensatory growth, or both after pneumonectomy during childhood and adolescence. J Thorac Cardiovasc Surg 1987; 93: 570–576.

23. Werner HA, Pirie GE, Nadel HR, Fleisher AG, LeBlanc JG. Lung volumes, mechanics, and perfusion after pulmonary resection in infancy. J Thorac Cardiovasc Surg 1993; 105:737–742.

24. Yee NM, Hyatt RE. Effect of left penumonectomy on lung mechanics in rabbits. J Appl Physiol 1983; 54:1612–1617.

25. Bennett RA, Addison JL, Rannels DE. Static mechanical properties of lungs from adrenalectomized pneumonectomized rats. Am J Physiol 1987; 253:E6–E11.

26. Burri PH, Sehovic S. The adaptive response of the rat lung after bilobectomy. Am Rev Respir Dis 1979; 119:769–777.

27. Thet LA, Law DJ. Changes in cell number and lung morphology during early postpneumonectomy lung growth. J Appl Physiol 1984; 56:975–978.

28. Rannels DE, Stockstill B, Mercer RR, Crapo JD. Cellular changes in the lungs of adrenalectomized rats following pneumonectomy. Am J Respir Cell Mol Biol 1991; 5:351–362.

29. Langston C, Sachdeva P, Cowan MJ, Haines J, Cyrstal RG, Thurlbeck WM. Alveolar multiplication in the contralateral lung after unilateral pneumonectomy in the rabbit. Am Rev Respir Dis 1977; 115:7–13.

30. Burri PH, Pfrunder HB, Berger LC. Reactive changes in pulmonary parenchyma after bilobectomy: A scanning electron-microscopic investigation. Exp Lung Res 1982; 4:11–28.

31. Hislop AA, Odom NJ, McGregor CGA, Haworth SG. Growth potential of the immature transplanted lung. An experimental study. J Thorac Cardiovasc Surg 1990; 100:360–370.

32. Weibel ER. Stereological Methods: Practical Methods for Biological Morphometry. New York: Academic Press, 1972.

33. Sterio DC. The unbiased estimation of number and sizes of arbitrary particles using the dissector. J Microsc 1984; 134:127–136.

34. McBride JT. Postpneumonectomy airway growth in the ferret. J Appl Physiol 1985; 58:1010–1014.

35. Ford GT, Galaugher W, Forkert L, Fleetham JA, Thurlbeck WM, Anthonisen NR. Static lung function in puppies after pneumonectomy. J Appl Physiol 1981; 50:1146–1150.

36. Brody JS. Time course of and stimuli to compensatory growth of the lung after pneumonectomy. J Clin Invest 1975; 56:897–904.

37. Karl HW, Rannels DE. Compensatory hyperplastic growth of the lung. In: Cantor JO, ed. CRC Handbook of Animal Models of Pulmonary Disease. Boca Raton, FL: CRC Press, 1989:111–128.

38. Cagle PT, Langston C, Goodman JC, Thurlbeck WM. Autoradiographic assessment of the sequence of cellular proliferation in postpneumonectomy lung growth. Am J Respir Cell Mol Biol 1990; 3:153–158.

39. Rannels SR, Rannels DE. Alterations in type II pneumocytes cultured after partial pneumonectomy. Am J Physiol 1988; 254:C684–C690.

40. Uhal BD, Hess GD, Rannels DE. Density-independent isolation of type II pneumocytes after partial pneumonectomy. Am J Physiol 1989; 256:C515–C521.

41. Uhal BD, Rannels SR, Rannels DE. Flow cytometric identification and isolation of hypertrophic type II pneumocytes after partial pneumonectomy. Am J Physiol 1989; 257:C528–C536.

42. Rannels DE, Rannels SR. Acute changes in pulmonary uptake of polyamines following partial pneumonectomy. Chest 1987; 91(suppl):25S–26S.

43. Evans MJ, Cabral LJ, Stephens RJ, Freeman G. Renewal of alveolar epithelium in the rat following exposure to $NO_2$. Am J Pathol 1973; 70:175–198.

44. Adamson IYR, Bowden DH. The type II cell as progenitor of alveolar epithelial regeneration: a cytodynamic study in mice after exposure to oxygen. Lab Invest 1974; 30:35–42.
45. Fisher JM, Simnett JD. Morphogenetic and proliferative changes in the regenerating lung of the rat. Anat Rec 1973; 176:389–396.
46. Brody JS, Burki R, Kaplan N. Deoxyribonucleic acid synthesis in lung cells during compensatory growth after pneumonectomy. Am Rev Respir Dis 1978; 117:307–316.
47. McBride JT. Lung volumes after an increase in lung distension in pneumonectomized ferrets. J Appl Physiol 1989; 67:1418–1421.
48. Morgan HE, Gordon EE, Kira Y, Chua BHL, Russo LA, Peterson CJ, McDermott PJ, Watson PA. Biochemical mechanisms of cardiac hypertrophy. Ann Rev Physiol 1987; 49:533–543.
49. Russo LA, Morgan HE. Control of protein synthesis and ribosome formation in rat heart. Diabetes Metab 1989; 5:31–47.
50. Kira Y, Kochel PJ, Gordon EE, Morgan HE. Aortic perfusion pressure as a determinant of cardiac protein synthesis. Am J Physiol 1984; 246:C247–C258.
51. Grove B, Zak R, Nair KG, Aschenbrenner V. Biochemical correlates of cardiac hypertrophy. IV. Observations on the cellular organization of growth during myocardial hypertrophy in the rat. Circulation Res 1969; 25:473–485.
52. Ryan TJ. Biochemical consequences of mechanical forces generated by distension and distortion. J Am Acad Dermatol 1989; 21:115–129.
53. Watson PA. Function follows form: generation of intracellular signals by cell deformation. FASEB J 1991; 5:2013–2019.
54. Gabella G. Hypertrophic smooth muscle. I. Size and shape of cells, occurrence of mitoses. Cell Tissue Res 1979; 201:63–78.
55. Peterson CM, Gross RJ, Atryzek V. Hypertrophy of the rat urinary bladder following reduction of its functional volume. J Exp Zool 1973; 187:121–126.
56. Cullen BM, Harkness RD. Collagen formation and changes in cell population in the rat's uterus after distension with wax. Q J Exp Physiol 1968; 53:33–42.
57. Davies PF. Endothelial cells, hemodynamic forces, and the localization of atherosclerosis. In: Ryan US, ed. Endothelial Cells. Boca Raton, FL: CRC Press, 1988:123–139.
58. Ingber D. Integrins as mechanochemical transducers. Curr Opin Cell Biol 1991; 3:841–848.
59. Ingber D, Folkman J. Mechanochemical switching between growth and differentiation during fibroblast growth factor-stimulated angiogenesis in vitro: Role of extracellular matrix. J Cell Biol 1989; 109:317–330.
60. Bissell MJ, Ram TG. Regulation of functional cytodifferentiation and histogenesis in mammary epithelial cells: role of the extracellular matrix. Environ Health Persp 1989; 80:61–70.
61. Rannels DE, Rannels SR. Influence of the extracellular matrix on type 2 cell differentiation. Chest 1989; 96:165–173.
62. Townsley MI, Parker JC, Korthuis DJ, Taylor AE. Alterations in hemodynamics and Kf,c during lung mass resection. J Appl Physiol 1987; 63:2460–2466.
63. Karl HW, Russo LA, Rannels DE. Inflation-associated increases in lung polyamine

uptake: role of altered pulmonary vascular flow. Am J Physiol 1989; 257:E729–E735.

64. Friedli B, Kent G, Kidd BSL. The effect of increased pulmonary blood flow on the pulmonary vascular bed in pigs. Pediatr Res 1975; 9:547–553.

65. Simnett J, Fisher JM, Heppelston AG. Tissue-specific inhibition of lung alveolar cell mitosis in organ culture. Nature 1969; 223:944–946.

66. McBride JT, Kirchner KK, Russ G, Finkelstein G. Role of pulmonary blood flow in postpneumonectomy lung growth. J Appl Physiol 1992; 73:2448–2451.

67. Rabinovitch M, Bothwell T, Mullen M, Hayakawa BN. High pressure pulsation of central and microvessel pulmonary artery endothelial cells. Am J Physiol 1988; 254:C338–C343.

68. Tozzi CA, Poiani GJ, Harangozo AM, Boyd CJ, Riley DJ. Pulmonary vascular endothelial cells modulate stretch-induced DNA and connective tissue synthesis in rat pulmonary artery segments. Chest 1988; 93(suppl 3):169S–170S.

69. Bartlett D Jr, Remmers JE. Effects of high altitude exposure on the lungs of young rats. Respir Physiol 1971; 13:116–125.

70. Burri PH, Weibel ER. Morphometric estimation of pulmonary diffusing capacity. I. Effect of $PO_2$ on the growing lung, adaptation of the growing rat lung to hypoxia and hyperoxia. Respir Physiol 1971; 11:247–264.

71. Cunningham EL, Brody JS, Jain BP. Lung growth induced by hypoxia. J Appl Physiol 1974; 37:362–366.

72. Brody JS, Lahiri S, Simpser M, Motoyama EK, Velazquez T. Lung elasticity and airway dynamics in Peruvian natives to high altitude. J Appl Physiol 1977; 42:245–251.

73. Karl HW, Wolpert EW, Rannels DE. Minimizing intraoperative hypoxemia has no effect on postpneumonectomy lung growth. Am J Physiol 1982; 55:E65–E69.

74. Hitchcock KR, Harney J, Reichlin S. Hormones and the lung: Thyroid hormones in the perinatal rat lung. Endocrinology 1980; 107:294–299.

75. De Troyer A, Desir D, Copinschi G. Regression of lung size in adults with growth hormone deficiency. Q J Med 1980; 49:329–340.

76. Bartlett D. Postnatal growth of the mammalian lung: Influence of excess growth hormone. Respir Physiol 1971; 12:297–304.

77. Brody JS, Buhain WJ. Hormone-induced growth of the adult lung. Am J Physiol 1972; 223:1444–1450.

78. Gaultier C, Harf A, Girard F. Lung mechanics in growing guinea pigs treated with growth hormone. J Dev Phys 1986; 8:315–321.

79. Kleinberg DL, Frantz AG. Human prolactin: Measurement in plasma by in vitro bioassay. J Clin Invest 1971; 50:1557–1568.

80. Amit T, Barkley RJ, Guy J, Youdim MBH. Specific binding sites for prolactin and growth hormone in the adult rabbit lung. Mol Cell Endocrinol 1987; 49:17–24.

81. Labbe A, Delcros B, Dechelotte P, Nouailles C, Grizard G. Comparative study of the binding of prolactin and growth hormone by rabbit and human lung cell membrane frations. Biol Neonate 1992; 61:179–187.

82. Ben-Harri RR, Amit T, Youdim MBH. Binding of oestradiol, progesterone and prolactin in rat lung. J Endocrinol 1983; 97:301–310.

83. Brody JS, Buhain WJ. Hormonal influence on post-pneumonectomy lung growth in the rat. Respir Physiol 1973; 19:344–355.

84. Khadempour MH, Ofulue AF, Sekhon HS, Cherukupalli KM, Thurlbeck WM. Changes of growth hormone, somatomedin C, and bombesin following penumonectomy. Exp Lung Res 1992; 18:421–432.

85. Mendelson CR, Johnston JM, MacDonald PC, Snyder JM. Multihormonal regulation of surfactant synthesis by human fetal lung in vitro. J Clin Endocrinol Metab 1981; 53:307–311.

86. Farrell PM. Fetal lung development and the influence of glucocorticoids on pulmonary surfactant. J Steroid Biochem 1977; 8:463–470.

87. Hitchcock KR. Lung development and the pulmonary surfactant system. Anat Rec 1980; 198:13–34.

88. Motoyama EK, Orzalesi MM, Kikkawa Y, Kaibara M, Wu B, Zigas CJ, Cook CD. Effect of cortisol on the maturation of fetal rabbit lungs. Pediatrics 1971; 48:547–555.

89. Carson SH, Taeusch HW, Avery ME. Inhibition of lung cell division after hydrocortisone injection into fetal rabbits. J Appl Physiol 1973; 34:660–663.

90. Kotas RV, Mims LC, Hart LK. Reversible inhibition of lung cell numbers after glucocorticoid injection. Pediatrics 1974; 53:358–361.

91. Adamson IYR, King GM. Postnatal development of rat lung following retarded fetal lung growth. Pediatr Pulmonol 1988; 4:230–236.

92. DeLemos RA, Shermata DW, Knelson JH, Kotas R, Avery ME. Acceleration of appearance of pulmonary surfactant in the fetal lamb by administration of corticosteroids. Am Rev Respir Dis 1970; 102:459–461.

93. Frank L, Roberts RJ. Effects of low dose prenatal corticosteroid administration on the premature rat. Biol Neonate 1979; 36:1–9.

94. Kotas RV, Avery ME. The influence of sex on fetal rabbit lung maturation and on the response to glucocorticoid. Am Rev Respir Dis 1980; 121:377–380.

95. Shimizu H, Miyamura K, Kuroki Y. Appearance of surfactant proteins, SP-A and SP-B, in developing rat lung and the effects of in vivo dexamethasone treatment. Biochim Biophys Acta 1991; 1081:53–60.

96. Ellington B, McBride JT, Stokes DC. Effects of corticosteroids on postnatal lung and airway growth in the ferret. J Appl Physiol 1990; 68:2029–2033.

97. Picken J, Lurie M, Kleinerman J. Mechanical and morphological effects of long-term corticosteroid administration on the rat lung. Am Rev Respir Dis 1974; 110:746–753.

98. Abe M, Tierney DF. Lung lipid metabolism after 7 days of hydrocortisone administration to adult rats. J Appl Physiol 1977; 42:202–205.

99. Liebowitz D, Massaro GD, Massaro D. Adrenalectomy and surfactant in adult rats. J Appl Physiol 1984; 56:564–567.

100. Nijjar MS, Chaudhary KC. Effects of adrenalectomy and thyroidectomy on postnatal rat lung development and cytoplasmic factors modulating adenylate cyclase activity. Lung 1987; 165:115–127.

101. Bennett RA, Colony PC, Addison JL, Rannels DE. Effects of prior adrenalectomy on postpneumonectomy lung growth in the rat. Am J Physiol 1985; 248:E70–E74.

102. Gallaher KJ, Wolpert E, Wassner S, Rannels DE. Effect of diet-induced sodium deficiency on normal and compensatory growth of the lung in young rats. Pediatr Res 1990; 25:455–459.

103. Rannels DE, Karl HW, Bennett RA. Control of compensatory lung growth by adrenal hormones. Am J Physiol 1987; 253:E343–E348.

104. Lindenberg JA, Brehier A, Ballard PL. Triiodothyronine nuclear binding in fetal and adult rabbit lung and cultured cells. Endocrinology 1978; 103:1725–1731.

105. Morishige WK, Guernsey DL. Triiodothyronine receptors in rat lung. Endocrinology 1978; 102:1628–1632.

106. Thompson ME. Lung growth in response to altered metabolic demand in hamsters: influence of thyroid function and cold exposure. Respir Physiol 1980; 40: 335–347.

107. Bartlett D. Postnatal growth of the mammalian lung: Influence of exercise and thyroid activity. Respir Physiol 1970; 9:50–57.

108. Gross I. Regulation of fetal lung maturation. Am J Physiol 1990; 259:L337–L344.

109. Sosenko IRS, Frank L. Thyroid Hormone depresses antioxidant enzyme maturation in fetal lung. Am J Physiol 1987; 253:R592–R598.

110. Wu B, Kikkawa Y, Orzalesi MM, Motoyama EK, Kaibara M, Zigas CJ, Cook CD. The effect of thyroxine on the maturation of fetal rabbit lungs. Biol Neonate 1973; 22:161–168.

111. Smith BT, Sabry K. Glucocorticoid-thyroid synergism in lung maturation: A mechanism involving epithelial-mesenchymal interaction. Proc Natl Acad Sci USA 1983; 80:1951–1954.

112. Nichols KV, Floros J, Dynia DW, Veletza SV, Wilson CM, Gross I. Regulation of surfactant protein A mRNA by hormones and butyrate in cultured fetal rat lung. Am J Physiol 1990; 259:L488–L495.

113. Ikegami M, Jobe AH, Pettenazzo A, Seidner SR, Berry DD, Ruffini L. Effects of maternal treatment with corticosteroids, T$_3$, TRH, and their combinations on lung function of ventilated preterm rabbits with and without surfactant treatments. Am Rev Respir Dis 1987; 136:892–898.

114. Smith CI, Searls RL, Hilfer SR. Effects of hormones on functional differentiation of mouse respiratory epithelium. Exp Lung Res 1990; 16:191–209.

115. Rodriguez MP, Sosenko IRS, Antigua MC, Frank L. Prenatal hormone treatment with thyrotropin releasing hormone and with thyrotropin releasing hormone plus dexamethasone delays antioxidant enzyme maturation but does not inhibit a protective antioxidant enzyme response to hyperoxia in newborn rat lung. Pediatr Res 1991; 30:522–527.

116. Tian J, Smorgorzewski M, Kedes L, Massry SG. Parathyroid hormone-parathyroid hormone related protein receptor messenger RNA is present on many tissues besides the kidney. Am J Nephrol 1993: 13:210–213.

117. Urena P, Kong XF, Abou-Samra AB, Jüppner H, Kronenberg HM, Potts JT Jr, Segre GV. Parathyroid hormone (PTH)/PTH–related peptide receptor messenger ribonucleic acids are widely distributed in rat tissues. Endocrinology 1993; 133: 617–623.

118. Jüppner H, Abou-Samra AB, Uneno S, Gu WX, Potts JT Jr, Segre GV. The para-

thyroid hormone–like peptide associated with humoral hypercalcemia of malignancy and parathyroid hormone bind to the same receptor on the plasma membrane of ROS 17/2.8 cells. J Biol Chem 1988; 263:8557–8560.

119. Rizzoli R, Ferrari SL, Pizurki L, Caverzasio J, Bonjour JP. Actions of parathyroid hormone and parathyroid hormone-related protein. J Endocrinol Invest 1992; 15(suppl 6):51–56.

120. Rubin LP, Kifor O, Hua J, Brown EM, Torday JS. Parathyroid hormone (PTH) and PTH-related protein stimulate surfactant phopholipid synthesis in rat fetal lung, apparently by a mesenchymal-epithelial mechanism. Biochim Biophys Acta 1994; 1223:91–100.

121. Benedict JH, Rannels DE. Postpneumonectomy lung growth following thyro-parathyroidectomy. Exp Lung Res 1994; 20:13–25.

122. Obata T, Cheng S-Y. Regulation by thyroid hormone of the synthesis of a cytosolic thyroid hormone binding protein during liver regeneration. Biochem Biophys Res Commun 1992; 189:257–263.

123. Rixon RH, McManus JP, Whitfield JF. The control of liver regeneration by calcitonin, parathyroid hormone and 1-alpha,25-dihydroxycholecalciferol. Mol Cell Endocrinol 1979; 15:79–89.

124. Sekhon HS, Thurlbeck WM. A comparative study of postpneumonectomy compensatory lung response in growing male and female rats. J Appl Physiol 1992; 73: 446–451.

125. Faridy EE, Sanii MR, Thliveris JA. Influence of maternal pneumonectomy on fetal lung growth. Respir Physiol 1988; 72:195–210.

126. Smith BT, Galaugher W, Thurlbeck WM. Serum from pneumonectomized rabbits stimulates alveolar type II cell proliferation in vitro. Am Rev Respir Dis 1980; 121:701–707.

127. Thurlbeck WM, D'Ercole AJ, Smith BT. Serum somatamedin C concentrations following pneumonectomy. Am Rev Respir Dis 1984; 130:499–500.

128. Bishop JE, Mitchell JJ, Absher PM, Baldor L, Geller HA, Woodcock-Mitchell J, Hamblin MJ, Vacek P, Low RB. Cyclic mechanical deformation stimulates human lung fibroblast proliferation and autocrine growth factor activity. Am J Respir Cell Mol Biol 1993; 9:126–133.

129. Faridy EE, Bucher S, Sanii MR. Relationship between maternal and fetal lung growth. Respir Physiol 1988; 72:171–186.

130. McAnulty RJ, Guerreiro D, Cambrey AD, Laurent GJ. Growth factor in the lung during compensatory growth after pneumonecomy: evidence of a role for IGF-1. Eur Respir J 1992; 5:739–747.

131. Bozzola M, Ravagni-Probizer MF, Guidoux S, Morretla A, Valtora A, Grenier J, Roger M, Bolis PF, Schimpff RM. Variation of growth factors in pregnant women during labor and in newborns at delivery. Biol Res Pregn 1987; 8:60–64.

132. Cheung WY. Calmodulin plays a pivotal role in cellular regulation. Science 1980; 207:19–27.

133. Sasaki Y, Hidaka H. Calmodulin and cellular proliferation. Biochem Biophys Res Commun 1982; 104:451–456.

134. Ofulue AF, Sekhon H, Cherukupalli K, Khadempour H, Thurlbeck WM. Morpho-

metric and biochemical changes in the lungs of growing rats treated with a calmodulin antagonist. Pediatr Pulmonol 1991; 10:46–51.

135. Ofulue AF, Matsui R, Thurlbeck WM. Role of calmodulin as an endogenous initiatory factor in compensatory lung growth after pneumonectomy. Pediatr Pulmonol 1993; 15:145–150.

136. Ofulue AF, Nijjar MS. Calmodulin activation of rat lung adenylate cyclase is independent of cytoplasmic factors modulating the enzyme. Biochem J 1981; 200: 475–480.

137. Nijjar MS, Thurlbeck WM. Alterations in enzymes related to adenosine 3',5'-monophosphate during compensatory growth of the rat lung. Eur J Biochem 1980; 105:403–407.

138. Russo LA, Rannels SR, Laslow KS, Rannels DE. Stretch-related changes in lung cAMP after partial pneumonectomy. Am J Physiol 1989; 257:E261–E268.

139. Starnes VA, Oyer PE, Bernstein D, Baum D, Gamberg P, Miller J, Shumway NE. Heart, heart-lung, and lung transplantation in the first year of life. Ann Thorac Surg 1992; 53:306–310.

140. Goldsmith MF. Mother to child: first living donor lung transplant. JAMA 1990; 265: 2724.

141. Demmenhayn L, Haverich A, Demertzis S, Reimer P, Kemnitz J. Growth of lung allografts after experimental transplantation. Thorac Cardiovasc Surgeon 1991; 39: 40–43.

142. Haverich A, Dammenhayn L, Demertzis S, Kemnitz J, Reimers P. Lung growth after experimental pulmonary transplantation. J Heart Lung Transplant 1991; 10:288–295.

143. Jennings RW, Lorenz HP, Duncan BW, Bradley SM, Harrison MR, Adzick NS. Adult-to-neonate lung transplantation: anatomic considerations. J Pediatr Surg 1992; 27:1285–1290.

144. Kern JA, Tribble CG, Flanagan TL, Chan BBK, Scott WW, Cassada DC, Kron IL. Growth potential of porcine reduced-size mature pulmonary lobar transplants. J Thorac Cardiovasc Surg 1992; 104:1329–1332.

145. Thomas DD, Standaert TA, Anton WR, Jones DR, Godwin JD, Raghu G, Hodson WA, Allen MD. Growth potential of the transplanted lung in the infant primate. Ann Thorac Surg 1993; 56:1274–1278.

# AUTHOR INDEX

*Italic numbers give the page on which the complete reference is listed.*

### G

# SUBJECT INDEX

## A

Acetyl-CoA carboxylase, role in surfactant biosynthesis, 498
Acetylcholine (Ach), 249
Acetylcholinesterase, 250
ACTH, 401, 448-449
    and compensatory lung growth, 642-643
Activating transcription factor-1 (ATF-1), 517
Adrenalectomy and compensatory lung growth, 643-645
Airway glands:
    development of, 164
    differentiation of, 169-170
    epithelial-mesenchymal interactions in, 169-170
    growth factors and growth of, 165-166
    morphogenesis of, 164
    overview, 163
    precursor cell for, 164
    proteinases in development of, 166
Airway obstruction, reversible
    and respiratory infections, 288-289
    and cystic fibrosis, 289
    relationship to inflammation, 288

Alkaline phosphatase as a marker for type II cells, 138
α-smooth muscle actin expression, 271
Alveolar ducts, innervation of, 259
Alveolar epithelium
    differentiation of, 618
    physiological role of, 119-123
    response to lung injury, 133
Aminopeptidase N as marker for type II cells, 139
Androgens:
    and fibroblast-pneumocyte factor, 621
    as a regulator of surfactant expression, 531
Angiogenin and vascular development, 382
146-kDa Antigen (see Aminopeptidase N)
α1-Antiproteinase in bronchopulmonary dysplasia, 584
Apoptosis, 20
Atropine, 276
Axonal growth, guidance by target tissues, 248
Azetadine-2-carboxylic acid and branching morphogenesis, 337

.

Printed in the United States
112002LV00001B/1/P

T - #1066 - 101024 - C0 - 234/156/35 [37] - CB - 9780824797720 - Gloss Lamination